A Textbook of Clinical Pharmacy Practice

Second Edition

A TEXTBOOK OF CLINICAL PHARMACY PRACTICE
Essential Concepts and Skills

Second Edition

Editors

G Parthasarathi
MPharm PhD Grad Dip Clin Pharm
Director, Post Marketing Surveillance and Control of Clinical Trials
Botswana Medicines Regulatory Authority, Gabarone, Botswana

Karin Nyfort-Hansen
BPharm Grad Dip Ed(Health) CGP
Clinical Trial Co-ordinator
Adelaide Medical School, The University of Adelaide, Australia

Milap C Nahata
PharmD MS
Director, Institute of Therapeutic Innovations and Outcomes
Professor Emeritus of Pharmacy at the College of Pharmacy
Professor Emeritus of Pediatrics and Internal Medicine
College of Medicine, Ohio State University, Columbus, Ohio

A TEXTBOOK OF CLINICAL PHARMACY PRACTICE (SECOND EDITION)

UNIVERSITIES PRESS (INDIA) PRIVATE LIMITED

Registered Office
3-6-747/1/A & 3-6-754/1, Himayatnagar, Hyderabad 500 029, Telangana, India
info@universitiespress.com, www.universitiespress.com

Distributed by
Orient Blackswan Private Limited

Registered Office
3-6-752 Himayatnagar, Hyderabad 500 029, Telangana, India

Other Offices
Bengaluru / Chennai / Guwahati / Hyderabad / Kolkata /
Mumbai / New Delhi / Noida / Patna

First published by Orient Blackswan Private Limited 2004
Reprinted 2005, 2006, 2007
First Universities Press Impression 2008
Reprinted 2009, 2011
Second Edition 2012
Reprinted 2013, 2014, 2015, 2016, 2017, 2018 (twice), 2020, 2021, 2022, 2023, 2026

502291

ISBN 978 81 7371 756 7

Typeset in Life 10.5/13.3

Printed in India by
The Print Park, Chennai 600 117

Published by
Universities Press (India) Private Limited
3-6-747/1/A & 3-6-754/1, Himayatnagar, Hyderabad 500 029, Telangana, India

Contributing Authors

Christopher P Alderman
BPharm PhD FSHP BCPP CGP
Director of Pharmacy
Repatriation General Hospital, Adelaide, Australia
Associate Professor, Quality Use of Medicines and Pharmacy Research Centre
University of South Australia

Gitanjali Batmanabane
MBBS MD(Pharmacology) PhD
Professor of Pharmacology & Officer-in-charge
Department of Pharmacology
Jawaharlal Institute of Postgraduate Medical Education & Research, Pondicherry, India

Shobha Churi
MPharm
Lecturer and Clinical Pharmacist
Department of Pharmacy Practice
JSS College of Pharmacy, JSS University
Mysore, India

David Cosh
MAppSci FPS FSHP BCPS
Clinical Pharmacist, Private Practice
Adelaide, Australia

Christopher Doecke
BPharm PhD
Director of Pharmacy
Royal Adelaide Hospital, Adelaide, Australia
Associate Professor of Pharmacy Practice, School of Pharmaceutical, Molecular and Biomedical Sciences, University of South Australia

Thomas R Einarson
BSc Pharm MS(Hosp Pharm) MEd PhD
Associate Professor, Faculty of Pharmacy
University of Toronto, Toronto, Canada
Division of Clinical Pharmacology
Department of Pediatrics, Hospital For Sick Children, Toronto, Canada

Rohan A Elliott
BPharm BPharmSc(Hons) MClinPharm FSHP FASCP CGP
Senior Pharmacist, Austin Health
Melbourne, Australia; Clinical Senior Lecturer
Faculty of Pharmacy and Pharmaceutical Sciences
Monash University, Melbourne, Australia

Ruth Ferguson
Dip Pharm MSc PhD Dip Art(Indust. Psych)
Clinical Pharmacist, Dunedin Hospital
Dunedin, New Zealand
Honorary Clinical Lecturer
School of Pharmacy, Otago University
Dunedin, New Zealand

Duska Franic
PharmD PhD
Associate Professor, College of Pharmacy
University of Georgia, Athens, USA

Johnson George
MPharm PhD Grad Cert Hr Edu
Lecturer, Centre for Medicine Use and Safety
Department of Pharmacy Practice
Faculty of Pharmacy and Pharmaceutical Sciences
Monash University, Melbourne, Australia

Jeffrey Hughes
MPharm PhD
Professor and Head, School of Pharmacy
Curtin University of Technology, Perth, Australia

Grant Kardachi
BPharm FPS
President, Pharmaceutical Society of Australia, Adelaide, Australia

Stefan Kowalski
BPharm MAppSci CGP
Senior Lecturer, School of Pharmacy
University of South Australia, Adelaide, Australia

Anandi V Law
BPharm PhD
Associate Professor and Chair
Department of Pharmacy Practice and Administration, Western University of Health Sciences, Pomona, USA

PA Mahesh
MBBS
Associate Professor, Department of Pulmonology
JSS Medical College Hospital, Mysore, India

BG Nagavi
BSc MPharm PhD
Dean, RAK College of Pharmaceutical Sciences
RAKMHS University, UAE

Milap C Nahata
PharmD MS
Director, Institute of Therapeutic Innovations and Outcomes
Professor Emeritus of Pharmacy, College of Pharmacy
Professor Emeritus of Pediatrics and Internal Medicine, College of Medicine
Ohio State University, Columbus, Ohio

Roger L Nation
PhD
Professor of Drug Disposition and Dynamics
Monash Institute of Pharmaceutical Sciences
Faculty of Pharmacy and Pharmaceutical Sciences
Monash University, Melbourne, Australia

Karin Nyfort-Hansen
BPharm Grad Dip Ed(Health) CGP
Clinical Trial Co-ordinator
Adelaide Medical School
The University of Adelaide, Australia

Sten Olsson
MSc Pharm
Head of External Affairs
Uppsala Monitoring Centre, Uppsala, Sweden

Vinita Pai
PharmD MS
Assistant Professor of Clinical Pharmacy Practice and Administration, College of Pharmacy
The Ohio State University, Columbus, USA

G Parthasarathi
MPharm PhD Grad Dip Clin Pharm
Director, Post Marketing Surveillance and Control of Clinical Trials
Botswana Medicines Regulatory Authority
Gabarone, Botswana

Dev S Pathak
DBA
Emeritus Professor
The Ohio State University, Columbus, USA
Affiliate Professor
University of South Florida, USA

A Ramesh
BSc MPharm PhD
Professor, Department of Pharmacy Practice
JSS College of Pharmacy
JSS University, Mysore, India

M Ramesh
MPharm PhD FICP Dip Clin Pharm (SHPA)
Professor, Department of Pharmacy Practice
JSS College of Pharmacy
JSS University, Mysore, India

Craig R Rayner
BPharm BPharmSc(Hons) PharmD
Clinical Pharmacologist (Virology)
Pharma Research and Early Development
Roche Products Pty Ltd, Australia

Renee Robinson
PharmD MPH
Pediatric Clinical Pharmacist
LCDR, United States Public Health Services
Alaska Native Medical Center, USA

Jayashri Sankaranarayanan
BPharm MPharm PhD
Assistant Professor
College of Pharmacy
University of Nebraska Medical Center, USA

BS Sathvik
MPharm
Assistant Professor
Department of Pharmacy Practice
RAK College of Pharmaceutical Sciences, UAE

Philip J Schneider
MS FASHP
Clinical Professor and Associate Dean
College of Pharmacy
The University of Arizona, USA

Urmila Thatte
Professor and Head
Department of Clinical Pharmacology
Seth GS Medical College and KEM Hospital
Mumbai, India

Katy E Trinkley
PharmD
Fellow, Pharmacotherapy
College of Pharmacy, The Ohio State University
Columbus, Ohio, USA

Graeme Vernon
BPharm BA FSHP
Senior Drug Information Pharmacist
Austin Health, Melbourne, Australia

Krisantha Weerasuriya
MBBS MRCP PhD(Clinical Pharmacology)
Medical Officer, Medicines Access &
Rational Use (MAR), Essential Medicines &
Pharmaceutical Policies (EMP)
World Health Organization, Geneva

CONTENTS

Foreword

The introduction of clinical pharmacy education and practice in India in the late 1990s heralded an exciting new era for the pharmacy profession. The enthusiasm of students for careers in pharmacy practice has more recently resulted in the Pharm D programme, now offered by over 70 pharmacy colleges throughout the country. It is important that these students, the clinical pharmacists of the future, receive high-quality, patient-focused teaching from well-trained teaching faculty.

This new edition of *A Textbook of Clinical Pharmacy Practice: Essential Concepts and Skills* is prepared keeping their needs in mind and will make a major contribution towards achieving this goal. The book is the result of an international collaboration between editors and authors from India and many other countries.

The authors of this book are known for their expertise in the field. Their contributions ensure that teachers, students and practising pharmacists have a comprehensive reference on the concepts and skills of clinical pharmacy practice. It is my great pleasure to commend this textbook, as it will help take forward the ongoing role of strengthening pharmacy practice in our country.

B Suresh
President
Pharmacy Council of India

Foreword to the Second Edition

The introduction of clinical pharmacy education and practice in India in the late 1990s heralded an exciting new era for the pharmacy profession. The enthusiasm of students for careers in clinical pharmacy practice has more recently resulted in the Pharm D programme, now offered by over 200 pharmacy colleges throughout the country. It is important that these students, the clinical pharmacists of the future, receive high quality, patient-focused teaching from well-trained teaching faculty.

This new edition of the *Textbook of Clinical Pharmacy Practice: Essential Concepts and Skills* is prepared keeping their needs in mind and will make a major contribution towards achieving this goal. The book is the result of an international collaboration between editors and authors from India and many other countries.

The authors of this book are known for their expertise in the field. Their contributions ensure that teachers, students and practising pharmacists have a comprehensive reference on the concepts and skills of clinical pharmacy practice. It is my great pleasure to commend this textbook, as it will help take forward the ongoing task of strengthening pharmacy practice in our country.

B Suresh
President
Pharmacy Council of India

Preface to the Second Edition

Growing numbers of people throughout the world are living healthier and longer lives, in part due to the availability and use of medicines to treat or prevent a variety of health conditions. This progress, however, is uneven for many reasons, including a marked variability in therapeutic knowledge and practice skills, resources and affordability, adherence to practice guidelines, and team approach to patient care.

The concepts and skills of clinical pharmacy practice are relevant to all pharmacists as members of healthcare teams concerned with the effective, safe and economic use of medicines. Pharmacists working in hospital pharmacy, community pharmacy, drug or medicines information, clinical research, government and non-government organisations, teaching and research will all find this book of relevance to their work. The authors seek to answer the question 'How do clinical pharmacists practice?' rather than 'What do clinical pharmacists need to know about drugs and therapeutics?'. As such this new edition of *A Textbook of Clinical Pharmacy Practice: Essential Concepts and Skills* complements other textbooks, which focus on applied therapeutics, and both types of text are needed to prepare pharmacists for clinical practice. The book is a recommended text for the M Pharm, Pharmacy Practice and Pharm D programmes.

New chapters in this second edition include **Community Pharmacy Practice, Medication Use in Pregnancy and Lactation, Poison Information** and **Ethical Issues in Clinical Research**. A number of other chapters have been completely revised, including Essential Medicines and Rational Drug Use, Drug Information and Therapeutic Drug Monitoring. All chapters begin with **learning objectives**, which should be reviewed again once the chapter has been studied. Many chapters include updated **case studies, practice scenarios** and **exercises** to illustrate the way concepts and skills may be applied in daily clinical practice. **Key messages** are summarised at the conclusion of each chapter and highlight important 'take home' messages and principles. **Reading suggestions** and relevant **websites** assist further study of each topic. A list of **medical abbreviations** is included and a comprehensive **glossary** and **index** can be found at the end of the book. **New appendices** include reference ranges for common laboratory investigations and how to take a medication history.

The most appropriate treatment approach in any specific clinical situation will vary between practice settings and as new evidence becomes available. The treatment regimens used in case studies, practice scenarios and examples are used to illustrate practice concepts and skills, and when applying these in clinical practice, readers should refer to the latest treatment guidelines.

As with the first edition, we have been fortunate that many highly respected Indian and international authors have contributed chapters, and we wish to sincerely thank them for their generous participation. The invaluable assistance of Madhavi Sethupathi at Universities Press is gratefully acknowledged, as is the support of our respective departments and colleagues.

Finally, we wish to thank all those who have utilised this book and provided feedback to us since publication of the first edition in 2004. We hope that this new edition fulfils your expectations.

G Parthasarathi, Karin Nyfort-Hansen & Milap C Nahata
Editors

Abbreviations

AAP	American Academy of Pediatrics
ACE	angiotensin converting enzyme
ACEI	angiotensin converting enzyme inhibitor
ADE	adverse drug event
ADH	anti-diuretic hormone
ADR	adverse drug reaction
AF	atrial fibrillation
AFB	acid fast bacilli
AIDS	acquired immune deficiency syndrome
AIIMS	All-India Institute of Medical Sciences
ALP	alkaline phosphatase
ALT	alanine aminotransferase
AMH	Australian Medicines Handbook
AR	absolute risk
ARB	angiotension receptor blocker
ARR	absolute risk reduction
ART	anti-retroviral therapy
AST	aspartate aminotransferase
ATC	Anatomical Therapeutic Chemical
b.i.d	bis in die (twice a day)
BGL	blood glucose level
BNF	British National Formulary
BUN	Blood Urea Nitrogen
CAP	community acquired pneumonia
CBC	complete blood count
CBP	complete blood picture
CCF	congestive cardiac failure
CEHAT	Centre for Enquiry into Health and Allied Themes
cfu	colony forming units
CHF	congestive heart failure
CI	confidence interval
CIOMS	Council for International Organizations of Medical Sciences
CMI	consumer medicine information
CMV	cytomegalovirus
CNS	central nervous system
COAD	chronic obstructive airways disease
COC	combined oral contraceptive
COPD	chronic obstructive pulmonary disease
COX-2	cyclo-oxygenase-2
CPE	cytopathic effect
CPI	consumer product information
CrCl	creatinine clearance
CRP	C-reactive protein
CSF	cerebrospinal fluid
CT	computed tomography
CYP P450	cytochrome P450
DBT	Department of Biotechnology
DC	differential count
DDD	defined daily dose
DIC	drug information centre
DMARD	disease modifying anti-rheumatic drug
DNA	deoxyribonucleic acid
DOT	directly observed therapy
DSMB	data safety monitoring board
DTC	Drug and Therapeutics Committee
DUE	drug utilisation evaluation
DUR	drug use review
DVT	deep vein thrombosis
EBM	evidence-based medicine
EC	Ethics Committee
ECG	electrocardiogram

EDL	Essential Drugs List
EIA	enzyme-linked immunoassay
ELISA	enzyme-linked immunosorbent assay
EML	Essential Medicines List
ESR	erythrocyte sedimentation rate
FBE	full blood examination
FBS	fasting blood sugar
FDA	Food and Drug Administration
FDE	fixed drug eruption
FiO_2	fraction of inspired oxygen
FIP	International Pharmaceutical Federation
FRE	Flesch Reading Ease
G6PD	glucose-6-phosphate dehydrogenase
GCP	good clinical practice
GFR	glomerular filtration rate
GOLD	Global initiative for Obstructive Lung Disease
GP	general practitioner
HAI	haemagglutination inhibition
HAV	hepatitis A virus
Hb	haemoglobin
HbA1c	glycosylated haemoglobin
HBV	hepatitis B virus
HCV	hepatitis C virus
HIV	human immunodeficiency virus
HMR	home medicines review
HSV	herpes simplex virus
hpf	high power field
IB	Investigator's Brochure
ICD	informed consent documents
ICF	informed consent form
ICH-GCP	International Conference on Harmonisation-Good Clinical Practices
ICMR	Indian Council for Medical Research
ICS	inhaled corticosteroids
ICU	Intensive Care Unit
IF	immunofluorescence
Ig	immunoglobulin
IgM anti-HAV	immunoglobulin M antibodies to hepatitis A virus
IM	intramuscular
INR	international normalised ratio
INSA	Indian National Science Academy
IP	inpatient
IV	intravenous
LAR	legally acceptable representative
LDH	lactate dehydrogenase
LFTs	liver function tests
MAC	*Mycobacterium avium* complex
MBC	minimum bactericidal concentration
MCHC	mean cell haemoglobin content
MCV	mean cell volume
MHI	medication history interview
MIC	minimum inhibitory concentration
MOR	medication order review
MRI	magnetic resonance imaging
MUE	medication use evaluation
NAPLEX	North American Pharmacy Licensure Examination
NKA	nil known allergies
NNH	number needed to harm
NNT	number needed to treat
NSAIDs	non-steroidal anti-inflammatory drugs
OBRA-90	Omnibus Budget Reconciliation Act of 1990
OPD	Outpatient Department
OR	odds ratio
ORCA	OpeRational ClassificAtion
OTC	over the counter
p	probability of an outcome arising by chance
$PaCO_2$	partial pressure of carbon dioxide
PaO_2	partial pressure of oxygen

PBS	Pharmaceutical Benefits Scheme (Australia)
PCC	poison control centre
PCI	Pharmacy Council of India
PCR	polymerase chain reaction
PCT	procalcitonin
P-gp	P-glycoprotein
PHC	primary health centre
PHQ-9	nine-point depression assessment survey
PI	poison information
PIC	poison information centre
PIL	patient information leaflet
PIS	patient information sheet
PML	promyelocytic leukaemia
PMN	polymorphonuclear neutrophils
PO	per oral
PPBS	postprandial blood sugar
PSI	pneumonia severity index
QA	quality assurance
QCPP	quality care pharmacy program (Australia)
QUM	quality use of medicines
RBC	red blood corpuscles
RCT	randomised controlled trial
RDT	Rapid Diagnostic Test
RDU	rational drug use
RMMR	residential medication management review
RNA	ribonucleic acid
RR	relative risk
RRR	relative risk reduction
SAE	serious adverse event
SC	subcutaneous
SD	standard deviation
Se Cr	Serum Creatinine
SG	specific gravity
SIADH	Syndrome of Inappropriate Anti-diuretic Hormone secretion
SNRI	serotonin–norepinephrine reuptake inhibitor
SOPs	standard operating procedures
SSRI	selective serotonin reuptake inhibitor
STG	Standard Treatment Guideline
TB	tuberculosis
TCA	tricyclic anti-depressant
TCR	treatment chart review
TDM	therapeutic drug monitoring
UNESCO	United Nations Education, Scientific and Cultural Organization
UPS	uninterrupted power supply
UTI	urinary tract infection
VZV	varicella zoster virus
WBC	white blood corpuscles
WCC	white cell count
WHO	World Health Organization (WHO)
WMA	World Medical Assembly
ZDV	zidovudine

1 CLINICAL PHARMACY IN INDIA

BG Nagavi

Learning Objectives

Upon completion of this chapter, the reader should be able to:

- Explain the need for clinical pharmacy in India
- Describe how clinical pharmacy can contribute to improved medication use at different levels of the healthcare system
- List the criteria used to assess educational programmes for clinical pharmacy and pharmacy practice
- Describe some of the future challenges for the pharmacy profession

It is now more than 75 years since the establishment of India's first degree in Pharmacy at Banaras Hindu University, under the able leadership of Professor Mahadeva Lal Schroff. The Pharmacy Act was drafted in 1948 under the aegis of the Pharmacy Council of India, the statutory body established to control the standards of the pharmacy profession. As a result of the first Education Regulation in 1953, the Diploma in Pharmacy (D Pharm) became the minimum qualification required to practise pharmacy in India, either in community or in hospital pharmacies. The Education Regulations were subsequently revised in 1972, 1981 and 1991.

For the fifty years following Independence, the degree pharmacist's education and practice was oriented towards the pharmaceutical industry. Most graduates traditionally found employment in this sector, primarily in the areas of production, formulation, quality control and marketing.

The growth of the pharmaceutical industry means that India is self-sufficient in its pharmaceutical needs, an outcome which has been made possible by the availability of skilled pharmacists. Over 100,000 different formulations, including various types of dosage forms, are currently manufactured and marketed by the Indian pharmaceutical industry. This achievement has not been duplicated in the development of pharmacy practice in India.

The first recognition of this was in 1991 when the Education Regulations were amended to include the subjects of hospital and clinical pharmacy, community pharmacy and health education, and drug store and business management in the Diploma of Pharmacy curriculum.

During the 1980s and '90s, the consequences of drug misuse, such as poor health outcomes from drug treatment, antibiotic resistance, adverse drug reactions (ADRs) and economic loss to patients and the wider healthcare system, were acknowledged not just by the pharmacy profession, but also by the medical profession, consumer and patient organisations and the government. The 1990s were a period of awakening, when the profession clearly recognised the urgent need for pharmacists to contribute to improving medication use in the community.

Having recognised the need for pharmacists to assume new responsibilities in healthcare, a problem remained. The existing education of degree pharmacists emphasised knowledge and skills in pharmaceutics, pharmaceutical chemistry, pharmacology and industrial pharmacy. However, a different set of knowledge and skills is required by pharmacists wishing to contribute to patient care. These include pathophysiology, applied therapeutics, clinical pharmacokinetics and practice skills such as patient counselling, drug information and drug therapy review. The early development of pharmacy practice and clinical pharmacy was hampered by a lack of teaching personnel with this background.

Determined to solve this problem, academic leaders of the profession examined options including the possibility of support from overseas. As a result, the first Masters in Pharmacy Practice programmes were offered by the JSS Colleges of Pharmacy at Mysore and Ooty in 1997 with the support of Australian institutions. Most significantly, these teaching programmes were based at local hospitals, with students participating in patient care activities on a daily basis using case-based learning.

Other pharmacy practice programmes quickly followed. In the southern Indian state of Tamil Nadu, a programme was initiated in 1998 at Sri Ramakrishna Institute of Paramedical Sciences, Coimbatore, and its attached hospital. The KLE College of Pharmacy, Belgaum, began a clinical pharmacy practice and education programme in 1999 using the KLES Hospital as a teaching base. In 2001, similar programmes were established by Manipal University through the Manipal College of Pharmaceutical Sciences in the Kasturba Medical College Hospital; Al-Ameen College of Pharmacy, Bangalore, using the Victoria Hospital (a government hospital); and by Annamalai University in Tamil Nadu at their Institute of Pharmaceutical Sciences and university hospital.

The following year, in Kerala, the Government College of Pharmacy, Trivandrum, commenced a pharmacy practice programme using the Trivandrum Medical College Hospital as a teaching site, and the Vishwesharapuram College of Pharmaceutical Sciences initiated clinical pharmacy services at the Kempegowda Institute of Medical Sciences in Bangalore. The National Institute of Pharmaceutical Education and Research (NIPER) in Mohali, Punjab, also established a new Department of Pharmacy Practice.

As of 2011, 23 institutions are offering postgraduate programmes in pharmacy practice. This has helped produce pharmacists with skills in patient and pharmaceutical care. The recent commencement of Doctor of Pharmacy (Pharm D) programmes in many institutions and Pharm D post-baccalaureate programmes in some colleges for the benefit of B Pharm graduates will help produce more pharmacists who are able to take on patient-focused roles in primary healthcare in rural and urban settings, nursing homes, hospitals and community pharmacies.

The result of this expansion is that the pharmacy profession in India is in transition. It is moving from a technical, industry-oriented profession to one that also has a significant role to play in patient care.

Need for Clinical Pharmacy in India

Clinical pharmacy practice is concerned with the promotion of effective, safe and economical drug therapy. Pharmacy practice is a broader term which includes clinical pharmacy and other patient care–related activities performed by pharmacists in the hospital and community settings. These include dispensing and drug distribution, drug information, health promotion, patient counselling, pharmacovigilance, medication reviews, academic detailing and sterile and non-sterile manufacturing. Clinical pharmacy has its origins in hospital pharmacy, but in some countries, clinical activities which in the beginning were restricted to hospitals are now well-developed in the community setting.

India is a country with many drug use problems. This is a result of complex socioeconomic, medical and political factors. Drug-related problems occur at various levels of the medication use process and involve prescribers, patients, pharmacists, nurses, the pharmaceutical industry and the government. Clinical pharmacy practice in the hospital and community settings, as seen in other countries, can improve the drug use process by promoting the quality and safe use of medicines.

Pharmaceutical industry: Around 100,000 formulations are available in the market today. Many of these formulations are irrational drug combinations and non-essential medications such as vitamin preparations. Many doctors use the promotional material from pharmaceutical companies as their main source of drug information. This information may be biased and does not provide doctors with independent advice regarding indications for treatment and safety issues. Most pharmaceutical companies in India do not have good medical information departments. The package inserts provided by them may contain only technical information about drugs, and are not useful to patients. Consumer product information is not provided. Clinical pharmacy can address these industry-based problems by providing unbiased, independent drug information to medical practitioners and by counselling patients at various levels of the healthcare system.

Prescribers: The patient load on medical practitioners is very high irrespective of the practice setting. A busy practitioner may spend only around 5–10 minutes per patient. Outpatient departments (OPD) in government hospitals are always overcrowded. It is often very difficult to make a clear diagnosis of the disease in a short time.

Some doctors tend to write a prescription or 'a pill for every ill', which may lead to unnecessary drug-related problems such as adverse drug reactions (ADRs). This is because many medical practitioners do not receive adequate pharmacotherapeutic training in the medical curriculum and often rely on pharmaceutical companies for drug information. Most doctors prescribe drugs by brand names with the risk of duplication of therapeutic equivalents. Infectious diseases at primary and secondary healthcare levels are often treated empirically. Definitive therapy after assessing culture and sensitivity data is not regularly practised. Broad-spectrum antibiotics are used for simple infections at the primary and secondary healthcare levels because of widespread antibiotic resistance. Clinical pharmacists can help by providing doctors with advice and information to achieve safer and more effective drug therapy.

Pharmacists: Pharmacists in pharmacies do not offer any professional services to patients such as patient counselling, labelling of medication with directions for use or advising patients regarding their disease or the use of their medications. Their interaction with doctors about possible drug interactions or other prescription problems is very limited. This is mainly because of a poor knowledge base, lack of training, lack of confidence and no financial benefits. The control on pharmacies by statutory bodies is far from satisfactory. Pharmacies may be managed by non-pharmacists and community pharmacies in the true sense do not exist in India. The concept of pharmacy chains is emerging in India, but this has been more for economic reasons than for reasons of professional development.

Hospital pharmacists manage drug inventory, drug dispensing at OPD dispensaries and record-keeping in Indian hospitals. With appropriate education and training, graduate pharmacists can help improve medication use, by providing services such as drug therapy monitoring, patient counselling, drug information services, ward round participation and ADR reporting and monitoring.

Government: The government's drug policies are mainly aimed at the pharmaceutical industry rather than at the patient. Technical and commercial matters such as price control and licensing of manufacturers have taken precedence over initiatives to ensure that medications are used wisely. Advertising and promotional claims by the pharmaceutical industry are not well regulated. A functional national ADR reporting system lacks continuity and remains to be established.

ADR monitoring and reporting is an important role for clinical pharmacists and will improve medication safety, especially among paediatric and geriatric patients. Much can be done by the government to develop pharmacy practice in India so that pharmacists can play a meaningful role in the healthcare system.

Patients: The majority of literate Indians cannot read and understand English, the language used for medicine labels on containers and closures. Clinical pharmacists can assist medication adherence through patient counselling in the local language and by identifying and helping to resolve factors which contribute to non-adherence. Patient information leaflets (PILs) and advisory labels provided in local languages will also help improve medication use, and PILs can be developed by clinical pharmacists in consultation with other healthcare providers. The low income of many Indian patients means that every rupee used to purchase a medicine should be well spent. Clinical pharmacists can advise patients and their doctors on the most cost-effective medications for a particular condition, and help reduce expenditure on unnecessary and irrational medications.

Scope for Clinical Pharmacy Practice in India

There is tremendous scope for clinical pharmacy practice at various levels of the pharmacy profession. This has been clearly demonstrated by the enthusiastic support of medical staff in the pioneering institutions where clinical pharmacy was introduced. Based on physician surveys at the JSS Hospital, Mysore, the services that are most appreciated by medical staff include:

- Drug information services
- Clinical pharmacy input on ward rounds
- Information about new drugs
- Patient counselling and advice on individual patient management

In the last category, the most common issues identified related to the detection and management of ADRs, choice of antibiotics, dose adjustment in renal/hepatic impairment and in geriatric patients, drug interactions and choice of therapy. Other areas where clinical pharmacists have contributed are preparation of treatment guidelines or protocols, education of nurses about the preparation and administration of parenteral drugs, interventions to reduce medication errors and support for clinical research activities.

In community pharmacy, knowledge of clinical pharmacy can be used to counsel patients about their medications, identify drug interactions and other drug-related problems, and provide advice regarding the management of minor ailments with referral of patients back to their doctors if necessary. While there is tremendous scope for community pharmacists to contribute to improved medication use in the country, there are also obstacles which must be overcome. In particular, diploma pharmacists must be trained to provide these services, and the public must be educated to expect a professional service from the pharmacist whenever a prescription is filled. If this happens, pharmacies which employ unqualified staff who cannot provide these services will eventually lose customers to pharmacies where these professional services are offered.

Clinical Pharmacy Education

The postgraduate programmes in pharmacy practice offered by Indian pharmacy colleges are designed to prepare pharmacists for an expanded role in the healthcare system. There is significant focus on pathophysiology, applied therapeutics and pharmacy practice, which are the foundations upon which clinical pharmacy practice is built. The following subjects are taught in the Master of Pharmacy Practice programme:

- **Pathophysiological basis of various diseases**
- **Patient data analysis,** to enable the student to understand the significance of laboratory tests and other biological values, and to interpret clinical data

with respect to the patient's disease condition and treatment

- **Applied therapeutics,** to understand the role of various classes of drugs in particular diseases and conditions, with an emphasis on the safety, efficacy and rational selection of drugs
- **Clinical pharmacokinetics,** to understand the kinetics of drugs and how this affects their selection and dosage; in particular, when used in patients with renal or hepatic impairment
- **Communication skills,** to support clinical pharmacy practice, particularly in the areas of patient counselling and communication with physicians and other healthcare professionals

Administrators of various pharmacy and medical colleges are interested in offering clinical pharmacy/pharmacy practice programmes. However, properly trained and skilled academic staff is essential. The Pharmacy faculty should be teacher–practitioners with sufficient training in clinical practice. They should have adequate knowledge and understanding of pharmacy practice–related subjects. Practical experience of ADR reporting and monitoring, providing drug information services, patient counselling and drug therapy review are essential. The minimum qualification should be a postgraduation in Pharmacy Practice or a first-class Doctor of Pharmacy degree.

The primary focus of clinical pharmacy is the optimisation of drug therapy in individual patients. The knowledge and skills needed to do this require hospital-based training, where students have the opportunity to directly observe the effects of drug therapy, both beneficial and adverse, in individual patients. Participation in patient care activities enables students to develop an understanding of the process of medical diagnosis, the role of treatment options other than drug therapy, and the use of laboratory data and other relevant information in the selection and monitoring of drug therapy.

Training in the hospital setting also allows students to develop the communication skills required to educate patients and develop good professional relationships with prescribers and other healthcare staff. Familiarity with the way doctors communicate with each other and with patients engenders confidence in their own professional communications. A teaching hospital is the ideal place for clinical pharmacy training, as staff and students can take advantage of the learning opportunities on medical teaching ward rounds and academic medical meetings.

Hospital Infrastructure and Resources

Though clinical pharmacists spend most of their time in the wards, they must have a department where administrative, educational and other professional activities can be based and where documentation about clinical pharmacy services is stored. The department should be located in a central place in the hospital to provide easy access to wards, patients, doctors and nurses. General requirements include an office area for each faculty member, an area for library and drug information resources, a teaching area and an area where students can study with access to library resources and the internet. Adequate books, journals and electronic databases are essential for teaching and to address drug information needs. Significant computer resources are required to support the activities of the department.

Relationship with the Medical Profession

The acceptance and advancement of clinical pharmacy practice depends on a good professional relationship with the medical profession. In most hospitals, this depends on individual pharmacists establishing good working relationships with individual doctors, where mutual support and respect for the other person's role is a key element. Support and respect for the clinical pharmacist's role cannot be assumed and must be earned, and Indian pharmacists need to be diligent in pursuing this goal. They need to demonstrate through their actions a commitment to patient welfare and respond to the needs of patients and hospital staff in a timely and professional manner.

There has been enthusiastic support for clinical pharmacy in hospitals where these principles are combined with an excellent knowledge of therapeutics. The pharmacy profession must nurture support from the medical profession carefully, particularly in these early years when clinical pharmacy is an unknown concept to many doctors, and the skills and experience of the clinical pharmacists are still being developed.

Future Challenges

As clinical pharmacy practice and education are in the formative stages in India, there are significant challenges for pharmacy educators and the pharmacy profession in general. The provision of pharmaceutical care to patients in the community and in hospitals will be uneven because of our large population and the shortage of trained clinical pharmacists. There is no short-term solution to this, and it will take many years to integrate pharmaceutical care into all parts of our healthcare system. The process can be hastened by teaching and training pharmacy students in pharmaceutical care skills.

In the meantime, it is important that where clinical pharmacy practice is established, the services provided are of high quality. This will depend on the qualifications, experience, skill and commitment of each individual pharmacist, together with support from academic leaders and hospital administrators. Newly-established departments of pharmacy practice and clinical pharmacy require appropriate infrastructure, information technology and equipment, drug information resources and provision for training and research. The opportunity to travel within the country and abroad for training and knowledge sharing is also a priority. These pre-requisites and the need for patient-focused teaching were acknowledged by the profession's leaders when they signed the Mysore Declaration on Clinical Pharmacy Practice and Education in 1999.

Co-operation and networking between existing pharmacy practice centres can help speed up the progress of clinical pharmacy, with the opportunity to share experiences and progress in common areas of interest. Creating a separate association of pharmacy practitioners in India to organise regular meetings and conferences and to publish newsletters on updates in the practice arena will be very useful. The profession must ensure that clinical pharmacists engage in a programme of continuing professional development to maintain their competency to practise. The publication of a professional journal exclusively in the area of community, hospital and clinical pharmacy is another challenge. The Association of Pharmacy Teachers of India has made an attempt in this direction with the publication of the Indian Journal of Pharmacy Practice.

Clinical pharmacy research has enormous potential to identify and address drug use problems relating to the Indian scenario, and at the same time raise awareness about clinical pharmacy in the medical community. Additional training in clinical research methodology and biostatistics is needed to support the potential of clinical pharmacy in this area.

The Kelkar Committee recommended that a professional or dispensing fee be paid to practicing pharmacists. For this to happen, such pharmacists need to demonstrate their ability and commitment to providing professional services such as labelling of medications with directions, and counselling of patients about their medication.

A few issues that need continuous monitoring and development are:

- **Quality of pharmaceutical education**: Building, monitoring, reviewing and upgrading the quality of Pharm D and M Pharm (Pharmacy Practice) programmes in private and public institutions is a major challenge and concern. Developing and managing relevant, needs-based and practice-oriented programmes requires expertise, transparency and professionalism at every level, including but not limited to admissions, delivery of courses, examinations and hospital-based training.
- **Accreditation of institutions and services**: To maintain international standards in education, training and examination, a mechanism should be put in place in the regulatory and professional bodies to review, approve and accredit institutions and services by the most competent professionals in the field. Graduates of the programmes may work in India or overseas and will need to compete at a global level. Hence, the quality of education and training are critical to achieve excellent standards.
- **Employment opportunities in hospitals**: Today, most postgraduates work for clinical research organisations, medical literature development companies, the pharmaceutical industry or overseas. A lack of hospital-funded positions for clinical pharmacists has slowed the uptake of clinical pharmacy in the healthcare system. Employment opportunities relating to patient care, clinical pharmacy and hospital pharmacy are necessary to sustain growth in the area and to provide practice-based services.

Conclusion

The introduction of clinical pharmacy education and practice has been one of the most significant developments in the history of the Indian pharmacy profession. Young pharmacists can now pursue rewarding and satisfying careers within the healthcare system. The future progress of clinical pharmacy rests with current and future postgraduates in pharmacy practice. With support from our profession's leaders, more and more pharmacists will take their place in the healthcare team and may contribute to the improved quality use of medications in the country.

KEY MESSAGES

- Pharmacists are under-utilised in the Indian healthcare system.
- High-quality postgraduate, Pharm D and doctoral programmes in pharmacy practice are essential to prepare pharmacists for clinical practice.
- Teaching of clinical pharmacy should be patient-focused and provide students with the opportunity to participate in the provision of clinical pharmacy services.
- Excellent relationships with the medical profession are needed to ensure the progress of clinical pharmacy.
- Clinical pharmacy is a rewarding career path with opportunities to contribute to improved medication use through employment in hospitals, teaching, drug information, pharmacovigilance, clinical research and medical information.

Further Reading

Dowling H. 2001. Achieving better quality health care through clinical pharmacy and managing the quality use of medicines. *Ind J Pharm Edu* 35(2):54–56.

Miglani BD. 2001. Pharmaceutical care vis-à-vis hospital and community pharmacy. *Ind J Hosp Pharmacy* 35(1):15–22.

Nagavi BG, Parthasarathi G and Nyfort-Hansen K. 1998. Post graduate clinical pharmacy education: Minimum requirements. *Ind J Pharm Edu* 32(1):8–11.

Parthasarathi G, Ramesh M, Nyfort–Hansen K and Nagavi BG. 2002. Clinical pharmacy in a South Indian teaching hospital. *Ann Pharmacother* 36:927–932.

Patel H. 1999. Health care for humanity – through pharmacy education. *Ind J Pharm Edu* 33(4):196–201.

Revikumar KG, Mohanta GP, Veena R and Sekhar S. 2009. Genesis, Development and Popularization of Doctor of Pharmacy (Pharm D) Education Program at the Global level - A study based on the story from 1955 to 2009. *Indian J Pharm Pract* 1(2):8–17.

The Mysore Declaration on Clinical Pharmacy Practice and Education in India. *Proceedings of the National Seminar on Clinical and Hospital Pharmacy, Oct 1999*. JSS College of Pharmacy, Mysore 14–16.

2 Clinical Pharmacy: An International Perspective

Christopher Doecke

Learning Objectives

Upon completion of this chapter, the reader should be able to:

- Define the terms clinical pharmacy and pharmaceutical care
- Describe the origins of clinical pharmacy practice
- List the factors that influence the development of clinical pharmacy in different countries
- Describe how clinical pharmacists can develop a good working relationship with the medical profession

The Origins of Clinical Pharmacy

The term clinical pharmacy has its origins in the hospital pharmacy practised in the United States in the early 1960s. Clinical pharmacy has been defined as the services provided by pharmacists to promote rational drug therapy that is safe, appropriate and cost-effective. While the timing of the emergence of clinical pharmacy practice has varied from country to country, the reasons for its emergence have been remarkably consistent worldwide. In many Western countries, a number of related issues coincided to stimulate the demand for a more 'clinical' practice of pharmacy. These included:

- A reduced requirement for pharmacist-prepared products
- An increase in the number of pharmaceuticals
- An increased awareness of drug-related morbidity and mortality

Since the 1960s, the requirement for pharmacists to design and prepare elaborate pharmaceutical formulations has declined as the pharmaceutical industry took over this role. This left the pharmacist with the role of dispensing finished products. This is an important and essential role, but has limited impact on the patient's health outcome. Further, much of this dispensing function could be efficiently and safely undertaken by pharmacy technicians or, more recently, automated systems under the supervision of a pharmacist. This was seen as an opportunity for pharmacists to use their professional training in more clinical ways, rather than an opportunity to reduce pharmacist numbers.

Secondly, the number of pharmaceutical products available for human consumption has expanded at a dramatic rate since the 1960s. This has resulted from general advances in medicine, science and technology, with improved drug screening and production methods. These general advances have resulted in great improvements in disease diagnosis and monitoring, along with a rapid expansion in therapeutic options. Together, this progress has greatly increased the complexity of information in areas such as pharmaceutical formulation, pharmacokinetics, dosing, pharmacodynamics, adverse effects, drug interactions, patient compliance and pharmacoeconomics.

The volume of new drugs and the complexity of information associated with their use have made it very difficult for the medical profession to maintain expertise in drug therapy as well as disease state diagnosis and management. Pharmacists were thus a logical professional group to meet this clinical need and work with the medical practitioner to achieve safer and more effective use of drugs in patients, which consequently may result in better patient health outcome.

Finally, as drug therapy has expanded, so has the opportunity for, and incidence of, drug-related morbidity and mortality. While the understanding that drugs can harm as well as benefit has been known for centuries, the focus was originally always on chemicals as 'poison'. Over the last 50 years, it has become clear that it is not just the drug, but the way in which a drug is used that influences both its effectiveness and its potential for harm. Again, pharmacists were a logical professional group to guide and assist prescribers and patients in the optimal use of drugs to minimise adverse effects and maximise efficacy.

In summary, the decline in the pharmacist's traditional role in compounding, occurring at the same time as an explosion in drug availability, increased complexity of therapeutic options and increased awareness of the potential for harm related to drug therapy, all coincided to create the environment for the evolution of the clinical pharmacist.

Pharmaceutical Care and Clinical Pharmacy

During the evolution of clinical pharmacy in the United States, it was recognised by some pharmacists that clinical pharmacy was often practised as a series of services, without a clear uniting philosophy or ideal. The term *pharmaceutical care* was first used by Mikeal et al. in 1975 to define the care a patient requires to assure safe and rational drug use. Brodie et al. further elaborated the term in 1980 before Hepler and Strand in 1990 published a paper providing a conceptualisation of pharmaceutical care that has ultimately been widely accepted in the pharmacy and medical professions.

In essence, pharmaceutical care has the patient as the central focus and the pharmacist directly interacting with the patient and medical practitioner to care for the patient's drug-related needs. The other central theme of pharmaceutical care is that the pharmacist takes direct responsibility for the quality of this care. This provides a strong framework for specific clinical pharmacy activities to be coordinated towards the common goal of enhancing the care of the individual patient.

Development of Clinical Pharmacy Practice

The reasons why the pharmacy profession has moved towards clinical practice are clear. It is also clear that this development has not been consistent. This uneven development applies not only among countries, but also between regions within a country, between individual hospitals within a region and between pharmacy practice settings. This latter point is often overlooked when clinical pharmacy is discussed. Often, only hospital- or institution-based pharmacy services are considered. Clinical pharmacy is relevant to all practice settings; however, it may evolve in different ways, as can be illustrated by the development of pharmacy practice in Australia.

The majority of pharmacy practice in Australia is based in the community setting, with pharmacist-owned retail shops offering a drug distribution service by dispensing and selling medicines. This service mostly relates to the dispensing of drugs subsidised by the Australian government. The income for pharmacies has predominantly been from government-funded dispensing fees and from profit margins on the products sold.

Hospital pharmacy is a much smaller practice area in terms of pharmacist numbers. While funding comes again predominantly from the government, it is not linked to the volume of drugs issued, as in the community pharmacy setting. The significance of this fundamental difference has been that, as the need for a more clinical practice of pharmacy arose, community pharmacists were hampered in the development of clinical services because they were not paid for anything other than drug distribution. On the other hand, hospital pharmacists were able to respond by internal re-allocation of staffing resources to support clinical pharmacy activity.

For example, a greater utilisation of pharmacy support staff freed up pharmacist time in many hospitals. Variations in the ability to re-allocate resources from hospital to hospital means that some differences do exist in the level of services provided, but almost all Australian hospitals, both government and private, provide at least basic clinical pharmacy services.

While the issue of payment is key to explaining why clinical pharmacy has evolved in Australian hospitals at a much greater rate than community practices, it is certainly not the only reason. Greater access to patient information in hospitals, opportunities to develop relationships with medical and nursing staff, and the teaching and research culture within hospitals have all played a major role. In community pharmacy, the reason for prescribing is often unclear, and other information that is necessary to ensure proper drug use recommendations, such as the patient's laboratory results, are unavailable. Basic patient medication counselling is the most widely available clinical service in Australian community pharmacies, because general advice regarding medications can be offered without knowledge of the patient's medical history.

In Australia and other countries, clinical pharmacy initially developed to a much greater extent in the acute tertiary care hospital setting; however, this is now changing. Since 1997, the Australian government has provided funding for some clinical pharmacy services in community settings. Medication management services, such as the review of medications prescribed to patients in geriatric homes, are now funded independently of drug distribution. While these new services are still evolving, the practice models currently being established require significant collaboration between the patient's primary care doctor and pharmacist. With these changes and advances in information technology, it is likely that the differences between clinical pharmacy roles in the community and hospital pharmacy practice settings will gradually reduce.

Variations in the development of clinical pharmacy among different countries have also resulted from many related and unrelated factors. The balance between public and private health services, the relationship between the medical and pharmacy professions, the education focus of pharmacy undergraduate and postgraduate programmes and the willingness of individual pharmacists to relinquish or delegate their established role in distribution or manufacturing and adopt patient-focused clinical practice, have all contributed to the speed of adoption of clinical pharmacy in different countries. Despite these differences, it is clear from clinical pharmacy development throughout the world that the stimulus and need for the services in different countries are the same. When and wherever drugs are used therapeutically, there is a need for pharmacists to work with medical practitioners to assist and facilitate optimal and safe drug use.

In the United Kingdom, clinical pharmacy practice in hospitals has developed along similar lines to that in Australia. In some other major European countries, such as Germany, pharmacy education has retained a strong chemistry and pharmacognosy focus, which has slowed the advancement of clinical pharmacy practice. Undergraduate pharmacy students in some European countries now have the opportunity to complete electives overseas, and some of these students are choosing to complete clinical placements in countries such as Australia. With time, this should assist the development of clinical pharmacy in Europe.

Similarly, in some Asian countries such as India, Japan, Malaysia, Singapore and Thailand, there is increasing appreciation of the role of pharmacists in healthcare and increasing interest in clinical pharmacy practice. Some undergraduate and postgraduate students from these countries study in Australia and other countries, which increases their understanding of the pharmacist's role in healthcare. In 2000, the World Health Organization sponsored the clinical training of pharmacists from Malaysian government hospitals in Australia. These pharmacists are now passing on their skills in clinical pharmacy to other pharmacists in Malaysia.

Clinical Pharmacy in Hospitals

As mentioned earlier, clinical pharmacy had its origins in hospitals, where distribution functions could be delegated to technicians under the general supervision of pharmacists. This enabled pharmacists to leave the dispensary and enter wards where they could directly interact with medical staff, nursing staff and patients. In many cases, this was driven by the enthusiasm of individual pharmacists with a desire and ability to expand the role of the pharmacist within a medical team. This transition often initially involved a service called 'ward pharmacy' rather than clinical pharmacy.

Ward pharmacy has been defined as a system where the pharmacist visits wards regularly to monitor for completeness and accuracy of prescriptions, is available for consultation by medical and nursing staff and ensures that the drug distribution system is operating correctly. Often, this is an important stepping stone to a more extensive clinical pharmacy service, particularly in a setting where less experienced and/or less educated pharmacists are the only ones available to undertake ward-based services.

As the education, training and experience of ward-based pharmacists grew, so did the breadth of and demand for their services. At a local level, the appreciation of the value of the experienced and knowledgable clinical pharmacist by medical and nursing staff was often a key reason for the development and expansion of services in individual hospitals. Over time, participation in medical ward rounds, medication history taking, drug therapy selection, therapeutic drug monitoring services, provision of drug information, adverse drug reaction monitoring and prevention, drug use evaluation and research and teaching have become activities that now form the basis of contemporary clinical pharmacy practice.

Given the complexity of modern drug therapy, it was not surprising that clinical pharmacy practice across the full range of medical and surgical patients soon became too much for a generalist pharmacy practitioner. This has resulted in a variety of specialist clinical pharmacy practitioners in areas such as oncology, psychiatry, geriatrics, cardiology and nephrology, to name but a few. In countries such as the USA, these specialty practices are now endorsed by professional and registering bodies with defined accreditation criteria.

As the practice of clinical pharmacy has grown and developed in hospitals, so has the evidence of the benefits to patients and to hospitals. Studies have clearly shown that clinical pharmacy improves drug therapy and overall patient health outcome, reduces drug-induced illness and the length of hospital stay, and reduces both drug costs and total health costs. Despite this, the need for the cost justification of clinical pharmacy services has not diminished as the models of health system funding continue to change. However, the justification of services is dependent on the financial frame of reference for an individual hospital or health service. Results of financial benefit obtained in one country may not always be applicable in another country with different cost structures. However, the benefits of clinical pharmacy services to improved drug use, patient well-being and health outcome are likely to be similar between health services and different countries.

Clinical Pharmacy in the Community

As outlined earlier, the expansion of clinical pharmacy services to community patients in Australia was limited by the lack of reimbursement for these services. The same has been true in other Western countries. This situation is now changing, in response to evidence that pharmacist involvement in drug therapy review and management could improve the health outcome. The Australian government now pays accredited pharmacists to undertake a formal review of medication regimens for patients living either in the community or in homes for the elderly. Pharmacists must undertake additional study to become accredited to provide this service, and a referral from the patient's doctor is required. The pharmacist then conducts a Home Medicines Review (HMR) by visiting patients in their own home to identify and help resolve any medication-related problems. These are then summarised in a written report to the patient's doctor. The service requires no payment from the patient as the government covers the full cost.

Other areas where clinical pharmacy may extend into the community setting in the future include collaborative prescribing and the management of anti-coagulation for patients taking warfarin.

Relationship with the Medical Profession

One of the most important aspects of practice for clinical pharmacists is their relationship with medical practitioners. While many clinical pharmacy activities such as counselling can be undertaken directly with the patient, other interventions rely on a co-operative working relationship between the pharmacist and the prescriber. For example, co-operation from the medical practitioner is required to enable the implementation of significant changes to therapy recommended by the clinical pharmacist. Good collaborative relationships with the medical profession depend on mutual respect, and on the pharmacists demonstrating clearly their commitment to the welfare of patients under the physician's care. Individual relationships can also be strengthened by participation in non–patient care activities, such as research and educational activities. Specialist clinical pharmacists have the opportunity to strengthen relationships with specialist medical practitioners in their fields by providing high-level clinical support and specialised drug information.

From a historical perspective, the factors that resulted in the need for clinical pharmacists were also recognised by the medical profession and resulted in the creation of a new medical specialist, the clinical pharmacologist. The American College of Clinical Pharmacology was founded on September 11, 1969 by a group of eminent physicians who recognised the need for a new medical specialty to bridge the gap between the well-established discipline of basic pharmacology and drug use in humans.

While the evolution of clinical pharmacists and clinical pharmacologists commenced at about the same time in the 1960s with similar broad goals, differences have emerged with time. Clinical pharmacology remains a small but important discipline of medicine. Its influence on individual patient outcome, however, relies on consultation requests from other medical practitioners. Most specialist medical groups are often well-informed about the range of medications they regularly use. The need for another medical opinion from a pharmacology specialist is often not considered necessary. The clinical pharmacist, on the other hand, is able to identify problems and issues without specific consultation and is therefore in a significantly better position to contribute positively to individual patient care.

While it has been difficult for clinical pharmacologists to have a broad impact at the patient level, they have excelled in many areas. These include drug utilisation at the hospital or regional level through their involvement in drug committees, establishment of drug use guidelines, therapeutic drug monitoring services and clinical toxicology services. These valuable services coupled with their critical role in medical research and education has meant that clinical pharmacologists have had a major impact on improved drug use globally.

The overlap in focus and interest between clinical pharmacologists and clinical pharmacists has the potential for conflict between the two professional groups. In most cases, however, collaboration between clinical pharmacologists and clinical pharmacists is mutually beneficial.

An important milestone in the history of clinical pharmacy development in the United States was the publication of an editorial by Lundberg, entitled 'The clinical pharmacist', in the Journal of the American Medical Association in 1983. The editorial traced the history of the development of clinical pharmacy and endorsed the role of clinical pharmacy in patient care. This public endorsement from a conservative medical body was of huge assistance in legitimising clinical pharmacy in the eyes of the broad medical profession.

More recently, the American College of Physicians and the American Society of Internal Medicine jointly published a position paper on their current perspective on the scope of pharmacist practice in the United States. The paper supports collaborative practice between physicians and pharmacists but opposes independent pharmacist prescribing rights. The paper also provides the reader with a useful overview of United States legislation, defining responsibilities for pharmacists in the United States.

In Western countries, the healthcare needs of an ageing population have resulted in a shortage of doctors, nurses and other healthcare professionals. In the United Kingdom and some other countries, this shortage has resulted in nurses and pharmacists taking on supplementary or independent prescribing roles within their specialised area of practice. UK pharmacists who wish to do this must complete a university-based course recognised by the Royal Pharmaceutical Society of Great Britain. They must also undertake a programme of practice-based learning under the supervision of a medical practitioner. The goal is to ensure that pharmacist prescribers are competent to practise as specified by the National Prescribing Centre, UK.

In Australia, nurse practitioners are permitted to prescribe certain drugs and under certain conditions, and it is possible that in the future, pharmacists with appropriate training may follow their UK colleagues in this area. High-quality accreditation programmes and careful negotiation will be essential to ensure that this extension of the pharmacist's role does not adversely affect good relationships with medical colleagues.

Clinical Pharmacy Education

The change in pharmacy practice focus from a product to a patient would not have occurred without parallel changes in the pharmacy undergraduate and postgraduate curriculum. In fact, it was essential that pharmacy educators embraced the vision of clinical pharmacy very early in its origin. The inclusion of therapeutics and clinical pharmacy as core subjects was fundamental to the continued progress of clinical pharmacy. Again, there has been variation from country to country in this regard, which has also influenced the speed of clinical pharmacy development in some countries.

As well as course content, the course length and style of teaching has also evolved with time to meet the needs of the profession. In the United States, a Doctor of Pharmacy degree, which requires four years of education beyond the minimum two years of pre-pharmacy study, has become the standard for hospital clinical practice. These undergraduate programmes are supported by postgraduate general residencies, specialty residencies and fellowships to further prepare clinical pharmacists for practice. In addition, and to complement this, certification for selected areas of specialty practice may also be required.

In other countries such as the United Kingdom, Australia and New Zealand, the duration of undergraduate programmes has increased to a minimum of four years, with a clear focus on clinical pharmacy and therapeutics. These undergraduate changes are complemented by structured postgraduate clinical pharmacy programmes ranging from diploma to doctorate levels. In addition, a period of supervised pre-registration experience is required before practice registration.

The style of teaching is also an important consideration when preparing clinical pharmacy practitioners. While pharmacology and the basis of therapeutics can be effectively taught didactically, practical therapeutics and clinical pharmacy require significant practice-based training to be taught optimally.

The Future

Clinical pharmacy has been evolving for over 50 years. One of the most exciting recent developments is the introduction of clinical pharmacy education and practice in countries such as India, where these services have previously been limited. In countries where clinical pharmacy services have predominantly been located within hospitals, we are now seeing them adopted in other healthcare settings.

The key to the continuing development of clinical pharmacy services internationally will be demand from patients for safer and more effective drug therapy, coupled with greater recognition of the pharmacist's expertise in evaluating drug information and evidence from medical literature. The opportunity exists for significant expansion of existing clinical pharmacy services. The concept that a healthcare team is required to meet all the complex health needs of patients is now well-established. The clinical pharmacist should be a primary member of such teams.

The level of uptake internationally will depend on many factors. These include the willingness of pharmacy educators to provide courses that prepare practitioners for clinical work, the willingness of pharmacists to delegate drug distribution to technician support staff, the support of medical colleagues and recognition by healthcare funders that clinical pharmacy is a fundamental and cost-effective core health service that independently improves patient healthcare outcome.

KEY MESSAGES

- Clinical pharmacy has evolved in many countries around the world for similar reasons.
- These reasons include a large increase in the number of drugs available, an increase in the complexity of therapy and a need for the safe and effective use of drugs. These demands have occurred as the requirement for pharmacists to prepare elaborate formulations has diminished, thus freeing them to undertake clinical pharmacy activities to improve the quality use of medicines.
- This evolution has been varied, resulting in differences in the level of clinical pharmacy practice among countries, and within countries between different hospitals and other practice settings.
- Clinical pharmacy is most effective when it is practised within a healthcare team in close collaboration with the medical and nursing professions.

Further Reading

American College of Physicians and American Society of Internal Medicine. 2002. Pharmacist Scope of Practice. *Ann Intern Med* 136:79–85.

Bond CA, Raehl CL and Franke T. 2001. Clinical pharmacy services, pharmacy staffing, and the total cost of care in United States hospitals. *Pharmacotherapy* 20(6):609–21.

Boyko WLJ, Yurkowski PJ, Ivey MF, Armitstead JA and Roberts BL. 1997. Pharmacist Influence on Economic and Morbidity Outcomes in a Tertiary Care Teaching Hospital. *American Journal of Health-System Pharmacy* 54:1591–1595.

Brodie DC, Parish PA and Poston JW. 1980. Societal Needs for Drugs and Drug-Related Services. *Am J Pharm* 44:276–8.

Gattis WA, Hasselblad V, Whellan DJ and O'Connor CM. 1999. Reduction in heart failure events by the addition of a clinical pharmacist to the heart failure management team; results of the Pharmacist in Heart Failure Assessment Recommendation and Monitoring (PHARM) Study. *Arch Intern Med* 159:1939–45.

Hepler CD and Strand LM. 1990. Opportunities and Responsibilities in Pharmaceutical Care. *Am J Pharm* 53:75–155.

Hughes J, Donnelly R and James-Chatgilaou G. 2001. *Clinical pharmacy: a practical approach*. The Society of Hospital Pharmacists of Australia.

Johnson JA and Bootman JL. 1997. Drug-Related Morbidity and Mortality and the Economic Impact of Pharmaceutical Care. *American Journal of Health-System Pharmacy* 54:554–558.

Kaboli PJ, Hoth AB, McClimon BJ and Schnipper JL. 2006. Clinical Pharmacists and Inpatient Medical Care. A Systematic Review. *Arch Intern Med* 166:955–964.

Leape LL, Cullen DJ, Clapp MD, Burdick E, Demonaco HJ, Erickson JI et al. 1999. Pharmacist participation on physician rounds and adverse drug events in the intensive care unit. *JAMA* 282:267–70.

Lundberg GD. 1983. The Clinical Pharmacist. *JAMA* 249:1193.

McMullin ST, Hennenfent JA, Ritchie DJ, Huey WY, Lonergan TP, Scaiff RA et al. 1999. A prospective, randomised trial to assess the cost impact of pharmacist-initiated interventions. *Arch Intern Med* 159:2306–9.

Mikeal RL, Brown TP, Lazarus HL and Vinson MN. 1975. Quality of Pharmaceutical Care in Hospitals. *Am J Hosp Pharm* 32:567–74.

Raehl CL and Bond CA. 2000. 1998 National Clinical Pharmacy Services Study. *Pharmacotherapy* 20:436–460.

Schumock GT, Meek PD, Ploetz PA and Vermeulen LC. 1996. Economic Evaluations of Clinical Pharmacy Services: 1988–1995. The Publications Committee of the American College of Clinical Pharmacy. *Pharmacotherapy* 16:1188–1208.

Stewart S, Vandenbroek AJ, Pearson S and Horowitz JD. 1999. Prolonged beneficial effects of a home-based intervention on unplanned readmissions and mortality among patients with congestive heart failure. *Arch Intern Med* 159:257–61.

World Health Organization. 2006. *Developing pharmacy practice*. A focus on patient care.

3 Community Pharmacy Practice

BG Nagavi, Ramesh Adepu and Grant Kardachi

Learning Objectives

Upon completion of this chapter, the reader should be able to:

- Explain the importance of community pharmacy in healthcare
- List medication use problems which are common in India
- Summarise the professional responsibilities of community pharmacists
- Discuss the findings and implications of research studies on community pharmacy practice in India

Ccommunity pharmacy is the term used to describe the provision of pharmaceutical care by pharmacists in primary healthcare settings. In India, a community pharmacy is a drug store or medicine shop used by people residing in the nearby area. It may be located in a remote village, district centre or busy metropolitan city. In other words, it is a pharmacy set up in a community to meet the public's medicine and other healthcare needs. This includes stocking and dispensing prescription and over-the-counter (OTC) medicines, and professional services such as patient counselling and health screening services. Depending on the location, some community pharmacies may also provide medicines to nearby hospitals and nursing homes.

The World Health Organization (WHO) has identified community pharmacists as the healthcare professionals who are most accessible to the public. They supply medicines in accordance with a prescription or sell them without prescription when legally permitted. Depending on the location, the responsibilities of community pharmacists include processing prescriptions, making up extemporaneous preparations, manufacturing medicines on a small scale, supplying traditional and alternative medicines, responding to symptoms of minor ailments, monitoring medication use, providing drug information to healthcare professionals and to the public, aiding health promotion, offering domiciliary services and referring customers to other healthcare professionals. In rural areas, they may also supply veterinary medicines. The International Pharmaceutical Federation (FIP) has also identified similar responsibilities for community pharmacists.

All over the world, community pharmacists are respected and appreciated for their preventive and curative care of the ailing public. Every day, millions of people across the world visit community pharmacies for their healthcare needs. Due to easy accessibility without a need for an appointment and free advice, pharmacists are often the first point of contact in the healthcare system. This means that community pharmacies and pharmacists have enormous potential to play a positive and useful role in the public healthcare system.

Community Pharmacy Practice in the United Kingdom, North America and Australia

Pharmacy first appeared as an independent profession in Europe in the thirteenth century, when the Emperor Frederick II separated the practices of medicine and pharmacy. However, in England, this division was lost over succeeding centuries. In 1617, the independence of London apothecaries from grocers was established by a royal charter, and in 1815 the apothecaries were recognised in law as medical practitioners, alongside physicians and civil and military surgeons. However, the Apothecaries Act excluded chemists and druggists from the control of apothecaries, allowing this separate occupational group to buy and sell drugs and medicines. This became the early foundation for community pharmacy as we know it today.

In the twentieth century, the government assumed greater control and regulation of pharmacy and healthcare in general. The Nuffield report in the United Kingdom (1986) recommended that pharmacists accept extended responsibilities to improve patient health, leading to a shift in focus from the product to the patient. Thus community pharmacists became engaged in drug information services to both patients and doctors, health screening services, monitoring of drug therapy and counselling of patients.

In the United States of America (USA), the Omnibus Budget Reconciliation Act of 1990 (OBRA-90) established the pharmacist's responsibility to ensure that drug therapy is as safe and effective as possible. The pharmacist is required to actively resolve medication use problems by conducting a thorough review of the patient's prescription at the time of dispensing, to maintain patient case records and to provide counselling services.

Community pharmacists in Canada are engaged in professional dispensing, patient counselling and medication management review for senior citizens, care for patients with diabetes, hypertension and those who want cease smoking cigarettes. In Australia, community pharmacists are engaged in professional dispensing, patient counselling, monitoring patients' health through screening services and offering drug information services. Accredited community pharmacists also offer home medicines review (HMR) services to patients in consultation with General Practitioners.

In all these countries, a Bachelor of Pharmacy (B Pharm) or Doctor of Pharmacy (Pharm D) degree is the minimum qualification required to register and practise as a community pharmacist. In some countries, courses for pharmacy technicians are also available, which may lead to non-registrable qualifications.

Community Pharmacy Practice – Indian Scenario

In pre-Independence India, community pharmacies were opened as Chemists and Druggists based on the English model. Chemists from Britain established businesses in Calcutta (Kolkata), Madras (Chennai) and Bombay (Mumbai). They carried out compounding activities under the supervision of qualified persons from the UK and with the help of local untrained staff. As chemists and druggists, these early community pharmacies were predominantly traders, and no importance was given to professional services.

After Independence, the Pharmacy Council of India (PCI) was constituted in 1949 under Section 3 of the Pharmacy Act, to regulate pharmacy education and practice in India. A two-year Diploma in Pharmacy (D Pharm) was established as the minimum qualification necessary for an individual to register and practise as a pharmacist. Every year, about 34,000 students pass out with the D Pharm certificate and more than 60,000 B Pharm students graduate from various universities across the country. As B Pharm education is more focused towards the industry, community pharmacies in India are managed by registered pharmacists with a D Pharm qualification. As per the latest statistics, more than 600,000 community pharmacists are registered in various state pharmacy councils.

In India, more than 500,000 retail medical stores (community pharmacies) are functioning. The legal requirements to start a community pharmacy are a qualified person, a practice site area of 120 sq ft, suitably designed racks for storing medicines of all schedules and special storage facilities for biological preparations such as vaccines and sera. Most of these pharmacies are managed by pharmacists with a D Pharm qualification.

Many community pharmacists consider community pharmacy as a trade rather than a profession. In a study conducted by Ramesh et al. in 1999 in Mysore, it was observed that more than 65% of pharmacies are managed by non-pharmacists who 'hired' the practising licence of registered pharmacists. The situation is more or less the same in other parts of the country. In 2001, the same author investigated the public's perception of pharmacists, finding that 92% of the respondents rated community pharmacists as drug traders. In 2002, Ramesh and Nagavi found that more than 50% of surveyed pharmacists were unaware of their professional responsibilities. The main reasons for this were lack of adequate training and knowledge, non-legislation of professional services, lack of professional fees and doctor dispensing.

India is a country with significant drug-related problems due to polypharmacy, drug duplication, underdosing, potential drug interactions, illiteracy and inadequate information about medication use. Due to heavy patient load, a doctor's consultation is limited to the issue of prescriptions to patients with very limited or no information about the prescribed medications and their use. Community pharmacists, who should be the information providers and act as a vital link between patients and prescribers, remain as prescription fillers. Many articles have been published in various national journals explaining the reasons for poor recognition of pharmacists by the public and by other healthcare professionals.

In recent times, considerable changes have taken place in the practice of community pharmacy in India. Newly graduated pharmacists today accept the responsibility of maintaining patient medication records, counselling patients about their medication, diet and other lifestyle modifications, and offering health screening services.

In the next few years, the situation is expected to change for the better. A new professional degree, Doctor of Pharmacy (Pharm D) was introduced in 2008–09 in many pharmacy colleges and universities. This is expected to prepare a new breed of competent and qualified practising pharmacists who will take up the challenge of offering professional and pharmaceutical care services in the community and hospital practice settings.

Country Example: Community Pharmacy Practice in Australia

Community pharmacy practice varies between different countries depending on history, government regulations, funding sources, professional education and the overall healthcare system. To illustrate this, the community pharmacy scenario in Australia is described in more detail below.

Pharmacy in Australia has always had a dispensing/retail mix and this varies from pharmacy to pharmacy. The retail component has evolved to support the income derived from the dispensing side, thus making the pharmacy more viable. This blend of retail versus dispensing often also depends on the setting of the pharmacy – rural area, in a large shopping complex or small suburban shopping centre.

The retail component is a combination of products and services depending on the pharmacy, but generally consists of Scheduled Medicines that can be purchased directly by consumers, complementary medicines, vitamins, weight loss products, baby needs, skin care, first aid products and cosmetics.

Regulation: Community pharmacy in Australia is governed by a number of regulations. An overview of this is necessary to understand the Australian landscape.

Ownership: Pharmacies in Australia can only be owned by pharmacists. The number that can be owned by one pharmacist is restricted and that number varies from state to state. The aim in keeping the number small is that the pharmacist is able to be involved and to oversee the operations of each pharmacy that he or she owns.

Location rules: These exist so that established pharmacies serving the local community are protected against unreasonable competition, which may result in the pharmacy becoming unviable. A new pharmacy can only gain approval to operate based on community need.

Registration of premises: A pharmacy must be registered with the Pharmacy Board. This register allows contact with the pharmacy in case of any unprofessional pharmacy practices that may occur and also in the event of drug recalls that may need to be made. It is able to maintain contact with pharmacies to ensure that good practice standards are adhered to at all times.

Registration of pharmacists: At least one pharmacist registered for practice with the Pharmacy Board of Australia must be present on the premises during opening hours. To maintain competency, the Pharmacy Board ensures that pharmacists participate in ongoing education (at least 20 hours per calendar year) in the area that they mainly practice.

The Pharmaceutical Benefits Scheme (PBS): Most of the medicines dispensed in Australia are subsidised under the Pharmaceutical Benefits Scheme (PBS). The aim of this government-funded programme is to make all essential medicines available to all residents of Australia at an affordable price. Patients make a co-payment to the pharmacy at the time of dispensing and the balance is paid to the pharmacy by the government. In other words, it means that concession card holders (patients who receive social security benefit from the government or the Department of Veterans' Affairs, such as the elderly, the unemployed or people with some disability) pay $5.60 per prescription while general patients pay a maximum of $34.20.

Supporting this arrangement is a Safety Net Scheme whereby patients pay a maximum yearly amount if they buy a significant number of medicines. Patients who hold a concession card pay for a maximum of 60 prescriptions per calendar year. Once this limit is reached, they are not required to make any co-payment for the remainder of the year. General patients pay up to a maximum of $1317.20 per calendar year, and once this threshold is reached, they only pay $5.60 per prescription for the remainder of that year.

Not all drugs approved for marketing in Australia are listed on the PBS. To be listed, a medicine must first pass through a rigorous screening process to ensure that the drug is cost effective relative to other listed therapies for the same condition. In this way, the PBS acts as a de facto national formulary. Medicines which are not listed are generally more expensive for the patient than listed drugs, and as a result are prescribed infrequently.

Dispensing and counselling: The core business for most pharmacies involves dispensing prescription medicines. It is a legal requirement that each dispensed medicine is labelled with directions for use, the patient's name and the name of the pharmacy. In addition, the pharmacist may attach small cautionary and advisory labels to advise the patient about possible side effects or interactions. In many pharmacies, dispensary technicians dispense medications ready for final checking by a pharmacist. For each prescription dispensed, the government pays the pharmacy a dispensing fee and also a mark up on the cost of each medication. This process facilitates the appropriate and safe use of medicines by the public.

The pharmacist is expected to counsel the patient so that they obtain maximum benefit from the medications. To support this process, pharmacists use Consumer Medicine Information (CMI) leaflets that give the patient a plain language summary of important information about a particular medication, including how best to take it, the mechanism of action and effect of the medication and any adverse side effects. CMIs are prepared by the manufacturer, and pharmacists are reimbursed by the government when a CMI leaflet is supplied to a patient.

Staffing: The pharmacy undergraduate programme in Australia is a four-year course with an internship or pre-registrant year as its fifth year. Those who spend it in community pharmacy work under the direct supervision of a preceptor pharmacist whose responsibility it is to oversee this important practical developmental year. The intern pharmacist is exposed to all operations and services within the pharmacy and learns to be an active member of the pharmacy team.

The support staff in an Australian pharmacy are integral to the effective operation of the pharmacy. Pharmacy assistants can undergo formal training and obtain certificates according to their responsibility in the pharmacy. This may vary from a general pharmacy assistant involved in sales, to a retail manager overseeing a number of staff and being responsible for purchasing stock for the pharmacy, and to a dispensary technician supporting the pharmacist in the dispensary. Pharmacy assistants must now verify some of their educational activities according to Quality Care Pharmacy Program (QCPP) guidelines.

Quality Care Pharmacy Program (QCPP): This has been an initiative of the pharmacy profession in recent years to illustrate to the government and consumers that community pharmacy maintains appropriate standards and quality of practice.

The programme ensures that the pharmacy meets professional standards with regard to dispensing and any professional services that it might offer. These may include services to aged care facilities (nursing homes), HMRs in the community, methadone programmes and other screening programmes. QCPP ensures that a pharmacy has appropriate policies and procedures for all activities undertaken in it. All staff must maintain a portfolio that includes employment contracts, education activities and performance reviews.

An important component of QCPP is the cold chain procedure. All pharmacies are required to have an industry-standard vaccine fridge which is temperature-monitored for the storage of vaccines and other refrigerated products. This fridge is used for the sole purpose of storing medications. All refrigerated items received into and dispensed from the pharmacy must be transported in appropriate storage bags and maintained at a certain temperature, that is, the 'cold chain' must be maintained.

Accreditation for HMRs and residential medication management reviews (RMMRs): The last decade in Australia has seen the development of clinical services in community pharmacy. Pharmacists can now undergo an accreditation process to become eligible to conduct medication reviews for patients in their own homes (HMRs) or in aged care facilities (RMMRs).

This has been an exciting development for the profession and has clearly added another dimension to community practice. Financial incentives were introduced for pharmacists both to become accredited and to then maintain accreditation. This payment was funded by the Federal Government under the Medicare Scheme. This accreditation process is a competency based assessment and further details are available from the Australian Association of Consultant Pharmacy (AACP) website.

Home Medicines Review (HMR): This is a collaborative process which is initiated by a general practitioner (GP) referral to the patient's preferred community pharmacy.

The pharmacy organises for an accredited pharmacist to conduct the interview in the patient's home. This setting has been chosen because the pharmacist can more readily access all the patient's medicines and look at the equipment used by the patient such as nebulisers, asthma spacers and blood glucose meters.

In their own home, the patient is more comfortable and relaxed, and the pharmacist will often gain much more information and therefore achieve better health outcomes. The service involves the pharmacist assessing how the patient is managing their medicines. Issues that arise centre around compliance and the potential need for a dosage administration aid (DAA), side effects and benefits of medications and the use of medicines including complementary medicines that have been purchased without a prescription. In reviewing the patient's medicines, the pharmacist will look at the appropriateness of each medicine for the patient's medical conditions.

A report is compiled and sent to the patient's GP who then develops a care plan for future management of that patient and discusses any issues raised in the report from the pharmacist. The service is free to the patient while both the GP and pharmacist are paid by the government. This model is being reviewed to give the process more flexibility to meet patient needs in a more timely manner, including hospital discharge and patients living in rural and remote areas.

Residential medication management reviews (RMMR): These reviews are conducted in aged care facilities and can currently be initiated by a pharmacist or a GP. As with the HMR service, all patients are eligible for one review per year unless circumstances indicate that another review is warranted. In this setting, the pharmacist has access to more patient information such as nursing progress notes, laboratory data and care plans. In reality, it is a more clinical review compared to an HMR, where the focus is more on medication management.

The payment to the pharmacist by the government for conducting reviews in aged care facilities assumes that the pharmacist is involved in quality use of medicines (QUM) activities. These activities include being a member of the facility's Medication Advisory Committee (MAC) and focuses on medication issues such as medication incidents, drug use evaluation and nurse-initiated medication lists. Part of the QUM activities includes developing education sessions for nursing staff and protocols on how to manage crushing of medications for patients with swallowing problems. Pharmacists can be paid directly for undertaking RMMRs as opposed to the HMR service where the payment is made to the pharmacy.

Other professional services: Now that the HMR and RMMR services are established, other professional services are being implemented in pilot projects around Australia. These include diabetes and asthma management, vaccination services, supply of dosage administration aids, and patient medication profiles.

All these programmes give pharmacists the opportunity to show greater focus on patient care and health outcomes. They enable pharmacists to become respected members of the healthcare team and to work more closely with other health professionals, particularly GPs.

Community Pharmacy Agreement (CPA): The Pharmacy Guild of Australia has negotiated with the government to put in place a Community Pharmacy Agreement which is reviewed every five years. The Fifth Agreement was signed in 2010. It is through these agreements that the pharmacy profession negotiates funding arrangements for dispensing and professional services.

A component of the Agreement is focused on research grants which lead to the development of new programmes. It is clear that community pharmacy in Australia is highly dependent on the government for funding for these services once they are developed and introduced. There are, however, other initiatives that are developed by the pharmacy profession that are not government funded. These include programmes for weight management, smoking cessation and sleep apnoea.

Future direction and opportunities for Australian community pharmacists: Clear emphasis has been laid on the importance of developing professional services for the sustainability of the pharmacy profession in the community setting. Some Australian pharmacies use automated dispensing systems, and further developments in this technology will clearly redefine the dispensing process as time evolves. This means that pharmacists will need to use their skills in different ways.

In Australia, the government has set up a number of superclinics at different sites around the country with the aim of taking the load off an already stressed public hospital system. These clinics provide healthcare relevant to the area in which they are situated; for example, paediatrics, the elderly or sexual health. These clinics employ medical specialists, GPs and allied health practitioners. There are also opportunities for pharmacists in these multi-disciplinary settings, either working in a pharmacy setting within the clinic or as clinical pharmacists. Pharmacists can also work in GP practices and, occasionally, some have been employed on a private basis to coordinate care plans for patients and conduct medication reviews.

Another opportunity for pharmacists is in the area of non-medical prescribing. Other health professionals are moving into this area, including optometrists and nurses. The challenge for pharmacy will be to clearly separate supply and prescribing. There are some niche areas for pharmacy where this may soon occur, for example, methadone prescribing and the management of patients on warfarin therapy.

Scope of Community Pharmacy in Healthcare

Pharmacists in many developing countries are confined to prescription filling and stores management. With the changing scenario of pharmacy practice and the introduction of clinical pharmacy programmes in India, pharmacists have started to promote patient education, drug therapy monitoring, unbiased drug information, and monitoring and reporting of adverse drug reactions. Private pharmacies have also shown interest in providing counselling services to their clients.

Many professional organisations including the International Pharmaceutical Federation (FIP), Pharmaceutical Society of Australia (PSA) and the Royal Pharmaceutical Society of Great Britain stress that patient counselling is the pharmacist's responsibility. In a study conducted by Ramesh et al. surveying members of the public, respondents from Karnataka in India opined that patient counselling is a shared responsibility of both doctors and pharmacists, whereas respondents from Kerala viewed patient counselling as the pharmacist's responsibility.

Whatever the type of medication, patients need basic information regarding the administration technique, storage conditions, possible side effects associated with use and possible drug–drug and drug–food interactions, together with suitable strategies to overcome these. Next to drug dispensing, patient counselling is probably the most widely accepted professional responsibility of pharmacists in most developed countries. In the United States, legal standards such as OBRA-90 require that pharmacists should offer patient counselling. Pharmacists have a duty to inform patients about the risks of prescribed drugs.

Many pharmacies maintain patient medication records. This helps the pharmacist understand and identify drug-related problems like non-adherence, drug interactions and adverse drug reactions. Especially in elderly patients, non-adherence is very common due to polypharmacy, adverse effects and forgetfulness. In the UK and Australia, there is increasing involvement of community pharmacists in the management of anti-coagulation and diabetes. Some pharmacists provide point-of-care measurement of International Normalized Ratios (INRs) for monitoring warfarin therapy and screening services for the detection of diabetes.

Community Pharmacist's Role in Preventive and Therapeutic Care

Pharmaceutical care is a patient-centred, outcome-oriented pharmacy practice that requires community pharmacists to work in concert with the patient and other healthcare providers to promote health, prevent disease and to assess, monitor, initiate and modify medication use to ensure that drug therapy is safe and effective. The ultimate goal of pharmaceutical care is to optimise the patient's health-related quality of life.

Pharmaceutical care in communities includes both preventive and therapeutic approaches. In the preventive area, they can actively participate in health education, health promotion, immunisation and vaccination programmes with other healthcare providers. Many research studies have been published showing the impact of pharmaceutical care in improving the symptoms, decreasing the number of hospital visits, and reducing the healthcare costs in chronic diseases such as arthitis, diabetes, hypertension and migraine.

On the therapeutic side, pharmacists can be involved in professional dispensing, counselling, drug information services, ADR reporting and monitoring, drug utilisation review (DUR) and HMR. Counselling and drug therapy monitoring services offered by pharmacists in community pharmacies can improve medication adherence and therapeutic outcomes, and have a positive impact on the patients' quality of life.

Community Pharmacy Practice Research

Community pharmacies are the places where community pharmacists have the opportunity to offer patient care services. Development of these services should ideally be evidence-based and corroborated by research studies conducted in community pharmacies. In the international scenario, many authors have published research studies pertaining to the effectiveness of patient counselling on therapeutic outcomes, medication adherence and quality of life.

Community pharmacy practice has gained momentum in recent years in India. Many Indian universities are now offering masters programmes in pharmacy practice and several research studies have been published in Indian journals in the area of community pharmacy practice. In a study by Ramesh et al. in 2001 regarding the attitudes and behaviours of community pharmacists towards patient counselling in the state of Karnataka, around 80% of the respondents agreed that patient counselling was a primary professional responsibility. However, this service was not provided for a number of reasons including lack of renumeration, non-co-operation by patients and lack of knowledge and confidence. The main strategy suggested for updating their professional skills and knowledge was through continuous professional development programmes.

Ramesh et al. showed the positive impact of community pharmacist-provided patient education on glycaemic control and improved therapeutic outcomes. Another study conducted by Ramesh et al. showed that counselling by community pharmacists had a significant impact on health-related quality of life in diabetic patients. In a study published by Raja Rakesh Chandra et al., trained community pharmacists actively participated in detecting adverse drug events in patients visiting their pharmacy and reported 45 ADRs in three months after receiving appropriate training. The ADR reports were found to be valid, and on the WHO causality assessment scale, many ADRs were rated in the 'possible' category. Carvalho et al. showed the impact of pharmacist-provided patient counselling on quality of life in hypertensive patients and Anjan Kumar et al. investigated the influence of patient counselling on therapeutic outcomes in asthma patients. Counselling improved the patients' understanding of the disease and improved inhaler technique. In a study conducted by Ramesh et al., 65% of prescriptions received in selected community pharmacies contained drug–drug interactions and among them 15% were assessed as moderate in nature.

A 2010 bibliometric review of the research articles published in various national and international journals pertaining to research in community pharmacy practice in India indicated that the main focus of research has been on the professional responsibilities of pharmacists and the impact of patient counselling on quality of life. Areas that need attention are pharmacovigilance, health screening activities and drug utilisation evaluation in community pharmacies.

Community pharmacy can provide a vital ground for retrospective and prospective research on drug and healthcare utilisation, disease management and outcomes of medication use. Research can provide useful information to professional and policy-making bodies and governmental agencies. Research findings can also help professionals, politicians and policy-makers recognise the value of community pharmacy services and thereby strengthen the healthcare system.

Future Directions

Over the next decade, a large number of Pharm D, M Pharm (Pharmacy Practice) and PhD holders will change the landscape of pharmacy practice in India. The quality and quantity of services provided will improve in favour of patients and the public. Research outcomes will provide new inputs to decision-makers to improve medication systems and policy; however, this future development depends on the quality and commitment of practicing pharmacists. There is a need to upgrade position descriptions together with commensurate salary packages to attract the best talent in the field. The long-pending issue of providing a professional fee for dispensing needs to be considered. Regulations are needed to ensure that employers provide facilities and the environment for pharmacists to practice. Health screening services in community pharmacies will attract more customers and improve business as well as healthcare. Pharmacists shall be involved in the planning and delivery of pharmaceutical care services, especially those concerning medication safety issues. Pharmacists have an important role to play on policy-making committees and in key positions along with other healthcare professionals to give their expert opinions about medicines policy and medication use.

There may be a need to conduct an entry-level qualifying exam before pharmacists can register and practice. This will ensure a minimum competency level for registered practitioners. These exams may be conducted once or twice a year regionally or nationally, as is done for North American Pharmacy Licensure Examination (NAPLEX) in the USA. Quality is the only engine for success. Hence, only competent and skilled pharmacists should be allowed to practise to protect patients and the public interest.

KEY MESSAGES

- Community pharmacists are often the first point-of-contact in the healthcare system and have enormous potential to play a positive and useful role in patient care.
- A wide variety of factors determine how community pharmacy is practised in different countries.
- Government funding, strictly enforced regulation and patient-focused education for pharmacists have assisted the development of professional services in community pharmacy practice in Australia and other countries.
- Changes in pharmacy education in India will equip pharmacists to introduce new professional services in community pharmacies in India.
- Excellent working relationships with the medical profession will assist community pharmacists during the transition to patient-focused care.
- Research into medication use in India should be used to provide evidence for new initiatives in patient care in the community pharmacy setting.

Further Reading

Anjan Kumar DS, Ramesh A, Parthasarathi G and Mahesh PA. 2009. Impact of community pharmacist provided patient education on treatment outcomes in community pharmacies. *Indian J Pharm Educ Res* 43(2):125–133.

Basak SC and Sathyanarayana D. 2010. Community Pharmacy Based Research Activity in India. A bibliometric study of the past ten years. *Southern Med Review* 3(1):7–10.

Carvalho S and Nagavi BG. 2007. Impact of community pharmacy-based patient education on the quality of life of hypertensive patients. *Indian J Pharm Education* 41, 2, (164–169).

Raja Rakesh Chandra P and Ramesh A. 2009. Design, implementation of adverse drug reaction reporting system in community pharmacies. *Indian J Pharm Pract* 2(2): 31–37.

Ramesh A and Karthik S. 2009. Study of impact of patient education on health related quality of life in benign prostatic hyperplasia (BPH) patients in a South Indian teaching hospital. *Asian Journal of Pharmaceutical and Clinical Research* 2(4):97–103.

Ramesh A and Nagavi BG. 2003. Public perception of Community Pharmacists in the State of Karnataka, India. *Indian J Pharm Sciences* 45(2):15–18.

Ramesh A and Nagavi BG. 2009. Attitudes and behaviors of practicing community pharmacists towards patient counseling. *Indian J Pharm Sciences*. 71(3): 285-–289.

Ramesh A, Babu BA and Nagavi BG. 2009. Impact of community pharmacy based patient education on quality of life in type 2 diabetes mellitus. *Indian J Pharm Pract* 2(2):43–51.

Ramesh A, Nagavi BG and Mahendra Kumar BJ. 2003. Karnataka state practicing community pharmacists perception about their professional responsibilities – A study. *Indian J Pharm Sciences* 45(2):65–69.

Ramesh A, Nagavi BG and Mahendrakumar BJ. 2004. Patient Counseling - practicing community pharmacists perception from two south Indian states. *Indian J Pharm Sciences* 66, 10, 44–48.

Ramesh A, Nagavi BG and Ramanath KV. 2000. Critical review of community pharmacies (Drug stores) in Mysore city. *Indian J Hosp Pharm* May–June 91–93.

Ramesh A, Rasheed A and Nagavi BG. 2007. Influence of patient counseling on quality of life in type 2 diabetes mellitus patients in two selected South Indian community pharmacies – a study. *Ind J Pharm Sciences* 69(4):519–524.

Ramesh A, Singhal R and Nagavi BG. 2008. A study of potential drug–drug interactions in prescriptions received at selected community pharmacies. *Ind J Pharm Edu Res* 42(2):184–189.

Ramesh A and Somashekar A. 2010. Influence of structured patient education on therapeutic outcomes in diabetes and hypertensive patients. *Asian J Pharm Clin Res* 3(3):174–178.

Roberts A, Benrimoj C, Dunphy D and Palmer I. 2007. *Community Pharmacy – Strategic Change Management*, McGraw-Hill Australia Pty Ltd.

Tipnis HP. 2009. *Community Pharmacy.* Career Publications, India.

Websites of Interest

International Pharmaceutical Federation
www.fip.org

The Pharmaceutical Benefits Scheme
www.medicareaustralia.gov.au

The Quality Care Pharmacy Program (QCPP)
www.guild.org.au/qcpp

The Australian Association of Consultant Pharmacy
www.aacp.com.au

The Pharmacy Guild of Australia
www.guild.org.au

The Community Pharmacy, Scotland
http://www.communitypharmacy.scot.nhs.uk

4 Key Competencies for Clinical Pharmacy Practice

David Cosh and G Parthasarathi

Learning Objectives

Upon completion of this chapter, the reader should be able to:

- List the key competencies for clinical pharmacy practice
- Describe how these competencies can be acquired
- Understand the importance of clinical acumen and evidence-based medicine when formulating opinions about drug therapy

A description of the competencies required for any activity calls for a clear definition of the activity in question. One way of defining clinical pharmacy practice is to describe scenarios that represent the core roles of a clinical pharmacist, and then use these to reflect upon the competencies needed to perform them effectively.

In the first scenario, a clinical pharmacist attending a ward round suggests a drug treatment regimen designed to improve a patient's health outcome. In doing so, the pharmacist uses his knowledge of the disease being treated, the recommended drug(s) and their role in disease management, results of relevant investigations and procedures, a knowledge of the patient's medical history and current co-morbidities, patient demographics and an understanding of the patient's own wishes and attitude to his illness. The pharmacist then communicates his conclusions to the medical team in a clear and logical manner.

In the second scenario, the same pharmacist explains to the patient or carer why the selected drug has been chosen, what effects, both beneficial and adverse, might be expected from taking the drug, and ensures that the patient or carer has a clear understanding of how to take or use the drug, thereby ensuring the best chance of effective, safe and economic drug use.

With these very straightforward scenarios in place, it can be seen that a competent clinical pharmacist needs a sound knowledge of therapeutics and disease state management, good communication skills and the ability to formulate an opinion on drug treatment strategies in a logical manner using a variety of information sources.

Therapeutics

Knowledge of therapeutics is an essential prerequisite for effective clinical pharmacy practice. Therapeutics can be simply defined as the use of drugs to treat disease in a rational, safe and cost-effective manner. There are two elements in therapeutics: the drug and the disease. Knowledge of disease state management is essential if therapeutics is to be practised well. Knowing when a drug is indicated is just as important as knowing when the reverse applies.

The oft-quoted phrase 'pharmacists are drug experts' is so broad as to be of little relevance in the clinical setting. Many pharmacists may be 'drug experts' from the perspective of chemistry, formulation, chemical class and principal mode of action, but when confronted with a real-life patient, it is not uncommon for pharmacists to be unsure of how effective a drug might be in treating the disease(s) for which it is intended in that patient.

Most pharmacy undergraduate courses attempt to provide links between drugs and disease. However, the bewildering array of drugs and the increasing complexity of disease management mean that teaching therapeutics at anything other than a basic level can be difficult in any undergraduate curriculum, whether it be medicine or pharmacy. Problems arise because of time and resource constraints, together with the need for adequate patient contact time. The latter is usually obtained at the bedside in the teaching hospital environment, though ambulatory settings are also suitable teaching environments for many clinical situations, for example, dermatology.

Traditionally, ward rounds have been used to teach junior doctors, aspiring physicians and medical students a whole range of medical skills, not the least of which is therapeutics. In the early days of clinical pharmacy practice in Western countries, medical practitioners became surrogate teachers of therapeutics to pharmacists as the latter joined formal ward rounds. Clinical pharmacists have been able to benefit from teaching activities intended for medical students and junior doctors, and these educational opportunities are now available to many clinical pharmacists who practise and train in Indian teaching hospitals.

The ward round provides an unrivalled opportunity for the clinical pharmacist to see, first hand, what a disease means to a patient. The textbook descriptions of disease that may be difficult to remember for exams take on a whole new dimension when supplemented with exposure to a person suffering from the disease in question. The observation of pain and distress and, hopefully, the alleviation of these when treatment is successful provide a level of education and understanding that can never be supplied by a classroom or computer.

Participation in ward rounds is an important activity for clinical pharmacists in terms of their contribution to patient care. It enables pharmacists to offer advice and suggestions at the time when prescribing decisions are made, and thereby contribute to rational drug use. Adverse drug reactions

(ADRs) are common and can mimic diseases, and hence be difficult to detect. Expertise in this area is extremely useful, and may reduce the need for additional investigations and treatment. It must be remembered that diagnosis is a cornerstone of medical practice, and if one is restricted to one piece of advice to an aspiring clinical pharmacist, it might profitably be *"with some exceptions, avoid the temptation to diagnose."* The exceptions are possible drug-related illnesses where pharmacists may be able to offer relevant advice.

Communication Skills

On ward rounds or clinic visits, clinical pharmacists see and hear how medical practitioners approach their task of diagnosis and treatment, and through this they gain an understanding of how medical practitioners communicate with each other and their patients. This exposure to the 'medical language' used to communicate decisions and treatment plans enables clinical pharmacists to communicate with medical practitioners in their own language.

The competent clinical pharmacist counsels patients to ensure that they understand why they have been asked to take a drug, how to take it and what they might expect in terms of outcomes and side effects. This is one of the most important responsibilities of a clinical pharmacist, and many medical practitioners welcome the support of the pharmacist in reinforcing messages that may have been given during a medical consultation. Effective communication underpins the pharmacist–patient relationship, whether it takes place in the pharmacy, clinic or at the bedside. Many undergraduate pharmacy programmes are now paying particular attention to the need for their graduates to be well-trained in communication skills and patient counselling.

The Importance of Clinical Acumen

Exposure to a broad range of treatment options teaches pharmacists that drug treatment is not necessarily the panacea for every ill, and that for many illnesses, drugs are either inappropriate or may even make matters worse. They realise that choosing an appropriate, efficacious and safe drug for the correct indication, a suitable dose and formulation administered at the correct intervals for the required duration is important to ensure rational and safe drug use.

They learn to recognise that, while identifying potential drug interactions is important, many of the potential interactions may be of minimal clinical significance for individual patients. Drug use that appears to be the accepted course of action according to textbooks may be seen to fail, and what may appear to be misguided prescribing in theory may be surprisingly effective. This emphasises that even in the era of evidence-based medicine, medicine remains an art as well as a science, and that clinical acumen remains a highly valued attribute for both the medical practitioner and the pharmacist.

Formulating Opinions

Clinical pharmacists must use a variety of information sources to formulate an opinion on the drug treatment for a patient. These include information gathered through taking the patient's medication history, reviewing the patient's drug therapy and the results of relevant laboratory investigations.

Clinical pharmacists must understand the role that laboratory monitoring can play in both the diagnosis of disease and the monitoring of drug therapy. Drugs affect physiological processes and these effects, both desired and not, may be reflected in parameters that are amenable to measurement. Clinical pharmacists need to know what test(s), in an ideal situation, would be appropriate, and how such investigations may be used to improve the efficacy and safety of a particular drug regimen.

For example, if a drug that may impair renal function is prescribed, then monitoring renal function by determining serum urea and creatinine levels may be useful. A competent clinical pharmacist would recognise the need for testing to take place, know how often to test and be able to relate the results obtained to ongoing treatment decisions. Equally important in many situations is an opinion on whether it is safe to use the drug in the absence of facilities to determine renal function. Here, knowledge of the clinical signs that may indicate renal impairment is essential. Similarly, the ability to understand and interpret other laboratory results that provide information on liver function, thyroid function, pulmonary function, haematological parameters, cardiac function, microbiology and culture sensitivity data are essential for the practice of clinical pharmacy.

Therapeutic drug monitoring (TDM) has made it easier and safer to use drugs of narrow therapeutic index. However, it needs to be remembered that many of the drugs for which TDM is used to guide dosing can be used effectively and safely by experienced clinicians who do not have access to modern laboratory facilities. Both the prescriber and the pharmacist who work without the resources of a modern hospital laboratory need to be able to establish safe dosing regimens based on available information; for example, the patient's age, weight, concurrent drug therapy, co-morbid conditions and whatever relevant laboratory data might be available. In such a setting, an awareness of clinical signs that may indicate lack of efficacy or toxicity is very important.

Providing drug information to other health professionals and the public is a core activity of clinical pharmacy practice. The explosion in biomedical information makes it difficult for prescribers to stay up-to-date with the latest advances in drug therapy. Clinical pharmacists need to know where to find reliable information on drug use and how to formulate a written or verbal response to queries. They also need to be able to critically evaluate published studies in biomedical literature and to extrapolate the results of these studies to the patients they see. Once again, we notice that an essential skill for clinical pharmacy practice is the ability to formulate an independent opinion on drug treatment strategies in a logical manner using a variety of information resources, and to clearly communicate the conclusions to the doctor or patient.

Specialised Practice Versus General Practice

It has become common for clinical pharmacists to find themselves attached to specialist units such as respiration, psychiatry, nephrology and oncology. In some institutions, clinical pharmacy practice evolved from an initial attachment of a pharmacist to a specialist unit. Such attachments often happened because of the desire of the medical or surgical head of the unit to have a pharmacist on the team to assist in educating both the patients and the junior medical staff, and to act as a resource person for more general therapeutic information in a very specialised setting.

Debate continues over the need for specialist pharmacists versus generalists but there is room for both, as is the case in medicine. However, the first step to be taken by a pharmacist in acquiring competency in therapeutics and disease state management is to recognise the need to be a generalist, in the same way that an aspiring cardiologist will undertake a training programme that allows for the development of general physician skills. The special considerations needed when drugs are used in the very young and the elderly means that both generalist and specialist clinical pharmacists should have an awareness of the important principles of drug use in these age groups.

Conclusion

The role that a trained clinical pharmacist can play in today's healthcare environment is well recognised. Aspiring clinical pharmacists need to acquire skills in disease state management, therapeutics, communication, biomedical statistics and literature evaluation to complement their undergraduate training. Before making treatment recommendations, they also need to use a variety of practice methods and skills to gather patient-specific information. The rapid pace of developments in therapeutics means that all clinical pharmacists must make a commitment to continuing education throughout their career. Clinical practice provides opportunities for ongoing education and professional development, especially for pharmacists who work closely with medical colleagues in teaching hospitals.

KEY MESSAGES

To develop and maintain effective clinical pharmacy practice, one needs:

- Sound undergraduate education
- High-quality postgraduate education incorporating bedside learning
- A good working knowledge of therapeutics, disease state management and laboratory medicine
- Good communication skills
- The ability to arrive at a considered opinion on how drug treatment might be instituted or improved upon using a variety of information sources
- A commitment to continuing professional development

5
Communication Skills for Pharmacists

Ruth Ferguson

Learning Objectives

Upon completion of this chapter, the reader should be able to:

- Identify the key elements for successful communication
- Explain the processes by which information is sent and received
- Identify the communication methods required in clinical situations
- List the requirements for different forms of professional communication
- Choose appropriate and effective communication methods for a variety of audiences, including those with special needs
- Develop their communication skills through exercises, reflective practice and role play

When pharmacists take on clinical roles like identifying and reviewing patients' medication, providing medication counselling, offering information about medicines or an adverse drug reaction (ADR) monitoring service, interpersonal communication skills are critical for effective practice. Clinical situations can be challenging; for example, informing a senior consultant that a medicine they have prescribed may cause a potentially fatal interaction or counselling a family about the management of analgaesia for their dying loved one. Such situations require skill and a very high level of sensitivity to the circumstances. To be professionally effective, pharmacists will need to be aware of:

- The different messages they are sending
- How these could be perceived
- The messages others send
- How to interpret these and how misunderstandings can occur
- How to adapt communication to suit the audience and situation

While some people seem to be inherently good communicators, all pharmacists through education, training and practice can develop and improve their abilities.

This chapter provides a brief introduction to communication theory and discusses the common types of communication required of clinical pharmacists, with examples to illustrate key messages and exercises to assist skill development.

COMMUNICATION THEORY

Communication is, at its most basic, the sending and receiving of messages. The physical senses of sight, hearing, touch, smell and taste are part of day-to-day communication but in pharmacy practice, sight, hearing and occasionally touch are used. Individually, our communicating style is shaped by our experience of language, culture, social status, personality, interests, abilities and disabilities. When working as a pharmacist, we modify our personal style of communicating to fit the culture and language of the pharmacy profession. In this section, the importance of empathy, developing rapport and verbal and non-verbal aspects of communication are discussed.

Empathy

At the heart of all effective communication is empathy. *Empathy* is defined as the ability to see and feel the way another person does. For example, a pharmacist may need to discuss paracetamol dosing with a mother who is anxious about her child's illness. If this pharmacist can understand how frightening it may be to have a febrile, distressed infant who has been refusing to eat, then they are likely to be more attentive and sympathetic to the mother's concerns. This would enable the pharmacist to choose suitable words and non-verbal messages to provide support to the mother.

When feelings are not shared and empathy has not developed, communication can be impaired. If, for example, a hospital pharmacist is not able to identify a patient's fear of hospitals, they would be unlikely to obtain a reliable medication history. If this pharmacist could identify with and acknowledge the patient's concerns, they would be more likely to obtain the required information.

While some people are naturally empathetic, for others, it is an attribute that needs to be developed through awareness and practice. Every individual is unique and special, and it takes effort, patience and practice to develop the skills to react suitably to the uniqueness of every person we meet. Careful listening, close observation and reflecting on our interactions with others, especially those we find more challenging, can help develop our understanding of others and our ability to share with and understand others.

The significance of empathy is that it enables rapport (a sympathetic relationship based on understanding) to develop and this is an important first step in establishing successful and interactive communication.

Non-verbal Communication

Non-verbal messages begin to be received and interpreted as soon as something catches our attention. For example, when two people first meet, before a word is spoken, impressions are formed from information gained through sight, sound, smell and sometimes touch, such as through shaking hands. What is the expression on their face? How are they dressed? How old are they? What perfume are they wearing? Do they appear hostile or friendly? and much more.

These usually unconscious impressions are compared with information from past experiences and can quickly lead to judgments, forming an initial impression. This can have a significant impact on how people react during new encounters. Further contact with an individual will augment and support this first impression or may lead to modification, as more information is received and processed.

For example, if two young, blonde, well-tanned women come to a pharmacy, the pharmacist could assume that they are tourists visiting India and could be seeking treatment for gastroenteritis. These assumptions may or may not be accurate. At an emotional level, the pharmacist may be embarrassed by the clothing of these women, which seems more suited to a beach resort than to a respectable neighbourhood.

Strong emotional reactions are associated with prior experience and prejudice. Unless recognised and understood, these reactions can be a significant barrier to effective communication. Our pharmacist decides his customers have recently arrived in India and need his professional assistance.

Non-verbal communication includes messages conveyed through body posture. For example, someone who is sitting with their legs and arms crossed in front of their body signals a 'closed' body posture and this will hinder the flow of communication. A stance with feet together and uncrossed legs and arms (an open body posture) tends to ease communication. A very casual stance, for example, slouching, would suggest lack of interest and inattention. Other non-verbal signals such as looking away, fidgeting, being preoccupied with another activity or allowing other people to interrupt can also signal inattentiveness and inhibit communication. In *Exercise 1*, the influence of non-verbal information is explored.

Facial expression is an important indicator of emotional state. People instinctively observe the face to gain information which is not provided verbally. For example, does the person look angry, happy, worried, relaxed, friendly, and so on. Eye contact (or eye avoidance) can indicate the level of attention, and suggest honesty or confidence, but this may vary in different cultures.

The meaning of spoken language is modified by non-verbal information like loudness, the pitch, tone or how rapidly the message is delivered. For example, the statement 'what a day' spoken lightly in a higher pitch would mean that something unexpectedly positive has occurred, while spoken slowly and emphasising 'what' suggests a difficult time.

It is important that pharmacists are aware of the non-verbal messages they are transmitting to others, especially if these are likely to inhibit communication. Being able to recognise personal internal psychological states, being aware of how these states may be communicated non-verbally and then being able to modify non-verbal information is a useful approach to develop. *Case Study 1* provides an example of how personal awareness can be used to modify non-verbal communication.

In a professional setting, the interpretation and use of non-verbal messages can assist our work. By interpreting non-verbal signals from others and then modifying our approach to take account of their feelings, we can improve the opportunities for effective interaction. For example, if someone is restless, looking down and avoiding our eyes, we may interpret this as being embarrassed or ill-at-ease. We could change our style of language, soften our voice, adopt an open body posture, smile more to try to make the other person feel more comfortable. Verbally acknowledging the discomfort of another and offering an option to improve a delicate situation can be helpful. For example 'I'm sorry there is not much privacy here to discuss such a personal matter. If you like, I can see if an office is free.'

Non-verbal mannerisms vary from culture to culture, region to region, country to country. What is common and widely accepted in one place may be offensive or mean something quite different in another. There are inter-gender differences in the meaning of non-verbal messages and differences between people of different age groups. Being aware of potential differences can help avoid misinterpretation or causing offence. This is especially important when working away from our home territory or culture.

Diagrams are another form of non-verbal messages used to convey information. Pictograms (a picture which represents a concept or object) have recently been developed to communicate medical and medication information to people who are illiterate. The US Pharmacopeia website provides examples. Pictograms could be used in place of medicine labels (*see Exercise 2*) or to show how to administer a dosage form such as eye drops. Examples of advice sheets for different pharmaceutical products are provided in the PharmWeb website (listed at the end of this chapter). As there may be differences in interpretation of diagrams between cultures and countries, the interpretation should be checked with the recipient.

Verbal Communication

Verbal communication occurs through the meaning of words which may be spoken or written. Meaning can be subtly modified by non-verbal qualities; for example, the tone of voice or the typeface used. This is one aspect of spoken communication which we are usually least aware of and least in control of. We can, for example, convey irritation through voice tone without realising it. Interpretation of a message can be confusing when word meaning and non-verbal qualities conflict. If, for example, a very jaundiced patient responds to a standard query 'How are you feeling today?' with 'I'm fine, thank you', the meaning of the words is likely to be discounted. Emphasis too can create differences in meaning. For example: 'Did YOU remember to take your medicine this morning?' is likely to sound accusatory, but if spoken without emphasis, becomes a neutral inquiry.

Writing is less sensitive to non-verbal modification than spoken language, but differences in writing style can be used to modify meaning. For example, an informal and personal style is commonly used in email messages, while for business letters, the presentation and style is formal. Written fonts can convey subtle messages and do differ in their ease of reading. For example, a writing style like *italics* suggests the personalised style of handwriting, while a format like Arial is considered one of the more legible font styles. With written materials, all aspects of the composition such as word selection, writing style and presentation should be carefully selected for the audience.

Language: To be reliable, communication should be in a language which both the speaker and the audience are fluent in and comfortable with. For example, someone whose primary language is Urdu but who also speaks some Hindi and English may need to speak in English to communicate with someone who lives in Tamil Nadu and whose mother tongue is Tamil. Dialects modify spoken language and both pronunciation and meanings of words can differ greatly. For example, referring to someone as a Hindu in India is likely to refer to their religion, while in Australia this could mean someone from the Indian subcontinent.

Medicine and pharmacy have a shared professional language that uses Greek and Latin terms which are very different from everyday terms with the same meaning. Choosing the appropriate terms is important to both communicate effectively and to convey suitable verbal messages. For example, most patients would not understand the term 'myocardial infarction' but they will know what is meant by a 'heart attack'. Similarly, but in reverse, a pharmacist discussing a patient's alopecia with a doctor is more likely to be respected as a fellow health professional than one who discusses a patient's hair loss. Developing vocabularies for both professional and everyday terms is useful for sucessful professional pharmacy communication.

A website reference for common medical terms is provided at the end of this chapter. It could also be used as a base to prepare a dictionary specific to the local language and dialects or culture.

Differences in the pronunciation of medical terms and medicine names can cause confusion and is a source of error. Pharmacists have an important role to help promote, teach and standardise pronunciation. Both spoken dictionaries (*see the Merck website*) and phonetically spelt ones (*see the drugs.com website*) are available for medicine names.

The abbreviations and terms used for prescribing medicines represent a specialised type of communication shared by the medical and pharmacy professions. However, prescribing terms can be interpreted differently, and this has led to dosing errors and, in some cases, death. The notation 'qd' is commonly used in North America to mean 'once daily', but has been confused with 'qds' which in other countries means four times a day. Some health organisations provide a dictionary of prescribing terms and abbreviations to be used by their staff to reduce the risk of interpretational errors. Identifying confusing terms or abbreviations and checking the meaning with the author is the safest method to avoid these potential fatal errors.

Interactive communication: Two activities are principally involved in communication: the sending and the receiving of messages. A passive, one-way verbal process, like a traditional lecture, is considered an inefficient communication and learning method in most situations. (In reality, it is a two-way process, with the audience sending non-verbal messages such as listening attentively or yawning and chatting to neighbours, which may influence the lecturer). Effective communication and learning sessions are essentially two-way, interactive processes. Both parties will actively participate in speaking and listening in turn, interpreting the meaning of what is happening and comparing this to their personal experience.

At its simplest, when sending a message, the sender first forms a concept in their mind of what they want to communicate. This image will be based on the many and varied aspects of their personality and experience. They then form the concept into a verbal message and speak. The listener will then receive the words, the tone, emphasis and other non-verbal messages such as facial expressions, body position and hand movements and interpret the message within the framework of their experience.

We assume that if a message we have communicated seems clear to us it will be interpreted correctly by the listener. However, when people come from different language, cultural or educational backgrounds, interpretations can vary a great deal. Even two people from similar backgrounds will experience misunderstandings from time to time. The best way to ensure that a message is correctly understood is to ask the listener to repeat the message using their own words. If this differs from the intended meaning, then through discussion, a common understanding can be reached.

Listening skills: Developing good listening skills is important to promote clear interactive communication and to obtain reliable information. Good listeners are able to maintain their attention and not be distracted by external preoccupations (for example, the telephone) or internal diversions (thoughts on an unrelated topic such as an assignment due tomorrow). Non-verbal cues such as maintaining eye contact (but not staring or gazing) can demonstrate attention, as can nodding, verbally echoing the person's significant words or asking questions.

Good listeners will also use statements which back up and support the speaker, for example 'Ah, now I see what you mean', and this helps keep the conversation interactive and flowing. If a speaker wanders off the topic, it may be appropriate to politely interrupt and re-introduce the topic from the point of departure. When giving key information, it is an important practice to check for correct understanding by asking the listener to identify the main points of the message. While this may appear like an interrogation or be demeaning, if the purpose is carefully explained then the listener will not be offended and can assure the speaker that their message has been correctly understood (*see Case Study 2*).

Stages in verbal communication: In pharmacy practice, communication is usually short, often lasting only a few minutes. It is important that the time available is used well. The communication structure described below and demonstrated in *Case Study 2* shows how time can be used to good effect.

The purpose of the INTRODUCTION is to establish a connection between the parties who are communicating. It can promote rapport, build empathy and trust, engage interest and encourage an open interaction. The introduction involves the exchange of everyday courtesies and general enquiries. If a patient or caregiver appears distressed, this can be acknowledged and discussed to build up rapport and gain commitment and attention.

During the OPENING, the topic to be covered is introduced and briefly explained.

The BUSINESS stage is when the main messages are delivered or information is obtained.

It is important that a personal RE-CONNECTION is made as a preparation for ending the interaction. It is helpful at this point to make sure the details and relevance of the material are understood and clarification provided if needed.

During the CLOSURE, non-verbal messages can be important in signalling the end of a session (for example, gathering up papers or packing medicines and handing them over). Concluding courtesies will round off the encounter positively, and both parties will then separate.

Written Communication

There are different writing styles which are appropriate for different purposes. For example, a paper published in a professional journal must conform to the format required by that journal in order to be accepted for publication. Patient information leaflets (PILs) for medicines require a detailed and precise style in easily understood terms. Notation on a patient's medication chart, for example, 'take with food', is required to be concise and legible and may need to conform to local standards.

All forms of professional writing require clarity and precision. Short sentences and paragraphs, unambiguous words or statements and precise sentence structure are important qualities. Words need to be carefully chosen, with correct spelling and grammar, and presented in an easy-to-read handwriting or font.

Written messages require a logical structure. There should be a brief, clear introduction outlining the purpose of the article, statement or paragraph. The body should present ideas in a clear, logical structure. A concluding summary will repeat the main messages and clarify any action to follow.

Pharmacists are trained to use a particular style for the dosage instructions written on medication labels. While these may be second nature to us, they can be unclear or confusing for patients. The common expression 'Take one tablet daily' gives no indication about the time at which the tablet should be taken or when in relation to food. 'Take two tablets daily' does not identify whether the tablets should be taken together or spaced apart. Using more complete instructions and verbally checking understanding can prevent potentially dangerous misunderstandings.

Special Situations

Face-to-face interviewing: Interviews can be used to obtain information, for example, to obtain medication history, to assess a student's understanding of a subject during an oral examination or for screening job applicants. *Case Study 3* describes the use of interview techniques to obtain medication history. In any interview situation, there is a power difference between the interviewer and the interviewee (person being interviewed) which can be intimidating. The interviewee is also likely to be in unfamiliar surroundings while the interviewer is in a known environment, often of their choice. To obtain reliable information, it is important that the interviewee is at ease with both the environment and the interviewer. Spending time to develop rapport is important.

During an interview, NON-VERBAL MESSAGES conveyed through body posture are influential. Sitting at the same level as an interviewee is less intimidating than standing over them, especially if they are seated or lying in bed. Sitting also enables the interviewer to present an open body posture, and side-by-side seating is less threatening than face-to-face. The physical environment is important and in hospitals the provision of privacy can be challenging.

During the introduction, the PURPOSE of the interview is clearly identified. Sometimes it may be necessary to obtain consent from a patient to proceed. OPEN QUESTIONS are helpful to capture a wide range of information and are less likely to be influenced by the expectations of the interviewer. CLOSED QUESTIONS are suitable for verifying information. When used excessively, closed questions can make an interviewee feel they are being interrogated, while open questions give the interviewee the opportunity to express themselves in their own way.

When the information to be gathered appears complete, it is important that the content is CHECKED. A common and useful approach is to verbally summarise the information for the interviewee to confirm and comment on. If there is a large quantity of information or if it is complex, providing a written copy for the interviewee may be appropriate. If this is not suitable, then organising the information under different topics and providing a brief account of each may be helpful.

During an interview, difficult situations may occur which can be challenging for the interviewer. If, for example, an interviewee attempts to divert the discussion away from the topic, a skilled interviewer will politely interrupt and re-introduce the topic. If after further attempts the interviewee continues to digress, it may be more productive to politely stop the interview and perhaps return at a later time when the interviewee may be more co-operative. When topics which may be threatening or embarrassing to the interviewee are covered, the conversation may cease to flow. It may be necessary to DIGRESS to a subject the interviewee will be comfortable with for a short time or provide reassurance and supportive comments.

Encouraging a reluctant interviewee or controlling a vociferous one requires skill. Sometimes pharmacists may be placed in particularly difficult situations such as facing an angry, disturbed or threatening patient. Ways to handle less familiar or particularly challenging situations can be explored through role plays with classmates or colleagues. This provides a process which is safe for all, can provide useful insights and can be fun. In professional practice, the opportunity to interview in a wide range of situations and then to reflect on these (what went well, what didn't work and how performance could be improved) is a most useful life-long learning approach.

Providing information: Providing information about medicines is a common role for clinical pharmacists. Messages can be verbal, written, pictorial or a demonstration with verbal support. Actively engaging the client will aid their learning.

The first stage in the successful delivery of information is to CHECK the client's knowledge level and their information requirements. Information can then be adapted to maintain the client's interest, be relevant, complement information given by another health professional or to address inaccurate perceptions.

The length or AMOUNT of information required to be provided is important. Most verbal messages provided in pharmacy practice are short, often five minutes or less. Written information can be used to provide detail and to serve as a record of the verbal information. Well-presented medicine information will cover the most important points for treatment safety and effectiveness. For health professionals, an in-depth explanation based on current medical literature may be required.

The structure of the message should be PLANNED. If a person has a particular interest or concern, this is best acknowledged early to enhance rapport and arouse interest. People are more likely to remember information that is delivered early and late in a session. Placing key messages at the beginning and end of a session is a useful technique. Repetition of information using different words helps to reinforce learning.

Messages should be clearly delivered using language suitable for the recipient. Short sentences are more easily understood and encourage interaction and discussion. If complex information needs to be communicated, this is best built up gradually with frequent checks to ensure client understanding.

The final step is to check if the client understands the message and then reinforce the key points by SUMMARISING them. While this may seem repetitious, it is a well-established sucessful learning technique.

Case Study 4 provides an example of how information can be given to a patient and illustrates the different steps explained above.

COMMUNICATION IN PROFESSIONAL PRACTICE

People interact best when they feel comfortable with their surroundings and are at ease with and feel respected by those they are communicating with. Hospital wards or busy dispensary counters are very difficult environments for effective communication. Small attempts to increase privacy such as drawing the curtains or lowering the voice so that others can't overhear are important.

Clothing and presentation are important to convey non-verbal messages that have an impact on the development of first impressions. A clean, pressed, white coat gives the appearance of professionalism and, if other clinical staff dress similarly, this may promote better inter-professional communication. To a patient, the coat may emphasise a difference in status, education or wealth and could act as a communication barrier. It may be best to use your white coat for medical meetings but leave it in the office when interviewing patients.

Communication with Medical and Health Professionals

During the establishment of a clinical pharmacy service, inter-professional communication can be challenging. Once a service is well-accepted, pharmacists may be required to establish their credibility with new staff members or with a ward area in which they do not usually practice.

An important but difficult role faced by pharmacists is that of reviewing the prescribing of medical staff. It is important to avoid giving the impression of a pharmacy police force. Resolving or preventing medicine-related problems and carefully handling the potential friction this role may cause can be challenging to a new pharmacist or a new clinical pharmacy service. To gain acceptance requires a courteous approach and willingness to help, the provision of well-presented and reliable medicine-related information when needed and being effective as a team player. Patient welfare is the focus of any medical team and one which pharmacists need to share.

Pharmacists can represent an unwelcome intrusion in wards or clinics. Doctors and nurses who are unfamiliar with clinical pharmacy may feel that the pharmacist is a threat to some of their own roles and power. Focusing on the needs of patients, adding pharmaceutical/pharmacological value to an established service, acknowledging the abilities of other staff and supporting their roles are effective diplomatic approaches to help overcome resistance and barriers.

When interacting with any busy health professional, it is important to avoid trivia and focus on the most significant issues in patient care. If, for example, a pharmacist discussed with a physician the importance of administering an analgaesic dose of aspirin with food, but omitted to discuss a potentially fatal interaction with the patient's coumarin anti-coagulant, he or she would be unlikely to earn the respect of the medical team.

Spoken messages: Spoken messages can occur in person or over the telephone. Commonly, they are used to obtain information about a patient or their treatment, to provide medicine information to a practitioner or to clarify or recommend modifications in a patient's therapy. Skills and confidence in handling difficult situations can initially be developed through role plays. *Role Play 1* aims to explore and develop the student's information gathering skills.

Telephone skills are an important aspect of professional life. Telephone conversations differ from face-to-face contact as there are fewer non-verbal cues which can represent a distraction. The skill and confidence required to manage spontaneous situations like answering the telephone can be developed through practice with self-reflection. For more difficult situations, seeking the advice of a skilled mentor or colleague can be helpful.

When initiating a telephone conversation, an effective skill is to maintain some control of the process by keeping the content focused and ending the call when the purpose is achieved. Preparation may be useful, for example, jotting down the main points on a piece of paper or preparing a structure for the call. *Role Play 2* can be practised as a telephone conversation and covers a potentially challenging situation.

Case note annotation: Comments in a patient's case notes convey important information to those caring for the patient and provide a record of the patient's hospital management. In a busy ward, when a pharmacist records important information, this can be easily overlooked. Alerting the appropriate staff member verbally is important. This provides an opportunity for discussion and clarification of a complex message and reduces the possibility of misunderstanding. Case note entries can be of legal importance when prescribing could harm the patient.

In some countries, pharmacists who do not identify and document potentially harmful therapy carry an equal or greater legal blame than the medical professional who prescribed the treatment.

Entries into case notes are required to conform to standards for clarity and precision. The entry should be dated and have a short informative heading. Short, clear statements should identify the issue, provide reasoning or an explanation, and the recommendation of any action which may be required. The author's name, position and contact telephone, cell phone or pager number should be included. Sometimes, journal articles or printed information can be attached to the notes to support an entry. In many hospitals, pharmacists use a coloured pen (green is traditional) or an identification mark to distinguish their entries. *Case Study* 5 gives an example of a case note annotation with a verbal interaction.

Communication with Patients

Medication history interviews: To review current medical treatment and identify suitable additional treatments, medical professionals will require complete and reliable medication history. Research has established that in routine practice, pharmacists provide the most accurate history when compared to other health professionals. It is an important role that pharmacists are well-prepared to fulfil.

A well-prepared, structured approach helps to obtain relevant complete information and avoid omissions. The following information is commonly recorded:

- currently or recently prescribed medicines
- medicines purchased without prescription (OTC)
- vaccinations
- alternative or traditional remedies
- description of reactions and allergies to medicines
- medicines found to be ineffective
- adherence to past treatment courses and the use of adherence aids

An example of a form used to structure and collect medication information is provided in the UK Psychiatric Pharmacy Group website.

Reliable medication history is the foundation of the medicine reconciliation process. The information obtained can then be compared to the medicines presented by the patient and information obtained from other sources such as the medical notes or a practitioner's file.

Labelling medicines: Medicine labels are concise messages to identify and aid the effective and safe use of medicines. A common standard is that all containers of medicines should be clearly labelled to identify:

- the medicine (by generic or trade name)
- dosage form, number of dosage units supplied, strength
- number of dose units to be taken at a time and its frequency
- any specific administration guidance or precautions; for example, take at least 30 minutes before food
- the patient's name
- date of dispensing
- batch numbers and expiry dates for non-prescription medicines and medicines not likely to be used immediately

Standards and guidelines for medicines labels are required in many countries. An example of the guidelines for American pharmacists is shown on the Institute for Safe Medicines Practices website.

Patient information leaflets (PILs): Patient information leaflets are used to outline key information to assist patients and their caregivers in the effective and safe use of a medicine. Where computer technology is available, PILs can be customised for individual patients or be prepared for groups of patients. The following information is commonly included:

- trade and generic names
- indications for which the medicine is being taken
- precautions or contraindications
- administration advice
- information on the action required if a dose is missed
- common and serious side effects
- medicine interactions
- action to be taken if a side effect is experienced
- storage information
- name and contact details of the institution providing the information
- author and date of publication

PILs should include all essential information without making a document too lengthy or the typeface too small. Common usage terms should be used for medical indications and written to be understood by people with basic (for example, newspaper) reading ability. All sheets need to be regularly reviewed and updated to reflect current knowledge and practice. Examples of PILs are those provided by the US National Library of Medicine and from a pharmaceutical company on the Xenical website.

Patient medication sheets or cards: When patients are taking several medicines, a handwritten or computer-generated medication summary can improve compliance and understanding (an example is provided in Fig. 6.1 *Chapter 6, Patient Counselling*). A tabular form presents the information clearly. The dose timing can be identified as a specific time (for example, 7:00 AM), a meal time (breakfast) or a phase of the day (morning). Other information such as the purpose of the medicine, when treatment is to stop, specialised advice (for example, take with food) as well as information specific to the person, such as adverse reactions experienced or the use of adherence aids, can be recorded. Keeping medication sheets up-to-date and accurate is a common problem, especially when a patient is attending different clinics or medical practitioners.

Medication counselling for patients: Effective patient counselling can help patients use their medicines safely and reliably. All the principles of effective verbal communication are important to the success of an encounter and are covered in *Chapter 6, Patient Counselling*.

Developing Communication Skills through Practice

The best way to develop professional communication skills is by observing others, regular practice with reflection and discussion with colleagues. Role plays are useful to develop confidence and to practice specific skills or situations before approaching patients or health professionals. As competence develops, a pharmacist can move from lower skilled tasks like obtaining information to the higher skilled activity of giving information. For example, a recently qualified pharmacist may start by taking medication history under supervision, then on their own. When competent, they could start providing medication counselling, initially under supervision and then alone. They may progress to working in a medicine information service, providing in-depth information for the medical profession.

A structured approach with supervision until competency is achieved helps foster skills and develops confidence. It also helps in maintaining service quality and value. Throughout their professional lives, a reflective learning approach enables pharmacists to reflect on areas for improvement, and identify and adopt approaches to achieve new learning, before incorporating them into practice and evaluating the effect.

Special Considerations for Indian Pharmacists

Pharmacists in India face considerable communication challenges which require innovation and creativity to manage successfully. Lack of familiarity with modern therapy may prevent some patients from benefitting from their medicines unless clearly explained and discussed. For example, they may not understand that a course of antibiotics must be completed even though the symptoms have resolved.

There may be problems with contaminated or counterfeit medicines, expired or poorly-stored batches, unpredictable supply, and so on. All of these require the greatest degree of vigilance and, often, considerable communication skills to resolve.

There are other great challenges which are encountered with an educationally and culturally diverse population. Examples are finding appropriate symbols or diagrams to support verbal messages for illiterate and innumerate patients, communicating with patients when a common language is not shared or the provision of patient medicine information in the local language.

Pharmacists have a critical role to play in ensuring the safe and effective use of medicines. The more skilled a pharmacist is as a communicator, the more influence he or she will have and the greater their contribution will be to the health and welfare of those for whom they provide a service.

CASE STUDY 1: MODIFYING NON-VERBAL MESSAGES

Feroz Haroom works as a pharmaceutical representative for a well-respected pharmaceutical company. This day has been particularly frustrating. Early in the morning, a workers demonstration caused traffic delays so he missed his first appointment and is now 15 minutes late for the next. He is feeling stressed, angry and frustrated. When Feroz telephoned ahead to confirm his delay, the pharmacy manager said he could not spare more time so the visit would be for five minutes.

Feroz identifies the key points he needs to cover and nearing the hospital, he checks his appearance in the car mirror. His face looks pinched and tense. Knowing it is important to appear confident and relaxed, Feroz takes several deep breathes and remembers the warm welcome of his last meeting with the pharmacy manager. He checks his appearance again as he leaves the car, nods, straightens his tie and feels confident the meeting will go well.

CASE STUDY 2: STRUCTURE OF COMMUNICATION: DISCHARGE MEDICATION COUNSELLING

INTRODUCTION

Raj Good morning, Mr S. We haven't met before, but I am Raj, the pharmacist covering this ward. How are you this morning?

Mr S I'm feeling much better, thank you. Dr Ramesh has said I can go home today.

OPENING

Raj Now I am here to tell you about the medicines you are to go home with. I have them here with me. I understand that chest pain has been troubling you, is that right?

Mr S Yes it has. That's why my family brought me to the hospital.

BUSINESS

Raj Well, these tablets can stop the pain when it occurs. They are called glyceryl trinitrate.

explanation When you get the pain, you need to place one under the tongue and let it dissolve there. It.........

checking Does this all seem clear to you, Mr S?

Mr S Yes, but I'm rather bothered about only keeping the tablets for a month.
They are rather expensive.

Raj Well, it is important to maintain the effectiveness of the tablets. If the tablets are too old, they will not be very effective and will not work to relieve your chest pain.

re-capping Also, I may not have explained things clearly before, but if you have taken at least three tablets over 30 minutes and your chest pain is not relieved, this may indicate you are having a heart attack and should come to the hospital straightaway. Now if you were using old tablets which have lost their strength, you may come to the hospital unnecessarily.

Mr S Ah, now I see.

Raj Now I just need to check I have explained things clearly to you.

confirming Can you tell me when you would use these tablets?

Mr S ....

RECONNECTING

Raj Well, Mr S, these tablets will really help you in managing chest pain. I expect you are looking forward to getting back to your family and resuming work again.

Mr S Yes, certainly.

CLOSURE

Raj Well, Mr S, I wish you all the best. If I can be of any further assistance, please contact me at the hospital. Here is a card which gives you my contact details.

CASE STUDY 3: INTERVIEWING: OBTAINING MEDICATION HISTORY

ST is a pharmacist who is to obtain medication history from BN who has recently been admitted to the hospital with severe abdominal pain.

ST Good morning, Mr BN. My name is Siri T and I am a pharmacist on this ward.

opening purpose I have come to ask you about the medicines you are taking. Now before we start, I would just like to make sure you are comfortable. Is it all right if I sit here?

Mr BN Hello, Miss ST. Yes, I can see you well there. I'm comfortable now, thank you. The nurse gave me an injection and that has helped with the pain.

ST I'm sorry there isn't much privacy in this ward. Now, if I talk like this, will you

environment be able to hear me clearly?

Mr BN Yes, that is fine

ST That's good. Now I need to find out about the medicines you have taken recently, to check if any of them could have caused your pain.

open question Could you tell me what medicines you have been prescribed by your doctor recently?

Mr BN Well about a week ago, I hurt my ankle and the doctor gave me something for it. I think they were called 'indo' something.

ST Would that be indomethacin? It is sometimes know as Indocin.

Mr BN Yes, that's it, it was Indocin.

ST Now what about any other medicines?

Mr BN Well I regularly take these medicines here. They are glucoformin and chlorthalidone.

ST Can I see the containers please, Mr BN. I need to note down the doses.

closed question Now I assume you take these for diabetes and fluid overload.

Mr BN	Yes, that is right
ST	Now have you bought any other medicines at all recently?
Mr BN	No, nothing.
ST *prompting*	Do you ever take anything for headaches or other aches and pains, Mr BN?
Mr BN	Well I have this special remedy that my wife gets from the ayuvedic clinic.
ST	Hmmm, that's very interesting. Could you get your wife to bring it and any other remedies you could have taken in the last few weeks so I can make note of them.
Mr BN	Yes, certainly. I will ask her this afternoon. I don't think many of them have labels though.
ST *permission*	Well Mr BN, that shouldn't be a problem. Would you be happy if I contacted the clinic to try and identify what they contain?
Mr BN	Yes, certainly.
ST	Thank you, Mr BN. Now I would just like to check that what I have noted down is correct and I have a complete list of your medicines.
checking	Now you normally take .... and about a week ago ..... and you also take...
Mr BN	Yes, that is so.
ST	Thank you, Mr BN. I will place a list of your medicines in your hospital notes with information about these medicines for the doctors to see. Thank you for your help, Mr BN.

CASE STUDY 4: DELIVERING A MESSAGE: MEDICATION COUNSELLING IN A COMMUNITY SETTING

RT is a pharmacist who is to explain to the mother of an eight-year-old child, Chandra, how to administer an iron mixture to her daughter.

MESSAGE LENGTH

RT recognises that the message needs to be short (about five minutes) and must cover only the main points.

MESSAGE STRUCTURE

RT identifies the main points to be covered as:

- purpose of treatment
- dose
- measuring the dose
- administration times
- avoiding teeth staining
- length of treatment
- monitoring for effectiveness

RT then identifies that the dose and avoidance of teeth staining needs to be emphasised, and so places information on the dose early in his message with repetition at the end, and information on teeth staining towards the end. He decides he will not give information on the length of treatment as this was not clear from the prescription or from the mother's comments.

CHECKING UNDERSTANDING

RT has introduced himself to Mrs VK, established rapport and identified the purpose of the discussion. He has also identified that Mrs VK will be administering Chandra's medicine and that she can communicate well in English.

RT (*open question*) Do you know what Chandra's medicine is for, Mrs VK?

Mrs VK The doctor said it is to add iron to her blood as she has anaemia and this is why she is lacking in energy.

MESSAGE DELIVERY

RT Yes, that is right, Mrs VK. Chandra is to have one spoonful of this mixture three times each day. (RT shows Mrs VK a measuring spoon). It can be an irritant to the stomach so it is best taken with food. I would suggest you give Chandra a dose with her breakfast, lunch and dinner.

Mrs VK nods

RT (*closed question*) Now iron can stain the teeth, so I suggest you give it to Chandra through a straw. Do you have any straws at home, Mrs VK?

Mrs VK Yes, I do. Chandra and the younger children like to have milkshakes.

RT (repetition for emphasis) That's good. I would suggest you keep one straw just for giving Chandra her iron mixture with each meal.

CHECKING

RT Is there anything you would like to ask, Mrs VK?

Mrs VK No, everything is quite clear, thank you.

RT Now I would just like to check that I have explained about Chandra's medicine clearly to you. When will you be giving Chandra her iron mixture?

Mrs VK Well, I will give her a spoonful with each meal.

RT That's right, Mrs VK, but do remember to use a straw to prevent staining Chandra's teeth.

SUMMARISING

RT I would just like to go over everything one more time. Now to treat Chandra's anaemia, you are to give her one 5 ml spoonful of this iron mixture three times each day at meal times. Using a straw will prevent Chandra's teeth from becoming stained by the mixture.

CASE STUDY 5: MEDICAL NOTES ANNOTATION WITH VERBAL COMMUNICATION

24/12/09 14.00 *Ciprofloxacin*

Ciprofloxacin prescribed 22/12/09 to treat chest infection. Sputum sample (22/10/09) grew *Pseudomonas aeruginosa* resistant to ciprofloxacin but sensitive to amikacin, tobramycin and ceftazidime. Recommend change to ceftazidime and add an aminoglycoside for synergism and secondary cover. For both amikacin and tobramycin, plasma level and renal function monitoring will be required.

G Patel (pharmacist) ext7774

G Patel spoke to the patient's doctor to draw attention to her note and to ensure that the doctor understood how aminoglycosides should be dosed and monitored. The doctor tells G Patel that although it is not written in the patient's notes, the patient developed an urticarial rash to penicillins in the past. G Patel then tells the doctor that there is about a 1:20 chance of cross-sensitivity to cephalosporins, so this patient should be carefully observed for signs of an allergic response after the ceftazidime has been given. If a reaction occurs, the laboratory should be contacted to run additional antibiotic sensitivity tests and so provide a wider range of treatment options.

Exercise 1: Subtle Non-verbal Messages

In the classroom form of this exercise, three people are involved:

- the experimenter (that is, the person purposely using non-verbal signals),
- the subject who will participate in the exercise but will not be aware or told that non-verbal communication is being explored,
- the observer who will report back to both participants what they have observed.

A topic that is familiar is chosen. For example, the experimenter could explain to the subject how to treat a headache with paracetamol. The experimenter should remain attentive throughout the explanation.

In the second part of the exercise, the subject will give information to the experimenter, for example, explain why flucloxacillin (or dicloxacillin) should be taken on an empty stomach. This time, part way through the explanation, the experimenter will signal non-attention. For example, they could obviously shift from an open to a closed body position by crossing their arms and their legs or focus on an object away from the experimenter, or change their facial expression, for example, from a smile to a frown.

When the exercise is complete, the observer then reports back to both the experimenter and the subject what they have noticed and then all three participants should discuss their experience.

This exercise could be undertaken during a conversation with a friend or family member. It is really important that the purpose of the exercise and what has occurred is explained to the subject after the exercise is complete, otherwise the experimenter may lose a friend!

Exercise 2: Non-verbal Communication of Medicine Information

Srimati DA is a 45-year-old villager who cannot read or write. You (as her pharmacist) need to explain the use and dosing of her medicine verbally but she would like something she could refer back to (*see example*).

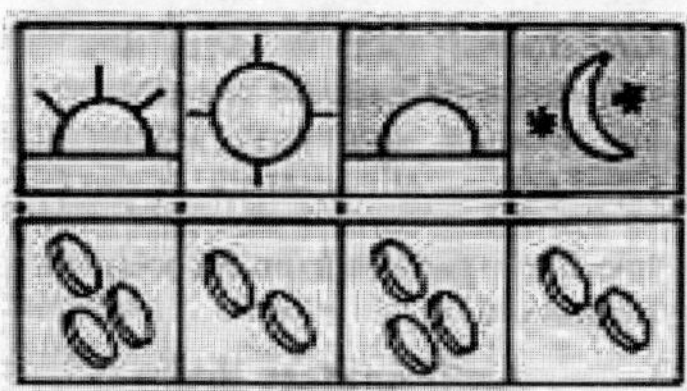

You are to explain the purpose and dosing of her medicine using a similar diagram, or other pictograms available on the US Pharmacopeia website (listed at the end of this chapter).

She has been prescribed:

Amoxycillin/clavulanic acid 500 mg, one capsule three times daily

You will also need to check that she understands the diagram you have used.

Role Plays

These provide valuable practice and can be used to help develop skills and confidence in communicating in different situations. For experienced pharmacists, role plays can provide the opportunity to explore and practise skills when preparing for particularly challenging situations. Role plays involve two people (the pharmacist and the patient, doctor or nurse). Using a third person as an observer/reporter to provide critical comments on the interaction is helpful.

One person will have the active role and practice their communication skills while the other responds. Briefing sheets are useful to define the roles being undertaken. Acting skills are not required, as students will become absorbed in their role as contact develops. A supervisor has copies of the briefing information and can guide particpants through the role play procedure and act as time keeper.

Procedure

When individuals have been assigned roles, a supervisor gives a verbal briefing to those in each role group and hands out the briefing sheets. The participants can develop their roles by imagining their character or role. Often people they have met in real life can form useful models.

If a telephone conversation is being enacted, then the actors can sit back-to-back (so they do not look at each other but can hear each other). If an interview is being practised, then they should sit facing each other or side by side. The observer sits where they can hear and fully observe the interaction but not be intrusive.

A time limit is set for the role play (usually about five minutes). As the role play proceeds, the supervisor observes the group and defines when the time is up. Each observer reports back to their group and comments on the interaction. The people in each role can then discuss how they felt about their roles and what they have learnt.

If undertaken as a class exercise, the main learning points from the exercise can be identified and recorded on a whiteboard.

Role Play 1: Obtaining Patient Information from a Nurse

Pharmacist's Briefing

TH is an elderly patient who has recently had a stroke (cerebral vascular accident or CVA). He is prescribed the following medicines:

- Slow-release potassium chloride tablets
- Frusemide tablets
- Paracetamol tablets

You are concerned that he may not be able to safely swallow these tablets and is at risk of choking on them. You are to ask the nurse about this.

Nurse's Briefing

You are taking care of Mr TH, an elderly man who has recently had a stroke (CVA). He is unable to speak but appears to understand what you say to him. This morning you noticed he choked on his food. You have not attempted to give him his medicines.

Role Play 2: Reporting a Prescribing Error to the Prescriber

Pharmacist's Briefing

You have received a prescription for BT, a two-year-old boy, for paracetamol tablets 500 mg every four hours. The dose of paracetamol for young children in the Paediatric Drug Information Handbook is 15 mg/kg/dose. BT weighs 10 kg. You are to telephone the prescriber to discuss this dose.

Doctor's Briefing

You have a very busy practice and although you remember some patients, you cannot recall most. You have records for a patient BT. These state that you saw him yesterday, a day when you saw at least 10 children with similar symptoms. He had fever and aches and pains so you prescribed paracetamol. BT is two years old. You do not like being interrupted.

Role Play 3: Obtaining a Medication History from an Elderly Patient

Pharmacist's Briefing

You are working in a hospital clinic and are required to identify the medicines currently being taken by Mrs MR.

Patient's Briefing

You are Mrs MR who is in her 80s and quite deaf. You take the following medicines regularly:

- Glyceryl trinitrate tablets, when required for all types of pain although you haven't found them useful for headaches. You don't know the strength.
- A tablet to get rid of water from your body. You can't remember the name.
- A tablet for blood pressure, you think the name is aten-something.
- Four days ago, the doctor prescribed tablets for a chest infection but your family didn't have enough money to obtain these.
- About a month ago, a friend gave you some pain relief tablets she had left over and you think these have helped you. The name begins with I.

Role Play 4: Giving Information about Taking an Oral Contraceptive

Pharmacist's Briefing

You have received a prescription from a young woman, AT, for a combined oral contraceptive. This is the first prescription she has had for an oral contraceptive. You need to provide her with advice on how to take this medicine and any important adverse effects she should be informed of.

Patient's Briefing

You are AT, an 18-year-old woman who will shortly be getting married and moving to another town. You are waiting for your prescription for an oral contraceptive to be filled. You are rather shy and anxious; having your bossy mother waiting outside doesn't help.

KEY MESSAGES

- ❖ A critical aspect of a clinical pharmacist's work is to effectively communicate with a wide range of people.
- ❖ Professional communication involves both obtaining and giving information to assist others to use medicines effectively and safely.
- ❖ An understanding of communication theory, practice through role plays and the use of reflective learning practices will enable pharmacists to become highly effective communicators of medicine information.

Further Reading

Berger B. 1999. Effective patient counselling. *US Pharmacist* 24(Feb): 64, 66, 69, 73.

Berger B. 2000. Types of verbal communication. *US Pharmacist* 25(Jan): 61–62, 64, 66–67.

Berger B. 2000. Guidelines for physician interaction. *US Pharmacist* 25(Feb): 88, 90, 92.

BA Berger. 2009. Communication Skills for Pharmacists, 3rd edition. American Pharmacists Association, Washington DC.

Dickson DA, Hargie O and Morrow NC. 1996. Communication Skills Training for Health Professionals, 2nd ed. Nelson Thornes Ltd, London.

Northouse PG and Northouse LL. 1985. Health Communication, Strategies for Health Professional. Prentice-Hall, Englewood Cliffs, New Jersey.

Websites of Interest

Drugs.com
http://www.drugs.com

Heymans Institute of Pharmacology
http://allserv.UGent.be/~rvdstich/eugloss/EN/lijst.html

Merck
http://www.merck.com/mmhe/resources/pronunciations/index/a.html

PharmWeb
http://www.pharmweb.net/pwmirror/pwz/patient/pharmwebpatinf.html

UK Psychiatric Pharmacy Group
http://www.ukppg.org.uk/site-map.html

US Institute for Safe Medicines Practices
http://www.ismp.org/tools/guidelines/labelFormats/comments/default.asp

US National Library of Medicine
http://www.nlm.nih.gov/medlineplus/druginformation.html

US Pharmacopeia
http://www.usp.org/audiences/consumer/pictograms

Xenical™
http://www.online-xenical.com/consum_info.html

6 PATIENT COUNSELLING

Ramesh Adepu

Learning Objectives

Upon completion of this chapter, the reader should be able to:

- Understand the need for patient counselling
- Identify outcomes of effective patient counselling
- Discuss the verbal and non-verbal communication skills required by a good counsellor
- Describe the steps in the counselling process
- Identify the barriers to patient counselling and strategies to overcome them
- List the main points of medication use which may be discussed during counselling
- Identify patient groups who require counselling

The safe and effective use of drugs depends on patients being well informed about their medication. In India, healthcare is provided at the primary, secondary and tertiary levels, and at each level, most patients receive medications as part of their treatment. Due to heavy patient load, most prescribers have little time to explain the use of these medicines to their patients. Pharmacists in community pharmacies and hospitals have not been trained for this role, and serve largely as prescription-fillers or dispensers. Many patients do not get enough information about their medication, including how and when to take it, how long to take it, what to do if side effects occur or if a dose is missed.

Lack of information may result in the patient not taking the medication the way it was intended to be used, which in turn may result in therapeutic failure, adverse effects, additional expenditure on investigations and treatment or even hospitalisation. The inappropriate use of antibiotics by patients may contribute to antibiotic resistance within the community in general. Thus, patient education can address many drug use problems and their consequences.

What is Patient Counselling?

Patient counselling refers to the process of providing information, advice and assistance to help patients use their medications appropriately. The information and advice is given by the pharmacist directly to the patient or to the patient's representative, and may also include information about the patient's illness or recommended lifestyle changes. The information is usually given verbally, but may be supplemented with written material.

During counselling, the pharmacist should assess the patient's understanding about his or her illness and the treatment, and provide individualised advice and information which will assist the patient to take their medications in the most safe and effective manner. To provide accurate advice and information, the pharmacist should be familiar with the pathophysiology and therapeutics of the patient's disease. Good communication skills are required to gain the patient's confidence and to motivate the patient to adhere to the recommended regimen.

Effective patient counselling aims to produce the following results:

- Better patient understanding of their illness and the role of medication in its treatment
- Improved medication adherence
- More effective drug treatment
- Reduced incidence of medication errors, adverse effects and unnecessary healthcare costs
- Improved quality of life of the patients
- Better coping strategies for medication-related adverse effects
- Improved professional rapport between the patient and pharmacist

Communication Skills for Effective Counselling

The counselling process uses verbal and non-verbal communication skills. Verbal communication skills include language and paralinguistic features such as tone, volume, pitch and rate of speech. Paralinguistics, or the way we say words, accounts for 40% of how a message is received, so the way in which we speak has an impact on patient understanding.

Language: When speaking to patients, use simple language and avoid unnecessary medical terminology. If possible, speak the patient's own language.

Tone: During counselling, the tone of our voice has a great impact on patient understanding. Changes in the level and range of pitch convey information about the feelings and attitudes of the person speaking. When counselling, the tone of the voice should be caring and reassuring.

Volume: Many people speak with wide variations in volume, depending on the situation, and where and to whom they are speaking. Ideally, counselling should be conducted in a quiet, private setting where it is unnecessary to raise one's voice. Although it may be necessary to speak more loudly to patients with a hearing problem, most deaf patients gain more benefit if the speaker moves closer, and directs their voice towards the patient's ear.

Speed: The clarity of our communication depends on our rate of speech. Patients may be reluctant to interact with a pharmacist who speaks quickly because they may feel the pharmacist is too busy. This may happen if the pharmacist is nervous or is uncertain about the information being given. In contrast, a person who speaks too slowly may lose the interest of the listener. For good verbal communication, the pharmacist should present clear, relevant messages in a logical sequence, and at a speed which gives the patient time to think about what is being said. This will help the patient understand and remember the concepts more easily.

Non-verbal communication: This includes body language such as the movement and position of the head, limbs and body, and other aspects such as whether the pharmacist is dressed in a professional manner. During any interaction, approximately 50% of the way a message is conveyed comes from body language. Aspects of non-verbal communication include proximity, touch, eye contact, facial expressions, head movements, gestures with hands and arms and body postures.

Proximity: This refers to the distance that people maintain between themselves during the counselling process. This space has been classified into four zones: intimate (45 cm or less), personal (45 cm to 1.2 m), social (1.2–3.6 m) and public (>3.6 m). Generally, counsellors and healthcare professionals use intimate or personal proximities.

Eye contact: The amount that people look at one another during conversation varies depending on whether they are speaking or listening. Listeners look at the speaker more often and for longer periods of time. For cultural or personal reasons such as timidity, sadness or depression, some people may avoid looking into the counsellor's eyes.

Facial expression: These can be used during counselling to demonstrate empathy towards the patient. Head movements such as nodding, hand gestures and body posture also can be used to advantage.

Steps of Patient Counselling

Counselling is a two-way communication process, and interaction between the patient and the pharmacist is essential for counselling to be effective.

Preparing for the session: The success of counselling depends on the knowledge and skill of the counsellor. The pharmacist should know as much as possible about the patient and his/her treatment details. In the hospital setting, this may be accomplished by referring to the patient's case notes. In the community pharmacy setting, sources of information include the patient and their prescription, and in some cases, a record of previous dispensing for the patient. If the patient is receiving a medication which is unfamiliar to the pharmacist, then a drug information reference should be consulted before counselling commences.

Another issue worth considering is the mental and physical state of the patient. If the patient is in a hurry, in pain or is not communicative, it is very difficult to counsel the patient effectively. In such situations, the aims of counselling may need to be modified, or with the patient's agreement, the session may be postponed to a later date.

Opening the session: The first phase of counselling is used for information gathering. The pharmacist should introduce him or herself to the patient and greet them by name. If help is required in pronouncing the name, ask colleagues or the patient directly. It is best to use titles such as Ms, Mrs and Mr and then switch over to the

Table 6.1 *Qualities of a good counsellor*

Be a good listener: Counselling is an interactive process. The pharmacist must listen attentively to the patient and observe both verbal and non-verbal behaviour. This gives the pharmacist an opportunity to assess the patient's knowledge about their disease and medications.
Be flexible: The pharmacist should be flexible and provide advice and information which is tailored to the individual patient's needs and capabilities.
Be empathetic: The pharmacist should try to understand the patient's personal suffering and situation as if the problem was his or her own.
Be non-judgemental: The pharmacist should not judge the behaviour of the patient based on their illness or the group he or she belongs to.
Be tolerant: During the course of counselling, patients may become agitated, unreasonable or hostile. The pharmacist should acknowledge the patient's feelings and be tolerant of these.
Communicate confidently: The pharmacist should speak confidently as this will improve the patient's acceptance of the pharmacist's advice.

first name. The pharmacist should identify the purpose of the session very clearly. For example, 'Hello, Mr Sreenivas! I am Vinod, your pharmacist. I would like to tell you about your medication. Do you have a few minutes to spend with me?'. Patients who visit community pharmacies are often in a hurry to go home with the medication, and this type of introduction mentally prepares the patient to spend some time with the pharmacist.

Next, the pharmacist gathers information from the patient about their understanding of the disease they are suffering from, drug treatment and use of alternative medications such as ayurvedic medications or home remedies. Other information which may be relevant includes previous drug allergies, past medical history and personal habits such as chewing pan masala, smoking cigarettes and consuming alcohol.

Using open-ended questions is a useful technique for gaining the confidence of the patient, and the answers allow the pharmacist to assess the patient's information needs. For example, 'What did your doctor tell you about your illness?', 'What do you know about your disease?', 'Can you tell me about the symptoms you have been experiencing?'. It can also be useful to ask, 'What did your doctor tell you about this medication?'. This enables the pharmacist to assess the patient's understanding of their medication and to avoid giving information which may contradict advice given by the patient's doctor. Reflective questioning is another useful approach for gathering information. This involves using the patient's own remarks to gather more information on certain important points. For example, 'So these tablets made you feel ill last time. Can you describe what happened?'.

Patients may be disturbed and distressed due to their illness, and this may reduce their ability to receive and understand information from both the doctor and the pharmacist. In these situations, a few kind words to demonstrate empathy and understanding will assist the counselling process. During counselling, the pharmacist should avoid asking questions in a direct or embarrassing way, show excessive curiosity, discuss the patient's personal problems, pass moral judgments, interrupt when the patient is speaking, make premature interpretations or argue with the patient. If the patient becomes hostile or aggressive despite the pharmacist's best efforts to calm him or her, it is preferable to terminate the counselling session.

Counselling content: The counselling content is considered to be the heart of the counselling session. During this step, the pharmacist explains to the patient about his or her medications and treatment regimen. Lifestyle changes such as diet or exercise may also be discussed. Topics commonly covered include:

- Name and strength of the medication
- The reason why it has been prescribed (if known), or how it works
- How to take the medication (how much and how often)
- Expected duration of treatment
- Expected benefits of treatment
- Possible adverse effects
- Possible medication or dietary interactions
- Advice on correct storage
- Minimum duration required to show therapeutic benefit
- What to do if a dose is missed
- Special monitoring requirements, for example, blood tests
- Arrangements for obtaining further supplies

Because of time constraints, it is often necessary to prioritise these points. Some patients are more interested in learning about their medication than others and the information which is given should be tailored to the individual patient. It is important that the pharmacist uses language which is understandable to the patient. Medical jargon and even simple medical terms will not be understood by most patients and should be avoided. This means developing fluency with a simple vocabulary which nevertheless can be used to describe medication use accurately. So instead of saying 'This medication is for hypertension' it is better to say 'This medication is for high blood pressure'.

In some situations it is important not to jump to conclusions about why a particular medication has been prescribed. For example, tricyclic anti-depressants are often used for conditions other than depression, such as neuropathic pain, incontinence or pruritis. Asking questions such as 'What has the doctor told you about this medication?' can help avoid misunderstandings in this type of situation.

Sometimes the patient's family may visit the pharmacy to collect the medication. They should be provided with suitable advice after gathering information such as their relationship with the patient and their awareness of the patient's disease and medication history.

Closing the session: Before closing the session, it is essential to check the patient's understanding. This can be assessed by feedback questions, such as 'Can you remember what this medication is for?' or 'For how long should you take this medication?'. During the discussion, some of the patient's information needs may have been cleared, but the patient may have new questions or doubts. It is therefore advisable to finish the session by asking the patient 'Do you have any questions?'. Before final closure and if time permits, summarise the main points in a logical order. If appropriate, the pharmacist can supply their telephone number to encourage the patient to make contact if they need further advice or information.

Getting Started

The idea of patient counselling can be daunting for beginners. It is important that students or young graduates have the opportunity to observe an experienced pharmacist provide counselling to a number of different patients. This prepares the student or pharmacist for the type of interactions which occur during a typical counselling session, and gives them confidence to make a start. For newly graduated pharmacists who lack confidence in counselling, a useful approach is to start by limiting counselling to a certain type of medication, for example, oral hypoglycemic medicines. As skill and confidence develop in one area, the pharmacist can gradually move on to other medications.

In hospitals and community pharmacies, time and the availability of staff often determine who one can counsel. High patient numbers means that pharmacists may need to identify and give priority to those patients who are most in need of counselling services. These may include:

- Patients receiving specific medications, such as antibiotics or drugs with a narrow therapeutic window such as warfarin, theophylline or methotrexate
- Patients receiving complex medication regimens, for example, anti-tubercular drugs
- Patients receiving medications through a specialised delivery system, for example, inhalers and rotohalers
- Patients with a history of poor medication adherence
- Elderly patients taking many medications
- Patients being discharged from hospital
- Patients referred by physicians

Counselling Aids

When information is provided to the patient verbally, there is a chance that the patient may forget the information over a period of time. A variety of teaching and educational aids have been developed to assist patient counselling. If information is provided in a printed format, the patient can go through the information at leisure as and when the information is required.

Medication cards can be a useful aid, particularly for patients on many medications on a long-term basis. A medication card is a written summary of a patient's medications, presented in a way which is easy for the patient to understand.

An example of such a card is shown in Fig. 6.1. Cards may be written by hand or generated by computer. Once a card is given to a patient, it can be used to assist the patient to organise their medication routines at home and to show to other healthcare providers. It is important that the card is updated when changes to the medication regimen are made.

Patient information leaflets (PILs) produced by drug manufacturers for their products are known as consumer product information (CPI) or consumer medicine information (CMI). PILs are written information leaflets in simple language about the patient's illness and its treatment, including medications and relevant lifestyle changes. Printed materials reinforce verbal advice and may result in improved understanding and acceptance of treatment recommendations.

Written information should be considered as a supplement to verbal counselling, rather than a replacement, and is of course only useful for patients who are literate.

Pharmacists can also develop useful PIL using their knowledge of therapeutics and the local language. However, it is essential that such materials are peer reviewed to ensure accurate and high-quality content. In a hospital setting, it is also wise to seek the input and approval of relevant medical staff.

While preparing PILs, reading ease, layout and design are very important. To assess the reading ease of any PIL written in English, the Flesch Reading Ease (FRE) formula can be used. The reading ease scores in FRE scale are 0–100. If the score is less than 60, the document is considered to be difficult for the general public to read. The ideal PIL should have a readability score of 70–80. The reading ease score can be calculated by using the following formula:

$$FRE = 206.84 - 0.85W - 1.02S$$

where W is the number of syllables per 100 words and S is the number of words in an average sentence. From this formula it can be seen that readability is improved if simple words are used in short sentences.

Patient Counselling and Medication Adherence

Medication adherence refers to the extent to which an individual's medication-taking behaviour coincides with medical advice. If patients do not adhere to the directions given by their doctor, the following may be the consequences:

- Treatment failure
- Increased chance of hospitalisation
- Increased medical and non-medical expenditure
- Decreased quality of life

Patients who are informed about their medications are more likely to take the medication as advised and avoid these problems.

Barriers to Patient Counselling

Patient counselling may not take place in community pharmacies due to various reasons, known as barriers. These barriers are classified as patient-based, provider-based and system-based barriers.

Patient-based barriers: In India, many patients are unaware that pharmacists may provide counselling and generally ask their prescriber about medication use. Gender and language differences may also inhibit patients from asking the pharmacist about medication use information.

Provider-based barriers: Many pharmacists lack the confidence to counsel patients due to lack of knowledge and counselling skills. A heavy patient load for prescription filling is also an important barrier in many practice situations.

System-based barriers: In India, counselling is not a mandatory legal requirement and officially pharmacists are not entitled to charge for dispensing or for the information provided to patients. These factors act as regulatory and financial disincentives to providing a counselling service. Lack of privacy in many busy community and hospital pharmacies can also be a problem.

Strategies to overcome barriers: By definition, provider-based barriers are the easiest to modify. Pharmacists can start by updating their knowledge and counselling skills. Confidence can be developed by initially focusing on one particular disease or group of drugs (for example, antibiotics). A good approach is to ask patients 'Have you used this medication before?' when they collect their prescription. Encouraging individual patients to ask questions about their medications or media campaigns will also improve counselling opportunities.

Recent Developments

Despite the above-mentioned barriers, some pharmacists in community pharmacies are showing interest in educating their patients about medication use. They also offer various health screening services such as blood pressure and blood glucose measurement. State pharmacy councils conduct continuing education programmes for practicing pharmacists to help update their therapeutics knowledge and counselling skills.

Conclusion

Patient counselling is an essential component of clinical pharmacy practice in hospitals and in community pharmacy settings. Counselling enhances the patients' understanding of their illness and its treatment, and may improve adherence and therapeutic outcome. It allows pharmacists to gain first-hand knowledge of medication use from the patient's perspective.

CASE STUDY 1

Mr SP is a 52-year-old businessman who recently consulted his physician for a burning pain in his feet. He is a known diabetic for four years, for which he has been following a diabetic diet. His social history reveals that he is a long-term smoker and drinks alcohol occasionally. On examination, his blood pressure (BP) was 160/95 mmHg. His doctor ordered a range of laboratory tests, including fasting blood sugar (FBS), postprandial blood sugar (PPBS), blood urea nitrogen (BUN) and serum creatinine. His FBS was found to be 8.42 mmol/L (normal is 3.9–6.1 mmol/L), PPBS 10.28 mmol/L (normal is 8.4 mmol/L), BUN 6.06 mmol/L (normal is 2.9–7.1 mmol/L) and serum creatinine 52 mmol/L (normal is 62–133 mmol/L). Mr SP was given an outpatient prescription for the following medications.

Rx

Cap. Gabapentin 300 mg one TID

Tab. Ramipril 2.5 mg one OD

Tab. Gliclazide SR 30 mg one OD

Tab. Metformin 500 mg one BD

How should Mr SP be counselled?

Discussion:

From the case records, you find that Mr SP's problems are peripheral neuropathy, hypertension and diabetes mellitus. The first step is to introduce yourself and confirm the patient's identity. This is an important step to avoid giving the medication to the wrong patient.

Figure 6.1 Example of a medication card

MEDICATION CARD
Patient name: Mr SP Valid from …20../…5…/…2011…..
Address: 202, Tank Bund Road

Name of medication	Strength	Brand name	Break-fast	Lunch	Evening meal	Bed-time	Further advice
Gabapentin	300 mg	Gabantin®	1	1		1	For pain
Ramipril	2.5 mg	Hopace®	1				For blood pressure
Gliclazide SR	30 mg	Azucon®	1				For diabetes – take after food
Metformin	500 mg	Diamet®	1		1		For diabetes – take after food

A good opening question is to ask Mr SP 'Have you taken these medications previously?' As he replies 'No, this is the first time', the next useful question could be 'What did your doctor tell you about these medications?'. Based on his answer, the counselling advice can be tailored to his information needs. Specific information which could be given to Mr SP includes:

❖ ***Gabapentin***: This medication relieves the burning nerve pain in your feet. The dose is 300 mg (one capsule) three times a day with or without food. The medication must be taken on a regular basis (every day) to be effective. Sometimes this medication may cause drowsiness or dizziness. If you experience any unwanted effects, do not stop the medication abruptly but please bring your symptoms to the notice of your doctor. Gabapentin may increase the effects of alcohol, so please avoid driving or operating heavy machinery.

❖ ***Ramipril***: This medication is for high blood pressure. Take one tablet each morning. The medication must be taken on a regular basis (every day) to be effective. Sometimes this medication can cause dizziness, particularly during the first few days. Getting up gradually when sitting or lying down will help minimise this problem. This medication occasionally causes dry cough. If this occurs and persists, let your doctor know.

❖ ***Gliclazide***: This medication is given to reduce your high blood sugar levels. The dose is 30 mg (one tablet) once daily, immediately after breakfast. This is a slow-release tablet so swallow the tablet whole. Do not take this medication without food or if a meal is missed, as your blood sugar levels may fall below normal. This can also occur after strenuous exercise. The symptoms of this include sweating, increased heart rate and confusion. If you experience such effects, eat some sugar candy or a spoonful of sugar.

❖ ***Metformin***: This medication is given to reduce your high blood sugar levels. The dose is 500 mg (one tablet) twice daily after the morning and evening meals. Sometimes this medication can cause nausea or diarrhoea. If this happens, let your doctor know.

At the end of the session, Mr SP's understanding can be assessed by asking questions such as 'Can you remember what this medication is for?' or 'What time do you think you will take this medication?'. The session should be concluded by asking 'Do you have any other questions?'. Each medication should be individually labelled with full directions. PILs (*see websites given at the end of this chapter*) would also be useful in this case as a number of new medications have been started concurrently.

If time allows, more general information about diabetes and associated risk factors could also be provided. For example, 'If these medications for diabetes are not taken as prescribed, blood sugar levels may remain high and may lead to damage to the heart, kidneys, eyes, blood vessels, and nerves. For patients with diabetes, diet and lifestyle changes are important. Regular exercise is recommended, and some changes to your diet may be needed. Avoid eating sweets, honey, jams and other foods with high sugar content. It is important to check your feet regularly and avoid cuts, blisters or other injuries. Smoking increases the risk of heart attack, stroke and blood circulation problems in the feet. Have you tried to quit smoking before? Quitting smoking is difficult but is strongly advised.'

CASE STUDY 2

Mr RV, a 22-year-old postal worker, presents a prescription to a community pharmacy following discharge from the local hospital. Mr RV's asthma was first detected when he was at school, when he became acutely short of breath during a football match. After initial treatment, he was free of symptoms, and he has not used his salbutamol inhaler for many years. Recently, he developed severe shortness of breath and was admitted to hospital. His current prescription lists the following medications.

Rx

Salbutamol MDI 200 µg four times a day and sos

Beclomethasone MDI 250 µg twice daily

Prednisolone tablets 10 mg every morning

What counselling would you give Mr RV ?

Discussion:

Mr RV appears to have had an acute exacerbation of asthma. Common reasons for this include respiratory infection, exposure to pollen or other allergens, and poor medication adherence. After introducing yourself to Mr RV and confirming his identity, you need to obtain medication history and assess his knowledge of asthma and its treatment. Mr RV tells you that he has been taking diclofenac on and off for relief from muscle aches.

You: "Can you tell me more about this. When was the last time you took diclofenac?"

Mr RV: "I took several tablets earlier this week before I went to hospital."

You: "Did you tell your doctor about this?"

Mr RV: "No, I wasn't taking it often so I didn't mention this to him."

You: "Some people with asthma develop asthma symptoms when they take aspirin or medications like the one you have taken for muscle ache. I would advise you to speak to your doctor about this, but in the meantime avoid taking aspirin, diclofenac tablets or other types of medication for muscle aches."

Based on the patient's knowledge and awareness, he should be educated about the inflammatory nature of asthma and the need to use both a preventer inhaler and a reliever inhaler.

- ***Salbutamol 200 μg MDI***: This is a reliever inhaler and opens up the air passages of the lungs. The recommended dose is two puffs four times daily. It works quickly and can also be used for fast relief from shortness of breath if needed. This is the inhaler you should use in an emergency when you have a severe asthma attack.
- ***Beclomethasone 250 μg MDI***: This is a preventer inhaler and reduces the inflammation or swelling of the airways. When used regularly every day, this medication decreases the number and severity of asthma attacks. The recommended dose is one puff twice daily. Use the salbutamol inhaler about 5–10 minutes beforehand as this will increase the amount of preventer medication that reaches your lungs. After using the beclomethasone inhaler, rinse your mouth with water and spit it out afterwards. This helps avoid infections in the mouth like thrush.

It is important that patients on inhalers are educated about the correct way of using them. You proceed to explain the following steps to the patient:

1. Remove the cap.
2. Shake the inhaler.
3. Breathe out gently.
4. Hold the inhaler upright and place your lips around the mouthpiece or two finger-widths from the mouth.
5. Start to inhale slowly immediately before actuation.
6. Actuate the inhaler while continuing to inhale.
7. Inhale completely and then hold your breath for as long as possible.
8. Breathe out.
9. Wait one minute and repeat the steps above if more than one inhalation is prescribed.

You then ask the patient to use the inhaler so that you can check their understanding of your directions. Most patients find this difficult in the first few attempts, so it is important to encourage the patient while you help them improve their technique.

- ***Prednisolone***: This is a strong medication used to reduce inflammation in the airways. It should be taken once daily after breakfast. Sometimes it can cause nausea and irritation in the stomach. Other side effects may occur but for you these should not be a problem with short-term use. 'Has the doctor told you how long to continue prednisolone? You should take this medication strictly according to your doctor's instructions'.

The information you give can be strengthened by providing a PIL about asthma and its treatment, if available. You can also suggest to the patient that he return to see you after one week with his inhaler, so that you can re-check his inhaler technique.

CASE STUDY 3

Mrs PV, a 25-year-old housewife, presented to her family doctor with a two-week history of frequent fever, productive cough and weakness. Her fever frequency did not decrease despite taking paracetamol 650 mg regularly. After examination, her doctor ordered a sputum test for acid fast bacilli (AFB) and the AFB test came back as positive. Her doctor prescribed the following medications and asked her to see him after two months.

Rx

AKT – 4 ® 1 Combipack a day for two months

(Each combipack contains 1 capsule of Rifampicin 450 mg + 2 tablets of Pyrazinamide 750 mg + 1 tablet of Ethambutol 800 mg + 1 tablet of Isoniazid 300 mg)

Benadone ® 40 mg. One tablet every day for two months

How should Mrs PV be counselled?

Discussion:

Mrs PV tells you that she has recently returned from her village where she cared for her father who was sick and suffering from a similar problem to her own. She started experiencing symptoms after she returned from the village. Her family physician confirmed TB infection, prescribed antibiotic therapy for two months and asked her to consult him after completing the course.

Given the complexity of her treatment, you ask her whether she has some time to discuss her condition and treatment with you. Mrs PV agrees and you provide the following information to her.

About the disease:

You tell her that TB is a serious lung infection caused by bacteria that are generally transmitted from person to person by the inhalation of cough droplets containing the bacteria. Symptoms include high fever, night sweats, weight loss, cough with sputum and chest pain.

To treat the infection, she will need to take four different antibiotics for two months followed by two antibiotics for the next six months.

You show her the combipack of AKT-4® and tell her that she needs to take the following medications each day for the next two months:

Isoniazid 300 mg one tablet per day

Rifampicin 450 mg one tablet per day

Pyrazinamide 750 mg two tablets per day

Ethambutol 800 mg per day

You tell her that she should take all four medications daily without fail to treat the infection successfully. Completing the course is also very important in the management of the disease.

- *Isoniazid*: One isoniazid tablet should be taken each day on an empty stomach for better absorption. If she experiences gastric irritation, you advise her to take the medicine with food.
- *Rifampicin*: One rifampicin tablet should be taken each day. This antibiotic should be taken one hour before or two hours after a meal for maximum effect. You warn her that rifampicin may change the colour of body fluids like urine, sweat and tears to orange or red, and that she should not panic if this happens. However, some types of contact lenses may be permanently stained. If Mrs PV is taking oral contraceptives, you advise her that these may be unreliable and that she should also use a non-hormonal method of contraception for the duration of rifampicin treatment and for eight weeks thereafter.
- *Pyrizinamide*: Two tablets of pyrazinamide should be taken each day after food. Mrs PV should report to her doctor if she experiences any unusual reactions.
- *Ethambutol*: One tablet of ethambutol should be taken every morning after food. Mrs PV should report any changes in her vision or eyesight to her doctor.
- *Benadone®*: Benadone® is a brand name of pyridoxine and is used to prevent nerve pain which may be a side effect of isoniazid. Mrs PV tells you that her doctor has also advised her to eat liver, wholegrain cereals, bananas and legumes.

Lifestyle modifications:

To help her body's immune system resolve the infection, you advise Mrs PV to eat a nutritious diet containing green leafy vegetables, eggs, milk, meat, fish and fruits.

Mrs PV should be advised to keep her rooms well-ventilated. Whenever she coughs, she should cover her mouth to prevent the spread of cough droplets in the air, and wash her hands afterwards. It is worth giving an information leaflet about TB and its treatment to help her remember the points you discussed with her.

Before closing the session, you ask her whether she has any doubts to be clarified.

KEY MESSAGES

- Educating patients about the safe and effective use of their medications is a core responsibility for both hospital and community pharmacists.
- Patient counselling requires therapeutic knowledge and good communication skills.
- Patient counselling aims to improve the safety and effectiveness of medications.
- Counselling involves two-way communication and must be tailored to the information needs of each patient.
- Open-ended questions help the pharmacist assess the information needs of the patient.
- Written information may be a useful supplement to verbal counselling for some patients.

Further Reading

Counselling, Concordance and Communication: Innovative education for pharmacists. 2005. FIP and PIPSF. Available at http://www.hrhresourcecenter.org

Baker SJ. 1997. Who can read Consumer Product Information. *Aust J Hosp Pharm* 27(2):126–131.

Barbanel D. 1994. Personal approach to patient counselling. *Pharm J* 253:742.

Gibbs S, Waters WE and George CF. 1989. Benefits of prescription information leaflets. *Br J Clin Pharmacol* 28:345–351.

Websites of Interest

National Prescribing Service
This Australian government-funded website provides consumer medicine information which may be downloaded or used as reference for counselling. Note that brand names are those available in Australia.
http://www.nps.org.au/consumers

Patient.co.uk
This independent UK website provides patient information leaflets on both medications and diseases. Some leaflets have been translated into other languages such as Hindi, Bengali, Gujarati and Punjabi.
http://www.patient.co.uk

The Pharmaceutical Society of Australia (see Professional Practice Standard 3: Counselling. 2010 Version 4)
http://www.psa.org.au

The Society of Hospital Pharmacists of Australia
Standard of Practice for the Provision of Consumer Medicine Information by Pharmacists in Hospitals, February 2007. Also in *J Pharm Pract Res* 2007; 37(1):56–8
http://www.shpa.org.au

7

MEDICATION ADHERENCE

PA Mahesh and G Parthasarathi

Learning Objectives

Upon completion of this chapter, the reader should be able to:

- Understand various determinants of medication non-adherence
- Explain the methods to detect medication non-adherence
- Summarise commonly-used intervention strategies to improve medication adherence
- Understand the role of the pharmacist in improving medication adherence

Medication adherence is defined as the extent to which a patient's medication-taking behaviour coincides with the intention of the health advice he or she has been given. Medication adherence is one of the most important factors that determine therapeutic outcomes, especially in patients suffering from chronic illnesses. Whatever the efficacy of a drug, it cannot act unless the patient takes it. Low medication adherence has assumed importance as it seriously undermines the benefits of current medical care and imposes a significant financial burden on individual patients and the healthcare system as a whole.

The term patient compliance was previously used when referring to the medication-taking behaviour of patients. The word 'compliance' can imply an authoritarian attitude on the part of healthcare professionals and may suggest yielding and submission by the patient. 'Non-compliance' is failure or refusal to comply with advice and can imply disobedience on the part of the patient. Hence, it has been replaced by the term medication 'adherence'. Recently, the Royal Pharmaceutical Society of Great Britain adopted the term 'concordance', which means agreement and harmony. The backbone of concordance is that the patient is the decision-maker.

Adherence to treatment is the key link between treatment and outcome in medical care. Many variables which may influence adherence have been studied, but none of them have been shown to consistently predict adherence. Research into medication adherence has been piecemeal, and as there is no gold standard for measuring adherence, it is difficult to draw conclusions from the studies which have been done. Further research is needed in this complex field, especially taking into account the various factors that can be controlled to improve adherence. Medication adherence richly deserves attention and much impetus is needed to develop new ideas and theories to improve it.

Medication Adherence Research

The problem of making sure patients follow prescriptions is as old as medicine itself. In the fifth century BCE, Hippocrates reminded physicians "... to check patient's behaviour because often they lie about having taken prescribed drugs. This unadmitted negligence may lead the physician into error...".

Some early research reports were presented in the 1950s. Sackett and Haynes were the pioneers in the recent interest in adherence research. The majority of adherence research has been carried out by healthcare providers and by the pharmaceutical industry, and has focused on patient determinants of non-adherence rather than on the shared responsibilities of the doctor and the patient.

The first three decades of compliance research, from 1970 to 2000, have yielded little information to improve medication adherence. The reasons for this include the lack of a gold standard to measure medication adherence, lack of experimental evidence for many models, failure of measurement methods to gather valid information on the extent of patient adherence, uncertain reliability and validity of some scales used in medication adherence research studies, lack of patient-centric information and lack of long-term follow-up data. High-quality research studies in this area would perhaps establish the causes of medication non-adherence, and suggest strategies to improve medication adherence.

When is Adherence Important?

There are many situations in clinical practice where adherence is extremely important for better therapeutic outcomes. These include:

a. *Replacement therapy*. For example, thyroxine and insulin are essential for maintaining the body's metabolism and must be used regularly as prescribed.
b. *Maintenance of pharmacological effect.* For example, anti-hypertensive and oral hypoglycemic agents. Control of blood pressure throughout the day and maintaining blood sugar levels within the normal range are necessary to obtain optimal treatment benefit.
c. *Maintenance of serum drug concentrations to control a particular disorder.* For example, anti-convulsants. Subtherapeutic levels of anti-convulsants may increase the risk of convulsions in an epileptic patient.
d. *Some diseases of public health importance where non-adherence is a major obstacle to achieving control.* For example, tuberculosis, human immunodeficiency virus and related opportunistic infections, hepatic infections, preventive strategies such as immunisation programmes.
e. *In chronic diseases such as diabetes and hypertension*, where adherence is important to prevent short- and long-term complications such as diabetes

ketoacidosis, and microvascular and macrovascular diseases due to longstanding diabetes and hypertension.

Extent of non-adherence: The extent of non-adherence in the general population in the outpatient setting can vary greatly from as poor as 33% with antibiotic treatment, to as high as 94% for hypertension in the first year of treatment. It is estimated that as many as 50% of prescriptions fail to produce the desired results because of improper use, and 14–21% of patients never even fill their original prescriptions. It has been noted that adherence tends to decrease with time, and prospective long-term studies should ideally be considered when evaluating the therapeutic efficacy of new drugs.

Cost of Non-adherence

Levine in 1983 studied non-adherence in the treatment of cardiovascular disease in the general population in an outpatient setting in the USA, and noted an excess of 125,000 deaths, several thousand hospitalisations per year, a loss of 20 million workdays and a loss of over $1.5 billion. Cowen in 1981demonstrated a definite link between non-adherence and increased utilisation of health resources in the community in an elderly population as evidenced by a larger mean number of clinic visits per patient (5.48 vs 1.86), a larger mean number of medications per patient (5.36 vs 1.96), and a larger number of dosage changes, hospital admissions and longer duration of hospital stay.

Ettenger in 1991 observed that poor adherence with post-transplant immune suppression regimens is a leading cause of rejected organ transplants. In a study involving paediatric cadaver renal transplants, 13% of 165 recipients lost their graft due to non-adherence.

Categories of Medication Non-adherence

Patients demonstrate medication non-adherence in many different situations. These have been categorised based on whether the prescription was honoured, the medication was underused or overused or whether non-prescription medicines were used. Non-adherence has been further categorised based on whether it was done on the patient's own volition. It is possible that each condition and each doctor–patient pair involves different motivating factors, which affect adherence.

Primary

Not having a prescription dispensed.

Secondary

- *Intentional:* The patient does not adhere to the prescription on his own volition. For example, the patient may take less than the prescribed dose with an assumption that the prescribed dose is high or may take more than the prescribed dose expecting quicker recovery from the disease. An asthma patient may not use the inhaled steroid (preventer medication) as he/she feels much better after a few weeks of using steroids, and does not understand the role of steroids in asthma management. Sometimes, the patient benefits from his action and that is termed 'intelligent non-adherence'. This term was coined by

Weintraub to describe patients who alter their therapy without suffering any adverse events. For example, a patient may cease taking a medication because it causes nausea and vomiting. The patient's non-adherence appears rational when analysed without any bias; for example, misdiagnosis, inappropriate prescribing.

- *Unintentional:* This typically occurs when the patient has misunderstood or forgotten the doctor's directions, or fails to adhere to the prescribed dosage regimen due to cognitive problems such as memory loss or confusion. For example, patients may cease to take antibiotics after two days or anti-tubercular drugs after two months if they forget that the doctor had advised them that a full treatment course should be completed. In both situations, there is a chance of treatment failure and an increased risk of drug-resistant organisms emerging.

Another way of categorising medication adherence is given below:

- Adherent
- Partially adherent
- Non-adherent

Partially adherent is defined as adherence to more than 70% of the medication regimen, while complying with more than 80% of the prescribed regimen is termed adherent. Most patients fall between the two extremes. Patient medication adherence may vary on a day-to-day basis, and may vary for different medications depending on the patient's beliefs about the need for and efficacy of a particular medication.

Methods to Detect Medication Non-adherence

Various methods to detect medication non-adherence have been described and are presented in Table 7.1. There is no gold standard yet for adherence measures. This is one of the important reasons why research in adherence is difficult and comparisons between different research results cannot be made. Each method has problems relating to generating valid and reliable data to give an accurate estimate of the extent of adherence. These aspects are discussed in the practice scenarios.

Determinants of Medication Adherence

Medication adherence or non-adherence is the result of complex interactions among many factors. Some of these factors are seen to improve medication adherence while others may negatively influence the medication adherence of a patient. The situation is almost unique to each patient and this is one of the reasons why it is so difficult to predict medication adherence.

The factors that may influence adherence, or for that matter any health-related behaviour, can be divided into three categories: predisposing, enabling and reinforcing. Pre-disposing factors include demographic factors, as well as the patient's knowledge, attitudes, beliefs and perceptions about illness and its severity, cause, prevention and treatment.

The Health Belief Model developed in 1974 attempts to predict adherence, or other health-related behaviour change, in terms of certain belief patterns. Under this model, the

Table 7.1 Methods to detect medication non-adherence

1. Direct – objective
▪ Measure blood or urine levels of drugs – gives indication of short-term adherence, unless the drug has a long half-life ▪ Measure blood levels of marker – add marker to medicines and measure levels in the body. The ethical issue of the safety of the given marker is a matter of concern. For example, low-dose phenobarbitone gives both quantitative and qualitative data over the preceding few weeks with little intra and interindividual variation.
2. Indirect – objective
▪ Pill count – count the tablets remaining in the container. Vulnerable to overestimates of adherence. ▪ Prescription refill – accurate data monitoring system required. ▪ Electronic medication containers – opening and closure times of container recorded on a microprocessor in the lid of the container.
3. Health outcome measures – assessing therapeutic efficacy, for example, blood pressure control, asthma severity, survival, hospitalisation, etc.
4. Utilisation of healthcare services
▪ Clinic attendance – opportunity to counsel patients. Clinic non-attenders are more likely to be non-adherent. ▪ Appointment making ▪ Appointment keeping ▪ Preventive visits
5. Indirect – subjective (methods of questionable reliability)
▪ Patient interview – asking patients if they have adhered to the prescribed regimens ▪ Diary keeping

sequence of belief events which must occur if the patient is to be adherent is as follows:

- The patient must believe that his or her health is in jeopardy.
- The patient must perceive the potential seriousness of the condition in terms of symptoms, time lost from work, economic difficulties and so on.
- On assessing the circumstances, the patient must believe that the benefits of treatment outweigh the costs, and are indeed possible and within his or her grasp.
- There must be a 'cue to action' that makes the patient feel the need to adhere to their medication.

Enabling factors are the skills and resources needed for adherence. The term 'skills' here refers to the patient's ability to adopt behaviours which will assist adherence; for example, making an appointment with the doctor to obtain a prescription. Resources include the availability and accessibility of healthcare facilities such as doctors, pharmacies, clinics or hospitals.

Reinforcing factors are those that determine whether adherence is supported by family members, peers, healthcare providers, the local community and society in general. The reinforcement may be positive or negative depending on the attitudes or behaviour of significant people, some of whom will be more influential than others.

An example of family and societal attitudes affecting adherence is illustrated in *Practice Scenario 1*. This scenario demonstrates how the identification of predisposing, enabling and reinforcing factors can assist pharmacists to more effectively address the underlying reasons for a patient's non-adherence.

Other examples of reinforcing factors are those associated with the treating physician, such as communication with the patient, the ability to resolve the patient's concern regarding their disease and medication, regular follow-up by the same physician, and quality and quantity of time spent with the patient and family members. Giving written instructions to the patients may also improve medication adherence. The social isolation associated with diseases such as tuberculosis and leprosy is also a reinforcing factor for poor medication adherence in these conditions.

Unlike other health-related behaviours, such as diet or lifestyle changes, factors associated with the medication itself are also very important. Long duration of treatment and adverse effects may lead to poor medication adherence. The complexity of the regimen is an important determinant of non-adherence and includes:

- *Number of medicines*: The fewer the medicines prescribed, the better the adherence. This is the reason for the availability of many combination products on the market today; for example, combinations of anti-hypertensives, anti-diabetic drugs, anti-tubercular drugs.
- *Frequency of dosing*: Better medication adherence may be expected for medicines administered once daily compared to more frequent administration.

Following are some of the factors that have been found in some studies to have no association to the patients' medication adherence:

- Age
- Sex
- Income
- Education
- Ethnicity
- Patient's intelligence
- Knowledge about the disease
- Illness being treated
- Actual seriousness of the disease
- Actual susceptibility to the disease
- Actual efficacy of treatment
- Physician's prediction of adherence
- Marital status
- Number of people in the household
- Clinical setting
- Features of the disease
- Referral process
- Therapeutic regimen

These findings are based on studies conducted in Western settings, and it is possible that some of these factors may be more influential among Indian patients.

How Can Medication Adherence Be Improved?

A large number of interventions to improve patient adherence have been studied. Most of these have been patient-oriented and educational. Oral instructions are the most frequently studied interventions, followed by written instructions and educational leaflets. Other commonly studied interventions are those directed at modifying patient behaviour. Very few studies have addressed the issue of provider-focused interventions. There is no evidence till date that any one method improves medication adherence better than another.

The interventional strategies can be provider-targetted or patient-focused. Provider-targetted interventions include the education of healthcare workers including the treating physician, community pharmacists and nurses. Patient-targetted interventions include various educational strategies with oral or written instructions, or audiovisual materials. Education can be imparted to patients individually or with their family members or in patient groups. Interventions which target the behaviour of patients are also useful. These include medication diaries, dosettes, verbal agreement with patients, tailoring the regimen to suit the patients' convenience and reminders by mail or telephone.

Affective strategies such as counselling patients in depth, home visits and generating family support may also improve patients' medication adherence. Pharmaceutical formulations such as sustained release and long-acting medications which decrease the frequency of dosing, transdermal medications and depot preparations may increase patient convenience and improve medication adherence.

An important factor that influences patient medication adherence is the nature of the doctor–patient relationship. Many adherence researchers feel that patients need to be involved as equal partners in decisions concerning their health, and doctors need to modify their role from being the sole decision-maker to an expert advisor.

Another important strategy aimed at improving adherence involves patient education, patient counselling and providing information. Information may benefit the following groups of patients:

- Those who want to comply but need more information to allow them to do so.
- Patients with misconceptions and fears, which can be dispelled by providing information and reassurance.

A number of studies claim to have improved knowledge and adherence; however, no significant effect was found in other studies. Massuea reviewed 30 studies of patient education in chronic disease. He concluded that increasing patient knowledge alone is rarely successful in improving adherence and that the most effective programmes involved a behavioural aspect as well.

Studies on the effect of patient counselling with checking for recall by pharmacists, doctors and nurses under the direction of a pharmacist have shown a positive benefit on adherence. The duration of counselling lasted from 5–15 minutes to one and a half hours. The overall evidence for effectiveness of counselling is equivocal (Level I). Levels of evidence are listed in Table 7.2.

Table 7.2 Levels of evidence for adherence studies

Level I	Meta analysis of randomised control trials with high power
Level II	Randomised control trials or meta analysis with low power
Level III	Non-randomised concurrent cohort studies
Level IV	Non-randomised historical cohort studies
Level V	Case series

There is evidence that individualised leaflets for diseases such as diabetes and hypertension are effective in improving adherence to lifestyle and diet changes, and are better than the standard patient information leaflet as they may incorporate a behavioural component. The evidence for giving patient information leaflets of varying kinds has been found to be equivocal (Level I).

Urquhart has provided a scale of interventions of increasing intensity to ensure good adherence with crucial medicines. The cost of these interventions increases disproportionately with intensity. The hierarchy begins with prescribing as usual and ends with admission to a nursing home. Incarceration is used as a last resort in tuberculosis treatment because of the public health hazards of incomplete or erratic treatment and the likelihood of the emergence of resistant micro-organisms. It is an extreme measure and may not be practical, at least in a democratic setting. The other measures can be used in a graded manner. Directly observed therapy (DOT) is used to improve medication adherence in patients with tuberculosis.

The patient education strategies that can help improve medication adherence are listed in Table 7.3. Many of the terms listed in the table are self-explanatory. A few important ones are discussed below.

Counselling: This involves providing verbal information to patients about their illness and its treatment. It may entail the use of various methods, but true counselling is a two-way process and involves listening as well as talking.

Tailoring or cueing: This involves matching the medicine regimen with a patient's normal daily routine such as mealtimes or usual time of retiring to bed.

Packaging: The use of a calendar pack with special packaging is an inexpensive option and is useful though it has its own drawbacks.

Table 7.3 Patient education strategies that can help improve medication adherence

• Present the most important instructions first.
• Reinforce a few simple, clearly stated instructions with easy-to-read, written instructions.
• Tailor medication regimen to the patient's daily schedule and lifestyle.
• Involve the family to assist and encourage adherence.
• Stress the importance of adherence at follow-up and recognise the patient's effort to comply.
• Schedule follow-up visits according to the patient's previous adherence record.
• Select medications which can be given once daily and with the least potential to cause side effects.
• Patients should not only be informed of possible side effects, but also what to do if the side effects occur; for example, stop the medicine, contact the doctor, take a simple remedy or persevere with treatment.
• Restrict information to four key points.
• Use simple language, short sentences and specific instructions.
• Check for recall.

Simplification of the regimen: This refers to the rationalisation of a patient's regimen to one that can be realistically managed, that is, a compromise between the ideal and one that can be achieved. This can in most situations be done without adversely affecting the patient's treatment outcome. For example, this may involve decreasing the number of medications being taken, reducing the frequency of dosing (for example, the same drug given as a once-daily slow release formulation) or synchronising the dose times of various medicines in the regimen.

A list of the important conclusions from research in this area is given below:

- As the comprehensiveness of the programme to improve medication adherence increases, the adherence also improves.
- Multiple interventions: Education, behavioural and affective components when used in combination have an additive effect. For example, oral instructions followed by written instructions (educational) coupled with maintaining a medication diary (behavioural) and in-depth counselling (affective) have a greater effect than either of them alone or two of them in combination. This has been demonstrated by meta analysis of various randomised control trials (Level I).
- There is no evidence to say that any one method is better than the other.
- Written instructions are less effective than other educational interventions to improve adherence.
- Group education improves both direct measures of adherence and utilisation, whereas telephone education improves utilisation.
- Telephone reminders are not more effective in improving utilisation than mailed reminders.
- Rewards for being adherent showed greater effect when combined with educational or affective components. The physician's communication skills is probably one of the most important factors in determining patient adherence.
- Adherence interventions were found to be more useful for patients with certain diseases, for example, more for diabetes, less for asthma, cancer, hypertension and mental illness, and even less for conditions such as otitis media and the use of antibiotics in routine general practice.

Role of Pharmacists

Pharmacists are in a unique position to improve medication adherence because they can actually show the medication to the patient and relate any information to the medication itself. Pharmacists often provide verbal education and written individualised information for the patient although the benefits of these strategies alone are unclear.

A few studies provide evidence of Level II or improved patient medication adherence as a result of patient education given by pharmacists. Macdonald studied the effects of patient education by pharmacists on medication adherence in post-discharge patients, which demonstrated a clear benefit in patients receiving education from pharmacists.

In an unpublished study by the authors, clear benefit was demonstrated in a randomised control trial in both asthma and COPD patients with a follow-up period of two months in improving medication adherence along with the inhalation technique following a pharmacist-based educational interventional programme. It was interesting to note that the improvement in the inhalation technique continued with each educational sitting. The patients received both oral education and written instructions in the local language about their disease, need for regular medication and the importance of each medication in an educational programme lasting 45 minutes in each sitting.

The information that patients need to know which pharmacists can impart includes:

- Name and purpose of the drug
- When and how to take the medication
- Possible side effects
- Precautions
- Interactions with food or other drugs
- Duration of therapy
- Action to take if a dose is missed
- How to tell if the medication is working or not working

Strategies to improve the patient–pharmacist relationship are presented in Table 7.4. Apart from patient education, a pharmacist may contribute towards improving medication adherence by other means including advice to prescribers on the simplification of drug regimens, providing patients with medication cards or medication aids such as a dosette, and by identifying the predisposing, enabling and reinforcing factors which may contribute towards medication non-adherence. In hospitals, clinical pharmacists have many opportunities to assess factors which may assist the patient's medication adherence. Through patient interviews, the pharmacist can assess the patient's knowledge of their drug therapy and usual medication habits. For example, does the patient have a set routine and is family support available to supervise medication use? The pharmacist is also able to identify if the patient has any specific problems with medication, such as a problem swallowing large tablets, or difficulty opening child-proof containers. The pharmacist can also assess the patient's ability to comprehend and recall information, and if an adverse drug reaction may discourage medication adherence.

Table 7.4 Strategies to improve the pharmacist–patient relationship

• Be friendly and approachable
• Improve communication skills
• Take into account the spiritual and psychological needs of the patient
• Improve patient education
• Encourage patients to discuss their main concerns without interruption or premature closing
• Elicit patient perception of the illness and associated feelings and expectations
• Learn methods of active listening and empathy
• Give clear explanations
• Check the patient's understanding
• Negotiate a treatment plan
• Check the patient's attention to medication adherence
• Simplify the therapeutic regimen
• Be aware of the patient's wishes
• Involve the patient in treatment decisions
• Improve home support
• Monitor beneficial effects
• Monitor side effects
• Provide long-term support to the patient and continuity of care
• Speak the same language
• Shorten the pharmacy waiting time

At the end of the process, the pharmacist should be able to determine the patients' own assessment of their adherence to medication and make a professional assessment of the ways in which this can be improved. For example, this may involve counselling for any specific problems with medication and preparation of individualised medication information sheets.

Medication Adherence – Indian Scenario

Several unique factors affect medication adherence in the Indian setting, which may be generalisable to any developing country. Some factors have a positive impact while others a negative one. Not many controlled studies are available that have looked at medication adherence in the Indian setting.

Factors with a positive impact on medication adherence include good family support. A joint family setting is especially important for children and the elderly as a carer is always present to administer the medicines. The other important factor is a good doctor–patient relationship. Western studies also have emphasised the positive effect on medication adherence of a good doctor–patient relationship. More than 80% of the Indian population resides in rural areas and medical help is usually far away. Family practice is the norm and specialists are rarely available. Patients are closely attached to their family doctor and discuss not only their medical problems but also family and social problems. The doctor also doubles as their philosopher and guide and offers solace and comfort. This relationship has a very positive effect on improving medication adherence.

Factors with a negative impact on medication adherence include illiteracy, poor understanding of the disease and its treatment, and poor socioeconomic status. Poor involvement of community pharmacists in providing patient education is another factor. A family practitioner in a town regularly treats about 150–200 patients in a single day and has little time for educating patients regarding disease and drug therapy. Many of the patients cannot afford medicines on a regular basis as they do not have any medical insurance. The knowledge, attitude and practices of the population are focused on symptomatic treatment rather than on preventive treatment. Though there is government support for communicable diseases through the provision of investigations and drugs, there is no such provision for non-communicable diseases such as diabetes and hypertension. This contributes to poor medication adherence as many patients do not have money to buy the drugs they need. It is not uncommon in urban metros to have an elderly patient with visual impairment, deteriorating cognitive function and poor health due to poor medication adherence staying alone. Lack of carers or community nurses providing home care adds to the problem.

One of the diseases for which adherence has been studied in some detail in India is tuberculosis. The national control programme to improve medication adherence has aggressively adopted the DOT strategy. In one of the first studies on medication adherence in the DOTS regime of the national control programme in Bangalore, certain factors were found to predict medication non-adherence. After two months of treatment, when patients started feeling better, they missed doses prior to travelling to their native place or moving to another part of the country; this led to them dropping out of the programme. The distance from the DOTS centre was found to be unimportant. More studies need to be done in the Indian scenario to investigate the factors that could be peculiar to this country, and the effect of various adherence improving measures on the Indian population.

Conclusion

Adherence is very important in medical care for three reasons. Medication non-adherence imposes considerable financial burden. Adherence to treatment and lifestyle changes is the key link between process and outcome in medical care. If adherence levels are not considered in clinical trials, it can have a major impact on conclusions drawn from clinical research, especially drug trials. Every effort must be made to develop new research methodologies which could be a gold standard for adherence measures and to develop new strategies and ideas to improve patient adherence.

Practice Scenario 1

You are working as a clinical pharmacist attached to a hospital. Dr SVS, a physician from the Department of Medicine, contacts you requesting patient education on the use of inhalers. The patient is an adolescent girl suffering from asthma for the last one year. She was started on inhalers (salbutamol and a combination of salmeterol plus fluticasone) two weeks ago by her family physician but continues to have symptoms. The physician feels that her medication adherence is poor and her inhaler technique needs correction.

Outline the approach you would adopt for this situation.

Discussion

The first step is to make a list of problems to be addressed in this patient:

1. Check assessment of medication adherence
2. Assess reasons for poor medication adherence
3. Assess inhaler technique
4. Provide patient counselling and education to improve medication adherence and inhaler technique

Check assessment of medication adherence: Medication adherence in patients using inhalers can be assessed by:

- **Patient interview**: Patient interview is one of the methods used for assessing patient medication adherence. Its advantages are that it is very simple and easy to perform, and may provide additional information about the patient's attitudes towards their illness and medication use. Its disadvantages are that it may not be very accurate if the patient is not forthcoming, and it is difficult to accurately assess medication adherence for longer periods of time due to recall bias. On patient interview, the patient tells you that she has been on inhalers regularly. On further questioning, you realise that she has been using salbutamol inhaler excessively (reliever medication) but has only occasionally used the inhaler containing salmeterol + fluticasone (preventive medications).

- **Diary keeping**: This is one of the common methods used in assessing patient medication adherence and treatment outcomes. It involves the patient maintaining a standard diary where the occurrence and severity of various symptoms and medication use is recorded. For example, in asthma, recording of daytime symptoms and nocturnal awakenings, and peak flow meter readings may be recorded. The diary is reviewed during every consultation. Its advantages are that it is easy and practical. The disadvantages are that some patients may find it too time-consuming, that patients need to be literate and that there is no objective measure that the patient has actually taken the drug.
- **Weighing of inhaler canisters**: This is an accurate, direct and objective measurement of medication use but it cannot tell you whether the patient has used it at the appropriate time or whether the patient has used it correctly. It is done by using an electronic balance and having a standard reference chart for all the inhalers available in the market with their weight at different doses left in the canister. You decide not to do that as poor medication adherence has already been clearly demonstrated.

Assess reasons for poor medication adherence: The next step is to assess the reasons for the poor medication adherence. You spend time getting to know the background of the patient and how she and her family have responded to her diagnosis of asthma. You realise that she is from a very conservative family and there is a lot of social stigma in her community if the girl is labelled an asthmatic, which may affect her future marriage prospects. There is also an intense steroid phobia and this is the reason she has hardly used the preventive medication. Because she spends most nights awake, she used her reliever medicines excessively to gain temporary relief from her symptoms.

Assess inhaler technique: The next step is to assess her inhaler technique. You ask the patient to demonstrate her inhaler technique and check it with a standard checklist you have prepared based on the standard resources or patient education published by the American Academy of Asthma, Allergy and Immunology in the Journal of Allergy and Clinical Immunology. You find that some important steps are not done correctly, specifically breathing out fully before inhalation and hand–mouth co-ordination.

Provide patient counselling and education: In the next step, you counsel the patient to improve her medication adherence and inhaler technique. By this time, you have established a good rapport with the patient and her family and they have taken you into their confidence. You briefly discuss asthma, the importance of using anti-inflammatory drugs regularly, the dangers of over-using relievers and the advantages of inhalers. You explain that they are the safest and most effective medications for asthma currently available. You alleviate the patient's steroid phobia by discussing normal steroid production in the body and how the small dose in micrograms she is currently taking will not interfere with her body's normal functions. You discuss the possible risk of side effects and alleviate her concerns in this regard. You give her patient information leaflets (PILs) to go through and ask her to return to see you regularly.

You educate the patient regarding the correct use of the inhaler by demonstrating this with a placebo inhaler, and re-checking her technique. You provide her with a PIL which summarises the technique. You ask her to practice in front of a mirror and give her a placebo inhaler for practice.

You give feedback to her regular doctor. You discuss the various reasons for poor medication adherence and also her poor inhaler technique. You also discuss the possibility of using spacers or dry powder inhalers if her inhaler technique continues to be poor.

To follow up, you try to obtain feedback both from the patient and from the doctor about the progress of the patient, her inhaler technique and her medication adherence.

Practice Scenario 2

You are a clinical pharmacist in a major teaching hospital and a team member implementing the National Tuberculosis Control Programme in your hospital. It is your responsibility to develop intervention strategies to improve medication adherence.

What would be your approach?

Discussion

As a first step, you need do a literature survey of all the intervention strategies which have been shown to improve medication adherence. You next need to see the strength of evidence for each of these intervention strategies. Ideally, you should choose strategies whose effectiveness has been demonstrated by meta analysis of Randomised Control Trials (Level I or Level II). You then need to assess which of these strategies can be implemented in your programme and devise the protocol.

There are various intervention strategies whose effectiveness has been proved by meta analysis of randomised control trials. Many of them can be easily implemented in a developing country.

After a literature survey, you come to the following conclusions:

- ❖ Combined focus interventions are more effective than single focus interventions. A combination of educational, behavioural and affective components would be the strongest intervention strategy.
- ❖ Directly observed treatment short course [DOTS] for tuberculosis has been adopted by most countries to improve medication adherence. However, non-adherence is seen in the DOTS programme too and studies are required to evaluate the effect of the addition of other intervention strategies to DOTS on medication adherence.
- ❖ Group education moderately improve direct measures of compliance and utilisation, and telephone education is very effective in improving utilisation.

- Telephone reminders of appointments are not any more effective in improving utilisation than mailed reminders.
- Packaging dose reminders improve compliance.
- The physicians' communication skills are important in determining patient compliance.
- Rewards are more effective if combined with educational or affective components than when offered in isolation.
- No single intervention strategy is consistently better than any other.
- Written materials are weaker than other educational interventions when given without oral instructions.

Based on the evidence in the literature, you decide to use a combined approach with three focus interventions: educational, behavioural and affective. You also decide to use a provider-based intervention and organise a symposium for physicians involved in the programme on communication skills and the doctor–patient relationship by an expert in the field.

As part of the educational strategies, you decide to use both the individualised approach and the group education approach. A 20-minute counselling session is planned for each patient and his/her family members, with verbal instructions in the patient's own language. Visual aids and PILs will also be used. A mailed reminder is sent to the patient to reach two days prior to the date on which the patient has his or her next appointment.

Three group education sessions are planned during the six-month course of treatment. These are also attended by physicians in the programme and free interaction among the participants is encouraged. A group of patients who have completed treatment and are leading a normal life is requested to attend the meeting so that they can share their experience with others.

As a part of the behavioural strategies to be incorporated in the programme, it is planned to include dosage tailoring to suit each patient, use of special packaging with instructions on the foil to simplify medication use, and the use of a medication diary for literate patients. The patients are also encouraged to note any adverse effects of the medications or write down any other doubts that need to be clarified.

The affective strategies that are planned include home visits by the treatment supervisors and involving all the family members to generate family support for the patient.

The patient is encouraged to freely discuss any problems they may have both with their physicians and their pharmacist and a patient-centred approach is used, where they are encouraged to participate as an equal partner in the decision-making process.

The PILs would also include brief information on the different drugs used and when to take them, possible side effects and the necessary action to take including when to contact a doctor, total duration of treatment, action to be taken if a dose is missed, interactions with food and other drugs and precautions to be taken. The PIL would also include brief information on tuberculosis and emphasise that it is a totally curable disease. The need for regular medication use is also emphasised.

Practice Scenario 3

Mrs YH, a 58-year-old, was admitted to hospital for ischaemic stroke. She is discharged with the following prescriptions for hypertension, COPD and a seizure during admission.

Tab. Nifedipine	10 mg three times a day
Tab. Aspirin	325 mg once daily
Tab. Phenytoin	100 mg three times a day
Tab. Prednisolone	5 mg three times a day
Inhaler Ipratropium	2 puffs three times a day
Inhaler Salbutamol	2 puffs three times a day

You are the clinical pharmacist working with the medical team looking after Mrs YH. On talking to her, you discover that she is confused about her medication and her aged husband is of little help.

What strategies would you adopt to improve Mrs YH's medication adherence when she leaves the hospital?

Discussion

One of the important strategies that you could use to improve her medication adherence is regimen simplification and the use of combination products. Mrs YH is being treated with nifedipine 10 mg three times a day, so switching to a long-acting dihydropyridine such as amlodipine 5 mg once daily is possible. The dose can then be titrated to achieve the 'target blood pressure'.

Phenytoin 100 mg three times a day is prescribed for Mrs YH. Phenytoin can be administered once daily as it has a long biological half-life (24 hours). Your advice would be to administer phenytoin 300 mg once daily.

Mrs YH is receiving prednisolone 5 mg three times a day for an acute exacerbation of COPD. Here, you recommend taking prednisolone 15 mg once daily in the morning, as this is the preferred dosing regimen for prednisolone therapy. Mrs YH is using inhaled ipratropium bromide and salbutamol three times a day as two separate inhalers. An inhaler which contains a combination of these agents will simplify her medication regimen.

As she is literate but has poor memory, you may decide to give her a medicine card listing the details of her medication and their dosage regimen.

KEY MESSAGES

- Medication adherence is one of the most important factors determining therapeutic outcomes.
- There is no gold standard for medication adherence measures.
- The direct objective method is the most reliable one to determine medication adherence but is not practical for routine clinical practice.
- Indirect objective methods are the most commonly used adherence measures in clinical trials.
- Multiple focus interventions are more effective in improving medication adherence than single focus interventions.
- Pharmacists have a very important role to play in improving medication adherence as they are at the interface between doctors and patients.

Further Reading

Interventions for enhancing medication adherence. 2008. *Cochrane Database of Systematic Reviews*, Issue 2. Art. No.: CD000011. DOI: 10.1002/14651858.CD000011.pub3.

Kripalani S, Yao X and Haynes B. 2007. Interventions to enhance medication adherence in chronic medical conditions. A systematic review. *Arch Intern Med*167:540–550.

Osterberg L and Blaschke T. 2005. Adherence to medication. *N Engl J Med.* 353:487–97.

Vermiere E, Hearshaw H and Van Royen P. 2001. Patient adherence to treatment: three decades of research. A comprehensive review. *J Clin Pharm and Therap*. 26:331–342.

8 Essential Medicines and Rational Drug Use

Gitanjali Batmanabane and Krisantha Weerasuriya

Learning Objectives

Upon completion of this chapter, the reader should be able to:

- Define the term essential medicines
- Describe how essential medicines are selected
- List the advantages of an Essential Medicines List (EML)
- Explain what is meant by the rational use of drugs
- List some common examples of irrational drug use and explain why these are a problem
- Describe the methods to monitor drug use
- List some drug use indicators for prescribing in primary healthcare facilities
- Discuss the strategies that can be undertaken to promote the rational use of drugs
- Define and understand the roles of Standard Treatment Guidelines and Drug and Therapeutics Committees
- Understand the role of a clinical pharmacist in promoting the rational use of drugs

Definition of Essential Medicines

The short definition of essential medicines according to the World Health Organization (WHO) is that they are medicines that satisfy the priority healthcare needs of a population.

How are they selected?

Essential medicines are selected based on public health relevance such as the disease prevalence in the region/country, scientific evidence of efficacy, safety and cost effectiveness. Selection also takes into account the treatment facilities available at the level of healthcare provided, the knowledge, skills and training of the healthcare personnel involved, ease of administration of medicines, storage facilities and patient acceptability. Thus, they are a mixture of evidence-based criteria and factors relating to the healthcare system.

WHAT IS THE IMPORTANCE OF ESSENTIAL MEDICINES?

They should be available at all times in the health facilities in adequate quantities in appropriate dosage forms, with assured quality and accompanied by appropriate information at a price the individual and community can afford. Essential medicines are expected to take care of the health needs of the majority of the population; it is difficult to give a figure but essential medicines should cover about 80–90% of healthcare needs.

WHAT IS THE CONCEPT UNDERLYING THE ESSENTIAL MEDICINES LIST (EML)?

The concept of an EML is to have a limited range of carefully selected core essential medicines, which will lead to better healthcare, better drug management and lower costs. These essential medicines should satisfy the priority healthcare needs of the population of the target country/state. They are selected with due regard to disease prevalence, evidence of efficacy and safety, and comparative cost effectiveness. This is a very vibrant and progressive concept, as the need to regularly update the selection of medicines on the list based on current evidence, changes in resistance patterns of organisms, emerging diseases, newer molecules as well as improved formulations are all taken into account.

IS THERE A DIFFERENCE BETWEEN THE EML AND THE ESSENTIAL DRUGS LIST (EDL)?

There is no difference between the two. Prior to 2000, the word 'drug' was used to indicate medicines. However, in some countries, 'drug' has become associated with narcotics and other substances of abuse. Hence, it has now been replaced with the word 'medicine' in most documents. In French, the word 'medicaments' was used from the beginning and continues today.

HOW DID IT ALL BEGIN?

The initial idea for essential medicines came from developing country requests to the WHO for a list of medicines and a report which was presented to the World Health Assembly in 1975. A committee was then set up which was given the task of defining essential medicines and producing a list which could help populations with limited access to medicines. In 1977, the first list of essential medicines was published. The Alma Ata declaration of 1978 outlined the eight components of primary healthcare, with essential medicines being one of them. The WHO has regularly updated the list every two years and in 2011, the seventeenth list was published. In October 2007, a model Essential Medicines List for Children (EMLc) was also published. This too was updated in 2009 and in 2011.

THE MODEL EML OF THE WHO

The model list of the WHO serves as a guide for national and institutional lists and is not meant as a global list. The method of selection however, can be applied by all countries. The essential medicines concept is more than three decades old and the process of selection of drugs into this list has undergone major changes. Initially, drugs were added or deleted based on the experience of the expert members of the committee. In 2003, an evidence-based approach was used.

To add or delete a drug in the list, an application form has to be filled and submitted. This form has 15 questions and the application is made available for public comment on the WHO website on medicines. The information available is very useful for healthcare professionals, especially for pharmacists and has detailed information (including references) both in the application and the comments. An expert international committee is constituted every two years. They evaluate the evidence that is submitted before reaching a consensus, and members must declare conflicts of interest. This transparent and rigorous exercise forms the key to the acceptance of the model EML of the WHO all over the world.

What are the advantages of having an EML?

In developing countries, most deaths occur from treatable causes such as diarrhoea, pneumonia, neonatal sepsis, and so on. If the medicines needed to treat these conditions were available in the health facilities at an affordable price, in sufficient quantity and in good quality, and reached those who needed them, then a large proportion of these deaths would be prevented.

Having a limited list also makes procurement easier. If there are too many medicines, procuring the correct formulation in appropriate quantities becomes difficult. Also, storage becomes unmanageable. Keeping track of a smaller number of medicines and preventing stock-outs becomes easier. If the public health facilities are spread over a large geographical area, transporting a smaller number of medicines in the required quantities is easier.

The question of assuring good quality is also linked to having a limited list, since testing the quality will be cheaper.

The most important advantage is to the doctors who prescribe the medicines and to the pharmacists who dispense them. With a restricted list, doctors and pharmacists can acquire an in-depth knowledge of the clinical pharmacology of the drugs and make sure that they are used appropriately. Pharmacists can counsel patients on the optimal use of the medicine. Studies have repeatedly shown that a prescriber uses a maximum of only about 50 drugs whether they be prescribers at primary healthcare level or hospital doctors, including consultants. If most of these drugs come from the EML and are therefore familiar to prescribers, it increases the efficiency of the healthcare system.

Since all the medicines listed in the Standard Treatment Guidelines (STGs) and national health programmes will be listed in the EML, patients will be treated according to accepted guidelines.

What are the disadvantages and controversies of having an EML?

It is difficult to see any disadvantage in a carefully selected list based on transparent criteria; the objections are based on criteria other than health. However, the EML is often perceived as a list for the poor, though it is not. Doctors may resent having to prescribe from the list and believe that their right to prescribe whatever they want is taken away. Ironically, doctors in low- and middle-income countries may have the freedom to prescribe what they want, from the medicines available in the country. However, doctors in high-income countries do not have this freedom and must prescribe from the list that has been approved by their healthcare system. The British National Formulary shows that only five benzodiazepines are available in the National Health Service in the UK, whereas many more are registered. The high income countries have adopted the principles of the Essential Medicines Concept as enthusiastically as the low and middle-income countries, though the lists themselves have other names.

Finally, the pharmaceutical industry has a strong commercial interest in having many medicines in the market. The industry obviously does not like limited lists, especially those based on transparent criteria. Hence, there has been persistent opposition from the very beginning to this concept. This is a classic example of the irreconcilable role of health and commerce in medicine.

HOW MANY LISTS DO WE NEED?

Since the EML reflects the healthcare needs of a population in a country, one national list is prepared. In countries with large and diverse populations such as India, there might be State Lists but generally there is one National List. However the countries usually indicate in these National Lists which medicine will be available at what level (primary, secondary and tertiary).

What Is Meant by the Rational Use of Drugs?

In 1985, the WHO conference of experts in Nairobi defined the rational use of drugs as one that 'requires that patients receive medications appropriate to their clinical needs, in doses that meet their own individual requirements for an adequate period of time, and at the lowest cost to them and to their community'. This means that the correct drug is chosen based on the efficacy, safety, suitability and cost for the appropriate indication, and that the drug is correctly dispensed in the most suitable dosage formulation with appropriate information that the patient can understand and that the patient adheres to the treatment. Medicine use is termed irrational when one or more of these conditions are not met.

WHAT ARE THE COMMON TYPES OF IRRATIONAL USE?

- Polypharmacy: The use of too many medicines in a single patient
- Inappropriate use of antibiotics, often in inadequate dosage (either strength or duration of treatment) or the use of antibiotics for non-bacterial infections like viral infections
- Over-use of injections when the oral route would be more appropriate
- Inappropriate self-medication, mostly with prescription-only drugs
- Failure to prescribe in accordance with STGs

WHY IS IRRATIONAL USE OF MEDICINES A PROBLEM?

It has been estimated that more than half the medicines used worldwide are prescribed, dispensed or sold inappropriately and that more than half of the patients do not take their medicines as prescribed by the doctor. Therefore, the irrational use of medicines is a very serious global public health problem costing countries and patients a large amount of money. It leads to an increase in adverse drug reactions, widespread antibiotic resistance, failure of treatment causing people to lose faith in the healthcare system and wastage of meagre resources. Irrational over-use of medicines can also stimulate inappropriate patient demand, leading to reduced access, poor patient attendance and frequent stock-outs.

The natural history of an illness also makes it difficult at times to separate the cause and effect, thus leading to irrational use. A person with a cold (which does not need antibiotics and resolves spontaneously in a few days) may take an antibiotic on the second day and be 'cured' on the fourth and think of the antibiotic-induced diarrhoea on the third day as a part of the illness.

There is also pseudo-logic in some decisions – a fever represents infections and therefore antibiotics should be taken. However, most community-acquired infections are viral and do not respond to antibiotics. Another belief is that antibiotics 'should' be taken to prevent secondary infections after a cold. All clinical trials of antibiotics in colds to prevent secondary infections have shown no such preventive effect.

Pharmaceutical advertising also plays a huge role in promoting irrational use and is a very effective driver of increased (mostly irrational) use of medicines. The ostensible goal of advertising medicines to prescribers is to provide information about the product and not to stimulate demand. This is very different from advertising for consumer products (for example, mobile phones) where the objective is to create demand. The number of patients with pneumonia (and, therefore, the medicines for it) will not increase because amoxicillin is advertised! However, pharmaceutical advertising rarely follows the principle of providing information and is about creating demand; a cursory glance at any medicine advertisement in a medical/pharmacy journal will demonstrate this. The unethical promotion of medicines (not limited to advertising) is a major factor in the epidemic of irrational use.

Prescribers often think that they are not influenced by advertising; however, they will give you many examples where their colleagues are influenced. However, this is a delusion, as a simple examination of their prescribing habits will show examples of irrational use brought about by promotion.

The unnecessary use of injections when the oral route is sufficient increases costs. This is because injections cost more than the oral formulation (for a given medicine). The cost of the needle and syringe and at times the fee that has to be given to the person injecting the medicine also add to the costs. Unsterile injections are known to lead to the spread of blood-borne infections like Hepatitis B and C and also HIV/AIDS, besides occasionally causing injection abscesses.

The preparation of STGs and their use at all levels of healthcare is one of the major policy decisions that can improve the rational use of drugs. By adhering to STGs and prescribing only the generic drugs listed in the EML, the cost of treatment can be reduced. While this can be implemented in government healthcare systems, it is impossible to implement in the private sector, which is where the majority of healthcare takes place in India. Implementation of STGs leads to a conflict of interest for the doctor and the pharmacist, who may gain financially only if expensive, unnecessary, branded drugs are prescribed.

How can rational drug use be monitored?

Aggregate medicine consumption data: This can be used to compare actual consumption against expected consumption (based on morbidity data). It is also used to determine whether costlier medicines of lower efficacy are being used for treatment. When done in a hospital, and consumption between wards is compared and made public, it can bring about decreased consumption and promote rational use remarkably quickly and effectively.

WHO drug use indicators: These are used to describe the prescribing pattern and the quality of care at primary healthcare facilities (Table 8.1).

Table 8.1 Selected WHO/INRUD* drug use indicators for primary healthcare facilities (WHO, 1993)

Prescribing Indicators:
Average number of medicines prescribed per patient encounter
% of medicines prescribed by generic name
% of encounters with an antibiotic prescribed
% of encounters with an injection prescribed
% of medicines prescribed from essential medicines list or formulary
Patient Care Indicators:
Average consultation time
Average dispensing time
% of medicines actually dispensed
% of medicines adequately labelled
% of patients with knowledge of correct doses
Facility Indicators:
Availability of essential medicines list or formulary to practitioners
Availability of clinical guidelines
% of key medicines available
Complementary Drug Use Indicators:
Average medicine cost per encounter
% of prescriptions in accordance with clinical guidelines

*International Network for the Rational Use of Drugs

(Source: How to investigate drug use in health facilities. 1993. Selected drug use indicators. *World Health Organization*, Geneva.)

The Anatomical Therapeutic Chemical (ATC) classification and defined daily dose (DDD) methodology: This is used to compare drug consumption patterns across institutions, regions and countries.

Drug utilisation review or focused drug use evaluation: This is useful especially in hospitals where the use of specific medicines or the treatment of specific diseases need to be documented for identifying problems associated with them.

Qualitative methods: Methods such as in-depth interviews, structured questionnaires or focus group discussions can be used to identify the causes of irrational drug use.

HOW CAN THE USE OF MEDICINES BE IMPROVED?

Even though a large amount of money is spent on procuring medicines, very little is spent on improving their use. More interventions to promote rational use, assessment of these interventions and frequent monitoring are all needed to sustain the rational use of medicines.

The following strategies can be used to improve the use of medicines:

- **Managerial**: This is done by supervising and guiding clinical practice. Doctors are persuaded to use STGs and prescribe medicines listed in the EML. Prescription audits can be used to obtain feedback on prescribing behaviour.
- **Economic**: Offering incentives to institutions, patients and providers. Many insurance agencies and some governments reimburse only if medicines are chosen from a restricted list. Once health insurance/managed care becomes a major factor,

pharmaceutical companies compete to get their products on the list by offering attractive prices.

- **Regulatory**: By restricting the choice of what can be prescribed by whom. There is a law that allopathic medicine cannot be prescribed by doctors belonging to other systems of medicines and vice versa. Licensing of doctors and pharmacists, scheduling of drugs and banning unsafe medicines are also examples of regulatory approaches. An important goal is the regulation of pharmaceutical promotion. Currently, there is very little (or no) regulation of promotion in India, which is a serious lacuna.
- **Educational**: Health providers can be persuaded to improve the use of medicines by regular educational and training sessions, use of formularies and clinical supervision. Patients should receive counselling from pharmacists. However, education by itself often has only a small effect unless it is accompanied by monitoring and feedback and ensuring compliance.

All of this requires funding which becomes a serious hurdle; however, if a small percentage of the medicines budget itself is used for this, the problem of funding can be solved. If 1% of the budget is used for these measures, it is likely to result in far more savings.

What are the National Strategies to Promote the Rational Use of Medicines?

Promoting the rational use of medicines requires medicines, trained healthcare professionals and money. The WHO recommends that the following strategies be undertaken at the national level (Table 8.2):

- Establish a mandated national body to co-ordinate medicine policies and to monitor them
- Prepare and use evidence-based clinical guidelines or STGs for training and clinical decision-making

Table 8.2 Core interventions to promote rational use of medicines at a national level

• A mandated multi-disciplinary national body to co-ordinate medicine use policies
• Clinical guidelines
• EML based on treatment of choice
• Drug and Therapeutics Committees in districts and hospitals
• Problem-based pharmacotherapy training in undergraduate curricula
• Continuing in-service medical education as a licensure requirement
• Supervision, audit and feedback
• Independent information on medicines
• Public education about medicines
• Avoidance of perverse financial incentives
• Appropriate and enforced regulation
• Sufficient government expenditure to ensure availability of medicines and staff

(*Source:* Promoting the rational use of medicines: Core components. 2002. WHO Policy Perspectives on Medicines, No.5. *World Health Organization*, Geneva. Available at: http://apps.who.int/medicinedocs/pdf/h3011e/h3011e.pdf)

- Prepare an EML based on the treatment of choice and use it for procurement and insurance reimbursement purposes
- Set up a Drug and Therapeutics Committee (DTC) at institutional and district levels
- Introduce and promote problem-based pharmacotherapy training in undergraduate medical courses

- Make continuing medical education a mandatory requirement for licensing to practice medicine
- Provide and promote the use of independent, unbiased drug information such as formularies and bulletins to healthcare providers
- Encourage the supervision of prescribing, drug audit and feedback based on audit results in healthcare facilities
- Educate the public about medicines
- Eliminate perverse financial incentives that would lead to irrational prescribing
- Enforce appropriate drug regulations and ensure that drug promotional activities are in keeping with the WHO ethical criteria
- Ensure adequate government spending for equitable availability of medicines and health providers

WHAT ARE STANDARD TREATMENT GUIDELINES (STGS)?

STGs are defined as a systematically developed statement designed to assist practitioners and patients in making decisions about appropriate healthcare for specific clinical circumstances.

They are clinical treatment protocols for a particular disease/condition prepared using the best available scientific evidence by a group of experts, which help health providers make decisions regarding the treatment of that condition. They list the preferred drug and non-drug treatments for common health problems. These are formulated taking into account the demographic, epidemiological, cultural and socioeconomic factors of the disease as well as the availability of medicines, storage facilities and professional expertise needed for treatment. Therefore, STGs can be prepared for different levels of healthcare providers.

STGs are one approach to promote therapeutically effective and economically efficient prescribing and have been proven to improve the rational use of medicines, provided:

- they have been formulated using a participatory approach including clinical decision-makers and end users from the country/region/healthcare setting
- they are easy to follow and read
- they are officially introduced with proper training and wide dissemination accompanying the launch – it is also necessary to ensure sufficient copies are printed and distributed to all who will be using them
- audit and feedback are a part of the use of STGs

WHAT ARE THE ADVANTAGES OF STGS?

The advantages of STGs are listed below:

- **To the patient**: STGs enable the patient to receive therapeutically effective treatments chosen based on the best available evidence. There is greater consistency of care.
- **To healthcare providers**: STGs provide expert consensus and quality of care standards and can form the basis for monitoring the care provided. They may also improve patient adherence.
- **To supply managers**: STGs make the demand for medicines and other medical equipment more predictable,

and allow time for ordering or preparing pre-packs.

- **To policy makers**: They provide a focus for the therapeutic integration of special programmes and promote the efficient use of funds by lowering the cost of treatment.

However, unless STGs are regularly updated, they will not be viewed favourably and be used by prescribers. Hence, adequate funds should be set aside for the formulation of guidelines, printing them, training users and auditing their use and disseminating the feedback.

What is a Drug and Therapeutics Committee (DTC)?

DTCs are also known as Medicine and Therapeutics Committees or Pharmacy and Therapeutics Committees. These are committees formed by an institution or hospital to facilitate the rational use of medicines by providing support to healthcare providers and hospital administrators. The DTC should comprise clinicians from different specialties, pharmacists and a representative of hospital administration. The responsibilities of a DTC are:

- Developing, adapting or adopting clinical guidelines for the health institution or district
- Selecting cost-effective and safe medicines (hospital/district drug formulary)
- Implementing and evaluating strategies to improve medicine use (including drug use evaluation, and liaison with antibiotic and infection control committees)
- Providing on-going staff education (training and printed materials)
- Controlling access to staff by the pharmaceutical industry with its promotional activities
- Monitoring and taking action to prevent adverse drug reactions and medication errors
- Providing advice about other drug management issues such as quality and expenditure

How can a pharmacist contribute towards promoting the rational use of drugs?

Pharmacists play a vital role in the promotion of the rational use of medicines. From the provision of pharmaceutical care and unbiased drug information to the selection, procurement and dispensing of essential medicines, the pharmacist is in a position to make a major difference to the manner in which medicines are prescribed. However, the full potential of pharmacists can only be realised within a well-regulated, rule-based healthcare system. Until then, it will be the efforts and commitment of individual pharmacists that will contribute to rational drug use (RDU). A brief description of the activities in which pharmacists play an important role is given below:

Member of the Drug and Therapeutics Committee: The input given by a pharmacist during the selection of essential medicines, preparation and implementation of the EML and in all other activities is vital.

Drug procurement: The pharmacist is involved in the procurement process and can ensure that only good-quality medicines are procured at reasonable cost. Since drug procurement is based on proper inventory control and forecasting, pharmacists should be well-versed in these modern methods. They should make sure that only those medicines listed in the EML are procured and that they are bought from reliable pharmaceutical suppliers, are of good quality and are delivered on time.

Drug storage: The pharmacist should be capable of indenting, receiving and storing medicines for the health facility. Good storage practices should be followed and prevention of stock-outs of essential medicines or undue pile-ups of medicines leading to their expiry should be prevented. Procurement or indenting should be made based on actual needs. Standard operating guidelines to deal with expired medicines, narcotic drugs and costly medicines should be in place and strictly followed.

Dispensing: One of the most important activities undertaken by the pharmacist is the dispensing of medicines. In large hospitals, pharmacists dispense to both inpatients and outpatients. If a restricted list is in place, the chances of error in dispensing medicines are limited. It is also important that pharmacists are vigilant and ensure that drugs are not pilfered. Careful accounting and checks should be done to prevent this.

Patient education: Counselling of patients and giving them proper advice on the optimal use of medicines is one of the key activities of a pharmacist. Patient adherence in chronic diseases can be improved by the pharmacist providing both verbal and written information.

Pharmacovigilance: The monitoring and reporting of adverse effects is a major responsibility of pharmacists. They should be familiar with the monitoring forms and methods of reporting and should be actively engaged in all pharmacovigilance activities.

Drug information service: Pharmacists can provide information to prescribers, patients, the general public and other healthcare workers. Unbiased up-to-date drug information is part of the rational use of medicines, and the knowledge and skills of pharmacists are ideally suited to providing this service.

Pharmaceutical care: One of the more recent definitions of pharmaceutical care is 'a patient-centered practice in which the pharmacist assumes responsibility for a patient's drug related needs and is held accountable for this commitment'. This concept was started in the early 1990s in the United States of America, and focuses on the responsibility of the pharmacist to meet all of the patient's medicine-related needs. The pharmacist is responsible for helping the patient achieve his/her health goals by collaborating with other healthcare providers. It has been shown that pharmaceutical care activities improve the rational use of medicines.

The pharmacist must also inform the prescribers if any change in medication or a dosage modification is required. In many hospitals in the developed countries, the selection of appropriate antibiotics is done in collaboration with a pharmacist. However, there are many barriers to this concept, mainly from the medical profession who see it as a threat to their right to prescribe.

Some of these activities have a routine component which can be assisted by computer systems. Increasing use of computers in the management of medicines will be both cost-effective and increase the job satisfaction of pharmacists.

The Indian Scenario

The Central Government spends around 12% of the total health budget on drugs. The amount spent by the different states varies from 2% (Punjab) to 17% (Kerala). In many households belonging to the economically weaker sections of society, a large part of household expenses goes towards medicines. Low government investment in health coupled with the high cost of medicines often leads to non-availability of essential medicines at primary healthcare facilities. The lack of trained and motivated staff, incorrect prediction (and, therefore, inappropriate procurement) of the quantity and type of medicines needed, poor storage conditions coupled with problems such as corruption, lack of transparency and lack of accountability have contributed to the rather gloomy picture in the country.

In 1994, Delhi took the lead to develop a comprehensive drug policy with the main objective of improving the availability and accessibility of essential medicines. A list of essential medicines for Delhi was prepared and pooled procurement of medicines was initiated in Delhi State in 1996. The Tamil Nadu Medical Services Corporation (TNMSC) was also established in 1994 by the state government with a mandate to procure, store, distribute and dispense good-quality essential medicines to people accessing all levels of healthcare. To this day, TNMSC stands as an example of the advantages of the essential medicines concept when it is implemented in word and spirit.

Many states in India have prepared EMLs and have updated them. The first national EDL was brought out in 1996 and was last updated in 2003. It is slated to be revised shortly. Though the implementation of the EML in India leaves much to be desired, there is growing awareness and demand for the need to put in place the necessary infrastructure and technical personnel to successfully promote this concept.

Given that 80% of healthcare occurs in the private sector and that both health and medicines are very imperfect markets (World Bank reports), there are enormous inefficiencies, the cost of which is borne by the people of India. When there is an imperfect market in medicines, it has been said that 'If the one who decides (the prescribers) does not pay and the one who pays (the patient/consumer) does not decide, then can health be served?'

A managed healthcare system would ensure cost-effective care and benefit both the patient and the community, as well as provide a reasonable return to the commercial interests in the system. Given the current knowledge of healthcare systems in the world, it is likely that factors outside medicine use (such as health insurance) will play a bigger part in improving the use of medicines.

Pharmacists in India working in pharmacies and hospitals will therefore see major changes in their role in the healthcare system. Promoting the rational use of medicines could and should become an important part of their duties.

EXERCISE 1

List the essential medicines (generic name, formulation and strength) that will be required to be stocked in a primary health centre (PHC). The centre has erratic power supply and no facilities to store medicines in the refrigerator. The following is the mean percentage of cases seen at the PHC in the last year.

Diagnosis/Condition	***Percentage***
Abdominal pain	04
Anaemia	03
Asthmatic bronchitis	02
Bacillary dysentery	04
Cough/Cold	13
Cuts/Wounds	10
Diabetes	03
Diarrhoea	10
Epilepsy/Seizures	04
Fever	09
Gastritis	08
Headache	07
Hypertension	05
Insecticide poisoning	02
Muscle/Joint pain	08
Snake bite	04
Weakness	04

Compare your EML with that of others. Keep the number of medicines on your list to the minimum.

EXERCISE 2

Discuss various measures and specific activities that can be undertaken at (a) national level, (b) institutional level (tertiary care) and (c) community level to improve and promote the rational use of drugs. Discuss the merits and limitations of each activity with your group.

KEY MESSAGES

- Essential medicines are those that satisfy the priority healthcare needs of the population.
- Essential medicines should be available at all times in the health facilities in adequate quantities in appropriate dosage forms, with assured quality, accompanied by appropriate information and at a price the individual and community can afford.
- Standard Treatment Guidelines (STGs) promote therapeutically effective and economically efficient prescribing.
- Pharmacists play a vital role in the promotion of the rational use of medicines.
- The concept of pharmaceutical care focuses on the responsibility of the pharmacist to meet all of the patient's medicine-related needs.

Further Reading

Application form containing information to be included with an application for inclusion, change or deletion of a medicine in the WHO Model List of Essential Medicines. Available at: http://www.who.int/selection_medicines/committees/expert/17/application/EML17_AppForm.pdf

Chetley A, Hardon A, Hodgkin C, Haaland A and Fresle D. 2007. How to improve the use of medicines by consumers. *World Health Organization*, Geneva. Available at: http://www.who.int/medicinedocs/index/assoc/s14229e/s14229e.pdf

Fresle D, Hardon A and Hodgkin C. 2003. How to investigate the use of medicines by consumers. *World Health Organization*, Geneva. Available at: http://www.who.int/medicinedocs/en/d/Js6169e/#Js6169e

Green T and Holloway K. 2003. Drug and therapeutics committees – A practical guide. *World Health Organization*, Geneva. Available at: http://www.who.int/medicinedocs/en/d/Js4882e/#Js4882e

How to investigate drug use in health facilities. 1993. Selected indicators. EDM Research Series No. 7. *World Health Organization*, Geneva. Available at: http://www.who.int/medicinedocs/en/d/Js2289e/#Js2289e

Medicines use in primary care in developing and transitional countries: Fact book summarizing results from studies reported between 1990 and 2006. 2009. *World Health Organization*, Geneva. Available at: http://www.who.int/medicines/publications/primary_care_8April09.pdf

Promoting rational use of medicines: Core components. 2002. WHO Policy Perspectives on Medicines, No.5. *World Health Organization,* Geneva. Available at: http://apps.who.int/medicinedocs/pdf/h3011e/h3011e.pdf

The rational use of drugs. 1985. Report of the Conference of Experts. *World Health Organization*, Geneva.

WHO Ethical criteria for medicinal drug promotion. 1988. *World Health Organization*, Geneva. Available at: http://www.who.int/medicinedocs/collect/edmweb/pdf/whozip08e/whozip08e.pdf

9

ADVERSE DRUG REACTIONS AND PHARMACOVIGILANCE

Sten Olsson and G Parthasarathi

Learning Objectives

Upon completion of this chapter, the reader should be able to:

- Understand the classification of adverse drug reactions (ADRs)
- Describe the mechanisms of type A and type B adverse drug reactions
- Identify and interrelate the predisposing factors of ADRs
- Establish the causality relationship between a suspected drug and a reaction
- Document and communicate reported adverse drug reactions
- Monitor patients who are at high risk of developing an ADR
- Assist healthcare professionals in preventing and managing ADRs
- Understand the role of pharmacists in detecting, assessing and managing ADRs

Medicinal substances are used because of their ability to affect biological processes in the body. Using such substances always carries a certain risk of unwanted or unintended effects. The readiness of the patient and healthcare provider to use a medication depends on the extent of the expected benefit of the remedy balanced by the magnitude of the risk and seriousness of possible unwanted effects. The patient and his/her doctor also need to assess this risk in relation to how incapacitating, serious and durable the ailment to be treated is. Accordingly, patients and health professionals who advice patients need to know as precisely as possible the frequency and magnitude of the risks involved in medical treatment, as well as the magnitude and duration of the expected beneficial effects.

Every occasion that a patient is exposed to a new medicinal product is a unique situation, and we can never be certain exactly what will happen. However, we can learn from previous experience when patients under similar conditions have been exposed to the same or a similar medicine.

During the development phase of new medicines, both beneficial and unwanted effects are recorded in clinical trials. In this way, knowledge is accumulated which allows health professionals to make a reasoned prediction of the benefits and harm to all patients taking the medicine. Observation and recording of treatment outcomes should never stop. By observing the positive as well as negative effects of medicines as they are routinely used, and by reporting our observations to colleagues and specific monitoring centres, we can contribute to better knowledge and better medical treatment of future patients.

This is part of the professional duty of every healthcare professional. Pharmacovigilance is, according to the WHO, the science and activities relating to the detection, assessment, understanding and prevention of adverse effects and other possible drug-related problems.

Definition and Classification

The WHO defines an adverse drug reaction (ADR) as 'any response to a drug which is noxious and unintended, and which occurs at doses normally used in man for prophylaxis, diagnosis or therapy of disease, or for the modification of physiological function'. Thus, this definition excludes overdose (accidental or intentional), drug abuse, treatment failure and drug administration errors.

Often, the terms 'adverse drug reaction' and 'adverse drug event' are used synonymously, although they are not. An adverse drug event (ADE) is a broader term and includes 'any untoward medical occurrence presenting during the administration of a drug'. Thus, an ADR can also be considered as an ADE, but not all ADEs are ADRs.

Traditionally, ADRs are classified into two categories: type A and type B reactions. Type A (augmented) reactions are usually the exacerbation of the pharmacological effects of a drug and are thus dose-dependent. An example is insulin-induced hypoglycemia. These reactions are usually predictable due to the known pharmacology of a drug and are thus preventable. Although the incidence of type A reactions is high, they are generally associated with less morbidity and mortality. Because of their high incidence, the public health impact is large.

In contrast, type B (bizarre) reactions are hypersensitivity reactions and are not dose-dependent. An example is a penicillin-induced hypersensitivity reaction. These reactions are often not predictable and preventable in the individual case (unless the patient has a known history of this type of reaction). This type is associated with high morbidity and mortality but its occurrence in the clinical setting is low.

Recently, newer classifications have been proposed. One of these includes, in addition to type A (augmented) and type B (bizarre), a type C (continuous) and a type D (delayed effects). Type C reactions are diseases that occur at a higher frequency among exposed patients than those unexposed, although the exact mechanism is unknown. One example is the higher frequency of cardiovascular events among patients exposed to the COX-2 inhibitor rofecoxib compared with an unexposed control group.

Epidemiology of ADRs

The frequency of adverse drug reactions and other drug-related problems in society is not known. Many studies have been carried out in several parts of the world on the incidence in hospitalised patients and of hospital admissions that result from adverse reactions and other drug-related problems. In a recent analysis of 25 different studies of admissions to internal medicine departments, 4.2–6.0% of admissions were due to adverse reactions, with a median of 5.8%. A much-cited study from the USA demonstrated that the incidence of serious adverse drug reactions among hospitalised patients was 6.7%, and in 0.3% the outcome was fatal. This makes ADRs between the 4th and 6th leading causes of death in the USA.

A detailed study from the UK showed that 6.5% of hospital admissions were related to ADRs. These patients accounted for 4% of the hospital bed capacity. Approximately 70% of the reactions were considered avoidable. The most commonly implicated medicines were widely used ones like NSAIDs, diuretics, warfarin and ACE inhibitors. A similar study in 2007 carried out in Mumbai, India, demonstrated that 6.9% of hospital admissions were caused by ADRs, 60% deemed avoidable. The average hospital cost was calculated to be Rs 6197 (US$150/patient). Although the overall incidence of ADRs was similar to the UK study, the most commonly suspected medicines were different: anti-tuberculosis drugs, anti-epileptics, anti-malarials and anti-coagulants.

In an older Indian study, Malhotra et al. (2001) assessed 4764 consecutive visits to the medical emergency department at the Postgraduate Institute for Medical Education and Research, Chandigarh for adverse drug events. They reported that 5.9% of all such visits were deemed to be drug-related. Adverse drug reactions accounted for 45% of events.

Many studies are being reported from different parts of the world, most of them from industrialised countries. Knowledge is accumulating to demonstrate that ADRs are a considerable burden to society both financially and in terms of human suffering.

Predisposing Factors

Many factors can predispose a patient to the occurrence of ADRs. Patients who have one or more of the following predisposing factors are at high risk of developing an ADR:

- **Polypharmacy**: Patients on multiple drug therapy are more prone to develop an ADR either due to alteration of drug effect through an interaction mechanism or by synergistic effect. The amount of risk associated with multiple drug therapy increases with an increase in the number of drugs administered.
- **Multiple and intercurrent diseases**: Patients with multiple diseases are at increased risk of developing an ADR due to multiple drug use for their diseases. Similarly, patients with impaired hepatic or renal status are also at high risk of developing an ADR to drugs which are eliminated by these organs. For example, a patient with decreased renal function who is treated with aminoglycosides is at increased risk of developing nephrotoxicity unless appropriate dose adjustments are made.

- **Age**: Elderly and paediatric patients are more vulnerable to ADRs. Elderly patients are more susceptible to ADRs due to the physiological changes (pharmacokinetic and pharmacodynamic) which accompany ageing, and also because they often take many drugs for chronic and multiple diseases. Nitrate or an angiotensin converting enzyme inhibitor–induced postural hypotension in an elderly patient is an example, where the reaction may be exacerbated by age-related impaired baroreceptor response to a change in posture. Paediatric patients may develop serious ADRs to some drugs since all children, especially neonates, differ in their drug handling capacity compared to adults. An example of such a serious reaction is the grey baby syndrome with chloramphenicol.
- **Drug characteristics**: Some drugs are highly toxic in nature and patients who are treated with these agents are at an increased risk of ADRs. For example, nausea and vomiting is a common ADR seen in patients treated with cytotoxic anti-cancer drugs. Also, patients who are treated with drugs which have a narrow therapeutic range such as digoxin and gentamicin are more susceptible, as a slight increase in the serum concentration of these drugs may result in toxicity.
- **Gender**: Women are reported to be more susceptible to ADRs than men, for a number of reasons: physiological, pharmacokinetic, pharmacodynamic and hormonal. Chloramphenicol-induced aplastic anaemia and phenylbutazone-induced agranulocytosis are twice and thrice as common in women as in men, respectively.
- **Race and genetic factors**: It is evident that ADRs are more common in genetically predisposed individuals. For example, patients who are deficient in glucose-6-phosphate dehydrogenase (G6PD) are at higher risk of developing haemolysis due to primaquine than those who are not. Race and genetic polymorphism may account for alterations in handling of drugs and their end organ effects.

Mechanisms of Type A ADRs

A drug suspected to have caused an ADR in one patient may not necessarily cause a similar adverse reaction in another patient. This is due to inter-individual variability, which may predispose an individual to an ADR. Any type A reaction, which occurs in an individual, may be attributed to any one or more of the following mechanisms:

Pharmaceutical causes: The possible pharmaceutical causes which may be attributed to the occurrence of a type A ADR include changes in the drug quantity present in a particular product and changes in its drug release properties. A classic example concerns two brands of the poorly soluble anti-fungal agent griseofulvin having widely different particle size in the final dosage form. By switching patients stabilised on the brand with bigger particle sizes to the brand with the smaller size, the peak concentration of griseofulvin increased dramatically, leading to toxicity. Another example of a formulation factor being important for the risk of adverse reaction is doxycycline. Brands containing the hydrochloride salt have been associated with high frequency of oesophageal stricture and ulcers in patients lying down or who do not take the medicine with an adequate amount of water. The problem was avoided when the manufacturer introduced a formulation containing doxycycline carragenate resin instead of the corrosive hydrochloride.

Pharmacokinetic causes: Alterations in the absorption, distribution, metabolism and elimination of drugs may alter drug effects by changing the concentration of drug present at the site of action. The change in drug effect due to alterations in pharmacokinetic parameters may be experienced as therapeutic failure or as toxicity.

Absorption: Alterations in the rate and extent of drug absorption may result in adverse drug effects. The plasma concentration of a drug is partly determined by the rate at which the drug is absorbed after ingestion or injection. The plasma concentration of an orally administered drug in turn depends greatly on the gastric emptying rate. Similarly, the extent of drug absorption (the total amount of drug reaching general circulation) also plays an important role in altered response.

Following oral administration, many factors may influence the extent of drug absorption including drug formulation, gastrointestinal motility, first-pass metabolism, concomitant administration of other drugs and the absorptive capacity of gastrointestinal mucosa. Any alteration in the rate or extent of drug absorption may result in either therapeutic failure or toxicity.

Distribution: Several factors determine the extent of distribution of a drug, including regional blood flow, membrane permeability and protein/tissue binding. Changes in drug distribution may predispose to ADRs, although the clinical significance of such mechanisms is yet to be proved.

Metabolism: The drug handling capacity of an individual can greatly affect the drug effect. In an individual who has a reduced metabolic rate, accumulation of the drug in the body may be higher leading to increased risk of ADRs (especially type A reactions), while therapeutic failure may occur in an individual who has an enhanced metabolic rate. These changes are due to inter-individual variations in drug metabolising capacity, which in turn is greatly influenced by genetic, environmental and other factors.

For example, the oxidising enzyme, CYP3A4, responsible for the metabolism of a great variety of medicines (like nifedipine, erythromycin and cyclosporine) shows a genetically determined ten-fold difference in activity between individuals. This enzyme is irreversibly inhibited by grapefruit juice. Drinking a glass of grapefruit juice will dramatically increase the bioavailability of medicines metabolised by CYP3A4.

Elimination: The main routes of excretion for many drugs are the kidneys (excretion through urine) and liver (yields metabolites which are then excreted by the kidneys). One of the most important causes of type A ADRs is a change in the drug elimination rate. Drug accumulation due to reduced elimination may predispose to ADRs as a result of increased drug concentration in plasma and tissue. Conversely, reduced concentration of the drug in plasma and tissue due to enhanced drug elimination may lead to therapeutic failure.

Pharmacodynamic causes: Increased sensitivity of target tissues or organs may predispose a person to ADRs. Although the reasons why different individuals react differently to drugs are still not clear, evidence is accumulating to suggest that target tissue or organ sensitivity is influenced by the drug receptors themselves, by homeostatic mechanisms and by disease.

Drug receptors: Most drugs elicit their response by combining with receptors. These receptors are either protein molecules or enzymes. The amount and sensitivity of receptors of one individual may differ from those of another individual. Some individuals may have fewer specific drug receptors while others may have a higher number of less active receptors. This inter-variability between different individuals can greatly affect the drug effect when the drug acts through these specific receptors.

Homeostatic mechanisms: Many physiological factors may determine the extent of a drug's effect in an individual as drug effects occur within the environment of the body's physiological mechanisms. For example, intravenous atropine produces a variable increase in heart rate and some individuals develop tachycardia of 160 beats per minute at a dose which is almost ineffective in others. The magnitude of the observed effect is dependent on the balance between parasympathetic and sympathetic cardiac tone, which appears to be under genetic control.

Disease: The pharmacological effects of a drug which are not apparent in a healthy individual may be unmasked by intercurrent diseases. An example is an asthmatic patient who develops bronchoconstriction while taking non-selective beta blockers such as propranolol.

Mechanisms of Type B ADRs

Type B reactions are aberrant in terms of the normal pharmacology of the drug, and they are a heterogeneous group of unpredictable adverse effects. The causes of type B reactions may be pharmaceutical or pharmacokinetic, or may be determined by target tissue or organ response.

Pharmaceutical causes: The main sources for the pharmaceutical causes of type B reactions include decomposition of the active ingredient, effects of the non-drug excipients (additives, preservatives, colouring and solubilising agents) and synthetic by-products of active constituents. In most cases, the use of decomposed drug products may result in therapeutic failure. In some instances, though not all, the decomposed product may be highly toxic and lethal. Deaths have been reported due to decomposition of paraldehyde to acetaldehyde and its subsequent oxidation to acetic acid. There is clear recognition of ADRs caused by excipients. Many additives including propylene glycol and carboxymethylcellulose may cause hypersensitivity reactions. The eosinophilia–myalgia syndrome associated with L-tryptophan may be related to the use of preparations containing a contaminant, although a genetic factor may also be involved.

Many modern medicines are peptides or proteins produced in biological systems of great complexity, for example, colony stimulating factor and monoclonal antibodies. As the original products are getting old enough to lose their patent protection, competitor products, the so-called biosimilars, are entering the market. It is important to recognise that the competitor products will not be identical to the original since production conditions are inevitably different. It is well-established that patients are at risk of acquiring hypersensitivity reactions if they switch from one product to another. Patients prescribed a particular brand of a biological product should be kept on the same brand throughout their treatment.

Pharmacokinetic causes: Although changes in pharmacokinetic parameters such as absorption, distribution, metabolism and excretion may theoretically lead to type B reactions, there are no documented type B reactions that can be attributed to changes in absorption and distribution. However, the metabolism of a drug to unusual reactive metabolites may give rise to type B reactions either by a direct or by an immune-mediated mechanism. Examples of such reactions include phenacetin-induced methaemoglobinaemia and carbamazepine-induced hypersensitivity reactions. Individuals whose specific bio-inactivation pathways are either more active or less active and with immunological characteristics which render them highly responsive to immunogens/haptogens are more susceptible. However, the reasons for the occurrence of type B reactions in a particular individual are not clear.

Pharmacodynamic causes: Many factors including age, sex, body weight, medical condition and drug therapy influence the end response of a patient to an administered drug. As a result, individual patients may vary in their response to drug therapy. The qualitative differences in the target tissues or organ response to drugs may be due to genetic, immunological, neoplastic or teratogenic causes.

Genetic causes for abnormal responses: Until recently, many type B reactions were assumed to be due to some qualitative abnormality in patients and were labelled as an 'idiosyncrasy'. However, more recently, it has become clear that the mechanisms of many of these reactions may have a genetic basis. A well-known example is G6PD deficiency which affects over 100 million people worldwide. The deficiency of G6PD results in haemolysis, accompanied by a fall in haemoglobin level, fever and the formation of dark urine. It is postulated that deficiency of G6PD results in a corresponding deficiency in reduced glutathione, and under these conditions oxidising agents may denature the intracellular proteins including the globin part of haemoglobin.

Several drugs with oxidant properties are known to cause haemolysis in patients with G6PD deficiency, and these include primaquine, sulphones, sulphonamides, chloramphenicol, quinine and quinidine. Other genetically determined ADRs include methhaemoglobinemia (nitrates), porphyria (sulphonamides and barbiturates) malignant hyperthermia (halothane and suxamethonium), osteogenesis imperfecta (halothane) and familial dysautonomia (general anaesthetics and parasympathomimetics).

Immunological reasons for abnormal response: The primary cause of the most important group of qualitatively abnormal responses to drugs is immunological. If a drug is immunogenic in its own right (peptides of foreign origin such as streptokinase), the reaction is obviously a type A effect. Most allergic drug reactions are responses to immunologically mediated mechanisms. These reactions may vary from rash and serum sickness to life-threatening reactions such as anaphylaxis. Several factors (drug, patient and disease) influence the development of allergic reactions during therapy. However, patients with atopic or allergic disorders are at high risk of developing allergic drug reactions.

Some of the important features of allergic drug reactions are given below:

- Symptoms are not correlated with the known pharmacological effects of the drug
- There is usually a delay between first exposure to the drug and the development of a subsequent reaction
- If an allergy is established, very small doses of the drug may elicit the reaction
- The reaction disappears on cessation of therapy and reappears after re-exposure to the drug even with a small dose
- The illness is often recognisable and may include a rash, angioedema (angioneurotic oedema), serum sickness or anaphylaxis
- They usually occur in a very few patients receiving the drug
- There is a possibility of desensitisation

Teratological and neoplastic reasons for abnormal response: It is well known that there is a possibility that drugs can cause neoplastic or teratological changes. Also, it is important to consider the possibility of occurrence of qualitatively abnormal response to a drug in the presence of some potentially neoplastic and teratological tissues in the body. Administration of certain drugs such as oestrogen or an androgen may transform the pre-neoplastic condition into a frankly neoplastic state

Detection and Monitoring of ADRs

Pre-marketing studies: During the development of new medicines, their safety is tested in animal models. A great deal of risk information may be obtained from such tests, such as the level of acute toxicity, which organs will be affected in case of toxicity and the dose dependency of such tissue injuries.

Specific animal tests for carcinogenicity, teratogenicity and mutagenicity are also available. However, animals can only serve as approximate models for humans. We do not have sufficient knowledge to extrapolate information collected from animal studies directly into risks in humans. The predictive value of the different animal tests is in all instances uncertain. If animal tests do not reveal particularly worrying results, safety tests proceed onto testing in humans in clinical trial programmes.

Clinical trials are carried out in three different phases prior to the submission of a marketing authorisation application, with a stepwise increase in the number of individuals being exposed. Prior to the general release of a new product, not more than 4000 individuals would have normally been exposed to the new drug, often fewer. This implies that clinical trials normally only have the power to identify adverse reactions of a frequency greater that 0.5–1.0%.

Clinical trial programmes are designed to maximise the chance of demonstrating a therapeutic effect in relation to a control group. Children and the elderly are normally actively excluded from the studies. Once the drug is used in clinical practice, children, the elderly and patients with much more complicated disease situations and multiple drug exposures will be treated. For cost reasons, clinical trials often have a very short duration, which means they cannot generate information about longer term adverse effects.

The consequence of the above is that at the time of general marketing of a new medicine, only the most common, dose-related (type A) adverse reactions will be known.

Post-marketing surveillance: Since the experimental methods described above are inadequate for the identification of all drug-related risks, systems involving both passive and active pharmacovigilance methodologies have to be put in place for the detection of risks and for the collection of risk information from the healthcare system.

The most sensitive, powerful and cost-effective system for the identification of unknown drug-related risks is spontaneous adverse reaction reporting. Every healthcare practitioner should see it as a part of his/her professional duty to report any suspicion of a drug unexpectedly causing a risk situation for a patient under his/her care. Pharmacovigilance is, however, not limited to the reporting of classical adverse effects. It is also concerned with identifying product defects, intoxications and abuse and unexpected lack of therapeutic efficacy. An unexpected decrease in therapeutic effect could indicate interaction, resistance or inadequate product quality.

An important outcome of spontaneous adverse reaction reporting programmes is the creation of signals of previously unknown or insufficiently documented problems. To verify the hypothesis of a causal link between drug exposure and an adverse outcome, it may be necessary to employ epidemiological techniques. With such techniques, it is also possible to quantify the risk, which is not possible in spontaneous reporting programmes.

The two epidemiological methods that are most commonly used are cohort studies and case control studies. In cohort studies, patients exposed to a particular drug are followed up actively and systematically and adverse reaction frequencies are compared to an unexposed control population.

In case control studies, individuals affected by the adverse event being studied are identified (cases). Each case is matched with several disease-free control patients randomly recruited from the study base (controls). Both cases and controls are investigated regarding their exposure to possible causative agents prior to the occurrence of the event. The odds ratio is calculated on the basis of exposure data. Case control studies are particularly useful for the study of rare adverse reactions. For more information, see *Chapter 27, Pharmacoepidemiology*.

In the hospital set-up, healthcare professionals should be very vigilant in detecting ADRs. The possibility of an ADR should always be considered during differential diagnosis. ADRs may be detected during ward rounds with the medical team or during review of the patient's chart. Patient counselling, medication history interview and communicating with other healthcare professionals may provide additional clues, which may be useful in the detection of ADRs.

To assist the detection of ADRs, healthcare professionals should closely monitor patients who are at high risk. These include:

- Patients with renal or hepatic impairment
- Patients taking drugs which have the potential to cause ADRs, for example, those with a narrow therapeutic range
- Patients who have had previous allergic reactions
- Patients taking multiple drugs
- Pregnant and breastfeeding women

The first step in the detection of ADRs is collection of data. The data to be collected includes the patient's demographic information; presenting complaints; past medication history; drug therapy details including over-the-counter, current medications and medication on admission; and lab data such as haematological, liver and renal function tests.

Details of the suspected ADR such as time of onset and duration of reaction, nature and severity of reaction; details on the suspected drug including dose, frequency, time of administration, duration of treatment, plasma concentration of the drug; previous report on reactions; data on any other causes including risk factors and predisposing factors are useful.

All of the above can be obtained from the following sources of information:

- Patient's case notes and treatment chart
- Patient interview
- Laboratory data sources
- Communication with other healthcare professionals

Assessing causality: Causality assessment is the method by which the extent of the relationship between a drug and a suspected reaction is estimated. In eliciting a causality relationship, a temporal or possible association is sufficient for an ADR report to be made. The assessment of causality relationship is often highly subjective, based on an individual clinician's assessment. Thus, one clinician's 'possible' may be another clinician's 'unlikely'.

If an ADR is suspected, the assessment starts with collection of all the relevant data pertaining to patient demographics; medications including non-prescription drugs (OTC); comprehensive ADR details including a description of the reaction, time of onset and duration of the reaction, complications and/or sequelae; treatment of the reaction and outcome of the treatment; and relevant investigation reports. The collected data should be utilised to correlate and categorise the relationship between the suspected drug and the ADR. This can be done by using one or more causality assessment scales.

Methods for causality assessment of ADRs are classified into three groups:

- Opinion of experts, clinical judgment or global introspection methods
- Algorithms (with or without scoring) or standardised assessment methods
- Probabilistic or Bayesian approaches

In the first group, the causation is established based on the clinical judgment of the expert (clinical pharmacologist or physicians treating the patient) or panel of experts. The experts consider all the data available pertaining to the suspected ADR and express their opinion on the possibility of a drug causing the reaction. Such judgments are based on the knowledge and experience of experts. The tool developed by the WHO

Table 9.1 WHO causality assessment scale

Category	Criteria
Certain	➢ Event of laboratory test abnormality, with plausible time relationship to drug intake ➢ Cannot be explained by disease or other drugs ➢ Response to withdrawal plausible (pharmacologically, pathologically) ➢ Event definitive pharmacologically or phenomenologically (*an objective and specific medical disorder or a recognised pharmacological phenomenon*) ➢ Rechallenge (if necessary)
Unassessable/ Unclassifiable	➢ A report suggesting an adverse reaction ➢ Cannot be judged because of insufficient or contradictory information ➢ Report cannot be supplemented or verified
Probable	➢ Event or lab test abnormality, with reasonable time relationship during intake ➢ Unlikely to be attributed to disease or other drugs ➢ Response to withdrawal clinically reasonable ➢ Rechallenge not necessary
Possible	➢ Event or laboratory test abnormality, with reasonable time relationship to drug intake ➢ Could also be explained by disease or other drugs ➢ Information on drug withdrawal lacking or unclear
Unlikely	➢ Event or laboratory test abnormality with a time to drug value that makes a relationship improbable (but not impossible) ➢ Diseases or other drugs provide plausible explanations
Conditional/ Unclassified	➢ Event or laboratory test abnormality ➢ More data for proper assessment needed ➢ Additional data under examination

and the Uppsala Monitoring Centre (Table 9.1), Visual Analogue Scale method and Swedish Regulatory Agency method are examples.

Algorithms are usually in the form of a questionnaire that enables the user to gather adequate information while assessing the causal relation between the medication and the reaction. Some important algorithms include Naranjo's (Table 9.2), Karch and Lasagna's, Kramer's and the French imputation method. Most algorithms

Table 9.2 Naranjo's causality assessment scale*

	Yes	*No*	*Don't know*
1. Are there previous conclusive reports on this reaction?	–1	0	0
2. Did the adverse event appear after the suspected drug was administered?	+2	–1	0
3. Did the adverse reaction improve when the drug was discontinued or a specific antagonist was administered?	+1	0	0
4. Did the adverse drug reaction reappear when the drug was re-administered?	+2	–1	0
5. Are there alternative causes (other than the drug) that could solely have caused the reaction?	–1	2	0
6. Did the reaction re-appear when a placebo was given?	–1	+1	0
7. Was the drug detected in blood (or other fluids) in a concentration known to be toxic?	+1	0	0
8. Was the reaction more severe when the dose was increased, or less severe when the dose was decreased?	+1	0	0
9. Did the patient have a similar reaction to the same or similar drugs in any previous exposure?	+1	0	0
10. Was the adverse event confirmed by objective evidence?	+1	0	0

Definite ≥ 9; Probable 5–8; Possible 1–4; Unlikely ≤ 0

*Naranjo CA, Busto U, Sellers EM, Sandor P, Ruiz I, Roberts EA, et al. 1981. A method for estimating the probability of adverse drug reactions. *Clin Pharmacol Ther* 30 (2):239–45.

share common criteria to arrive at an objective conclusion. No single algorithm is accepted as a 'gold standard' because of the disagreements that exist between the various developed and published algorithms.

Bayesian methods involve the transformation of prior probability into a posterior probability of drug causation. The Australian method, Bayesian Adverse Reactions Diagnostic Instrument (BARDI) and MacBARDI are some methods that involve a Bayesian or probabilistic approach. A recent systematic review by Agbabiaka et al. concluded that there is still no universally accepted method for the causality assessment of ADRs.

When assessing causality, many factors need to be considered. These factors do not differ significantly between algorithms but the weight allocated to the different factors do. The common factors considered in causality assessment include:

- The temporal (time) relationship between the administration of the suspected drug and the reaction
- Dose and duration of drug treatment

- Possible alternative causes, other than the drug, for the occurrence of an ADR
- Outcome of the reaction upon cessation of drug (dechallenge)
- Outcome of the reaction upon re-introduction of drug (rechallenge)

Different scales categorise the causality relationship in different ways. For example, the WHO scale categorises the causality relationship into certain, probable, possible, unlikely, unassessable/unclassifiable and conditional/unclassified. The Naranjo scale categorises the reaction as definite, probable, possible or unlikely.

The assessment and establishment of causality relationship between suspected drugs and reactions has certain applications. These include:

- Patient treatment
- Signal generation
- Drug regulation
- Scientific publication
- Data exchange

Every suspected ADR should be assessed for its causality and documented in the patient's medical record. This serves as a useful reference to alert clinicians to the possibility of a particular drug causing a suspected reaction. Documentation should be made in the patient's medical and pharmacy records where appropriate.

Under-reporting

One of the major deficiencies of spontaneous reporting programmes is the failure of health professionals to identify and report drug-related injuries. It has been estimated that even in countries with a long tradition of adverse reaction reporting, less than 10% of drug-related unwanted events are notified to pharmacovigilance centres. The under-reporting could be compensated for if it was uniform. However, under-reporting varies with a number of factors:

- Reporting is higher for new drugs than for old
- Serious reactions are reported to a higher degree
- Type B reactions are reported more commonly than their share of events in practice
- Reporting is affected by promotional claims of the drug sponsor
- Publicity of a specific drug-related problem triggers further reporting, not necessarily related to the real frequency
- Reporting is affected by general publicity around the adverse reaction reporting scheme

The reasons given most often by health professionals for not reporting are:

- Lack of time
- Lack of knowledge on what, how or where to report
- The drug–reaction association is uncertain
- The reaction is already well known
- Guilt or fear of litigation
- Belief that all registered medicines are safe
- Non-availability of reporting forms

Managers of adverse reaction reporting programmes need to be active in order to maintain a high level of reporting and to involve all sectors of the healthcare system. Only if reporting is widespread and is maintained at a high level will the collected information give a fair representation of the actual problems that occur when medicines are used. Activities that may increase the reporting rate include:

- Ease of reporting, for example, by improving the design of reporting forms or by the use of online reporting, acknowledging the receipt of adverse reaction reports by personal letter or phone call
- Providing feedback to clinicians in the form of articles in journals, adverse reaction bulletins or newsletters
- Participation in pre-and postgraduate educational and scientific meetings
- Collaboration with local Drug and Therapeutics Committees
- Collaboration with professional associations
- The involvement of not only physicians but also pharmacists, dentists, nurses and patients in the reporting of suspected ADRs
- Integrating pharmacovigilance in public healthcare programmes

Communicating ADRs

As stated in the Introduction, it is essential that the health professional giving advice to the patient has access to information on the benefits and risks of available medicines. The present situation is, however, far from ideal. Knowledge about the benefits and risks of medicines, accumulated in reference books in medical libraries at adverse reaction monitoring centres, with pharmaceutical manufacturers or with regulatory authorities, often does not reach the users. Knowledge about the rational and safe use of medicines needs to be provided:

- During the basic training of health professionals
- Through continuous education programmes to health professionals
- By specially designated Drug Information Centres
- Through package inserts and patient counselling
- Through continuous mass media campaigns using newspapers, radio, television and the internet. This is of particular importance in countries with a high proportion of self-medication.

The messages given must be adapted to the needs of the specific target group and measures should be taken to record if the messages are received, understood and acted upon by the target audience. Resources should be set aside for the provision of unbiased information on the benefits and risks of medicines, since irrational drug use is the most frequent cause of adverse reactions. Preventing ADRs through rational use also prevents patient suffering and reduces spending in the healthcare system.

Safety Monitoring of Herbal Medicines

Traditional herbal medicines constitute a major part of the consumption of therapeutic remedies, often in combination with allopathic medicines. While ingestion of traditional medicines generally produces minimal toxicity, life-threatening events from severe intoxication may also occur. Herbal preparations are often complex mixtures of chemicals. Their composition may vary with regard to the constituents and their concentrations, depending on the part of the plant or the type of extract used, the origin of the plant, the climate or the season of harvesting. Many plants and their ingredients have not yet been chemically identified, classified and evaluated as regards their effects, toxicity and interactions. When an adverse reaction occurs, the identification of the causative factor may be difficult or impossible.

It is important that traditional medicines are also covered by the ADR reporting system. Such reporting has recently led to the identification of an interaction between *Hypericum perforatum* and allopathic medicines metabolised by the same enzyme system in the liver, market withdrawal of preparations containing *Kava-Kava* because of liver toxicity and remedies containing *Aristolochia* sp because of nephrotoxicity and carcinogenic potential.

The Problem of Counterfeit Medicines

The availability of counterfeit or fake medicines in the market has been documented in all parts of the world during the past decade. Counterfeit products normally contain nothing or very little of the active substance. They may also contain toxic ingredients. The most common outcome of the sale of counterfeit products is lack of the intended effect. This can have far-reaching consequences when contraceptive agents, vaccines or antibiotics are being counterfeited. If the fake medicine contains a toxic product, such as ethylene glycol instead of propylene glycol, serious toxicity might occur.

In 2008, the US Food and Drug Administration (FDA) received reports of clusters of acute hypersensitivity reactions in patients receiving heparin—in some cases with a fatal outcome. After a recall of heparin batches, investigation revealed widespread contamination of raw heparin imported from China with an over-sulphated form of chondroitin sulphate. This problem would not have been identified without a national pharmacovigilance system such as that provided by the FDA. Pharmacovigilance centres should also encourage the reporting of unexpected lack of therapeutic effect to identify cases of counterfeiting.

Patient safety: Pursuing the aim of pharmacovigilance, that is, preventing drug-related problems, leads to a concern not only about the safety of the pharmaceutical products themselves but also about the safety of processes in healthcare in which these products are being used. Medication errors are common and constitute an important part of avoidable medication-related problems. Information about medication errors and unsafe handling and use of medicines has become a part of pharmacovigilance. The focus is to find indications of system weakness rather than of individual mistakes. Root cause analysis of mistakes in prescribing, transcription, dispensing or administration often reveals working conditions for healthcare personnel that are unsafe for patients. Focus is shifted from medication safety to patient safety which is the ultimate aim of pharmacovigilance.

Role of pharmacists: Pharmacists with their immense knowledge of medication use can play a vital role in the detection, prevention and management of ADRs. Beyond doubt, the pharmacist's involvement in the ADR reporting system has had a positive impact. Pharmacists can assist busy medical practitioners in the better management of suspected reactions. Some of the important roles of pharmacists in the management of adverse drug reactions are presented in Table 9.3.

Table 9.3 Roles of pharmacists in the management of ADRs

Monitoring patients who are at greater risk of developing ADRs.
Monitoring patients who are prescribed with drugs highly likely to cause ADRs.
Assessing and documenting the patient's previous allergic status.
Assessing the patient's drug therapy for its appropriateness.
Assessing possible drug interactions in multiple therapies.
Assisting healthcare professionals in the detection and assessment of ADRs.
Encouraging/Stimulating healthcare professionals in reporting an ADR.
Documentation of suspected reported reactions for future reference.
Follow-up of patients to assess the outcome of the reaction and management.
Obtaining feedback about the reported reaction.
Educating healthcare professionals about the importance of reporting an ADR.
Educating patients.
Creating awareness about ADRs amongst healthcare professionals, patients and the public.
Preparation and utilisation of promotional materials.
Communication with other healthcare professionals such as nurses and community pharmacists.
Presentation of reports in meetings and conferences.
Conducting workshops/conferences/seminars on ADRs for healthcare professionals.
Dissemination of signals generated through publication of reports in bulletins or journals.

Exercise 1

A 25-year-old woman was admitted to a medicine ward complaining of 4–5 episodes of vomiting and epigastric discomfort. She had been diagnosed with type II diabetes mellitus and was receiving glimepiride (1 mg) with metformin (500 mg) once daily. Her blood glucose level was under control. On admission, she was prescribed oral pantoprazole 40 mg once daily and intravenous ondansetron 4 mg thrice daily. She continued to receive glimepiride with metformin at the same doses. Within a few minutes of receiving ondansetron, the patient developed urticaria and redness all over the body. She did not complain of pruritus. She was treated immediately with injection dexamethasone 4 mg and oral cetirizine 10 mg. The reaction abated within a few minutes.

1. What patient information pertaining to the ADR should be collected?

Collection of relevant information is the key step in ADR detection. Demographic details of the patient such as age, sex, medical and medication history including over-the-counter drugs, dosing regimen of the suspected drug, previous experience of the patient with the drug and allergy status of the patient would be useful in the detection of ADRs. In addition, information on temporal relationship, any dechallenge or rechallenge, outcome of accidental/intentional rechallenge, laboratory investigations related to the reaction and therapeutic drug monitoring (if relevant) need to be collected.

2. How do you establish the relation between the suspected drug and the reported reaction?

Collection of data*:* All the above mentioned data should be collected from various sources including patient/carer interview, medical records and laboratory reports.

Literature search: Literature search reveals many potential ADRs to ondansetron. The ADRs noted in this patient were similar to those reported in the literature:

Hypersensitivity reaction (rare), urticaria (4%), wheals, redness over the body, rash (6 %).

It is also necessary to consider the involvement of other drugs which the patient is taking. In this case, the symptoms started within a few minutes of receiving the injection. The patient had no similar experience in the past. These reactions were not suggestive of any other disease condition. The reaction subsided after receiving dexamethasone which suggests that there is an association between medication administration and the reaction.

Standard causality assessment scales are used to assess the causal relation between the suspected drug and the reported reaction. In this case, to assess the causality relationship of the suspected adverse drug reaction, Naranjo's ADR probability scale was applied. From the reactions observed and based on the available data, the reactions were probably related to the drug. Although impractical in most clinical situations, further details such as serum concentrations of ondansetron and rechallenge are needed to strengthen the causality relationship between the drug and the suspected adverse drug reactions.

3. What follow up actions do you consider in this case?

Patient education: The patient needs to be educated about the ADR and advised not to take ondansetron in the future. She should also be educated about how her symptoms can be managed further.

Alert card: The patient should be provided with an alert card as the causality relationship between the suspected drug and the reaction was probable in this case. This would help in preventing the future occurrence of similar reactions to the same drug or drugs belonging to the same class.

Education of healthcare professionals: Education of healthcare professionals may benefit both prescriber and patient in the effective management of suspected reaction in this patient.

Thank you note: Provision of a thank you note may encourage healthcare professionals not only to provide feedback on this reported reaction but also may stimulate them to report any further suspected adverse drug reactions.

Published literature: Any published case reports or any other information pertaining to this case may be produced in suitable form (printed or photocopied) and given to the reporter.

Dissemination of information: Exchange of information on reported adverse drug reactions amongst healthcare professionals may result in the cautious use of drugs causing severe and fatal reactions or drugs with high incidence rate of ADRs. Also the reported reaction may be considered for publication as a case report in a suitable medical/pharmaceutical journal.

EXERCISE 2

A 35-year-old woman was prescribed oral metronidazole 500 mg three times daily for seven days for recurrent trichomonal vaginitis. She was admitted to the dermatology ward with complaints of nausea and itchy lesions over her limbs. She had taken metronidazole on two separate occasions (45 days before hospital admission for a period of 7 days and 15 days before admission for a period of 7 days). Each time she had developed itchy lesions at the same sites. On examination, hyperpigmented macules were seen and a fixed drug eruption (FDE) was suspected. After obtaining written informed consent, topical provocation testing was performed using 0.8% metronidazole gel. It was applied to the sites of previous FDE and a positive reaction was noticed. Hydroxyzine 25 mg 4 times daily and betamethasone (0.08%) gel were prescribed. The reaction subsided within one week of treatment but the hyperpigmentation remained.

1. Could these signs and symptoms be an ADR?

Metronidazole can cause the symptoms present in the patient and an ADR should be considered in the differential diagnosis. ADRs for metronidazole occur most frequently during the two weeks of treatment. This patient developed these signs and symptoms during the first week of treatment.

2. What type of adverse drug reaction is it likely to be (type A or type B)?

The mechanism of metronidazole-induced fixed drug eruption is not dose dependent, that is, it is a type B reaction.

3. How should this patient be managed?

Fixed drug eruption is a serious ADR with low incidence. Causality relationship between adverse reaction and medication was found to be probable, according to Naranjo's scale. Patient education and provision of an alert card must be considered. The initial step that is needed to treat the fixed drug eruption is to withdraw the suspected drug and to avoid re-administering the same drug/similar class of medication. In this case, azithromycin or doxycycline can be used instead of metronidazole as the patient is experiencing recurrent trichomonal vaginitis.

4. What is the importance of rechallenge in ADR?

Rechallenge is defined as re-introduction of the suspected medication at the same dose, in the same route, frequency and dosage form. Reaction to the rechallenge is a strong indicator of causality. The temptation to use rechallenge as a diagnostic tool should be resisted unless clinically warranted and informed consent has been obtained. There must be a valid reason for the rechallenge.

KEY MESSAGES

- Adverse drug reactions (ADRs) are a significant cause of morbidity and mortality.
- They may mimic disease and should therefore be considered during differential diagnosis.
- They account for approximately 5% of all hospital admissions and occur in 10–20% of hospitalised patients.
- They increase healthcare costs and adversely affect the patients' quality of life.
- Multiple drug therapy, age and concurrent diseases are important general predisposing factors for ADRs.
- About 50% of drug-related problems in healthcare are estimated to be avoidable.
- Pharmacists can play a vital role in the detection, prevention and management of ADRs.

Further Reading

Dukes MNG and Aronson JK. 2006. *Meyler's side effects of drugs*, 15th ed. Elsevier.

Edwards IR and Aronson JK. 2000. Adverse Drug Reactions: Definition, Diagnosis and Management. *The Lancet* 356:1255–9.

Harugeri A, Parthasarathi G, Ramesh M, Sharma J and Padmini Devi D. 2008. Story of heparin recall: What India can do?. *J Postgrad Med* 54:222–4

KJ Patel, MS Kedia, D Bajpai, SS Mehta, NA Kshirsagar and NJ Gogtay. 2007. Evaluation of the prevalence and economic burden of adverse drug reactions presenting to the medical emergency department of a tertiary referral centre: a prospective study. *BMC Clinical Pharmacology* 7:8.

Lee A. 2006. *Adverse Drug Reactions*, 2nd ed. Pharmaceutical Press.

Websites of Interest

European Medicines Evaluation Agency, EMEA
http://www.ema.europa.eu/home.htm

International Society for Pharmacoepidemiology, ISPE
http://www.pharmacoepi.org

International Society of Pharmacovigilance, ISoP
http://www.isoponline.org

USA Food and Drug Administration
http://www.fda.gov/medwatch/safety.htm

WHO headquarters, Geneva
http://www.who.int

WHO Collaborating Centre for International Drug Monitoring, The Uppsala Monitoring Centre (UMC)
http://www.who-umc.org

10 DRUG INTERACTIONS

Ruth Ferguson

Learning Objectives

Upon completion of this chapter, the reader should be able to:

- Explain the mechanisms by which drugs interact
- Develop an understanding of the relative merits and shortcomings of the information sources available for identifying drug interactions
- Explain how to screen for potential interactions and to identify their clinical significance
- Explain how to provide advice for the management of drug interactions

All pharmacists working in a clinical setting, whether dispensing medicines or advice, require a well-grounded knowledge of drug interactions to prevent harm to patients from medicine combinations. This is an area in which a pharmacist's expertise is valued by other health professionals and where a pharmacist's knowledge of pharmacology can be recognised and appreciated.

Pharmacists play a valuable role in screening for interactions and advising on management when interactions occur. This may be at the patient's bedside, as part of the dispensing process or during the sale of a non-prescription medicine. Pharmacists have written many of the key texts and references on drug interactions and have documented many previously unrecognised interactions in the medical literature. A role of current and emerging importance is the detection of interactions between medicines and other pharmacologically active therapies, such as herbal and alternative remedies. Pharmacists, especially those practicing in India, are well placed to contribute significantly to the development of this knowledge.

Mechanisms for Pharmacokinetic Interactions

Drug Absorption

Important interactions that lead to the modification of drug absorption are largely associated with the gastrointestinal tract. There are, however, some interactions that have been used advantageously with parenteral formulations; for example, when the vasoconstrictor adrenaline is used to slow the absorption of a local anaesthetic to prolong analgesia. It is preferable, however, to use a long-acting molecule such as bupivacaine as this avoids exposing the patient to the risks associated with using another drug.

Interactions in the gastrointestinal tract can significantly reduce or increase the amount of a drug that is absorbed into the body. A variety of mechanisms for the modification of gastrointestinal absorption have been identified.

Chelation: Heavy metal ions such as iron, calcium, magnesium and zinc can bind anionic medicines like ciprofloxacin and tetracycline. This produces a poorly soluble salt form that does not dissolve significantly, and so the drug cannot be absorbed into the body in sufficient amounts for clinical activity. *Case Study 1* discusses a chelation type of interaction.

Ion exchange resins can also bind medicines and prevent absorption. For example, cholestyramine, an anionic resin that is used therapeutically to bind bile salts and lower serum cholesterol, can bind drugs such as thyroxine, digoxin and warfarin and reduce their absorption. Therapeutic failures have been reported with these medicines.

Changes in gastrointestinal motility: Some medicines can modify gastrointestinal (GI) motility and can thus alter the rate of passage of drugs through the GI tract. This commonly changes the rate of absorption, but there are examples where the extent of medicine absorption is affected. For example, metoclopramide increases GI motility and, more importantly for medicines absorbed under the basic conditions of the duodenum and jejunum, opens the pyloric sphincter at the stomach outlet. This will decrease the time a medicine like paracetamol takes to reach the small intestine. This will also increase the rate of absorption but not influence the amount absorbed. This is clinically important in migraine, where gastric emptying is delayed. By giving paracetamol with metoclopramide, a more rapid onset of analgesic action is achieved.

Alteration in GI motility is not usually of clinical importance for most drugs unless the drug is absorbed at one site in the GI tract (like paracetamol) or is poorly soluble, incompletely absorbed and has a low therapeutic index. Digoxin is an important example. It has a slow dissolution rate and, under normal GI conditions, about 20–30% of the tablet content will not dissolve during GI passage and is passed out in faeces. If the GI transit rate is increased, for example, by metoclopramide, then there is less time for digoxin to dissolve; therefore, less will be absorbed and therapeutic failure can occur. Drugs that slow intestinal transit, for example, anti-cholinergic agents, can increase the amount of digoxin absorbed and may precipitate toxicity.

Bowel flora effects: Some medicines can alter the normal microorganism population in the large intestines; these organisms play an important role in the kinetics and action of some drugs. Broad-spectrum antibiotics kill a wide range of bacteria and this may enable a few unsusceptible bowel bacterial species to dominate. With combined oral contraceptives (COCs), bowel bacteria cleave the conjugated metabolite of oestrogen to release free oestrogen for re-absorption into circulation. If the population of bond-cleaving bacteria is reduced, a lower quantity of oestrogen will be released, less absorbed and, especially with low oestrogen containing COCs, the levels may not be sufficient to inhibit ovulation and prevent conception.

The modification of bowel bacteria by broad-spectrum antibiotics can also indirectly affect the activity of coumarin anti-coagulants. These antibiotics can reduce the population of bowel bacteria that synthesise vitamin K and this will reduce the amount absorbed into the body. Vitamin K antagonises the action of the coumarin anti-coagulants. Reducing vitamin K absorption will increase the action of warfarin, increase bleeding time, and may place the patient in danger of haemorrhage.

Interactions Altering Drug Distribution

Interactions that affect the distribution of a drug are commonly associated with drugs that are bound to plasma proteins being displaced by another drug that binds more strongly.

Protein-binding displacement: Early references to interactions placed great emphasis on displacement from protein binding and it was used to explain many important adverse interactions. Today, protein-binding displacement as a mechanism for drug interactions is rarely of clinical importance. This is because when a drug is displaced by another drug, the concentration of free drug in the plasma will increase, exposing the drug to the normal elimination processes, and so levels are rapidly reduced.

The displacement of methotrexate or warfarin from protein binding by aspirin or other non-steroidal anti-inflammatories (NSAIDs) like phenybutazone was initially described as the mechanism for these important interactions. Subsequent evidence has shown that although displacement occurs, it is the alteration in metabolism with warfarin and renal excretion with methotrexate that are significant.

Interactions Affecting Metabolism

Some of the most important and interesting interactions occur through the induction or inhibition of drug metabolism. The continuing research on cytochrome P450 (CYP450) isoenzymes has helped identify and increase the understanding of the mechanism behind many interactions. The main drug-metabolising isoenzyme systems are CYP2D6 and CYP3A4, and also 2C9 and 2C19. Other CYP systems involved in drug metabolism are CYP1A2, 2B6, 2C8, 2E1, 3A5 and 3A7. While interactions most frequently occur with liver enzyme systems, other sites such as the intestinal wall are important.

For many metabolic interactions, the isoenzyme-based mechanism has not yet been identified. For example, several deaths have been reported from the inhibition of azathioprine metabolism by allopurinol but the actual mechanism is as yet unknown.

Metabolic induction: When one drug (the inducer) increases the metabolism of another (the substrate), this will decrease the levels of the substrate in the body and increase the levels of metabolites. If the pharmacological activity is due to the unmetabolised (parent) drug then the levels and effect of the parent drug will be decreased.

The anti-epileptic medicines phenobarbitone, phenytoin and carbamazepine are all potent inducers of cytochrome CYP3A4, other CYP isoenzymes and enzymes involved in Phase II metabolism (conjugation). These will interact with the combined oral contraceptive to reduce levels of the active oestrogen and progestogen constituents. With low-dose oral contraceptives (containing below 35 μg oestrogen), pregnancies have been reported in patients taking enzyme inducing drugs.

For most women, prescribing a high-dose combined contraceptive (oestrogen content of 50 μg or more) will provide sufficient hormone levels for the suppression of ovulation. The anti-tubercular drug rifampicin is such a potent inducer of CYP3A4 that no combined oral contraceptive can be considered reliable (*see Case Study 2*).

If the action or toxicity of a drug is caused by an active metabolite then increasing the rate of metabolism of the parent drug can increase the production of the metabolite. For example, paracetamol is metabolised by CYP2E1 to a hepatotoxic metabolite that is then conjugated with glutathione to an inactive form. The metabolic induction of paracetamol by a CYP2E1 inducer, such as ethanol or isoniazid, may result in high levels of the toxic metabolite which can exceed the amount of glutathione stored in the liver. Hepatic damage can result from persistently high metabolite levels.

Metabolic inhibition: The metabolic inhibition of a drug will increase its plasma levels with the potential for toxicity or enhanced risk of side effects if the parent drug is the active species. If the medicine is a prodrug that must be metabolised for activity, then inhibiting its metabolism can slow the onset or prevent the action of that drug.

Metabolic inhibition can be used to reduce the dose and cost of expensive medicines. For example, diltiazem which inhibits CYP3A4 has been used with cyclosporin (a CYP3A4 substrate) to reduce the dose and the cost of cyclosporin immunosuppression in organ transplantation.

Metabolic inhibition can place patients at risk of toxicity. For example, the inhibition of the metabolism of the active S-warfarin stereoisomer by analgesic doses of aspirin. (warfarin is a racemic mixture of the R and S isomeric forms). This is a complex interaction because aspirin also induces the metabolism of the less active R-warfarin. If total warfarin levels are measured then no change is seen, but the anti-coagulant activity is markedly increased due to the high levels of the active S-isomer, placing the patient at risk of haemorrhage.

Drug transporter interactions: Drug transporters carry drugs across cell membranes into cells (uptake) or out of cells (efflux). Research to date has concentrated largely on P-glycoprotein (P-gp), although as this is a new field, other transporters involved in drug interactions are likely to be identified. P-gp pumps drugs from the cell cytoplasm out of the cell. In the intestine, a drug such as digoxin diffuses through the intestinal enterocyte cells for absorption into the body. P-gp is present in the enterocytes and so will transport a proportion of the digoxin molecules out of the cells and into the intestinal lumen to be excreted in faeces. There are drugs that block P-gp to increase digoxin bioavailability (for example, macrolide antibiotics) and a few which can induce P-gp (for example, rifampicin) to decrease absorption.

P-gp is also located in other tissues like the renal tubule, bile canaliculi and blood–brain barrier. For the digoxin–erythromycin interaction, P-gp inhibition by erythromycin in the kidneys and liver can also modify digoxin excretion. Many drugs that are transported by P-gp are also substrates of CYP3A4. Colchicine is transported by P-gp and verapamil can inhibit the transporter, making higher cellular concentrations available for CYP3A4 metabolism. Verapamil is also an inhibitor of CYP3A4, so colchicine levels are further increased; toxicity has been reported. Cell transporters have been identified in the intestine, kidneys, liver, blood–brain barrier, testes, uterus and placenta. As more knowledge about this is gained, explanations for some previously unknown mechanisms are likely to emerge.

Genetic polymorphism and drug interactions: Within different populations and ethnic groupings, there are individuals who may have a different variant of an isoenzyme and so will metabolise substrates at a faster or slower rate than the majority of people. For example, someone who was a poor metaboliser through CYP2D6 would be at risk of toxicity when given the standard dose of flecainide (a CYP2D6 substrate) or would experience therapeutic failure with drugs requiring to be converted to a metabolite for activity, for example, codeine.

Genetic polymorphism occurs with CYP2D6, 2C9 and 2C19 but not CYP3A4 or 1A2. In India, different ethnic groups have different proportions of poor and extensive metabolisers. For example, between 2% and 5% of the Indian population are poor metabolisers of CYP2D6 substrates, with small regional differences reported. Data on genetic variation for other isoenzymes and in different ethnic groups in the Indian subcontinent are also available.

Metabolic status can explain some of the inter-individual variation that is seen with drug interactions. For example, if two patients, one who is a slow CYP2C19 metaboliser and the other an extensive metaboliser, were given a 5 mg dose of diazepam (a CYP2C19 substrate) then the slow metaboliser would experience more pronounced sedation while the extensive metaboliser would respond as anticipated. If both these patients had been given omeprazole (a CYP2C19 inhibitor) with the diazepam dose then both would respond with enhanced sedation, as both would experience metabolic inhibition of the diazepam, one from their genetic variation, the other from a drug interaction.

Interactions Affecting Renal Excretion

For water-soluble drugs that are eliminated by the kidneys, alteration in urinary pH, tubular secretion or the rate of glomerular flow can alter the amount of drug that is excreted.

Lithium is a drug that is excreted by the kidneys and there are many interactions associated with interference with lithium excretion. Thiazide diuretics will increase the renal tubular re-absorption of lithium and may cause toxicity. NSAIDs inhibit prostaglandins that maintain blood flow into the renal glomeruli. With reduction in blood flow, less lithium will be filtered out through the glomeruli and excreted in urine and so plasma levels are increased.

Some drugs are eliminated by active renal tubular secretion and others can compete for transporter sites. This is an important part of the story of the methotrexate–NSAID interaction discussed earlier in this chapter.

Change in the urinary pH is used clinically to increase the urinary excretion rate of some weak acids or weak bases in overdose situations; however, this may occur inadvertently. Sodium citrate is an alkalinising agent used to increase the urine pH and reduce the symptoms of urinary tract infection. It can increase the urinary excretion of acidic drugs like aciclovir, cephalosporins, penicillins and thiazide diuretics by increasing the amount of ionised drug in the renal tubule and so reduce tubular re-absorption. Sodium citrate can also reduce the excretion of basic drugs, for example, amiloride, cimetidine and ranitidine, by producing more un-ionised molecules which will be re-absorbed by the kidney tubules. Modification of urinary pH is rarely reported as the significant mechanism in adverse drug interactions.

Mechanisms for Pharmacodynamic Interactions

These occur when a drug has an additive or antagonistic effect on the pharmacological action of another medicine. Having a good knowledge of pharmacology makes it possible to predict many of these interactions. When patients are treated with a large number of medicines, the outcome can be difficult to predict.

Pharmacological Synergism

Synergism occurs when two drugs with a similar pharmacological or side effect are given together to produce an additive effect. This can be exploited for patient benefit or it may be hazardous. Combinations of medicines are frequently used for therapeutic advantage, for example, using different medicine classes such as opiates and tricyclic anti-depressants together to improve pain control. Some combinations can result in an increase in the incidence of side effects, for example, the additive potassium-sparing effects of an angiotensin converting enzyme (ACE) inhibitor with the aldosterone antagonist, spironolactone. Hyperkalaemia with this combination is difficult to predict but is potentially hazardous and requires regular monitoring.

A serious and life-threatening example of pharmacological synergism is the combination of a non-reversible MAO inhibitor (for example, phenelzine) with a serotonin re-uptake receptor inhibitor such as sertraline. This can result in an increase in the neurotransmitter, serotonin, and precipitate serotonin syndrome, a potentially fatal condition characterised by fever, shivering, confusion, ataxia, hypereflexia, diarrhoea or myoclonus.

Pharmacological Antagonism

This occurs when the effect of one drug prevents the pharmacological action of another. A common example is the reduction in the diuretic activity of a thiazide diuretic by an NSAID. The anti-prostaglandin action of the NSAID on the kidneys will reduce the glomerular filtration rate and so reduce sodium and water excretion. Another example is the prescribing of a tricyclic anti-depressant (for example, amitriptyline) with anti-epileptics. Tricyclic anti-depressants are known to lower the seizure threshold and so can counter the effects of the anti-epileptic. A further example is when a centrally active dopamine antagonist like metoclopramide is prescribed to treat nausea in a patient receiving levodopa treatment for Parkinson's disease. The metoclopramide can block the beneficial effects of the dopamine precursor, levodopa, thus exacerbating Parkinsonian ataxia and dyskinesia.

INFORMATION SOURCES ON DRUG INTERACTIONS

There are about 6000 drugs available worldwide along with traditional medicines and herbal remedies that can potentially interact. The range of possibilities is considerable. When evaluating interactions, it is important to consider both the theoretical potential of the interactions gained from pharmacological knowledge and the clinical information from the medical literature. In the 1970s, many interactions were predicted to occur, based on pharmacological knowledge, but have never been observed clinically.

Information is available from a wide range of sources such as in vitro and animal studies, case reports, clinical trials, review papers, handbooks, monographs in books, paragraphs in product data sheets and on the worldwide web. It is important that pharmacists are familiar with and use this information appropriately.

For example, if only case report data is used to evaluate the potential interaction between coumarin anti-coagulants and paracetamol, then patients may be prevented from taking a potentially useful analgesic. A small number of case reports show an increase in clotting time when paracetamol is given to patients stabilised on warfarin. Clinical trial results are inconclusive, with both no change and an increase in INR/clotting time reported. Several mechanisms for an interaction have been proposed. This is a complex situation for which further research is required to define the significance of what is most likely a rare event.

In Vitro and Animal Data

Information from in vitro studies and animal experiments is helpful in identifying the mechanism for an interaction. Recently, work on the cytochrome P450 isoenzyme system is an example of the value of in vitro experimentation. Animal and in vitro information cannot reliably predict that an interaction will occur in humans, as human pharmacokinetic and pharmacodynamic processes and physiology are not represented.

Case Reports

Interactions are often first identified as case reports or letters published in medical journals or reported to a pharmacy vigilance programme. The reliability of information in letters and case reports requires careful evaluation, as in most journals, this section does not undergo peer review. Table 10.1 presents a guide for evaluating case reports.

Table 10.1 Evaluating a case report

Timing: Can the reaction be related to the introduction of one medicine?
Dechallenge: Did the reaction cease when the suspect medicine was stopped?
Rechallenge: Did the reaction recur when the suspected medicine was re-introduced?
Other medicines: Can the reaction or interaction be explained by other medicines the patient was taking?
Other explanations: Are there other factors that could explain the reaction, for example, underlying disease, emergence of a new disease, dietary or lifestyle changes, dose changes?
Missing information: What information has not been given by the authors but would strengthen or weaken the evidence?

Case reports are a useful source for identifying interactions between infrequently used medicine combinations or for rarely occurring interactions. Clusters of reports can add further weight to verifying an interaction and may occasionally provide a concept of frequency. For example, ten cases reported for a very infrequently used combination of medicines would suggest this is likely to be a frequent and notable interaction when these medicines are taken together.

Clinical Trials

Clinical trials provide the most reliable evidence to support an interaction. Extraneous factors that could also explain the effect can be controlled and statistic tests can identify if the effect could have occurred by chance. To evaluate clinical trial quality, the CONSORT group has published guidelines (*see website references*).

With drug interactions, there are special considerations when considering trial data. Small numbers of subjects are commonly used to study drug interactions, so statistical significance can be underestimated (type II error). Also, most trials include only 'healthy, young males' and thus do not mimic the more at-risk patient population, who are likely to be elderly, include women and have active disease processes. Many of the trials reported are single-dose studies and these may overlook some of the effects that occur with chronic dosing. Furthermore, a statistically significant result does not imply a clinically significant result. For example, changes in the blood levels of a drug may be statistically significant but these may be so small as to not influence the clinical outcome.

Reviews, Monographs and Handbooks

Reviews on drug interactions are published in the pharmacy literature from time to time; for example, series have been published in the Pharmaceutical Journal (UK) for 1998–99 and are regularly published in the Annals of Pharmacotherapy. The purpose of these articles is to educate pharmacists about interactions, although some reviews will provide reliable lists for interaction screening. It is important to check for quality and completeness of a review. For example, a literature review that includes only information from medical journals could miss some important interactions reported in other journals or to pharmacovigilance organisations.

Some useful books that contain compilations of drug interactions are listed as key references. The reliability and completeness of any compilation should be verified. It is also important to check for recently published information in the medical literature, especially for recently introduced medicines and infrequent interactions or rarely used medicine combinations.

Tables, Charts and Datasheets

Quick reference sources available to screen for known drug interactions come in a variety of forms of which the British National Formulary (BNF) tables is one of the better known. There are also wall or pocket-sized charts and interaction warnings associated with dispensing computer programmes that can assist rapid identification of interactions. The currency and reliability of the information needs careful assessment. A particular disadvantage with many charts is that more in-depth information is required to assess whether the interaction is likely to be of significance and importance to a patient.

Product data sheets can provide useful information if they have undergone independent review. Approved data sheets from countries such as the USA, UK, Australia, Canada and New Zealand are reviewed by a local government health agency and may be published on the agency's web site.

Interaction Websites

There are a number of websites which contain information on drug interactions. Some sites cover specific classes of drugs or conditions; for example, herbal medicines or medicines used to treat HIV/AIDs. Some excellent references like Stockley's Drug Interactions are available through online subscription. For other web-based information, reliability needs to be considered with particular care.

Some sites like Dave Flockhart's cytochrome P450 isoenzyme site are accurate and current. This site is particularly useful for screening for suspected metabolic interactions but it does not predict clinical relevance and excludes many metabolised medicines for which the isoenzyme system involved has not been identified.

Working with Drug Interaction Literature

A wide range of information sources are available to pharmacists and familiarity with these is important. *Exercise 1* provides an approach to familiarising pharmacists with the drug interaction sources they are likely to use.

Guidance on Identifying an Adverse Drug Interaction

In a healthcare team, pharmacists are frequently asked to identify if an event experienced by a patient is likely to be medicine related. It is important that a systematic and reliable approach is used to identify likely interactions and to exclude other causes.

Medication and Reaction History

All medicines and therapeutically active substances the patient was taking before and at the time of the event should be identified. The starting and stopping dates, doses, formulations, when the event was first observed, a description of the reaction and the supporting laboratory tests should be noted. If one medicine has been stopped (dechallenge) or is re-introduced (rechallenge), the result should be described.

Most interactions will occur within a short time of commencing a combination, but the timing will depend on the type of mechanism and the medicines involved. For example, interactions resulting in a change in the blood concentration of a medicine will depend on the half-life of that medicine. Some interactions may, however, take months to appear. For example, interactions due to enzyme induction can take weeks to emerge as a new protein is laid down and the isoenzyme levels are increased.

When two or more medicines in combination are identified as potentially causing an event, the next stage is to check for literature support.

Using Drug Interaction Literature

Reliable drug interaction references are available but will not cover more recently published information. For screening well-recognised and researched interactions, these references may be sufficient. When screening for potential interactions that are omitted from a reliable text or when there are few reports, a search of the medical literature for more recent information or case reports is important. There are also differences in the medicines used among different countries, so books published for the American or European markets may not cover the range of medicines used in countries like India.

Managing an Adverse Interaction

The management of an interaction will depend on the severity and risk to the patient and on recognising if the dose or timing is likely to be important. A recently defined system for classifying and managing drug interactions according to the risk to the patient has been published, and this can help pharmacists identify an appropriate action. A reference for the OpeRational ClassificAtion of drug interactions (ORCA) is provided.

The interaction between erythromycin and terfenadine (a non-sedating anti-histamine) would be classified as Class 1; such a combination should be avoided as the risk outweighs the benefit. High terfenadine levels reported when combined with erythromycin has caused torsade de pointes, a potentially fatal type of cardiac arrhythmia. The options are to stop terfenadine and use an anti-histamine that does not cause arrhythmias at high plasma concentrations or to change to an antibiotic that does not interact with terfenadine and is not associated with modifying cardiac conduction.

Where an interaction has resulted in changes in plasma drug levels, these may be managed by changing the dose of the affected medicine. For example, when miconazole oral gel increases the bleeding time of warfarin, reducing the warfarin dose will bring the bleeding time back within range and reduce the risk of haemorrhage. It is important to re-titrate the dose of warfarin when the course of miconazole is complete. An alternative and simpler approach would be to use an anti-fungal agent such as nystatin that does not interact with warfarin.

Dose spacing is appropriate for interactions that involve inhibition of absorption in the GI tract. For example, to avoid the binding of ciprofloxacin by ferrous salts *(see Case Study 1)*.

Reporting New or Rare Interactions

Interactions for which there are no or few reports in the medical or pharmacy literature should be presented to a reputable journal as letters or case reports and be reported to a pharmacovigilance organisation with connections to the World Health Organization Programme. Ideally a rechallenge should be undertaken, but understandably most patients and their doctors are unwilling to participate. In thcsc situations, documentation of the outcome of the dechallenge (when the combination is stopped) will provide useful but less rigorous information.

Screening Patients' Medication to Prevent Drug Interactions

Reviewing therapy for potential interactions can occur as part of a medicine review process or before a patient takes a new medicine. Frail or malnourished patients, those with renal or hepatic impairment or multiple pathologies are at greater risk of developing adverse drug interactions. Some drugs pose a greater risk due to inherent toxicity, non-linear pharmacokinetics or potent enzyme inducing or inhibiting ability (Table 10.2). Ready reference systems like tables, pocketbooks or computer-based programmes can help with screening. The order in which medicines are added is an important consideration. For example, if bendrofluazide is added to lithium, there is a risk of lithium toxicity from competition for renal excretion. However, if lithium is added to bendrofluazide and the dose is titrated according to serum levels and the clinical response, the risk of toxicity is reduced.

Table 10.2 Medicines frequently implicated in clinically significant or serious interactions

Cancer chemotherapy and immunosuppressants (such as methotrexate, azathioprine)
Carbamazepine
Cholestyramine
Combined oral contraceptives
Cyclosporin
Digoxin
Lithium
MAO inhibitors (such as phenelzine, tranylcypromine)
Oral anti-coagulants (such as warfarin, dicoumarol)
Phenobarbitone
Phenytoin
Protease inhibitors (such as indinavir, ritonavir, saquinavir)
Rifampicin
Theophylline
Valproic acid and salts

Patient education can further help to avoid potential interactions. Patient information leaflets or a simple warning message printed on the tablet bottle label can be useful. For example, for a patient prescribed ciprofloxacin, the warning 'Do not take with iron' could be added to the label, or the patient could be advised verbally.

With newly introduced medicines, additional monitoring and care is required as clinical experience and exposure to potentially interacting medicines will be limited. Caution should be adopted when a newly introduced medicine is combined with medicines with a high risk of potentially serious side effects. This would include immunosuppressants (for example, methotrexate or azathioprine), anti-coagulants or drugs with a non-linear kinetic profile. For example, if a novel CYP3A4 inhibitor is given to a patient on cyclophosphamide (CYP3A4 substrate) then regular haematological monitoring could prevent serious and potentially life-threatening bone marrow suppression from elevated cyclophosphamide levels.

Interactions With Food and Herbal Medicines

There are some well-known and potentially dangerous interactions between medicines and food. A particularly dangerous interaction is that between monoamine oxidase inhibitors such as phenelzine and tyramine containing foods. The high levels of tyramine that result from metabolic blockade by phenelzine can precipitate a potentially fatal hypertensive crisis.

Some drug–food interactions have resulted in therapeutic failure; for example, when phenytoin is given with enteral feeding mixtures, leading to a decrease in GI absorption (considered to be caused by an interaction with calcium and other divalent cations). Other causes of toxicity include a high-fibre diet that increases warfarin activity by impairing the absorption of vitamin K. Grapefruit juice constituents are known to inhibit the gastrointestinal metabolism of medicines handled by the CYP3A4 isoenzyme. Some food ingredients may also exacerbate the side effects of medicines; for example, chili inhibits substance P and is reported to increase the incidence of coughing in patients on ACE inhibitors. Generally, however, medicines and food interactions are under-recognised and infrequently reported.

The importance of interactions between medicines and herbal remedies has recently been recognised and there are reviews and comments available for a limited number of remedies. In India, the very long and strong tradition of herbal and traditional medicine means that this is an important topic to be investigated.

Conclusion

The role of pharmacists in preventing and detecting interactions and providing reliable advice on interaction management can greatly add to the patient's safety and wellbeing. Pharmacists have a good educational base on which to develop expertise in drug interactions and so make a valuable contribution to patient management. While all practicing pharmacists need to develop basic skills in this area, there will be some who will develop a specialist interest and add to national and international knowledge pools.

CASE STUDY 1

TP is a young woman, who presents a prescription for doxycycline and quinine to a pharmacy to be filled. When giving out the prescription, the pharmacist checks whether TP takes any other medicines. TP explains that she takes an iron tablet each morning but nothing else. What advice should the pharmacist give?

Discussion:

The pharmacist identifies an interaction between doxycycline and iron. This interaction is well established and reduces the oral absorption of tetracyclines, leading to therapeutic failure. She recommends that TP take the doxycycline in the morning and at night with food and take the iron at lunch time. The pharmacist is aware that anaemia is commonly associated with malaria and recommends that TP discuss her iron self-treatment with her doctor. She also recommends that TP avoid taking antacid or drinking milk within two hours of doxycycline administration.

Heavy metal ions such as iron and calcium can chelate tetracyclines like doxycycline to produce an insoluble salt. As this will not dissolve, it is not absorbed from the gastrointestinal tract. The interaction could cause therapeutic failure of the antibiotic/anti-malarial. This can be avoided by taking doxycycline at least two hours before or after the iron or calcium. Taking the iron at lunch time and avoiding milk (which contains calcium) close to the tetracycline administration times will prevent this interaction. Calcium from other food sources in a normal diet is not usually of sufficient quantity to impair tetracycline absorption.

CASE STUDY 2

LW is a 35-year-old woman with three teenage daughters. She and her husband have been using a low-dose combined oral contraceptive (COC) for many years as their contraceptive of choice. After sustaining a head injury from a motorcycle accident, LW is prescribed carbamazepine to prevent seizures. She does not take any other medicines. The doctor asks the clinical pharmacist to provide advice about contraception management for LW and her husband. The pharmacist recommends a high oestrogen–containing COC for LW.

After five years of good health and good seizure control, LW's doctor contacts the clinical pharmacist again for advice. She is going to treat LW with prophylactic rifampicin as her nephew, who lives in the same household, has been hospitalised with bacterial meningitis. What should the pharmacist advise?

Discussion:

This time the pharmacist recommends that non-hormonal contraceptive methods such as condoms be used for the month after LW has taken the rifampicin.

The clinical pharmacist understands that carbamazepine is a cytochrome P450 enzyme inducer. Using reliable literature sources, he defines that the systems of importance in this situation are 3A4, as both oestrogen and progestogen are substrates, and 2C19 for progestogen metabolism. Carbamazepine induces the CYP450 2C19 and 3A4 isoenzymes and can reduce the plasma levels of both oestrogen and progestogen. A literature search identifies that using a COC containing at least 50 μg of oestrogen will maintain contraceptive effectiveness.

When asked about the use of a short course of rifampicin, the clinical pharmacist is aware that this medicine is a particularly potent inducer of several cytochrome P450 isoenzyme systems including CYP450 3A4. Rifampicin is such a powerful hepatic enzyme inducer that adequate hormone levels to suppress ovulation will not be maintained irrespective of the COC dose. A non-hormonal contraceptive method is therefore recommended.

As a final precaution, the pharmacist also checked for an interaction between rifampicin and carbamazepine. He does not find any monographs, studies or case reports. He decides that an interaction is unlikely to occur as both are reasonably common medicines and are likely to be prescribed together.

CASE STUDY 3

P is a frail 65-year-old man who is admitted to hospital with worsening congestive heart failure (CHF). He also has osteoarthritis. His medicines on admission are:

Digoxin	0.0625 mg	One tablet in the morning
Frusemide	40 mg	One tablet in the morning
Captopril	12.5 mg	One tablet twice daily
Diclofenac	75 mg long acting	One capsule twice daily with food

His doctor has read a recent review on the treatment of CHF and decides to prescribe spironolactone. What would the pharmacist recommend after reviewing P's medicines?

Discussion:

The clinical pharmacist considers that the doses and formulation of P's medicines are appropriate for him but drug interactions could compromise his wellbeing. As he is elderly and frail, P is at increased risk of experiencing an adverse interaction. She identifies a possible interaction between diclofenac and frusemide and also diclofenac and captopril.

The pharmacist suggests to the doctor that P may benefit by switching from diclofenac to paracetamol for relief of his arthritic pain. She also suggests that potassium levels be measured regularly and that P's renal function be assessed to exclude acute renal failure.

Diclofenac can counteract the diuretic effects of frusemide. The anti-prostaglandin effects of diclofenac reduce blood flow through the kidney glomeruli, and thus reduce the amount of fluid filtered into the renal tubule. This could lead to fluid retention which would increase the workload of the heart and worsen P's heart failure. Diclofenac could also precipitate acute renal failure when used in combination with an ACE inhibitor through an additive effect on reducing glomerula blood flow. Measuring P's urine output and serum creatinine levels will help establish if he has acute renal impairment. Removing the diclofenac and replacing it with a simple analgesic like paracetamol (for which there is good clinical trial evidence) will provide relief from his pain and prevent these interactions.

Digoxin toxicity is enhanced by hypokalaemia (low potassium blood levels) and, although electrolyte disturbances are less likely with loop diuretics than with thiazides, this should still be considered. A further complexity is that ACE inhibitors like captopril can increase potassium levels making the situation difficult to predict, so it is important that P's electrolytes are monitored regularly. The proposed addition of spironolactone, an aldosterone antagonist, may also increase the potassium levels. High levels of potassium can inhibit the action of digoxin.

Exercise 1: Evaluating and Comparing Different Sources of Drug Interaction Information

Select several different information sources that are available to you. If possible, select one source from each of the following types of references:

- Ready reference source (for example, BNF tables, a wall chart, the Drug Information Handbook, Stockley's Pocket Companion, Australian Medicines Handbook, Micromedex [a website])
- Product data sheets
- A specific drug interactions text; for example, Stockley or Hansten and Horne or specialised review articles published in reputable journals
- Clinical trials and case reports obtained through IOWA or a database like PubMed, MEDLINE, EMBASE

Compare the information (for example, is an interaction listed, what is the incidence, severity and mechanism for the interaction, is the onset immediate or delayed, what management advice is given) for the following interactions:

- Glibenclamide + Rifampicin
- Theophylline + Azithromycin
- Warfarin + Paracetamol
- Ritonavir + Simvastatin
- Tadalafil + Glyceryl trinitrate
- Digoxin + St John's Wort

Based on your findings, list what you consider are the benefits and the disadvantages of each type of information source.

Exercise 2: Literature Evaluation and Preparation of a Report

A pharmacist has been asked by a haematologist to investigate why a patient who was previously stabilised on warfarin has had a significant increase in their coagulation time. On obtaining an in-depth medication history, the pharmacist has not been able to identify any significant changes in dietary vitamin K intake or changes to the patient's regular medicines. As the patient appears to have a head cold, the pharmacist has questioned him on symptomatic management. This patient reports benefits from taking a strong tea prepared from ginger root which was started about three days before the first elevated test.

You are to undertake a literature search to identify if ginger could explain the change in coagulation time for this patient. Write a report for the doctor that he could use in the preparation of a case report to the Journal of the Indian Medical Association. He has asked you to be a co-author.

EXERCISE 3: SCREENING A PATIENT'S MEDICATIONS FOR MEDICINE INTERACTIONS

L is a 72-year-old male with a history of rheumatoid arthritis, chronic obstructive pulmonary disease and right-sided heart failure. He is stabilised on the following medicines:

Azathioprine	100 mg at night
Enalapril	20 mg twice daily
Frusemide	80 mg in the morning
Spironolactone	25 mg in the morning

He has recently been diagnosed with acute gout for which the following medicines have been prescribed:

Ibuprofen 400 mg three times a day and continued for 1 week

Allopurinol 300 mg in the morning, to be started two weeks after the ibuprofen

1. Identify each medication that has been prescribed and state why this patient may be taking it.
2. Identify any possible drug interactions which could arise.
3. Identify possible mechanisms for each interaction.
4. What is the potential risk of each interaction to the patient?
5. Which interactions would you would refer to the prescriber and what would you recommend? If you consider that a medicine combination should be avoided, identify alternative options.

KEY MESSAGES

Pharmacists have an important role in:

- detecting interactions
- providing advice on the management of interactions
- preventing adverse interactions from occurring

To do this proficiently, pharmacists require a good understanding of the:

- pharmacology of medicines and the mechanism of interactions
- reliability of different information sources
- likely clinical significance of an interaction
- risk compared to benefit for the patient

Further Reading

Adams P. 1998–99. Drug Interactions That Matter. *Pharmaceutical Journal*.

Articles on Cytochrome P450 published in the Australian Journal of Hospital Pharmacy in 2000, available at http://www.shpa.org.au/journal/P450.htm

Fugh-Berman A. 2000. Herb-drug Interactions. *The Lancet* 355:134–138.

Gardiner P, Phillips R and Shaughnessy AF. 2008. Herbal and Dietary Supplement-drug interactions in patients with chronic illness. *Am Fam Physician* 77(1):73–78.

Hansten PD, Horn JR and Hazlet TK. 2001. ORCA: OpeRational ClassificAtion of drug interactions. *J Am Pharm Assoc* 41:161–165.

Hansten and Horn's Drug Interactions: Analysis and Management. 2009. Hansten PD and Horn JR, eds. 4th edition. Lippincott, Williams and Wilkins: Philadelphia.

Horn JR and Hansten PD. Drug transporters: the final frontier for drug interactions Part 1 and 2 available at http://www.hanstenandhorn.com

Stockley's Drug Interactions. 2010. Baxter K ed. 7th edition. Pharmaceutical Press: London (also available via online subscription).

Stockley's Drug Interactions Pocket Companion. Baxter K ed. Pharmaceutical Press: London.

Uppsala Monitoring Centre. *Safety Monitoring of Medicinal Products*. 2000. WHO Collaborating Centre for International Drug Monitoring, London.

Websites of Interest

CONSORT Evaluation of Clinical Trials
http://www.consort-statement.org/

Dave Flockart's charts of CYP450 isoenzyme and drug metabolic sites
http://medicine.iupui.edu/flockhart/

Medscape Drug Interactions Checker (this site requires registration, which is free)
http://www.medscape.com/druginfo/druginterchecker

HIV/AIDs Medicines Interactions
http://www.hiv-druginteractions.org

11

Interpreting Laboratory Data: Biochemistry and Haematology

Christopher P Alderman

Learning Objectives

Upon completion of this chapter, the reader should be able to:

- Understand general principles relevant to the interpretation of laboratory data
- Interpret some biochemical parameters including serum creatinine, sodium, potassium, calcium and blood glucose levels
- Distinguish between different patterns of abnormalities in indicators of liver function
- Understand and interpret commonly measured haematological parameters that are reported in the complete blood picture, including haemoglobin, erythrocyte morphology, white cell count and differential and platelet count
- Recognise serious biochemical and haematological abnormalities and know when urgent intervention is required

To be able to practise effectively as a clinical pharmacist, it is essential to be able to interpret laboratory data for individual patients. Laboratory data provides a 'window' through which we gain an understanding of a patient's health and physiological function, and the ability to interpret this data with confidence is a skill that clinical pharmacists must use frequently in their work. Many specific and non-specific laboratory investigations are routinely used by clinicians as a means to assess patients, and although it is not necessary for pharmacists to be intimately familiar with all of these, it is important to have a working understanding of the tests that are frequently used, or which have a direct relevance to drug therapy.

The results of most laboratory tests are reported with a reference range – a numerical range of results that would be likely to be obtained if that investigation were performed for healthy subjects (in the absence of significant disease). A reference range may sometimes be misleading unless the pharmacist has an understanding of its meaning.

A result that falls outside a reference range does not always indicate the presence of disease or disordered organ function, but grossly abnormal results usually do signify serious problems. Conversely, if a result falls within the quoted reference range, this does not necessarily guarantee the absence of disease or abnormal organ function. Sometimes, results may appear to be abnormal because of an artefact effect, such as the factitious elevation of serum potassium that may be seen if erythrocytes in blood samples have undergone haemolysis prior to the analysis. Sources of error arising within the laboratory may also need to be considered in some practice settings. For these reasons, it is important that a clinical pharmacist interpret results with reference to the clinical status of the patient and other relevant information.

For example, an electrocardiograph may confirm myocardial damage in a patient with chest pain and an elevated serum concentration of creatine kinase, but clearly all three pieces of information are most useful when considered together rather than in isolation.

A clinical pharmacist must be able to interpret laboratory data for a number of reasons. Firstly, as part of an overall clinical assessment, laboratory data can assist review of the patient's current drug therapy. The results may suggest that a particular drug is not appropriate for the patient and should therefore be discontinued or avoided (for example, non-steroidal anti-inflammatory drugs [NSAIDs or metformin] for a patient with severe renal impairment). The results of an investigation may suggest the need for dose adjustment, most commonly a reduction that is necessary because of diminished renal or hepatic function. A laboratory test can also be used as a guide to determine the adequacy of drug response, with a good example being the measurement of blood glucose parameters when assessing the effectiveness of insulin treatment. As well as monitoring for the efficacy of treatment, laboratory tests can also be used to check for signs of serious drug toxicity that may be reflected by abnormal biochemical or haematological parameters or elevated liver function indices.

There is no simple way for pharmacists to familiarise themselves with the information needed to interpret laboratory data, but the investment of effort provides a good return when it enables a clinical pharmacist to play an active and informed role in patient care. In this chapter, some commonly encountered laboratory investigations are discussed, with particular focus on the implications for clinical pharmacists. The range of investigations covered is by no means exhaustive, but provides a starting point for clinical pharmacists involved in patient care activities.

Indicators of Renal Function

As many drugs and drug metabolites are dependent upon renal excretion for clearance, it is essential for a clinical pharmacist to be able to assess the renal function of a patient. In addition, some drug therapy may adversely affect the kidneys, and by monitoring the patient's laboratory data, it is possible to detect a drug-related decline in renal function. The laboratory data that provides information about the functional capacity of the kidneys includes serum creatinine concentration and serum urea concentration (and the closely related parameter, blood urea nitrogen).

Serum Creatinine (reference range 55–120 mmol/L or 0.6–1.35 mg/dL)

Creatinine is a metabolic byproduct of muscle metabolism that is formed at a relatively constant rate as a result of the degradation of creatine. Creatinine plays no significant physiological role and is eliminated by renal excretion with no active tubular secretion in the nephron. These unique features mean that the clearance of creatinine may be used as a surrogate marker of the *glomerular filtration rate (GFR)*, which in turn provides a basis for an estimation of the functional capacity of the kidneys as organs of elimination (the endocrine functions of the kidneys are much less closely correlated with serum creatinine concentration than the excretory functions).

Any event or noxious insult (including some drugs) that adversely influences kidney function can lead to an increase in serum creatinine concentration. Other factors such as muscle mass, gender and the period of time that has elapsed after the insult may also influence the extent to which diminished renal function is reflected by an elevation in serum creatinine concentration. A serum creatinine concentration below the reference range is generally not indicative of specific pathology, but may be encountered in patients with decreased muscle mass (for example, the elderly or in disabled people) or during the first or second trimester of pregnancy.

A significant elevation in serum creatinine is almost invariably associated with significant renal dysfunction, although elevation may not be observed in the early phase of renal disease. By the time serum creatinine is markedly and persistently elevated, other important electrolyte abnormalities such as increased serum urea, hyperkalaemia and hyperphosphatemia are quite common.

The relationship between the extent of elevation of serum creatinine concentration and the relative decline in renal function has been estimated using various methods, the most popular of which is that based on an equation proposed by Cockcroft and Gault. The *Cockcroft–Gault equation* (Fig. 11.1) incorporates an allowance for the influence of advancing age and diminished muscle mass on the rate of creatinine production, and is used to derive a rough estimate of the GFR. This formula is less reliable for very young and very old patients, when the patient is very emaciated or overweight, or when serum creatinine is changing rapidly.

Notwithstanding these limitations, the estimate of the GFR provides an approximate but useful guide to the extent of renal impairment (relative to the renal function of a young, healthy adult).

The GFR of a young person with no significant renal disease is generally of the order of 120–150 ml/minute, providing a value to compare against when assessing the renal function of patients. A patient

Figure 11.1 Cockcroft–Gault equation

$$\text{Estimated GFR}^{*} \text{ (ml/minute)} = \frac{(140 - \text{age}) \times \text{weight(kg)}}{\text{Serum creatinine (micromol/L)} \times 0.84}$$

* Multiply result by 0.85 if calculating for a female patient.

with an apparent GFR (estimated using the Cockcroft–Gault equation) of 50 ml/minute can generally be assumed to have a renal elimination capacity that is less than 50% of that expected from a young healthy subject.

In some cases, particularly among the elderly, renal function may be significantly impaired despite little or no elevation in serum creatinine concentration. Using the Cockcroft–Gault equation, the GFR of an 85-year-old woman weighing 55 kg and with a serum creatinine of 120 mmol/L (within the reference range) would bc cstimated at approximately 25 ml/minute, a level of renal impairment that would necessitate dose reduction for many drugs that are reliant upon renal excretion.

Note that in many cases, the elderly will have a serum creatinine concentration within the reference range despite significant renal impairment, even in the absence of specific renal disease or a nephrotoxic drug. This is because a progressive decline in the number of functional nephrons in the kidneys almost invariably accompanies advancing age. For this reason, it is important for clinical pharmacists to make a thorough and ongoing assessment of renal function for all elderly patients for whom they provide pharmaceutical care.

Using the GFR in Practice

Estimation of GFR is useful for many aspects of the work of a clinical pharmacist. If the estimated GFR declines from 80 ml/minute to 20 ml/minute after the introduction of a potentially nephrotoxic drug such as an NSAID, this suggests an adverse drug reaction and allows a clinical pharmacist to intervene by suggesting that drug therapy be suspended (thereby averting progression to even more serious renal impairment). Conversely, the estimated GFR can be used to monitor improvement in renal function after discontinuation of the drug therapy that has compromised renal function. After renal transplantation, an improvement in GFR is indicative of a functional allograft, whilst a decline in GFR can indicate early signs of rejection (or, in some cases, nephrotoxicity associated with immunosupressants).

Another very important use for estimating GFR is the reduction in drug dose for renally clcarcd drugs. In some cases (for example, digoxin, lithium, gentamicin), this approach can be used to select an appropriate maintenance dose and avoid toxicity from drug accumulation. In other situations, monitoring serum creatinine concentration (with GFR estimation, if necessary) can help identify a decline in renal function that requires a dose reduction. Impaired renal function identified during patient assessment by the clinical pharmacist may also influence drug selection. Potentially nephrotoxic agents may be avoided for patients whose renal function is already impaired, and drugs that accumulate (or with toxic metabolites that accumulate) may be replaced with alternatives that are cleared by other routes.

In end-stage renal disease, the excretory (and metabolic) functions of the kidneys are compromised to the extent that the patient requires dialysis or renal transplantation to sustain life. Although an expensive treatment that does not always deliver good quality of life, dialysis does serve to replace the excretory functions of the kidneys to some extent. This reduces the serum concentrations of creatinine and urea on a regular basis and assists in managing the dynamics of serum electrolytes such as potassium, calcium and phosphorus.

Serum Urea (reference range 3.0–8.0 mmol/L)

and

Blood Urea Nitrogen (reference range 2.9–7.1 mmol/L or 8–20 mg/dL)

Serum urea and Blood Urea Nitrogen (BUN) are the other secondary indicators of renal function that can be usefully monitored by a clinical pharmacist. As serum urea and BUN may be affected by the patient's hydration status and other factors, these parameters are less sensitive indicators of renal function than serum creatinine. BUN is a parameter that is closely linked to the serum urea concentration (urea forms a major component of BUN), and is most useful when considered together with serum creatinine. The ratio of BUN divided by serum creatinine (which must be calculated using comparable units) may provide some additional guidance about the possible causes of renal impairment. Marked elevation of serum urea or BUN with minimal or no elevation of serum creatinine suggests dehydration. Interested readers should refer to specialist text for further information about this.

Serum Electrolytes

Several serum electrolytes are of particular interest to clinical pharmacists, including serum sodium, potassium and calcium concentrations, although other electrolytes such as serum magnesium and phosphate may be of value in particular settings.

Serum Sodium (reference range 135–145 mmol/L)

Although mild abnormalities in serum sodium concentration are quite common, particularly in patients with multiple medical conditions or significant polypharmacy, clinically significant abnormalities are only encountered infrequently. Like many serum electrolyte abnormalities, disturbances in serum sodium concentration are not often accompanied by specific signs or symptoms unless the disturbance is considerable, and are generally of greater clinical significance in the very young or the very old, or in patients who are severely ill.

The serum sodium concentration is a function of available sodium and the water it is dissolved in. As the overall amount of sodium in the body is maintained within a relatively narrow range by the kidneys, the sodium concentration is most profoundly affected by the fluid volume status of the patient. When the sodium is present in a relatively excessive amount of water (for example, in some oedematous states), the sodium concentration is often reduced to a level below the reference range; this abnormality is called *hyponatraemia*. If there has been excessive fluid loss and the available sodium is dissolved in a relatively smaller volume of water than normal, the sodium concentration will be increased above the reference range, and this is called *hypernatraemia*.

An important concept for pharmacists to understand about the serum sodium value is that it bears little relationship to oral sodium intake, because if a patient consumes a large sodium load, this is offset by the thirst reflex. This means that the subject will normally drink sufficient fluids to enable the sodium load to be diluted until the kidneys are able to excrete the excess sodium load. Serum sodium and osmolarity are controlled by the interplay of the thirst reflex, anti-diuretic hormone action, the renin–angiotensin–

aldosterone system and renal tubular handling of filtered sodium.

Hypernatraemia: Severe hypernatraemia is an uncommon electrolyte abnormality that is most often observed in the context of haemoconcentration secondary to excessive loss of hypotonic fluids. Severe vomiting and/or diarrhoea may produce hypernatraemia because large volumes of fluids are lost and oral intake may be insufficient to compensate for this. Although hypernatraemia is not often of clinical significance until the sodium concentration exceeds 150 mmol/L, very high concentrations may cause central nervous system symptoms and must be addressed urgently. Equally important in most cases of hypernatraemia is the need to address underlying dehydration. This is achieved using fluid replacement, either orally or intravenously, as appropriate.

Other causes of hypernatraemia include osmotic diuresis such as that seen with poorly controlled diabetes mellitus, or in the recovery phase after some types of acute renal failure. Diabetes insipidus, where the kidneys produce inappropriately large amounts of dilute urine, may also cause hypernatraemia, and can be secondary to drug therapy with agents such as lithium or colchicine.

Hyponatraemia: Hyponatraemia is a relatively common electrolyte disturbance that may be associated with quite a broad range of underlying pathology. Early signs of hyponatraemia include lethargy, nausea, drowsiness and confusion. Hyponatraemia rarely assumes clinical significance until the sodium concentration is below 125 mmol/L, but urgent attention is needed if the level is below 120 mmol/L. Possible causes of hyponatraemia are outlined in Table 11.1.

Table 11.1 Possible causes of hyponatraemia

Pseudohyponatraemia – a laboratory artefact that is sometimes observed in patients with paraproteinemias (for example, multiple myeloma) and severe dyslipidemia. The sodium appears to be low but is not, serum osmolarity is normal.
Clinical fluid overload – may be observed in CCF, renal failure, cirrhosis, nephrotic syndrome.
Diuretic therapy – thiazide and loop diuretics may produce excessive loss of both sodium and water, reflected by an overall decrease in serum sodium.
Salt-wasting nephropathy – a rare cause of hyponatraemia that may be responsive to treatment with fludrocortisone.
Syndrome of Inappropriate Anti-diuretic Hormone (SIADH) – may be seen with several types of carcinoma (especially lung cancer), COAD, tuberculosis and stroke. Also associated with some drugs.

Hyponatraemia can be acute or chronic. The acute form is relatively uncommon and can be very serious, particularly when serum sodium concentration is less than 120 mmol/L. Acute hyponatraemia develops within 48 hours and requires rapid treatment. If left untreated, serious complications such as cerebral oedema, brainstem herniation and death may result.

Hyponatraemia may be caused by drug therapy in several different ways, with the most common being excessive salt/water loss associated with diuretics. Another cause of hyponatraemia that is of interest to clinical pharmacists is the Syndrome of Inappropriate Anti-diuretic Hormone (SIADH), where there is either production of excessive ADH (or an ADH-like compound), or the kidneys become abnormally responsive to normal ADH levels. The vast majority of SIADH cases is not drug-related, but in some, SIADH may be an adverse effect of drug treatment. Examples of drugs that may cause

SIADH include carbamazepine, selective serotonin re-uptake inhibitors (SSRIs) and other anti-depressants, narcotics and some anti-neoplastic drugs. The best management for SIADH is to address the underlying cause, and in drug-related SIADH this will require withdrawal of the implicated medication. Where the underlying cause cannot be reversed (for example, advanced lung cancer), treatment may involve fluid restriction or the administration of demeclocycline, a drug which antagonises the effects of ADH in the renal tubule.

Serum Potassium (reference range 3.4–4.8 mmol/L)

Hypokalaemia: Hypokalaemia is the term used to describe a situation where serum potassium concentration is below the lower limit of the reference range. Vomiting, diarrhoea and gastric suction are all common causes of hypokalaemia. Hypokalaemia may be drug related, with the most commonly implicated agents being thiazide and loop diuretics (which may also cause hypomagnesaemia). Overuse of laxative agents may also cause hypokalaemia. Patients treated with digoxin are particularly vulnerable to the effects of hypokalaemia, as a low serum potassium concentration accentuates the effects of digoxin upon the myocardium (this is particularly the case with digoxin toxicity).

If hypokalaemia is severe or persistent, or if the patient is treated with digoxin, some form of potassium replacement may be required. Intravenous potassium should always be diluted in a large volume of fluid and infused slowly, as the delivery of potassium chloride as a rapid intravenous push is likely to cause serious and dangerous cardiac arrhythmias. The conventional approach is to dilute 20–30 mmol of KCl in 1000 ml of infusion fluid (for example, normal saline or 5% dextrose) and infuse over six to eight hours. If intravenous replacement is not needed, another approach is to administer an oral potassium supplement or a potassium sparing agent such as amiloride. All potassium replacement therapy should be regularly monitored to ensure that serum potassium is maintained within safe limits.

Hyperkalaemia: Hyperkalaemia (serum potassium concentration higher than the reference range) is potentially a very dangerous electrolyte abnormality that may require urgent intervention. It is important to note that the red blood cells have very high potassium content, and if a blood sample has not been analysed promptly, lysis of the erythrocytes (haemolysis) may cause the factitious elevation of serum potassium. Even so, an urgent electrocardiogram should be obtained if there is any suspicion of significant hyperkalaemia – peaked T waves on the ECG are indicative of a need for urgent intervention.

Hyperkalaemia is a finding of interest for clinical pharmacists from several perspectives:

- Serious cardiac effects (described above) may require special attention if hyperkalaemia is significant.
- Pharmacists may be called upon to provide advice in relation to the management of hyperkalaemia, which may include the administration of intravenous glucose +/– insulin, treatment with a cation exchange resin, or even the use of haemodialysis.
- Hyperkalaemia may be drug related. The injudicious or combined use of

potassium supplements, potassium-sparing diuretics, ACE inhibitors, angiotensin receptor antagonists and NSAIDs is relatively commonly implicated.

- Hyperkalaemia is commonly present in acute renal failure, which in itself is an important finding for reasons described elsewhere in this chapter.

Serum Calcium (reference range 2.20–2.55 mmol/L or 8.8–10.2 mg/dL)

Approximately half of the serum calcium is bound to proteins; the remainder is unbound or 'ionised' calcium. The total serum calcium (bound plus unbound) can be misleading in the presence of hypoalbuminaemia, and it is sometimes necessary to consider the 'corrected' calcium value. The corrected calcium is reported to reflect the fact that there is an increased proportion of total calcium that is present as unbound (physiologically active) ions in the presence of hypoalbuminaemia. If the corrected calcium is not reported by the laboratory, it can be estimated as described in Figure 11.2.

In general, each 1 g/dL of albumin binds about 0.8 mg/dL (0.2 mmol/L) of calcium. To correct for hypoalbuminaemia, 0.8 mg/dL must be added to the total calcium concentration for each 1g/dL decrease in albumin concentration from the normal 4.0 g/dL.

Figure 11.2 Calculation of corrected serum calcium

$$Ca_{corr}\ (mg/dL) = \{(4.0 - \text{albumin g/dL}) \times 0.8\ mg/dL\} + Ca_{uncorr}\ (mg/dL)$$

Multiply result by 0.25 to convert to mmol/L.

Hypocalcaemia: Falsely low levels of calcium due to hypoalbuminaemia should be excluded by measuring ionised calcium. Common causes of decreased total serum calcium are Vitamin D deficiency, hypoparathyroidism and chronic renal failure. Vitamin D deficiency may be due to poor nutrition, inadequate exposure to sunlight or treatment with some anti-convulsant or anti-tubercular drugs. In chronic renal failure, decreased renal conversion of Vitamin D to its activated form 1,25-dihydroxyvitamin D_3 leads to reduced intestinal calcium absorption.

Hypercalcaemia: Hypercalcaemia may result from overuse of vitamin D therapy, or other drug-related causes such as thiazide treatment and the so-called 'milk alkali syndrome'. Symptoms of hypercalcaemia may include constipation, confusion, conjunctivitis, drowsiness, lethargy and polyuria. Probably the most common reason for seriously elevated serum calcium concentration is the release of calcium from bones in advanced malignancy as a result of paraneoplastic effects or bone lysis from metastatic spread. In these circumstances, adequate hydration (sometimes using intravenous fluids) may be effective, but in other cases it may be necessary to administer drugs such as disodium pamidronate to address the problem and provide symptomatic relief. Hypercalcaemia in the context of significant renal dysfunction with hyperphosphatemia is particularly significant because of the risk that calcium phosphate may precipitate in small blood vessels with catastrophic consequences.

Liver Function Tests

The term liver function tests is commonly used to describe a set of laboratory investigations that are performed to assess the state of health of the patient's liver. Liver function tests (LFTs) are not always an accurate indicator of the current functional capacity of the liver. Rather, elevation of LFTs is indicative of damage (and to some extent, malfunction) of liver cells (hepatocytes) or the liver's histological architecture (for example, the bile canaliculi).

The majority of the parameters that are used as LFTs are actually enzymes that are normally present in high concentrations within hepatocytes. The presence of elevated serum concentration of one or more of these enzymes suggests that hepatocytes have lysed in response to some form of noxious insult, releasing the cell contents to circulate in the blood.

The extent to which the serum concentrations of these enzymes are elevated above the upper limit of the reference range is proportional to the number of hepatocytes that have been damaged. Given the substantial functional reserve of the liver, the operating capacity of this organ may be maintained even when there has been substantial or acute damage.

Commonly used LFTs include gamma glutaryl transferase (GGT), alkaline phosphatase (ALP), lactate dehydrogenase (LDH), alanine aminotransferase (ALT) and aspartate aminotransferase (AST). Reference ranges for LFTs are summarised in Table 11.2.

The other indicator of hepatic function that is commonly examined is the serum bilirubin concentration. Elevation of serum bilirubin may reflect impaired movement of bilirubin through the biliary tree to the gall bladder, but may also be associated with haemolysis or with impaired removal of unconjugated bilirubin from circulation by the liver. Predominant elevation of ALP and GGT with or without a rise in bilirubin and ALT/AST is sometimes referred to as a '*cholestatic picture*' and may be caused by gallstones or obstruction of the common bile duct (for example, carcinoma of the head of the pancreas). Drugs may also cause cholestasis, with the implicated agents including some steroids (including contraceptives), chlorpromazine, erythromycin, flucloxacillin and others.

Table 11.2 Reference ranges for LFTs

Gamma glutaryl transferase	(GGT)	<30 u/L
Alkaline phosphatase	(ALP)	30–120 u/L
Lactate dehydrogenase	(LDH)	50–150 u/L
Alanine aminotransferase	(ALT)	<30 u/L
Aspartate aminotransferase	(AST)	<30 u/L
Bilirubin	(Bili)	0.1–10.0 mg/dL (2–18 mmol/L)

Predominant elevation of the hepatic enzymes AST and ALT in the absence of elevated bilirubin is often referred to as a '*hepatitic picture*' and may be due to a variety of causes including viral disease (especially viral hepatitis A, B or C), the toxic effects of many drugs (for example, some anti-convulsants, antibiotics and anti-tubercular agents) or chemicals, or the effects of alcohol. Occasionally, features consistent with both cholestasis and hepatitis may be present simultaneously, with this referred to as a '*mixed picture*'.

In the presence of severe and chronic liver damage, the synthetic capacity of the liver may be compromised. When this happens, the circulating concentrations of proteins produced by the liver are decreased. This may be reflected by low serum albumin concentration, although it is important to note that there are many other possible explanations for this finding (for example, malnutrition, urinary loss in the context of nephrotic syndrome). Similarly, the liver's capacity to produce clotting factors may be reduced if the extent of liver damage is severe. This may be reflected in prolonged clotting time (prothrombin time), a syndrome sometimes referred to as *coagulopathy*.

It is important for clinical pharmacists to monitor a patient's LFTs, mostly as a way to detect adverse effects of drugs, such as drug-induced hepatitis. LFTs are not commonly used as a basis for drug dose adjustment because drug clearance is one aspect of hepatic function that is usually preserved even in the context of moderately severe liver damage. Even so, in the presence of advanced liver disease (like cirrhosis) or acute severe hepatitis, it may be prudent to adjust the dose of drugs where hepatic clearance is the dominant elimination pathway. It is also advisable to select drugs that have uncomplicated metabolic clearance pathways that do not involve the formation of active metabolites.

Blood Glucose (reference range for fasting blood glucose 3.9–6.1 mmol/L or 70–110 mg/dL)

The blood glucose level (BGL) is an important biochemical parameter that is routinely measured in the course of patient assessment. By far the most common cause of an abnormal BGL result is diabetes mellitus, where abnormal glucose metabolism results in chronic elevation of BGL (hyperglycaemia) that may cause a wide range of serious complications such as cardiovascular disease, peripheral neuropathy, renal impairment and retinopathy resulting in damage to eyesight.

A BGL result above the reference range does not necessarily imply that the patient has diabetes mellitus. Because BGLs are influenced by the intake of carbohydrates and other energy sources, the result should be interpreted with reference to food intake. The fasting BGL is a more sensitive indicator of impaired glucose metabolism, and it is this result that is most commonly used to establish a diagnosis of diabetes mellitus. Alternatively, a glucose tolerance test may be used for this diagnosis: the patient consumes a standardised glucose load (often 75 g) and the BGL is measured subsequently.

Measurement of BGLs is routinely used as a means to monitor the response to treatment administered for diabetes. Even with drug treatment, it is often not possible to maintain BGLs within the usual reference range, but the aim of treatment is to maintain BGLs at a level close to the upper limit of the reference range. Particularly in older patients, it is unwise to pursue very tight control over BGLs, as overtreatment may results in low BGL (hypoglycaemia). Conversely, for younger patients (where there are substantial benefits to be gained from a reduction in risk of diabetic complications), clinicians often aim for tighter BGL control.

Long-term control of diabetes is usually monitored by measuring the proportion of haemoglobin present in the glycosylated form (HbA_{1c}), generally expressed as a percentage of overall haemoglobin. HbA_{1c} levels less than 7% of total haemoglobin indicate that control of BGLs over the three months preceding the test has been good.

Measurement of urinary glucose may also be used as an indirect marker of elevated BGLs. Not usually performed as a quantitative assay, this test is more commonly undertaken to demonstrate the presence of a significant amount of glucose in urine (glycosuria). Glycosuria may occur when BGL exceeds the renal threshold for reabsorption (about 10 mmol/L), a finding associated with chronic elevation of BGLs (for example, with diabetes mellitus).

However, urinary glucose testing provides no information about blood glucose levels below the renal threshold and so cannot be used to detect hypoglycaemia. It is not always an accurate marker of elevated BGL: other conditions may also result in glycosuria, with the most common example being glycosuria associated with normal pregnancy. For these reasons, blood glucose measurements have largely replaced urinary glucose testing, and are preferred because of their superior specificity and quantitative capacity.

Drugs may have a profound effect upon BGLs in some cases. The most common cause of drug-related hypoglycaemia is the use of anti-diabetic medications, including insulin. Particularly during acute illness and hospitalisation, oral intake (including food intake) may be significantly diminished; so if insulin or other anti-diabetic treatment is not modified, hypoglycaemia may result. When this situation can be anticipated (for example, around the time of major surgery), regular treatment may be suspended and an adjustable dosage regimen of a rapid acting insulin may be used together with regular BGL measurements – this is sometimes called a '*sliding scale*' insulin regimen.

Another increasingly popular approach is the so-called '*basal–bolus*' regimen, which can provide even better control of BGL. Here the basal insulin requirement is provided by a once-daily injection of a long-acting insulin, and post-prandial peaks in blood glucose are managed using regular injections of an ultra-fast acting insulin immediately before meals.

Drugs may also impair glucose tolerance and, in some cases, hyperglycaemia may result. Examples of drugs that may cause hyperglycaemia include corticosteroids and some diuretics. An episode of hyperglycaemia during treatment with a drug known to cause elevated BGLs does not constitute grounds for a diagnosis of diabetes mellitus. However, it is possible that such patients may have impaired glucose tolerance or sub-clinical diabetes.

Blood Picture

The blood picture – variously referred to as the complete blood picture (CBP), complete blood examination (CBE), full blood picture (FBP), full blood examination (FBE) and complete blood count (CBC) – is a panel of haematological investigations that provides information about the characteristics of blood cells in peripheral circulation. The individual elements of the CBP are described in detail below.

Haemoglobin (reference range 13.5–17.5 g/dL for men, 12.0–16.0 g/dL for women)

The haemoglobin (Hb) content of blood determines its oxygen carrying capacity and is of particular importance for patients with diseases such as obstructive airways disease or congestive heart failure, where a small decrease in the haemoglobin may have a major influence on functional capacity. The reference range for the concentration of haemoglobin in peripheral blood varies with age, with different ranges quoted for neonates and young children. The Hb concentration may be above the upper limit of the range in a condition called polycythemia rubra vera, but may also be elevated in patients who live at high altitudes or those with chronic hypoxic lung disease such as chronic obstructive pulmonary disease.

Of greater importance to the clinical pharmacist are the situations where the Hb is significantly below the lower limit of the reference range: a condition usually referred to as anaemia (the patient is said to be anaemic). The underlying cause of anaemia may sometimes be clarified by referring to other elements of the CBP that identify features of red cell morphology, with particular focus on the size of erythrocytes and their haemoglobin content (Table 11.3). Two important red cell parameters are the mean cell volume (MCV) and mean cell haemoglobin content (MCHC), which are described in Table 11.4.

Microcytic anaemia: One common form of anaemia is the type where low Hb occurs with low MCV (microcytosis) and/or low MCHC (hypochromic cells). Microcytic, hypochromic anaemia is the form that is most often associated with iron deficiency, which may itself occur through a number of mechanisms. Iron deficiency secondary to inadequate dietary intake is common in developing countries, but is uncommon in developed nations. This type of iron deficiency may be related to malnutrition or a vegetarian diet. Another cause of iron deficiency is malabsorption of iron, which may occur in coeliac disease, giardiasis or following gastric bypass surgery.

Iron deficiency with microcytic anaemia may also occur as a result of large and/or sustained blood loss, where the haemoglobin that has been lost to the patient represents a significant proportion of the total body stores of iron. This type of picture may be expected in the recovery phase after substantial blood loss secondary to trauma or major surgery, but may also follow chronic, low-level blood loss. The frequently encountered examples of this type of blood loss include chronic gastrointestinal bleeding (for example, bleeding gastritis or peptic ulcer, occult malignancy in the lower GIT), ongoing haemoptysis (such as that seen in tuberculosis), substantial haematuria or blood loss secondary to hookworm infection.

It is important to determine the underlying cause if possible, by testing for the presence of occult blood in the stool, as well as other investigations. If a significant cause can be identified, specific therapy can often be implemented, such as treatment of a peptic ulcer with acid-suppressive therapy. If the haemoglobin is very low, it may be necessary to provide a blood transfusion, particularly if the patient is symptomatic. Thereafter, it is necessary to administer long-term iron supplementation by mouth to replenish the iron stores. Drug therapy may contribute to the development of iron deficiency anaemia: warfarin, aspirin and NSAIDs may exacerbate bleeding and, in the case of the latter two examples, may also damage the gastrointestinal tract leading to GI bleeding.

Normocytic anaemia: When both the MCV and the MCHC are within the reference range, the condition is referred to as normocytic, normochromic anaemia. Sometimes referred to as anaemia of chronic disease, this condition

Table 11.3 Laboratory findings for microcytic, normocytic and macrocytic anaemia (↓ = decreased, ↑ = increased, → = no change)

	Microcytic anaemia	Normocytic anaemia	Macrocytic anaemia
RBC	↓	↓	↓
Hb	↓	↓	↓
MCV	↓	↓ →	↑
MCHC	↓	↓ →	→
Common causes	• Iron deficiency due to poor dietary intake, malabsorption of iron, or chronic blood loss	• Acute blood loss • Haemolytic anaemia • Anaemia of chronic disease	• Vitamin B_{12} deficiency • Folic acid deficiency • Drug-induced bone marrow toxicity

Table 11.4 Red cell morphology parameters

Mean Cell/Corpuscular Volume (MCV): Reference range 80–100 fL • Estimates the average volume of red blood cells • Calculated by dividing the packed cell volume/red cell count • Expressed in femtolitres (fL)
Mean Cell/Corpuscular Haemoglobin Concentration (MCHC): Reference range 33–37 g/dL • Estimates the weight of haemoglobin per volume of cells • Calculated by dividing haemoglobin/packed cell volume • Expressed in g/dL

may be associated with chronic infection, rheumatoid arthritis, hypothyroidism and some forms of malignancy. In chronic renal failure, the endocrine functions of the kidneys are also compromised, meaning that the production of erythropoietin (a hormone produced by the kidneys that stimulates the production of red blood cells by the bone marrow) is reduced. Although recombinant human erythropoietin and related products can be used to treat this anaemia, the drugs are expensive and not affordable for many patients.

Another important cause of normocytic anaemia is acute blood loss. This may occur after trauma or major surgery, or can be secondary to major acute internal bleeding such as that associated with bleeding peptic ulcer. The picture is usually characterised by reduction in haemoglobin with normal MCV and MCHC. The acute reduction in haemoglobin and accompanying loss of plasma volume mean that it is important to address the underlying cause of the blood loss, and then to replace the loss using a blood transfusion.

In the event that the patient is fluid overloaded, the transfusion may be given with packed red cells, rather than whole blood (so that the fluid load is reduced). Alternatively, the transfusion may be administered with an accompanying dose of frusemide, orally or intravenously (this approach is often used for patients with congestive heart failure). Subsequently, it may also be necessary to administer iron supplements for some time (see below).

Macrocytic anaemia: When the Hb is low and is accompanied by high MCV, this is referred to as macrocytic anaemia. Macrocytosis does occur in some forms of liver disease, but the most common underlying cause for this type of anaemia is deficient dietary intake (or malabsorption) of either folic acid or Vitamin B_{12}. Both serum folate and Vitamin B_{12} concentrations should be measured when investigating macrocytic anaemia, because undetected Vitamin B_{12} deficiency can cause serious neurological complications if left untreated. Certain drugs are sometimes associated with folate deficiency, with examples including methotrexate and phenytoin.

White Cell Count (reference range 4.5–10.5 x $10^3/\mu l$)

The white cell count (WCC) is used to describe the number (and in some cases, morphology) of leucocytes circulating in peripheral blood. Total WCC may be further subdivided to provide information about the count of granular white cells (neutrophils, eosinophils and basophils) and mononuclear cells (lymphocytes and monocytes). Elevation or depression of the overall number of a particular cell line or its proportionate contribution to the total WCC may provide important additional information for use in evaluating and interpreting the WCC.

Leucopaenia is the term used to refer to the situation when the WCC is significantly lower than the reference range. When a low count of a specific cell line is the major contributor to a low WCC, this may be specifically identified (neutropaenia and lymphopaenia are terms used to denote low neutrophil and lymphocyte counts, respectively). Leucopaenia is sometimes encountered in the context of neoplastic disease, where malignant cells infiltrate the bone marrow and compromise granulopoesis. Another important cause of a low WCC is the influence of noxious insults upon the functional capacity of the bone marrow.

A very wide range of drugs may cause leucopaenia as an adverse effect, with important examples including cytotoxic and immunosupressant drugs, antibiotics, anti-convulsants, disease modifying anti-rheumatic drugs (DMARDs) and some psychotropic agents such as clozapine. For a more comprehensive list of drugs associated with leucopaenia, readers should consult a reliable reference text dealing with adverse drug reactions.

Leucopaenia is very commonly encountered during aggressive chemotherapy for some forms of cancer, and clinicians may administer a granulopoeitic agent such as filgrastim to reduce the chance of opportunistic infection and associated morbidity. Exposure to ionising radiation or certain organic chemicals found in pesticides and herbicides is another important cause of a low WCC.

There are many causes for an elevated WCC, but by far the most important is illustrated in the association with various infections. When significant infections such as urinary tract infection, bacterial pneumonia, tuberculosis, cholangitis, meningitis or cellulitis are present, the patient mounts an immune reaction directed at overcoming the pathogen (most commonly, but not always, a bacterium). The result is that the number of leucocytes present in peripheral blood increases (leucocytosis), often with a marked increase in the neutrophil count (neutrophilia).

The presence of an increased WCC, particularly if accompanied by fever or specific signs of infection, is generally indicative that some form of infection is present, although some infections (for example, typhoid fever) are not associated with leucocytosis, and may in fact be accompanied by leucopaenia.

Clinical pharmacists may also monitor the WCC as a guide to the response to treatment of an infection – a decrease in the WCC often accompanies clinical improvement. Corticosteroids and lithium are two examples of drugs that may cause an iatrogenic increase in the WCC. Another important cause for a markedly elevated WCC is the presence of a haematological malignancy. Leukaemia and lymphoma are two examples where the total WCC may be up to ten times the usual upper limit of normal.

Eosinophilia is a condition where the absolute eosinophil count and perhaps also its proportionate contribution to the total WCC are unusually high. Although eosinophilia may be encountered as a result of allergic reactions (including drug allergy), the most common causes include parasitic infections. A very high eosinophil count is sometimes encountered in tropical eosinophilia, a condition associated with a pulmonary eosinophil infiltrate. Monocytosis is a large increase in the monocyte count, and may be seen in viral diseases or tuberculosis.

Platelet Count (reference range 150–450 x $10^3/\mu l$)

A minor to moderate elevation in platelet count is rarely of clinical significance, and is often regarded as a surrogate marker for inflammatory reactions/illnesses. Decreased platelet count (thrombocytopaenia) may be seen in severe iron deficiency and is also associated with some forms of liver disease, as well as fulminant infectious diseases.

Of interest to clinical pharmacists is drug-induced thrombocytopaenia, which may arise from several mechanisms. In some cases, thrombocytopaenia is caused by a generalised toxicity that compromises the synthetic capacity of the bone marrow. This type of toxicity may be secondary to drugs (for example, cytotoxic agents) or exposure to chemicals such as pesticides. In this context, thrombocytopaenia is often accompanied by anaemia and leucopoaenia, and the constellation of results is referred to as pancytopaenia.

Another type of thrombocytopaenia related to drug therapy is that which results from the accelerated destruction and removal of platelets from circulation. Examples of drugs that produce thrombocytopaenia through this mechanism include heparin, quinine and thiazide diuretics. The decline in platelet count may often be sudden and dramatic, falling from normal levels to a nearly undetectable count in a matter of days. It is important that the causative agent is promptly discontinued and that appropriate documentation is made to prevent subsequent inadvertent re-exposure.

Other Laboratory Data

Many other laboratory tests can be of considerable usefulness to clinical pharmacists in their daily work. The erythrocyte sedimentation rate (ESR) and C-reactive protein (CRP) are both inflammatory markers that may be used by pharmacists as sensitive markers of response to treatment. Serum amylase is a sensitive marker for acute pancreatitis. The concentration of creatine kinase in the serum provides an indication of damage to muscle cells – in some cases, myocardial damage from an infarction, but in other cases from rhabdomyolysis involving skeletal muscles. Microscopy, culture and sensitivity tests used to isolate and examine the characteristics of microbial growth in blood, urine and sputum, or other media can be used to guide the selection of anti-microbial therapy. Similarly, serological markers may reveal evidence of infections such as HIV, hepatitis and others. The concentration of glucose, sodium or proteins found in fluids other than blood/serum (for example, CSF, urine, pleural effusions) may also provide a great deal of information of relevance to pharmacists. A detailed discussion of highly specialised laboratory tests is beyond the scope of this discussion, and the interested reader should refer to a specialised reference source for further information.

CASE STUDY 1

A 67-year-old retired teacher has been treated for hypertension with chlorothiazide 500 mg daily and perindopril 10 mg daily for several years. He recently presented to his doctor complaining of joint pain, for which he was prescribed diclofenac 50 mg twice daily. Several days later he returned complaining of swollen ankles, shortness of breath, headache and decreased urine output. At that time, the results of serum electrolyte investigations were as follows:

Sodium	137 mmol/L	(135–145 mmol/L)
Potassium	6.7 mmol/L	(3.4–4.8 mmol/L)
Chloride	97 mmol/L	(95–110 mmol/L)
Bicarbonate	36 mmol/L	(22–32 mmol/L)
Urea	28.2 mmol/L	(3.0–8.0 mmol/L)
Creatinine	0.720 mmol/L	(0.055–0.120 mmol/L)

What significant abnormalities are present, and what is the underlying cause for these? What action needs to be taken now?

Discussion:

The elevation in serum creatinine and urea is consistent with acute renal failure, which in this case is almost certainly secondary to treatment with diclofenac. All NSAIDs are capable of causing acute renal failure, especially in elderly patients, those concurrently treated with ACE inhibitors or diuretics, and patients who are dehydrated. For this reason, the combination of a diuretic, an ACE inhibitor or angiotension receptor blocker and an NSAID is sometimes referred to as the 'triple whammy'. Hyperkalaemia is the other abnormality of particular importance in this case. Serum potassium appears to be elevated to an extent that places the patient at serious risk of cardiac arrhythmias.

An urgent electrocardiogram should be obtained as soon as possible to check for evidence of the possible effects of hyperkalaemia upon the heart. If T wave changes are present, it will be necessary to implement an intervention to reduce the serum potassium. This can be done by the oral or rectal administration of a cation exchange resin, or if cardiac effects are marked, by the intravenous administration of glucose 50% +/– a small intravenous dose of rapid acting insulin. Depending on the clinical state of the patient, the use of some form of dialysis may also be considered, and may assist in addressing underlying electrolyte abnormalities. The patient's blood pressure should be re-assessed and treatment adjusted if uncontrolled hypertension is present. The diclofenac should be discontinued immediately, and if further treatment for joint pain is required, alternatives such as regular paracetamol should be considered. The serum electrolytes should be urgently repeated to assess the effects of any interventions, and should be monitored several times over the next 7–10 days to ensure that renal function is recovering after discontinuation of the NSAID.

CASE STUDY 2

Within hours of attending a wedding, a 45-year-old woman developed symptoms of severe nausea, vomiting, fever and profuse, watery diarrhoea. Five days later she was brought to a clinic by her son. She had eaten little since the onset of her illness, and had often vomited after drinking. She was weak, drowsy and confused. On examination, her body weight was 41 kg, her mucous membranes were found to be dry, and there was markedly decreased skin turgor. Her blood pressure was 100/65 mmHg lying and 90/50 mmHg standing. Her serum electrolytes were as follows:

Sodium	153 mmol/L	(135–145 mmol/L)
Potassium	3.0 mmol/L	(3.4–4.8 mmol/L)
Chloride	90 mmol/L	(95–110 mmol/L)
Bicarbonate	36 mmol/L	(22–32 mmol/L)
Urea	17.5 mmol/L	(3.0–8.0 mmol/L)
Creatinine	0.420 mmol/L	(0.055–0.120 mmol/L)

What is the likely clinical assessment in this case, and what management is indicated?

Discussion:

Gastroenteritis with severe dehydration has almost certainly caused renal impairment in this case. The estimated GFR is approximately 10 ml/minute and indicative of severe (presumably acute) renal insufficiency. Other findings of note include hypokalaemia, hypochloremia and hypernatraemia. The low serum potassium is likely to be related to excessive loss of potassium because of diarrhoea, and hypochloremia is probably secondary to ongoing vomiting. Significant hypernatraemia is also present, reflecting haemoconcentration arising from volume depletion and decreased oral fluid intake (because of vomiting).

The most important clinical priority is to rehydrate the patient. In view of nausea and vomiting, it is unlikely that satisfactory rehydration will be achieved by the administration of oral fluids, although if parenteral fluids are not available, the oral administration of an electrolyte replacement solution may be attempted with anti-emetic drugs used to prevent further vomiting. Preferably, however, rehydration should be undertaken with the intravenous administration of fluids (for example, 5% dextrose 1000 ml every six to eight hours). In view of hypokalaemia, 20–30 mmol of KCl may be added to each litre of intravenous fluid. The serum electrolytes should be monitored every 24–48 hours to ensure that abnormalities are resolving, and to check that the serum potassium does not rise as a result of the renal impairment that is present. Anti-nausea and anti-diarrhoeal medication may be helpful, and it may be necessary to attempt to ascertain and address the underlying cause of the gastroenteritis.

CASE STUDY 3

A 21-year-old woman from a nearby village was brought to a hospital OPD by her husband, who was concerned that she had become increasingly weak over several months, and was unable to perform her usual home duties or to care for their young children. On examination, she was found to be tremulous, weak and very short of breath, with pale conjunctiva. She did not report any unusual gastrointestinal symptoms, and her usual diet was vegetarian. Her serum electrolytes were normal, and the results of her complete blood picture were as follows:

Haemoglobin	6.2 g/dL	(12.0–16.0 g/dL)
MCV	67 fL	(80–100 fL)
MCHC	27 g/dL	(33–37 g/dL)
WCC	3.3×10^3 / microL	($4.5–10.5 \times 10^3$/microL)
Platelets	122×10^3 / microL	($150–450 \times 10^3$/microL)

What do these findings suggest, and what possible underlying explanations should be considered? What action needs to be taken now?

Discussion:

The patient has severe, symptomatic anaemia, and an accompanying mild thrombocytopaenia. The microcytic, hypochromic picture reflected by the low MCV and MCHC in this case are suggestive of iron deficiency, even more likely because of her recent pregnancy and poor dietary iron intake. The absence of gastrointestinal symptoms means that occult GI blood loss is relatively unlikely as a cause, but testing of the stools for occult blood loss would be necessary to exclude this. Hookworm infestation may also need to be considered. Measurement of serum iron parameters may also confirm the diagnosis, but on the basis of the clinical evidence available, it would be reasonable to commence therapy for iron deficiency.

In view of the severity of the anaemia and its symptoms, one possible course of action, if available, would be to provide a blood transfusion as a way to raise the haemoglobin concentration over a relatively short period of time. However, it will also be necessary to commence treatment with an iron supplement such as oral ferrous sulphate. For a faster response, or where compliance may be in question, the use of parenteral iron may be considered. A repeat CBP should be undertaken later to assess the patient's response to treatment. The possiblity of other nutritional deficiencies should also be considered.

CASE STUDY 4

A 36-year-old farmer presented to a clinic complaining of nausea, lethargy, muscle and joint pains and generalised itch. On being questioned, he revealed that he had experienced a febrile illness about a week ago, for which he had taken some antibiotics. On examination, he appeared generally unwell and mildly dehydrated, with a tender and enlarged liver, and his eyes looked yellow. The results of his liver function tests were as follows:

ALP	550 u/L	(30–120 u/L)
AST	362 u/L	(<30 u/L)
ALT	425 u/L	(<30 u/L)
GGT	2220 u/L	(<30 u/L)
Total bilirubin	86 mmol/L	(2–18 mmol/L)

What do these findings suggest? What follow-up action is required?

Discussion:

The LFTs in this case are suggestive of a mixed cholestatic/hepatic picture, and are consistent with the clinical features of hepatitis in the history and physical examination. Although there are many causes for this type of mixed picture, some of the more common causes include viral hepatitis and exposure to organic solvents and other chemicals (such as some pesticides and herbicides). The possibility of antibiotic-related hepatotoxicity should also be considered.

Follow-up action should include obtaining a thorough clinical history of exposure to chemicals and drugs. An abdominal imaging technique such as ultrasonography may be used to ascertain if obstruction of the common bile duct (for example, by gallstones) has led to cholestasis. Ultrasound may be used to establish the size and echo-texture of the liver, spleen and pancreas. Viral serology may be used to determine if an infectious cause is present – if this is the case, it will have implications for other family members and contacts of the patient.

KEY MESSAGES

- Laboratory data must always be interpreted with reference to the clinical status of the patient.
- The clinical need for intervention should always be verified before acting on the basis of a laboratory result.
- A result that falls outside a reference range does not always indicate the presence of disease, nor does a result within a reference range guarantee the absence of pathology.
- The best way to accumulate knowledge about the interpretation of laboratory data is to continually check reliable reference texts to clarify any information that is not familiar.

Further Reading

Basic Skills in Interpreting Laboratory Data. 2009. Lee M ed. 4th edition. American Society of Health-System Pharmacists: Bethesda, USA. (*A comprehensive review of the interpretation of laboratory data, supplemented by numerous case studies of particular value. Specifically designed for use by pharmacists.)*

Harrison's Principles of Internal Medicine. 2008. Fauci AS, Braunwald E, Kasper DL, Hauser J and Jameson J (eds). 17th Edition. McGraw Hill: New York, USA. (*Probably the world's most respected textbook dealing with internal medicine. Many informative chapters that provide important information about the interpretation of laboratory data.)*

Websites of Interest

The Royal College of Pathologists of Australasia Manual

The online version of the fifth edition of the Manual of Use and Interpretation of Pathology Tests, produced by the Royal College of Pathologists of Australasia. A comprehensive guide to a wide range of laboratory tests and their interpretation.

http://www.rcpamanual.edu.au

The Internet Pathology Laboratory for Medical Education

Website from the University of Utah with an excellent range of resources including tutorials and case studies. Includes a useful section dealing with HIV/AIDs pathology.

http://www-medlib.med.utah.edu/WebPath/webpath.html#organ2

12 Interpreting Laboratory Data: Infectious Diseases

Jeff Hughes

Learning Objectives

Upon completion of this chapter, the reader should be able to:

- List the tests commonly used in the diagnosis of infectious diseases
- Use laboratory tests to assess the severity of selected infectious diseases
- Select laboratory tests which may be used in the monitoring of the appropriateness of anti-microbial therapy
- Use laboratory tests to monitor the toxicity of selected anti-microbials
- Develop plans incorporating laboratory tests to monitor the progress of patients with infectious diseases

The term infectious diseases covers all the diseases caused by bacteria, fungi, viruses and parasites. Infectious diseases are among the leading causes of death worldwide, and are also a leading cause of morbidity. This group of diseases is encountered in all areas of clinical pharmacy practice, and hence all clinical pharmacists must have a sound knowledge of the signs and symptoms, pathophysiology and treatment of common infections.

The clinical pharmacist can contribute to the management of patients with an infectious disease by ensuring the appropriate choice of anti-infective agent, that the correct dose and route of administration is used, and appropriate patient monitoring is performed. The pharmacist needs to understand the role of laboratory tests in the diagnosis and monitoring of patients with infections, and be able to use laboratory test data in the assessment of the appropriateness and effectiveness of anti-microbial therapy.

It is important to appreciate that the patient's clinical status (for example, temperature, blood pressure, heart rate, renal function, mental status) must always be taken into consideration when interpreting any laboratory test result. Laboratory test results can be used as markers of the severity of disease (for example, white cell count <4 x 10^9/L or >30 x 10^9/L is a marker of severe pneumonia) and as prognostic indicators. They may also be used to guide the appropriate choice of anti-microbial agents and to monitor progress of the infection and response to treatment.

Confirmation of Infection

One of the most difficult tasks in the diagnosis of infectious diseases is the differentiation between infection and colonisation. *Colonisation* may be defined as the invasiveness of an organism without disease in the host. *Infection* implies the presence of an organism within the tissues that evokes a *response* in the host's defence mechanisms.

Table 12.1 Examples of common colonising flora

Skin	**Upper Respiratory Tract**
Diphtheroids (for example, *Corynebacterium* sp)	*Bacteroides* sp *Hemophilus* sp
Propionibacteriaceae	*Neisseria* sp
Staphylococci	Streptococci
Streptococci	**Genital Tract**
Gastrointestinal Tract	*Corynebacterium* sp
Bacteroides sp	Enterobacteriaceae
Clostridium sp	*Lactobacillus* sp
Diphtheroids	*Mycoplasma* sp
Enterobacteriaceae (for example, *Escherichia coli, Klebsiella* sp)	Enterobacteriaceae
Fusobacterium sp	
Streptococc*i* (anaerobic)	

Table 12.1 lists some of the common colonising organisms and the associated sites. It should be remembered, however, that under the right conditions (for example, trauma to the skin, immunosuppression secondary to anti-cancer or immunosuppressive medications), colonising organisms may become pathogens.

Colonising organisms may also contribute to diagnostic problems, as specimen contamination may result in a false positive result. This is particularly important when samples are taken from the urinary tract, skin and soft tissue, blood and respiratory tract.

Non-specific Tests

White cell count and differential: The white cell count (WCC) represents the total number of leukocytes present in peripheral circulation (reference range 4–11 x 10^9/L), where the leukocytes are made up of neutrophils, lymphocytes, basophils, monocytes and eosinophils. The differential refers to the proportion of the total leukocyte count contributed by each of the above elements. When using the WCC as an indicator of possible infection, both the total count and those of the individual components must be taken into consideration. A patient may have a normal WCC, yet a change in the differential (for example, increased proportion of neutrophils) may be indicative of infection (Table 12.2).

Table 12.2 Normal white blood cell differential in an adult

	Absolute Count	Normal
Proportion		
Total (adults)	4–11 x 10^9/L	
Differential		
Neutrophils (PMNs*)	2.0–7.5 x 10^9/L	50–70%
Immature neutrophils (bands, stabs)		3–5%
Metamyelocytes		0–1%
Basophils	0–0.2 x 10^9/L	0–1%
Eosinophils	0.1–0.5 x 10^9/L	0–5%
Lymphocytes	1.5–4 x 10^9/L	20–40%
Monocytes	0.2–1 x 10^9/L	0–7%

* Polymorphonuclear leukocytes

Neutrophils are also known as granulocytes or segmented neutrophils, and are the main defender of the body against infection and antigens. High levels may indicate an active infection; a low count may indicate a compromised immune system or depressed bone marrow (low neutrophil production).

Neutrophilia (neutrophil count >7.5 x 10^9/L) may be caused by acute bacterial infection, trauma, myocardial infarction, chronic bacterial infection, leukaemia and certain drugs, notably corticosteroids, lithium and colony-stimulating factors. Neutropaenia (neutrophil count <1.5 x 10^9/L) and agranulocytosis (neutrophil count <0.25 x 10^9/L) place the patient at increased risk of infection. Depression of neutrophil count may occur due to drugs (for example, cytotoxic agents, ticlopidine, anti-thyroid agents, ganciclovir, clozapine), overwhelming bacterial infection, vitamin B_{12} and folate deficiency, salmonellosis or pertussis.

Lymphocytes are involved in protecting the body from viral infections such as measles, rubella, chickenpox or infectious mononucleosis, where elevations are seen. Lymphocytosis (>4 x 10^9/L) may also be encountered in tuberculosis, pertussis, toxoplasmosis, brucellosis, syphilis, lymphocytic leukaemias, and lead, carbon disulfide, tetrachloroethane and arsenical poisoning. Drugs may also cause elevations in the lymphocyte count; these include aspirin, griseofulvin, haloperidol, levodopa, niacinamide and phenytoin.

Lymphopaenia (<1 x 10^9/L) may occur in patients with HIV/AIDS, Hodgkin's lymphoma and aplastic anaemia, and following radiation exposure. Lymphocytes are highly sensitive to whole body irradiation. Drugs may also cause lymphopaenia, particularly corticosteroids, lithium, methysergide and niacin.

Lymphocytes are made up of a number of subtypes. CD4+ T cells act as regulators and 'helper' cells in the initiation and potentiation of immune reactions. Opportunistic infections (such as *Pneumocystis carinii* pneumonia) become more likely when the number of CD4+ T cells drops to or below a critically low value. Corticosteroids and cytotoxic drugs may both decrease CD4+ counts and consequently increase the risk of opportunistic infections. In addition, after intensive chemotherapy, regeneration of CD4+ T cell numbers is slow compared with other lymphocyte populations.

CD8+ cells are cytotoxic lymphocytes which regulate immune function but do not initiate or help immune response. They play important roles in the response to viral infections such as infectious mononucleosis, cytomegalovirus and herpes simplex virus II infections. The CD8+ T cell count may also increase rapidly after bone marrow graft, suggesting a role in graft-versus-host disease. CD8+ cells usually participate in T cell-mediated immune reactions and may therefore play a crucial role in some autoimmune diseases. The question of whether there is a critically low value for CD8+ cells below which normal immune function is not possible remains to be answered.

Monocytes are helpful in fighting severe infections and are considered the body's second linc of defence against infection. They are the largest cells in the bloodstream. Elevated levels (>0.8 x10^9/L) may be seen in the recovery phase of acute bacterial infection, as well as in diseases characterised by chronic granulomatous inflammation (tuberculosis, syphilis, brucellosis, Crohn's disease and sarcoidosis), ulcerative colitis, systemic lupus erythromatosus, rheumatoid arthritis, polyarteritis nodosa, and many haematologic neoplasms. Poisoning with certain agents such as carbon disulfide, phosphorus and tetrachloroethane, as well as administration of griseofulvin, haloperidol and ethosuximide, may cause monocytosis.

Eosinophilia (>0.5 x 10^9/L) is usually associated with allergic disorders (for example, asthma, drug reactions) and parasitic infections. A low eosinophil count (eosinopaenia <0.05 x 10^9/L) may be seen in the early phase of acute insults, for example, with shock, major pyogenic infections, trauma and surgery. Drugs such as corticosteroids, epinephrine, methysergide, niacin, niacinamide and procainamide may produce eosinopaenia.

Basophilic activity is not fully understood; however, basophils are known to carry histamine, heparin and serotonin. Basophils are probably involved in immediate as well as delayed hypersensitivity reactions. High levels are found in chronic inflammation and certain leukaemias.

Other Tests

Other non-specific tests that may be useful in confirming the clinical diagnosis of infection are shown in Table 12.3. The most commonly used test is C-reactive protein (CRP). It is the most useful of the acute phase reactants, rising sharply within cight hours of tissue damage by infection, infarction, inflammation or trauma. It returns to normal two days after disease activity has ceased. It is more useful than ESR, which rises and falls slowly. It can be used as an indicator of occult bacterial infection, suspected rheumatic fever, inflammatory bowel disease or other conditions where there is uncertainty whether symptoms are functional or due to organic disease. Chronic inflammatory diseases such as SLE can be monitored using serial CRPs and for this purpose it is a more useful test than ESR.

Mild elevation in CRP (10–40 nmg/L, reference range <5 mg/L) is suggestive of inflammatory conditions such as viral infections, rheumatoid arthritis and neoplasms. Marked elevations (40–300 mg/L) are highly suggestive of bacterial infections. However, there is considerable overlap in values between conditions, hence interpretation will depend on whether or not a baseline CRP has been established for the patient and on whether a series or a single CRP result is available.

The erythrocyte sedimentation rate (ESR) is often markedly elevated in acute or chronic infections, particularly endocarditis, chronic osteomyelitis and intra-abdominal infections.

However, the absence of an elevated ESR does not exclude the presence of infection. Serum complement concentrations, particularly the C3 component, are often reduced in serious infection due to consumption in the host defence processes. All other non-specific parameters may be used to monitor the efficacy of anti-microbial treatment.

Table 12.3 Some non-specific laboratory tests used in the diagnosis of infectious disease

White blood cell count
C-reactive protein
Erythrocyte sedimentation rate (ESR, sedimentation rate)
Procalcitonin
Serum complement
Other acute phase reactants (haptoglobin, α_1-anti-trypsin, fibrinogen)

Serum procalcitonin (PCT) levels may be used to estimate the probability that an infection is bacterial in origin, and hence direct antibiotic therapy. PCT, a protein precursor of the hormone calcitonin, is involved in calcium homeostasis, and is produced by the C cells of the thyroid gland. It is there that procalcitonin is cleaved into calcitonin, to form katacalcin and a protein residue.

In healthy individuals, it is not released into the bloodstream. However, in severe infections which elicit a systemic response, the blood levels of procalcitonin may rise to 1 μg/L. Results of a meta analysis suggest that elevated serum procalcitonin levels have 76% sensitivity and 70% specificity when used to diagnose bacterial infections. The following cut-off points have been suggested when using procalcitonin levels to assess the likelihood of bacterial infection: <0.1 mg/L – very unlikely, 0.1–0.25 mg/L – unlikely; 0.25–0.5 mg/L – likely and > 0.5 mg/L – very likely (See Figure 1. PCT algorithm for antibiotic stewardship–www.jama.com).

Identification of Pathogens

Identification of the infecting pathogens provides the definitive diagnosis of infection. Ideally, this is achieved by growth of the organism; however, in some cases, this may not be possible or desirable. In such cases, diagnosis is based on serological evidence.

Direct examination: One of the most rapid methods of identifying pathogens is the direct microscopic examination of body fluids or tissues thought to be infected. It is essential that the appropriate sample be taken and that potential contamination be avoided (for example, mid-stream urine sample to eliminate bacterial contamination in the lower urethra).

The Gram stain is the most commonly used differential stain for determining cell morphology. Differential stains allow for distinguishing certain characteristics of cells, and the stains commonly use two or more stains. The Gram stain, which divides most clinically significant bacteria into two main groups (Gram positives and Gram negatives) is the first step in bacterial identification. Certain other bacteria (for example, mycobacterium) and fungal pathogens may be identified microscopically using special stains or reagents. In the case of parasites, microscopy may be used to identify ova (for example, ancylostomiasis, ascariasis), larvae (aniskiasis, fasciolopsiasis) or the mature parasite (for example, malaria, fasciolopsiasis) depending on the infecting organism.

In the case of viruses, the clinical specimen may be examined directly for the presence of virus particles, virus antigens, viral nucleic acids and virus-induced histological changes. These direct examination methods have the advantage of being able to deliver a result in a short length of time, often within 24 hours. With the availability of specific anti-viral chemotherapy (for example, neuraminidase inhibitors), this is becoming an increasingly important consideration. These tests are often labour intensive and require experienced personnel. However, this is likely to change with the arrival of simple automated molecular biology techniques.

Current commercial examples include the PCR-based Roche Amplicor system, Abbott LCR system and the Chiron branched DNA system. Indeed, the Roche Amplicor and Chiron branched DNA systems are now widely used to determine HIV viral load. Currently the tests are very expensive. However, when the costs come down, they should gain widespread acceptance in the virology laboratory.

The importance of molecular techniques became evident with the SARS crisis in 2003 when PCR assays were rapidly developed and were the mainstay of diagnosis. It took several weeks before antibodies were detectable and serology was used to confirm infection and for epidemiological research.

Culture: Growth and subsequent identification of pathogens from body fluids or tissues remains the most frequently used method of determining the aetiology of infection. When culturing organisms, it is essential that the appropriate samples and the correct sampling and handling procedures are used to avoid contamination of the sample or possible death of the infecting organism.

Once growth of the pathogen is established, fermentation properties, morphology and staining and growth characteristics on selective media may be used to identify it. It is important to appreciate that a negative culture does not always imply no infection, as use of selective growth media may exclude unsuspected pathogens.

Indirect examination is one of three methods used in the diagnosis of viral infections (the other two are direct examination and serology). In this case, the virus in the clinical specimen is amplified by growing it in tissue culture, eggs or animals. Cell culture is by far the most commonly used method. Changes such as cytopathic effect (CPE) or the ability to haemadsorb may be used to reveal the presence of the growing virus. The identity of the isolated virus can be further confirmed by various tests, for example, virus neutralisation, immunofluorescence, complement-fixation, electron microscopy, etc.

The obvious disadvantage of virus isolation is the length of time required for the CPE or the ability to haemadsorb to become apparent, which may take a few days to a few weeks. It may take longer if confirmatory tests such as virus neutralisation are to be carried out. However, rapid culture methods such as the detection of early antigen fluorescence foci (DEAFF) tests for cytomegalovirus (CMV) are becoming available whereby the cell culture is examined for the presence of CMV early antigens by fluorescent antibody technique. Another problem with virus culture is that the sensitivity is often low and depends to a large extent on the quality of the clinical specimen received. Also, virus isolation would not be applicable to viruses which are difficult or cannot be cultivated such as hepatitis B and parvovirus. Moreover, there is considerable expense and expertise involved in setting up a cell culture facility, particular those that meet biosafety level II and level III standards.

Identification of pathogens allows targetting of anti-microbial therapy based on either local susceptibility patterns (empirical therapy) or further sensitivity testing (definitive therapy).

Immunological testing: In a number of instances, it is neither feasible nor possible to culture the infecting agent. In such cases, immunological testing is often used to confirm the clinical diagnosis. These techniques detect the presence of antibodies directed against specific pathogens, for example, human immunodeficiency virus – HIV/AIDS, *Helicobacter pylori* – peptic ulcer disease, Epstein–Barr virus – glandular fever, *Legionella pneumophilia* – Legionnaires', disease, Hepatitis B surface antigen – hepatitis B, Influenza virus – influenza.

These tests can be carried out on serum (serology) or on samples of body fluids or tissues. One limitation is that patients may have antibodies without clinical infection, thus it is normal practice to repeat serological tests two weeks after the initial test to determine whether there has been a rise or fall in the antibody titre. A rise is indicative of ongoing infection and a fall of convalescence.

Serology remains the bulk of the work carried out by a routine diagnostic virus laboratory. A large variety of serological tests are available; for example, complement-fixation (CFT), haemagglutination-inhibition (HAI), enzyme-linked immunoassay (EIA), radioimmunoassay (RIA), particle agglutination, immunofluorescence (IF), single radial haemolysis, Western blot, etc. The sensitivity and specificity varies greatly between different techniques. Most techniques will detect all classes of antibodies whereas some assays like RIA, EIA and IF can be made to detect one specific class only, that is, IgM, IgG or IgA.

The following virus infections are usually diagnosed by serology and are likely to remain so in the foreseeable future:

- **Hepatitis viruses:** Hepatitis A, B and C infections are usually diagnosed by serology as these viruses cannot be routinely cultured. Current serological tests including the test for HBsAg are well established and despite the availability of molecular biological techniques for the detection of viral nucleic acid, serology is unlikely to be challenged as the main means of diagnosis.
- **HIV:** HIV infection is normally diagnosed by serology. The only instance when serology cannot be relied on is in diagnosing HIV infection in the newborn.
- **Rubella and parvovirus:** Rubella and parvovirus infections are usually diagnosed by serology. The rubella virus is difficult to isolate and parvovirus cannot be isolated by routine cell culture. The onset of clinical symptoms for these infections coincides with the appearance of antibodies and thus there is little need for other means of diagnosis.
- **EBV:** Although EBV serology is reliable, the heterophile antibody test is usually used for diagnosing cases of infectious mononucleosis.

Some virus infections may be diagnosed by serology but it is not the method of choice. These include herpesviruses that reactivate from time to time to cause disease, and respiratory and enteroviruses where the illness has passed by the time the antibody is detectable. Direct and indirect detection methods are commonly used for these viruses and molecular biology techniques are likely to play an increasingly important role in the diagnosis of these viral infections.

- **Herpes simplex virus (HSV):** Although CFT and other serological tests are available for HSV, these infections are usually diagnosed by cell culture. Electron microscopy, immunofluorescence and PCR are available as rapid diagnostic methods. Serology is not very reliable for HSV infections, in particular, reactivations.
- **Cytomegalovirus (CMV):** Although serology is available for diagnosing CMV infections, it is not reliable as most cases result from reactivation/reinfection. Cell culture (including the DEAFF test) and rapid methods such as the CMV antigenemia test and PCR are preferred.
- **Varicella zoster virus (VZV):** Serology can be used to diagnose acute infection and also for immunity screening. Cell culture is difficult but rapid diagnosis may be reached in more severe cases by electron microscopy and immunofluorescence of the vesicle fluid.
- **Respiratory viruses:** Diagnosis of respiratory virus infections is more commonly made by cell culture or more rapidly by immunofluorescence of the clinical material. CFT and HAI techniques are usually used for serology and any diagnosis will be retrospective.
- **Enteroviruses:** Enterovirus infections are usually diagnosed by cell culture. Serology has a very limited role to play as available tests such as neutralisation are cumbersome to perform and in any case, the diagnosis would be retrospective. Serology is of some value in diagnosing cases of coxsackie B myopericarditis as it would be impractical to obtain biopsies of heart tissue.
- **Rabies:** Serology is used along with other direct detection methods in diagnosing rabies and it may be used to check for immunity after vaccination.
- **Arboviruses:** Arbovirus infections may be diagnosed by serology or virus isolation. Arboviruses will not usually grow in routine cell cultures and may require mosquito cell lines or animal inoculation.

Serology is of little value in the diagnosis of viral diarrhoea, papovirus infections and infections caused by poxviruses.

Use of Laboratory Tests in the Diagnosis of Infectious Diseases

Laboratory tests are used to provide direct and indirect evidence of infection, as discussed above. While signs (such as fever, redness, swelling, basal crackles) and symptoms (shortness of breath, urinary frequency, dysuria, cough) may be used to make the clinical diagnosis of infection, identification of the pathogen is required for a microbiological diagnosis to be made. The combination of clinical and laboratory data is often used to assess the severity of particular infections, which can influence prognosis and disease management. Discussed below are the laboratory tests used in the diagnosis of a number of common infections.

Pneumonia

Community acquired pneumonia (CAP) should be considered when a patient presents with two or more of the following symptoms:

- fever
- rigor
- new-onset cough
- change in sputum colour if there is chronic cough
- chest discomfort
- dyspnoea

However, such symptoms may occur in patients with acute bronchitis, a condition that generally does not require antibiotic therapy. Furthermore, CAP can present with fever without localising features, and some patients may have no fever (for example, elderly patients may present only with acute confusion).

In patients suspected to have pneumonia, a chest x-ray is needed to ascertain the presence of consolidation. Clinical signs, such as confusion, should be specifically noted because of their prognostic value.

Investigations

- **Chest x-ray**: This is the cardinal investigation. In the appropriate setting, a new area of consolidation on chest x-ray confirms the diagnosis, but x-ray is a poor guide to the likely pathogen. Other causes of a new lung infiltrate on chest x-ray include atelectasis, non-infective pneumonitis, haemorrhage and cardiac failure. Occasionally, the chest x-ray initially appears normal (for example, in the first few hours of *S pneumoniae* pneumonia and early in HIV-related *P carinii* pneumonia).
- **Sputum microscopy and culture**: Debate about the value of sputum samples in the diagnosis of CAP continues. Oral flora rather than the offending pathogen may dominate a sputum Gram stain and culture. Nevertheless, obtaining a sputum sample before beginning antibiotic therapy may provide the best opportunity to identify pathogens that require special treatment. Microscopy and culture for *M tuberculosis* should be requested for patients at high risk of tuberculosis.
- **Blood chemistry and haematology**: To assist in determining severity, all patients with CAP being assessed in emergency departments or admitted to hospital should have oximetry, measurement of serum electrolytes and urea levels, and a full blood count (Table 12.4). The pneumonia severity index (PSI) can be used to assess CAP severity and prognosis, and guide the selection of appropriate antibiotic therapy. Measurement of blood gases should also be undertaken, as it provides prognostic information (pH and PaO_2) and may identify patients with ventilatory failure or chronic hypercapnia ($PaCO_2$). If the patient has known or suspected diabetes mellitus, measurement of blood glucose also assists in assessing severity.
- **Blood culture**: Blood cultures are the most specific diagnostic test for the causative organism. They are, however, positive in only around 10% of patients admitted to hospital with CAP, with positive results more likely in patients with more severe pneumonia.
- **Other investigations**: In patients at risk of Legionnaires' disease, the Legionella

urinary antigen test is rapid, reliable and has a high degree of sensitivity and specificity. The test, however, only detects *Legionella pneumophila* serogroup 1, which accounts for only half of all cases of Legionella pneumonia.

Viral immunofluorescence testing of a nasopharyngeal aspirate is a valuable tool for detecting influenza or the respiratory syncytial virus, but does not exclude a secondary bacterial invader.

Serological diagnosis requires acute and convalescent serum samples and is therefore not useful in the acute management of CAP. Use of serology for the acute diagnosis of *M pneumoniae* lacks specificity.

Table 12.4 The pneumonia severity index (PSI)

PSI risk class I (lowest risk). Patient has none of the following:

- Age > 50 years;
- History of neoplastic disease, congestive cardiac failure, cerebrovascular, renal or liver disease; or
- Clinical signs – altered mental state, pulse rate ≥ 125 per minute, respiratory rate ≥ 30 per minute, systolic blood pressure < 90 mmHg, or temperature < 35 °C or ≥ 40 °C.

PSI risk classes II–V. Patients with any of the above characteristics are classified according to their PSI score, calculated according to the table below.

Calculation of PSI risk score

Factor	***PSI score***
Patient age	Age in years (male) or age – 10 (female)
Nursing home resident	+10
Co-existing illnesses	
Neoplastic disease	+30
Liver disease	+20
Congestive cardiac failure	+10
Cerebrovascular disease	+10
Renal disease	+10
Signs on examination	
Altered mental state	+20
Respiratory rate ≥ 30 per minute	+20
Systolic blood pressure < 90 mmHg	+20
Temperature ≤ 35 °C or ≥ 40 °C	+15
Pulse rate ≥ 125 bpm	+10
Results of investigations	
Arterial pH < 7.35	+30
Serum urea level ≥ 11 mmol/L	+20
Serum sodium level < 130 mmol/L	+10
Serum glucose level ≥ 14 mmol/L	+10
Haematocrit < 30%	+10
PO2 < 60 mmHg or O_2 saturation < 90%	+10
Pleural effusion	+10

Note: PSI risk scores: Class I not calculated, Class II ≤ 70, Class III 71–90, Class IV 91–130; Class V >130.

Source: Johnson PDR, Irving LB and Turnbridge JD. 2002. 3: Community-acquired pneumonia. *Med J Aust* 176: 341–7.

Urinary Tract Infections (UTIs)

Laboratory tests have traditionally been used to support the diagnosis of UTI. However, in a recent study of healthy young adult women with dysuria for less than one week without vaginal discharge, signs of pyelonephritis or predisposing conditions, empiric therapy guided by clinical presentation alone was the most cost-effective strategy; culture and treat-later strategies were significantly more expensive and, surprisingly, use of the dipstick alone was the most expensive approach. Further prospective clinical trials will be helpful in establishing the most cost-effective and clinically effective strategy, including patient-directed therapy.

Most patients with UTIs have pyuria equivalent to > 10 white blood cells (WBC) per high-power field (hpf). When a UTI diagnosis is suspected, the results of a simple urine dipstick test can be helpful. The presence of leukocyte esterase on a urine dipstick is equivalent to ≥ 4 WBC/hpf. A positive urinary dipstick for nitrites, leukocyte esterase or protein is usually always found in patients with signs and symptoms of UTI and a urine culture that is positive for bacteriuria. Table 12.5 highlights common urinalysis dipstick findings in UTI.

However, failure to detect nitrites does not exclude infection as some Gram-positive bacteria and *Pseudomonas* spp lack the enzymes to convert nitrate to nitrite, leading to false negatives. Further, false negative results may also arise in UTIs with low colony counts, or in recently voided or dilute urine. In cases where infection is suspected, a specimen should be sent to the laboratory for culture.

Microscopy and culture of a clean mid-stream urine sample are the gold standard for the diagnosis of UTI. Urinary bacteria counts of more than 10^5 cfu/ml indicate significant bacteriuria; however, this does not necessarily equate to clinical significance. Negative cultures in patients with persistent symptoms or pyuria require follow-up cultures for fastidious organisms. Fastidious organisms are those which require special growth media and/or conditions. In the case of UTIs, these include Mycobacterium, anaerobes, *Gardnerella vaginalis* and *Ureaplasma ureolyticum*.

Approximately 10–20% of women with acute uncomplicated pyelonephritis will have blood cultures positive for the offending pathogen. However, this is not predictive of a poorer outcome or need for protracted length of treatment in an otherwise healthy woman. Obtaining blood cultures during pyelonephritis will likely be of benefit only when there is evidence of complicated infection or suspicion of a multidrug-resistant pathogen.

HIV/AIDS

The enzyme-linked immunosorbent assay (ELISA) is used as a screening test for HIV infections. A positive result does not necessarily mean that the person has HIV infection, as there are certain conditions that may lead to a false positive result (for example, lyme disease, syphilis, lupus). The test may also be positive in babies born to HIV-positive mothers who carry the paternal antibody, but who themselves are not infected with HIV. Similarly patients receiving HIV vaccines may have positive antibody tests.

For this reason, a Western blot is carried out in all cases where the ELISA test is positive to confirm the diagnosis. While a positive Western blot is generally regarded as

Table 12.5 Common urinalysis dipstick findings in urinary tract infection

Finding	*Significance*	*Comment*
Colour	Typically pale yellow to colourless	Change in urine colour is not synonymous with urinary tract infection (UTI) or disease
Clarity	Typically clear	Pyuria causes urinary turbidity
Odour	Mild characteristic odour	Rancid or ammonia odour in urea-splitting organism
Specific gravity (SG)	Dilute urine = SG ≤ 1.008 Concentrated urine = SG > 1.020	Dilute or concentrated urine may influence the results of urine chemstrip testing
Leukocyte esterase (LE)	Test for enzyme present in white blood cell count (WBC)	Positive results indicated presence of neutrophils > 5 WBCs/hpf, an indicator of UTI, reported sensitivity of 75% to 90%. Results not valid in neutropaenic patient. Decreased sensitivity with increased urinary glucose concentration, high urinary SG, and presence of anti-microbial in urine.
Nitrites	Surrogate marker for bacteriuria. Presence indicates bacterial reduction of dietary nitrates to nitrites by select Gram-negative uropathogens including *Escherichia coli, Proteus sp* Normally absent in sterile urine and infection caused by enterococci, staphylococci	Best done on well-concentrated urine such as first AM void. For nitrites to be present, urine should be held in bladder for ≥ 1 hour for nitrate-to-nitrite conversion to take place; dietary nitrate intake must be adequate. False negative possible with low colony-count infections.
Protein	Dipstick testing most sensitive for albumin	Common in febrile response or represents presence of protein-containing substance such as white blood cells, bacteria, mucous. In UTI, usually trace to 30 g/L (1+), seldom ≥ 100 g/L.
pH	Average pH = 5–6 Acid pH = 4.5–5.5 Alkaline pH = 6.5–8	If alkaline urine is found in presence of UTI symptoms and positive leukocyte esterase, likely urea splitting such as *Proteus*, allowing urea to be split into CO_2 and ammonia, causing a rise in the urine's normally acid pH
Red blood cells (RBCs)	Low number of RBCs noted. Gross haematuria rare in uncomplicated UTI but may be present in infection complicated by nephrolithiasis	Microscopic haematuria common with urinary tract infection but not in urethritis or vaginitis

Source: M Fitzgerald and Lie D. 2002. Clinical Update http://www.medscape.com/viewprogram/1920

conclusive for an HIV infection, a negative test does not necessarily rule out HIV infection. The latter is true because there is a time interval between HIV infection and the appearance of measurable anti-HIV antibodies (the so-called 'window period'). During this window period, a negative HIV ELISA and Western blot do not rule out the possibility of HIV infection.

The antibody test is usually positive after three months; however, people at particularly high risk with a negative test are often retested at six months. It is uncommon for antibodies to develop after this time. During the window period, p24 antigen testing (detects actual viral protein in blood 1–4 weeks after exposure) or HIV viral load can be undertaken to exclude infection.

In patients who are HIV positive, CD4 T lymphocyte counts and HIV-1 RNA levels (viral loads) are used as markers of the likelihood of progression to AIDS, the risk of opportunistic infections and the need for treatment and its success. CD4 cell counts have been used to predict the likelihood of opportunistic infections and as a guide to when to commence anti-retroviral therapy and prophylaxis against opportunistic infections. More recently, several studies have indicated that the level of plasma HIV RNA is a more useful test in predicting the risk of progression to AIDS (Fig. 12.1).

In the Multicenter AIDS Cohort Study, men with a viral load greater than 100,000 copies/ml were found to have a 10-fold greater risk of progression to AIDS than those with a viral load less than 10,000 copies/ml. In this study, the viral load had a higher prognostic value than the CD4 lymphocyte count. HIV-1 RNA, and to a lesser extent CD4 cell counts, strongly predict the likelihood of disease progression, including

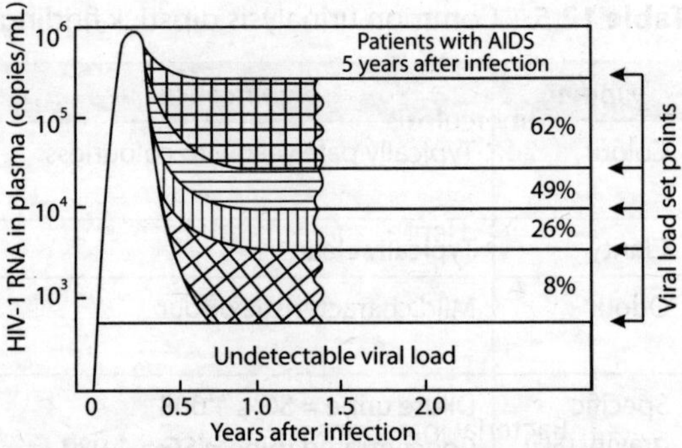

Figure 12.1 The level at which plasma HIV RNA stabilises after primary infection predicted subsequent progression to AIDS in a group of men in the Multicenter AIDS Cohort Study 4

Source: (Adapted with permission of Science © 1996 and David D. Ho. Viral counts count in HIV infection. *Science*. 1996:272:1124–1125)

death. Figure 12.2 illustrates the pattern of opportunistic infections dependent on the CD4 count. Therefore, the initiation of primary and secondary prophylaxis of such infections is guided by the CD4 cell count. For further information, readers should refer to the CDC website listed at the end of this chapter and to an HIV Carelink Newsletter article entitled 'Guidelines for Prevention and Treatment of Opportunistic Infections among HIV-Exposed and HIV-Infected Children, June 20, 2008'.

Commencing anti-retroviral therapy: When to commence anti-retroviral therapy remains controversial. Concerns about long-term adverse effects of therapy means the risks and benefits of starting treatment must be considered on a patient-by-patient basis. The strength of a recommendation to initiate treatment should be based on assessment of disease progression risk as determined by clinical, virologic and immunologic parameters and the individual's commitment

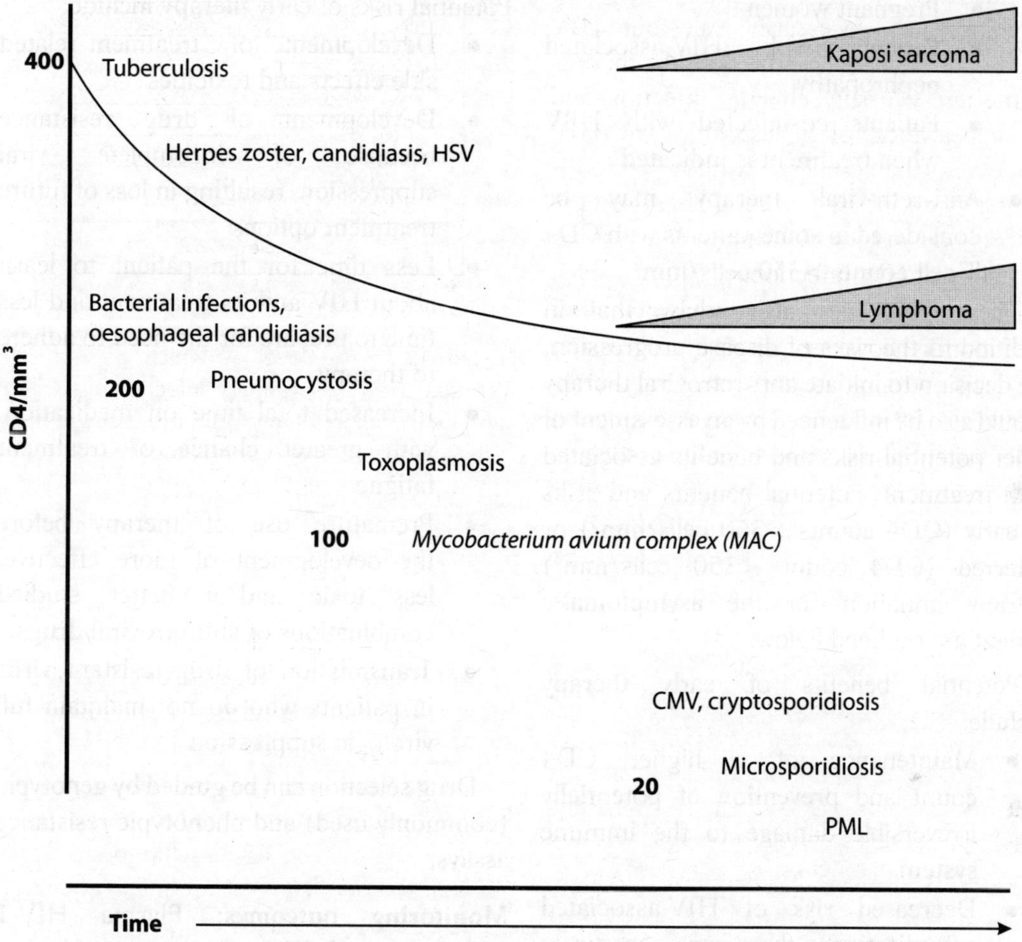

Figure 12.2 Major complications in the course of HIV infection related to CD4 counts

to therapy and willingness to adhere to a complex regimen.

According to the 2008 Guidelines for the use of anti-retroviral agents in HIV-1-infected adults and adolescents developed by the Department of Health and Human Services (DHHS) Panel on Anti-retroviral Guidelines for Adults and Adolescents (see websites at the end of this chapter):

- Anti-retroviral therapy should be initiated in patients with a history of an AIDS-defining illness or with a CD4 T-cell count <350 cells/mm^3. The data supporting this recommendation is stronger for those with a CD4 T-cell count <200 cells/mm^3 and with a history of AIDS than for those with CD4 T-cell counts between 200 and 350 cells/mm^3.
- Anti-retroviral therapy should also be initiated in the following groups of patients regardless of the CD4 T-cell count:

- Pregnant women
- Patients with HIV-associated nephropathy
- Patients co-infected with HBV when treatment is indicated

- Anti-retroviral therapy may be considered in some patients with CD4 T-cell counts >350 cells/mm^3.

These guidelines also advise that in addition to the risks of disease progression, the decision to initiate anti-retroviral therapy should also be influenced by an assessment of other potential risks and benefits associated with treatment. Potential benefits and risks of early (CD4 counts >350 cells/mm^3) or deferred (CD4 count <350 cells/mm^3) therapy initiation for the asymptomatic patient are outlined below.

Potential benefits of early therapy include:

- Maintenance of a higher CD4 count and prevention of potentially irreversible damage to the immune system
- Decreased risk of HIV-associated complications that can sometimes occur at CD4 counts >350 cells/mm^3, including tuberculosis, non-Hodgkin's lymphoma, Kaposi's sarcoma, peripheral neuropathy, HPV-associated malignancies and HIV-associated cognitive impairment
- Decreased risk of non-opportunistic conditions, including cardiovascular disease, renal disease, liver disease and non–AIDS-associated malignancies and infections
- Decreased risk of HIV transmission to others, which will have positive public health implications

Potential risks of early therapy include:

- Development of treatment-related side effects and toxicities
- Development of drug resistance because of incomplete viral suppression, resulting in loss of future treatment options
- Less time for the patient to learn about HIV and its treatment and less time to prepare for the need to adhere to therapy
- Increased total time on medication, with greater chance of treatment fatigue
- Premature use of therapy before the development of more effective, less toxic and/or better studied combinations of antiretroviral drugs
- Transmission of drug-resistant virus in patients who do not maintain full virologic suppression

Drug selection can be guided by genotypic (commonly used) and phenotypic resistance assays.

Monitoring outcomes: Plasma HIV-1 RNA levels and CD4 cell counts are the key laboratory parameters used in evaluating treatment response. Following initiation of therapy, HIV-1 RNA levels should decrease rapidly with a minimum 1.5–2.0-log reduction achieved by week 4 and the target level of less than 50 copies/ml reached by week 16–24.

The durability of the anti-retroviral response is indicated by the HIV-1 RNA nadir. Increase in memory CD4 cells occurs early in treatment, while increase in naive CD4 cells, essential for response to new antigens, occurs gradually following prolonged viral suppression. These increases

Table 12.6 Laboratory tests to be monitored prior to and after the intiation of anti-retroviral therapy

	Entry into care	*Follow-up before ART*	*ART initiation or switch*[1]	*2–8 weeks post-ART initiation*	*Every 3–6 months*	*Every 6 months*	*Every 12 months*	*Treatment Failure*	*Clinically indicated*
CD4 T-cell count	√	Every 3–6 months	√		√[2]			√	√
HIV RNA	√	Every 3–6 months	√	√	√[2]			√	√
HLA-B*5701 testing	√		√[3]					√	√
Resistance testing			√ (if considering ABC)						
Tropism testing								√ (if considering CCR5 antagonist)	√
Basic Chemistry[4]	√	Every 6–12 months	√	√	√				√
ALT, AST. T. bili, D. bili	√	Every 6–12 months	√	√	√				√
CBC w/ differential	√	Every 3–6 months	√	√ (if on ZDV)	√				√
Fasting lipid profile	√	If normal, annually	√	√ (consider after starting new ART)		√ (borderline or abnormal at last measurement)	√ (normal at last measurement)		√
Fasting glucose	√	If normal, annually	√		√ (borderline or abnormal at last measurement)	√ (normal at last measurement)			√
Urinalysis[5]	√		√			√ (patients with HIVAN)	√ (if on TDF)		√
Pregnancy test			√ (if starting EFV)						√

[1] Antiretroviral switch may be for treatment failure, adverse effects or simplification.

[2] For adherent patients with suppressed viral load and stable clinical and immunologic status for > 2–3 years, some experts may extend the interval for CD4 count and HIV RNA monitoring to every 6 months.

[3] For treatment-naive patients, if resistance testing was performed at entry into care, repeat testing is optional; for patients with viral suppression who are switching therapy for toxicity or convenience, resistance testing will not be possible and therefore, is not necessary.

[4] Serum Na, K, HCO_3, C1, BUN, creatinine, glucose (preferably fasting); some experts suggest monitoring phosphorus while on tenofovir; determination of renal function should include estimation of creatinine clearance using Cockroft–Gault equation or estimation of glomerular filtrations rate based on MDRD equation.

[5] For patients with renal disease, consult "Guidelines for the Management of Chronic Kidney Disease in HIV-Infected Patients: Recommendations of the HIV Medicine Association of the Infectious Diseases Society of America" (*Clin Infect Dis* 2005; 40: 1559–85).

Abbreviations: ART = anti-retroviral therapy; HIVAN = HIV-associated nephropathy; ABC = abacavir; TDF = tenofovir

Source: Panel on Antiretroviral Guidelines for Adults and Adolescents. Guidelines for the use of antiretroviral agents in HIV-1-infected adults and adolescents. Department of Health and Human Services. November 3, 2008; 1-139. Available at http://www.aidsinfo.nih.gov/ContentFiles/AdultandAdolescentGL.pdf.

in CD4 counts reflect at least partial immune reconstitution.

A median increase in CD4 cells of about 150 x 10^{12}/L generally occurs during the first year of therapy in patients whose viral load is less than 50 copies/ml. However, in some patients, less robust responses may occur. Failure of anti-retroviral therapy is defined as inadequate viral suppression, unsatisfactory increase in CD4 counts or clinical disease progression. The schedule of tests for monitoring prior to and during anti-retroviral therapy is shown in Table 12.6.

Tuberculosis

Diagnosis: As with other infectious diseases, the diagnosis of tuberculosis (TB) involves taking an accurate medical history together with a range of confirmatory tests, namely, a tuberculin skin test (Mantoux) or a blood test (Interferon–Gamma Release Assays [IGRAs]), chest x-ray and bacteriologic examination.

The medical history includes elucidating the person's contact with others with TB, the patient's symptoms, any history of TB, and the presence of any risk factors for developing TB. The symptoms of pulmonary TB disease include:

- cough
- pain in the chest when breathing or coughing
- coughing up sputum or blood (haemoptysis)

The general symptoms of TB disease (pulmonary or extrapulmonary) include:

- weight loss
- fatigue
- malaise
- fever
- night sweats

The site of extrapulmonary TB will influence the symptoms manifested.

Patients with symptoms of TB often undergo a **tuberculin skin test (Mantoux test)**; however, this may be negative despite active infection. Therefore, all patients with symptoms suggestive of TB should be evaluated for the disease regardless of their skin test results. In patients with a positive tuberculin test and those with symptoms suggestive of TB, the chest x-ray is used to assist the diagnosis of pulmonary TB, although the results cannot confirm that a person has TB disease.

Bacteriological examination is required to confirm the diagnosis. Sputum specimens are obtained from patients suspected of having pulmonary TB disease; other specimens are obtained from patients suspected of having extrapulmonary TB disease. These specimens are examined microscopically for the presence of acid-fast bacilli (AFB). When AFB are seen, they are counted. Patients with positive smears are considered infectious. The specimens are then cultured to determine whether they contain *M tuberculosis* or other mycobacterium. A positive culture for *M tuberculosis* confirms the diagnosis of TB disease. After the specimen has been cultured, it is tested for drug susceptibility. Drug sensitivities, however, are generally not available for 6–8 weeks and are therefore used for modifying empirical therapy.

Monitoring outcome: The incidence of drug-induced side effects is less than 1% overall, but baseline liver function tests and blood biochemistry should be performed and then monitored fortnightly. For patients receiving ethambutol, baseline visual acuity should be checked and the patient informed to report any changes in vision immediately.

Viral Hepatitis

The diagnosis of acute viral hepatitis depends on clinical and laboratory findings. The symptoms of viral hepatitis are general and vary greatly, and as such provide little help in identifying a specific viral cause. The majority of infections are totally asymptomatic, but common clinical features include anorexia, nausea, vomiting, right upper quadrant pain and raised liver transaminases (AST and ALT), bilirubin and to a lesser extent alkaline phosphatase.

In chronic hepatitis, clinical features vary. In many cases, the patients are asymptomatic, especially in chronic hepatitis C. Where symptoms do occur, the commonly reported ones are malaise, anorexia and fatigue; occasionally low-grade fever and non-specific upper abdominal discomfort may be reported. Jaundice is variable and is often absent. Development of the classical signs of chronic liver disease (splenomegaly, spider nevi, fluid retention) are often delayed, with many patients having subclinical infections for years. Manifestations such as acne, amenorrhoea, arthralgia, ulcerative colitis, pulmonary fibrosis, thyroiditis, nephritis and haemolytic anaemia may be seen in patients with the autoimmune variant. Patients who develop biliary cirrhosis may manifest predominantly cholestatic features.

Laboratory findings: Significant elevation in transaminase levels is the hallmark of acute viral hepatitis. Levels increase early in the prodromal phase, peak before jaundice is maximal, and fall slowly during the recovery phase. Levels of AST and ALT in the range of 500–2000 IU/L are typical; however, correlation with clinical severity is poor. Typically, in cases of viral hepatitis, ALT increases more than AST, with ALT being the last enzyme to return to normal. The presence of bilirubin in urine often precedes jaundice; its early detection is valuable for diagnosis.

The degree of hyperbilirubinemia is variable and alkaline phosphatase is only moderately raised unless cholestasis is severe. Coagulation abnormalities (elevated INR, prolonged prothrombin time) are uncommon in acute infections and may indicate severe disease. The white cell count is usually low–normal, and the differential shows a few atypical lymphocytes.

In chronic viral hepatitis, as with other forms of chronic liver disease (such as cirrhosis), elevations in ALT may not reflect the level of liver disease. One-third of patients with chronic hepatitis C infection have persistently normal serum ALT levels despite the presence of inflammation on liver biopsy. This is thought to be due to the fact that liver destruction occurs through apoptosis (programmed cell death), with the withering cells having few transaminases to release.

Diagnosis: Serological tests are used to diagnose most cases of viral hepatitis. The diagnosis of hepatitis A (HAV) is dependent on detecting the IgM antibody; while detection of IgG antibodies to the hepatitis A virus (IgG anti-HAV) is merely a marker of remote exposure and does not indicate current HAV infection. The presence of hepatitis B surface antigen (HbsAg) in serum is used to diagnose hepatitis B, with or without a concomitant antibody to the hepatitis B core antigen (anti-HBc). The test is, however, not 100% sensitive as antigenemia may be transient; therefore, in cases where hepatitis B is suspected, the isolated presence of IgM anti-HBc may establish the diagnosis.

The presence of serum antibody (anti-HCV) is used to diagnose hepatitis C infection. This antibody is not protective and its presence implies active infection. Anti-HCV often appears several weeks after acute infection, so a negative test does not exclude recent infection. Detection and quantification of HCV-RNA may also be used in the diagnosis of hepatitis C infections. Its detection in patient tissues provides evidence of active HCV infection and can be useful for confirming diagnoses and for measuring response to anti-viral therapy.

Monitoring outcome: In acute viral hepatitis, the following laboratory tests should be monitored:

- Serum transaminases (ALT, AST), lactic acid dehydrogenase, alkaline phosphatase
- Serum bilirubin
- Prothrombin time
- Full blood picture with differential
- Serological tests for HbsAg and IgM anti-HAV

In chronic viral hepatitis, additional monitoring should include:

- Serum albumin
- Serological tests for HbsAg and anti-HBc
- Polymerase chain reaction (PCR) for viral RNA (hep C)
- Viral load
- Viral genotyping for hep C

Patients with chronic hepatitis B or C infections started on interferon g (alone or with lamivudine) required baseline monitoring of their full blood picture (including differential and platelet count), electrolytes, renal and hepatic function, with follow-up tests every month. Thyroid function test should also be performed at baseline and repeated at three-monthly intervals.

Hepatitis B

In 25–40% of patients given interferon g loss of the hepatitis Be antigen (HbeAg) and normalisation of ALT occurred within the first year of treatment. The use of PCR testing for hepatitis B virus DNA has proved useful in monitoring the response to lamivudine treatment.

Hepatitis C

Monitoring patients after initiation of therapy may be done at 2–4-week intervals with serum ALT measurements. Determination of serum ALT levels and HCV-RNA after three months of treatment may help identify patients who are unresponsive to treatment with interferon alone. Further information may be obtained by measuring the baseline HCV-RNA viral load and by monitoring viral load periodically during treatment.

Malaria

There are four species of the genus *Plasmodium* responsible for the malarial parasite infections that commonly infect man: *P falciparum, P vivax, P malariae* and *P ovale*. The most important of these is *P falciparum* because it can be rapidly fatal and is responsible for most malaria-related deaths.

Diagnosis: In areas where malaria is endemic, the diagnosis of malaria is often made on clinical presentation alone, although ideally it should be made on the basis of blood film examination. The gold standard for the diagnosis of malaria is the examination of thick and thin blood films. Examination of a thick blood film is usually undertaken first as it concentrates the parasites 20-fold in comparison to a thin film, making detection of the parasite easier. However, distortion of the parasite makes species identification difficult. Hence, when parasites are seen, the species should then be confirmed by examination of a thin film. Blood samples are best taken when the patient's temperature is rising.

Various test kits (including ICT-Malaria Pf, OptiMALr and the Kat-Quick kits) are available to detect antigens derived from malaria parasites. The tests detect either the plasmodial histidine-rich protein-2 (HRP-2) or parasite-specific lactate dehydrogenase (pLDH) that is present in *P falciparum* infections. Such immunologic ('immunochromatographic') tests most often use a dipstick or cassette format, and provide results in 2–15 minutes. These rapid diagnostic tests (RDTs) offer a useful alternative to microscopy in situations where reliable microscopic diagnosis is not available. While malaria RDTs are currently used in some clinical settings and programmes, their widespread adoption is hindered by several issues including the need for improved accuracy, reduced cost and proven reliability under adverse field conditions. The World Health Organization's Regional Office for the Western Pacific (WHO/WPRO) provides technical information, including a list of commercially available malaria RDTs, at http://www.wpro.who.int/rdt/.

RDTs have the potential of enhancing the speed and accuracy of diagnosing *P falciparum,* particularly in non-specialised laboratories where inexperienced or junior staff may be involved. However, they do not eliminate the need for malaria microscopy. In some infections with lower numbers of malaria parasites circulating in the patient's bloodstream, RDTs may not be able to detect the parasite. Further, there is insufficient data available to determine the ability of these tests to detect the two less common species of malaria, *P ovale* and *P malariae*. Hence, at this time, all negative RDTs must be followed by microscopy to confirm the result.

In addition, all positive RDTs should also be followed by microscopy. The currently FDA-approved RDTs detect two different malaria antigens: one is specific for *P falciparum* and the other is found in all four species of malaria. Therefore, microscopy is required to determine the species of malaria detected by the RDT. Further, to assess patient prognosis, microscopy is needed to quantify the proportion of red blood cells that are infected.

Other tests that can be used to assist diagnosis include antibody detection using enzymatic immunoassays or immunofluorescence techniques, the QBC II system, Becton–Dickinson's Quantitative Buffy Coat (QBC) method and the relatively new polymerase chain reaction (PCR). The latter is used to detect parasite nucleic acids. The technique is more accurate than microscopy and can detect <10 parasites per 10 uL of blood. However, it is expensive, and requires a specialised laboratory (even though technical advances will likely result in field-operated PCR machines).

Monitoring outcome: The level of parasitaemia combined with the patient's clinical status is used to monitor patients with malaria. In patients with severe falciparum malaria who may have coma, jaundice, renal failure, hypoglycaemia, acidosis, severe anaemia, high parasite count and hyperpyrexia, close clinical and biochemical monitoring is essential. Blood sugar levels should be monitored in patients given quinine, particularly intravenous quinine. Primaquine, used for the treatment of vivax malaria, may induce haemolytic anaemia in patients with glucose 6-phosphate dehydrogenase (G6PD) deficiency, necessitating monitoring of haemoglobin levels.

Diarrhoea

The diagnosis of diarrhoea is usually self-evident. In young children, the elderly and the debilitated, diarrhoea can result in severe dehydration (elevated serum sodium and urea). Profound water loss associated with diarrhoea, particularly in the very young, can result in renal impairment, indicated by an elevation in both serum urea and creatinine.

Many cases of infectious diarrhoea are self-limiting and hence there is no need to identify the causative organism. Where a stool examination is carried out, the following can be looked for:

- blood
- white cells
- mucus
- toxins (particularly useful in cases of *Clostridium difficile*–associated diarrhoea)
- ova, larvae and mature parasites
- bacteria, fungi and viruses

Stool cultures use selective growth media to identify significant pathogens, such *Salmonella* spp, *Shigella* spp, *Campylobacter* spp and *Vibrio cholerae*. The stool culture report that states 'no growth' only eliminates those pathogens specifically cultured, and for that reason it is important to be aware of the pathogens routinely screened for. Whilst clinical manifestations may suggest typhoid fever, definitive diagnosis requires the isolation of *S typhi* from the patient. Where blood and faecal samples as well as bone marrow are cultured, *S typhi* is usually detected in more than 90% of cases. Culturing blood only reduces sensitivity to 50–70%. *S typhi* can exhibit multiple drug resistance. In cases where defervescence of symptoms does not occur, MIC testing is warranted; however, this may not be practical.

Sepsis

Sepsis is a systemic illness caused by the microbial invasion of normally sterile parts of the body. The term specifically serves to differentiate an illness of microbial origin from an identical clinical syndrome that can arise in several non-microbial conditions, pancreatitis being a classic example. The pathophysiology of both conditions involves cytokines, host-derived peptides released in response to a wide variety of stimuli. Sepsis is a clinical diagnosis, with up to 50% of cultures being negative. For this reason, anti-microbial therapy is given empirically, with positive cultures used as confirmation, and sensitivities to redirect treatment.

The signs and symptoms (Fig. 12.3) of sepsis are highly variable, being influenced by factors including the virulence and bioburden of the pathogen, the portal of entry, host susceptibility and the temporal evolution of the condition. Sepsis is the association of a variety of non-specific inflammatory responses with evidence or suspicion of a microbial origin. It becomes 'severe sepsis' when accompanied by evidence of hypoperfusion or dysfunction of at least one

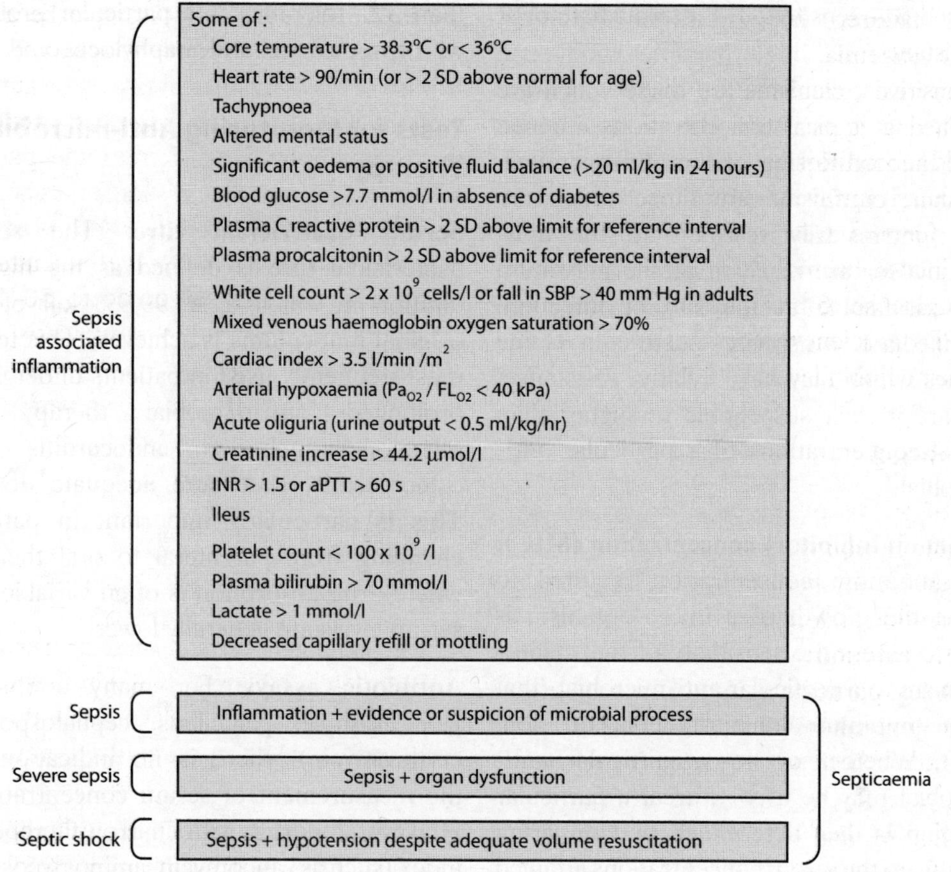

Fig. 12.3 Definitions of sepsis, severe sepsis and septic shock

Source: Lever A, MacKenzie I. 2007 Sepsis: definition, epidemiology, and diagnosis. *BMJ* 335: 879-83.

organ system. In cases where severe sepsis is accompanied by hypotension or the need for vasopressors, despite adequate fluid resuscitation, the term 'septic shock' applies. Previously, all three conditions were covered under the term septicaemia.

To date there is no specific test which can definitively prove the diagnosis of sepsis apart from visualisation by microscopy of the pathogens in tissue samples or, more commonly, culturing the pathogens from tissue, especially blood.

Assessing the Suitability of Anti-microbial Therapy using Laboratory Tests

Determination of anti-microbial sensitivities: Assessment of anti-microbial activity against a specific pathogen is an important guide for the selection of the appropriate anti-microbial therapy. Yet, it is important to realise that in vitro sensitivities do not always equate to therapeutic success and vice versa. Organism sensitivity may be deemed S – sensitive, I – intermediate or R – resistant.

Sensitive organisms are those which are inhibited at typical concentrations attained with standard dosing of the anti-microbial. Resistant organisms are those which are either intrinsically resistant to the anti-microbial or are resistant at the maximum levels attainable at the site of infection. Intermediate sensitivity occurs in some isolates which may have 'relative resistance' and are in fact susceptible to higher than typical concentrations of a particular anti-microbial.

Minimum inhibitory concentration (MIC): The minimum concentration required to inhibit the growth of a micro-organism is used to assess the sensitivity of that micro-organism to a particular anti-microbial (that is, the minimum inhibitory concentration, MIC). Whether or not a particular anti-microbial may be used to treat a particular infection is then determined by comparing the MIC to the serum concentrations attained when the normal dose of the drug is given. Using this method, organisms are classed as sensitive, moderately sensitive, conditionally sensitive or resistant.

Minimum bactericidal concentration (MBC): This is defined as the lowest concentration of a drug that results in a 99.9% reduction in the initial bacterial density. The bactericidal activity of an agent or combination of agents may be crucial in some infections, such as endocarditis. Here, the presence of tolerant organisms (those inhibited, but not killed by the drug(s)) may pose a major threat to the life of the individual. An organism is said to be tolerant if the MBC:MIC ratio is equal to or greater than 32. Tolerance is a particular problem with Streptococci and Staphylococci.

Tests for Monitoring Anti-microbial Therapy

Serum bactericidal titre: The serum bactericidal titre is defined as the highest dilution at which a ≥ 99.9% kill of the original innoculums is achieved. This test is most frequently used in patients undergoing prolonged anti-microbial therapy for infections such as endocarditis and osteomyelitis, to ensure adequate dosing. This is particularly important in patients changing from parenteral to oral therapy, where drug absorption is often variable and serum levels are generally lower.

Antibiotic assays: For many antibiotics (for example, penicillins, cephalosporins, erythromycin), there is no indication for the measurement of serum concentrations. However, for drugs with a narrow therapeutic index (such as vancomycin, aminoglycosides, chloramphenicol, flucytosine), routine monitoring of serum levels is recommended. In patients receiving oral flucloxacillin or cephalexin for the treatment of osteomyelitis, estimation of peak concentrations is recommended to ensure adequate drug dose.

Monitoring anti-microbial toxicity: Anti-microbial agents have a range of toxicity that may be manifested as abnormalities in laboratory tests. A monitoring plan for the progress of patients on anti-microbials should therefore incorporate monitoring of both disease progress and drug toxicity/efficacy based on clinical signs and symptoms together with laboratory monitoring. It is important

Table 12.7 Anti-microbial toxicity manifesting as abnormal laboratory tests

Adverse Effect	Laboratory Abnormality	Examples of Anti-microbials
Haematological		
Neutropaenia	Reduce white cell count (Neutropaenia < 1 x 109/L; agranulocytosis < 0.1 x 109/L)	Chloramphenicol, trimethoprim-sulphamethoxazole, beta-lactams, fluoroquinolones, glycopeptides, quinine, rifabutin, ganciclovir
Eosinophilia	Raised eosinophils (> 0.5 x 109/L or 5% of total count)	Nitrofurantoin, beta lactams
Anaemia	Reduced haemoglobin	Linezolid, amphotericin B, zidovudine, haemolytic anaemia - quinine, beta-lactams, primaquine, chloroquine
Thrombocytopaenia	Reduced platelet count (< 150 x 109/L)	Beta lactams, quinine, chloroquine
Monocytosis	Elevated monocyte count	Griseofulvin
Aplastic anaemia		Chloramphenicol
Elevated MCV	MCV > 100fL	Sulphonamides, trimethoprim
Biochemical		
Hyponatraemia	Reduced serum sodium (< 125 mmol/L)	Miconazole, fluconazole, itraconazole, quinupristin/dalfopristin
Hypokalaemia	Reduced serum potassium (< 3.3 mmol/L)	Aminoglycosides, beta lactams, amphotericin B
Hyperkalaemia	Elevated serum potassium (> 6.0 mmol/L)	Trimethoprim
Hypomagnesaemia	Reduced magnesium level (< 0.7 mmol/L)	Aminoglycosides, amphotericin B
Acute Renal Failure	Elevated creatinine (> 25% elevation above baseline)	Aminoglycosides, trimethoprim, beta lactams, fluoroquinolones, vancomycin, aciclovir
Hepatotoxicity	Abnormal LFTs	Flucloxacillin, dicloxacillin, amoxycillin/clavulanate, macrolides, streptogramins, minocycline, isoniazid, rifampicin, griseofulvin, ketoconazole
Gout/hyperuricaemia	Elevated serum uric acid	Pyrazinamide
Pancreatitis	Elevated serum amylase	Protease inhibitors
Diabetes mellitus	Elevated blood sugar	Pentamidine
Hypoglycaemia	Decreased blood sugar	Pentamidine (initial insulin release), quinine
Hyperlipidaemia	Elevated serum cholesterol	Protease inhibitors
Coagulation		
Hypoprothrombinaemia	Elevated INR	Cephamandole, cefotetan
Immunological		
	Positive anti-nuclear antibodies	Minocycline
Hypersensitivity reactions	Elevated IgE	Beta lactams

to appreciate that in some instances drug toxicity may be misinterpreted as a positive therapeutic response. An example of this is flucloxacillin-induced neutropaenia, where the initial fall in WCC may be interpreted as an improvement in the patient's infection. Examples of drug toxicity manifesting as abnormal laboratory tests are shown in Table 12.7. It is important to remember that some anti-microbials can interfere with certain laboratory tests, resulting in spurious test results. Some of the cephalosporins (like cefoxitin) can interfere with specific serum creatinine assays (Jaffe methods), resulting in falsely elevated levels.

CASE STUDY: COMMUNITY ACQUIRED PNEUMONIA

A 73-year-old man is admitted to hospital with increasing cough and pleuritic chest pain.

History of Presenting Complaint

Four days prior to admission, he developed a sore throat, which progressed to a dry cough. Two days later, he visited his local doctor who prescribed a course of amoxycillin/clavulanate. However, over the next two days, his cough became worse and he developed chest pain.

Past Medical History

- Aortic valve and mitral valve disease
- Transient ischaemic attacks
- Stroke
- Glaucoma
- Osteoarthritis
- Secondary epilepsy
- Fractures of L1 vertebra and the sacrum
- Hypertension
- Hypercholesterolaemia
- Peptic ulcer disease

Medications

Warfarin	4 mg daily
Amoxycillin/Clavulanate	875/125 mg 12-hourly (ceased on admission)
Prednisolone	5 mg daily increased to 37.5 mg daily (2 days prior to admission)
Simvastatin	10 mg at night
Sodium valproate	200 mg tds
Perindopril	5 mg daily
Omeprazole	20 mg twice daily
Alendronate	70 mg weekly

Nitrazepam	5 mg at night when required for sleep
Timolol Eye Drop	0.5% 1 drop both eyes twice daily

Laboratory and Other Tests

Patient looked flushed, afebrile T 39.8 °C, Pulse 142 bpm , BP 90/55 mmHg, bibasal crackles; Left > Right, wheeze +++, RR 32 bpm

Chest x-ray – left lower lobe consolidation

Urea and Electrolytes

Sodium	131 mmol/L (134–146 mmol/L)
Potassium	3.6 mmol/L (3.4–5 mmol/L)
Bicarbonate	28 mmol/L (22–32 mmol/L)
Urea	11.3 mmol/L (3–8 mmol/L)
Creatinine	92 mmol/L (50–90 mmol/L)

Liver Function Tests

Protein	67 g/L (60–80 g/L)
Albumin	35 g/L (35–50 g/L)
Calcium (corrected)	2.35 mmol/L (2.25–2.60 mmol/L)
Bilirubin	6 mmol/L (< 20 mmol/L)
Alkaline phosphatase	62 IU/L (<135 IU/L)
ALT	8 IU/L (< 40 IU/L)

Haematology

White cell count	5.40×10^9/L ($4.5–11 \times 10^9$/L)
Neutrophils	3.89×10^9/L
Lymphocytes	1.03×10^9/L
Haemoglobin	118 g/L (115–165 g/L)
Platelets	171×10^9/L ($150–400 \times 10^9$/L)

Diagnosis and Plan

Left lower lobe pneumonia

Sputum and blood cultures for microscopy, culture and sensitivities

Commence IV ceftriaxone 1 g daily and erythromycin IV 500mg four times daily

IV saline

Salbutamol nebules 5 mg 4-hourly

Oxygen

What features of this case suggest that the patient has severe pneumonia?

Based on the following findings, the patient's pneumonia would be classified as severe:

- Age
- Co-morbidities – cerebrovascular disease
- Systolic BP < 90 mmHg
- Respiratory rate > 30 breaths per minute
- Urea > 11 mmol/L

The patient's PSI score is >130 indicating a 30-day mortality rate of 27% (PSI risk class V). Further complicating this patient's pneumonia are his history of epilepsy secondary to his stroke and his use of warfarin (increased bleeding risk), prednisolone (immunosuppressive) and omeprazole (increased risk of pneumonia).

Is the choice of antibiotic appropriate?

In patients with severe pneumonia, hospital admission and the use of parenteral antibiotics is appropriate. Ceftriaxone is a broad-spectrum agent which will cover common causes of CAP, such as *Streptococcus pneumoniae and Haemophilus influenzae*. In such cases, the usual practice is to add a macrolide (like erythromycin, azithromycin, roxithromycin, clarithromycin) antibiotic to cover possible atypical organisms (for example, *Legionella, Mycoplasma*). However, erythromycin inhibits the hepatic clearance of warfarin and is likely to result in over-anticoagulation if the warfarin dose is not adjusted. A better choice would be azithromycin 500 mg once daily, which is less likely to interact with warfarin, and is usually better tolerated.

How can laboratory investigations assist the monitoring of antibiotic therapy?

The appropriateness of the use of antibiotics can be assessed based on the severity of his pneumonia, as outlined above. Serum procalcitonin levels could be taken to assess the likelihood that the patient was suffering from a bacterial infection until the results of sputum and blood are known. The results of the latter cultures, if positive, will allow targetting of the patient's antibiotic therapy. Erythromycin is known to cause cholestatic jaundice and liver function tests can be monitored if liver toxicity is suspected. In patients with pre-existing liver disease, erythromycin should be used with caution. Similarly, ceftriaxone can cause liver problems; it may also cause blood dyscrasias, so monitoring of the patients full blood picture may be appropriate in some cases. The effectiveness of antibiotic therapy can be assessed on the basis of improvement in his symptoms and signs, including normalisation of his white cell differential and reduction in his serum urea.

On Day 2 of the patient's admission, his sputum culture results become available. His sputum has grown *Pseudomonas aeruginosa*, sensitive to ciprofloxacin, ticarcillin, gentamicin and ceftazidime.

How should these results be applied in the clinical setting?

Based on these results, the patient's antibiotic regimen must be changed to contain two agents active against *Ps aeruginosa*. As fluoroquinolones may precipitate seizures and interact with warfarin, the use of ciprofloxacin would not be recommended. In this case, either ticarcillin plus potassium clavulanate or ceftazidime in conjuction with gentamicin should be started. Both erythromycin and ceftriaxone should be stopped.

How should the patient's progress now be monitored?

Monitoring of the patient's progress should now include:

- Clinical status – improvement in presenting symptoms (shortness of breath, pleuritic chest pain, cough and sputum production) and signs (x-ray changes; tachypnoea, hypotension, tachycardia and laboratory abnormalities) together with the development of possible complications (seizures, heart failure in light of his valvular heart disease)
- Signs and symptoms of antibiotic toxicity

KEY MESSAGES

- The patient's clinical status must always be taken into consideration when interpreting any laboratory test result.
- A patient may have a normal WCC, yet a change in the differential (for example, increased proportion of neutrophils) may be indicative of infection.
- Acute phase reactants such as C-reactive protein (CRP) and rheumatoid factor may be elevated and support the diagnosis of infection.
- The Gram stain is the most commonly used differential stain for determining cell morphology.
- The combination of clinical and laboratory data is often used to assess the severity of particular infections, which can influence prognosis and disease management.
- Urinary bacteria counts of more than 10^5 cfu/ml indicate significant bacteriuria, however this does not necessarily equate to clinical significance.
- In patients who are HIV positive, CD4 T lymphocyte counts and HIV-1 RNA levels (viral loads) are used as markers of the likelihood of progression to AIDS, the risk of opportunistic infections and the need for treatment and its success.
- Significant elevation in the aminotransferase level is the hallmark of acute viral hepatitis.
- The gold standard for the diagnosis of malaria is the examination of thick and thin blood films.
- Assessment of anti-microbial activity against a specific pathogen is an important guide for the selection of appropriate anti-microbial therapy.
- For drugs with a narrow therapeutic index (for example, vancomycin, aminoglycosides, chloramphenicol, flucytosine), routine monitoring of serum drug concentrations is recommended.

Further Reading

Beaman MH and Wesselingh SL. 2002. Acute community-acquired meningitis and encephalitis. *Med J Aust* 176:389–96.

Durrington HN and Summers C. 2008. Recent changes in the management of community acquired pneumonia in adults. *BMJ* 336:1429–33.

Centers for Disease Control and Prevention. 2010. Updated guidelines for using Interferon-Gamma Release Assays to detert *M tuberculosis* infection, United States. *MMNK* 59 (No. RR-5) (http://www.cdc.gov/mmwr/pay/rr/rr5905.pdf)

Hughes J (ed). 2009. Case Studies in Clinical Practice. Use of Laboratory Data: Process Guide and Reference for Healthcare Professionals. Pharmaceutical Society of Australia: Canberra.

Hughes J, Donnelly R and James–Chatgilaou G. 2001. Gastroenterology. In: Hughes J, Donnelly R and James–Chatgilaou G (eds). *Clinical pharmacy: A practical Approach*, 2nd ed, 171–207. MacMillan Education: Melbourne, Australia.

Hughes J. 2001. Infectious diseases. In: Hughes J, Donnelly R and James–Chatgilaou G (eds). *Clinical pharmacy: A Practical Approach*, 2nd ed, 208–49. MacMillan Education: Melbourne, Australia.

Johnson PDR, Irving LB and Turnidge JD. 2002. Community acquired pneumonia. *Med J Aust* 176:341–7.

Lee, M (ed). 2008. Basic skills in interpreting laboratory data, 2nd ed. American Society of Health System Pharmacists Inc.

Lever A and MacKenzie I. 2007. Sepsis: definition, epidemiology, and diagnosis. *BMJ* 335:879–83.

Schuetz P, Christ-Crain M, Thomann R, et al. 2009. Effect of procalcitonin based guidelines vs standard guidelines on antibiotic use in lower respiratory tract infections: the proHOSP randomized controlled trial. *JAMA* 302:1059–66.

Websites of Interest

Acute viral hepatitis. Merck Manual Online
http://www.merck.com/pubs/mmanual/section4/chapter42/42b.htm#A004-042-0340

Anon. Malaria diagnosis. Centers for Disease Control and Prevention, June 27, 2007.
http://www.cdc.gov/malaria/diagnosis_treatment/diagnosis.htm

Anon. Diagnosis of Tuberculosis Infection and Disease. NJMS National Tuberculosis Center, 1997.
http://www.umdnj.edu/~ntbcweb/tiddiag.htm

Centres for Disease Control and Prevention. Guidelines for Preventing Opportunistic Infections Among HIV-Infected Persons, 2002.
www.cdc.gov/mmwr/preview/mmwrhtml/rr5108a1.htm

Fitzgerald M and Lie D. 2002. Urinary Tract Infection Providing the Best Care. *Clinical Update*
http://www.medscape.com/viewprogram/1920

Guidelines for Prevention and Treatment of Opportunistic Infections among HIV-Exposed and HIV-Infected Children, June 20, 2008
http://www.faetc.org/PDF/Newsletter/Newsletter-Volume9-2008/HIVCareLink-Vol9-Issue-9-August-1.pdf

Medscape

http://www.medscape.com

Panel on Antiretroviral Guidelines for Adults and Adolescents. November 3, 2008. Guidelines for the use of antiretroviral agents in HIV-1-infected adults and adolescents. *Department of Health and Human Services*; 1–139.

http://www.aidsinfo.nih.gov/ContentFiles/AdultandAdolescentGL.pdf

The Royal College of Pathologists of Australasia Manual (Version 4. 12 March 2004)

http://www.rcpamanual.edu.au

World Health Organization

http://www.who.int/pub/en

13 MEDICATION REVIEW

M Ramesh

Learning Objectives

Upon completion of this chapter, the reader should be able to:

- Explain the role of medication review in patient care
- Outline the components of medication review
- Explain why evaluation of the patient's medical history, signs, symptoms, laboratory data and results of other investigations is central to medication review
- List the types of drug-related problems (DRPs) that are commonly identified during medication review
- Describe how an adverse drug reaction (ADR) is identified through routine medication review
- Describe important sources of information which are used to monitor the therapeutic outcome
- Describe the role of medication chart endorsement in medication review

Medication review involves the review of a patient's medication regimen to ensure that therapy is appropriate, safe, efficacious and cost-effective. This can be achieved by pharmacists attending ward rounds on a day-to-day basis and applying their knowledge of therapeutics in the management of specific diseases or conditions.

Daily review is desirable to keep up with any changes to drug therapy. Ideally, the pharmacist should follow the patient from the day of admission until the day of discharge. During each ward visit, the pharmacist should engage in clinical activities including identification of patient factors affecting medication management, assessment of drug therapy, monitoring outcome, intervening to prevent or resolve drug-related problems and education of the patient or carer.

Goal of Medication Review

The goal of medication review is to optimise drug therapy and patient health outcome by identifying and solving drug-related problems, and ensuring that all therapeutic objectives are being achieved.

Significance of Medication Review

Daily review of patients' drug therapy enables the pharmacist to:

- Assess whether desired therapeutic outcomes are being achieved
- Monitor for drug-related problems/ toxicity
- Ensure rational and quality use of medicines
- Assess patient compliance (medication adherence)
- Assess the completeness of medication charts

Components of Medication Review

The routine review of drug therapy for a specific patient or a specific condition includes a number of components:

- Medication order review (MOR)/ Treatment chart review (TCR)
- Clinical review/Daily progress review
- Detection and management of adverse drug reactions (ADRs)

Medication Order Review

Medication order review (MOR) is one of the fundamental responsibilities of clinical pharmacy practice as it is the basis for other clinical pharmacy activities such as medication counselling, therapeutic drug monitoring (TDM) and detection and management of ADRs.

MOR is a systematic review of a patient's drug therapy to ensure that the prescribed medication is appropriate for the patient. It involves the assessment of all current and recent medication orders, including routine medication and over-the-counter (OTC) drugs and the use of other systems of medicine (Unani, Ayurvedic, Siddha).

Goal of MOR

The goal of MOR is to optimise the patients' drug therapy by ensuring that patients receive the right drug, dose and dosage form for the right duration.

Steps

In reviewing a patient's drug therapy, any condition or drug-related problem that requires change in drug therapy or the management plan should be identified as an issue and discussed with the relevant medical practitioners.

A medication order should be reviewed for appropriateness by considering all relevant information including presenting complaints, clinical assessment, previous allergy status, laboratory investigation, treatment plans and the daily progress of the patient. The pharmacist should consider available data from sources such as the treatment chart, case notes, laboratory results and medication history obtained during patient interview.

The steps involved in MOR include:

- Collection and interpretation of patient-specific information, including medication history interview
- Assessment of therapeutic goals

- Identification of drug-related problems
- Individualising medication regimens
- Monitoring of treatment outcomes
- Medication chart endorsement
- Documentation

Collection and Interpretation of Patient-specific Information

Collection of patient-specific information is the first step in setting the therapeutic goal for a patient. Pharmacists need to collect information that will assist them to determine the appropriateness of drug therapy. This includes the patient's demographic details such as age, sex and body weight, social history, presenting complaints, past medical history, allergy and sensitivity status, current and recent medication, and results of relevant laboratory tests and other investigations.

This enables the pharmacist to understand the patient's disease condition, the reason why certain drugs are being administered and the patient's daily clinical progress. This understanding is the foundation for medication review. Relevant information can be obtained from a variety of sources including the patient, case notes, the medication chart, nursing notes, observational charts, laboratory results and through discussions with medical and nursing staff.

When a patient is admitted to hospital, medical staff document relevant information regarding the admission in the patient's case notes. This usually includes a list of medications which the patient is currently taking. This list may be inaccurate or incomplete, particularly in situations where medical staff are over-burdened with a high patient load. By speaking personally to patients about their medications, pharmacists can obtain further information which may be of importance to the ongoing medical management of the patient. This process is sometimes referred to as a *medication history interview (MHI)*.

The goal of the medication history interview is to obtain a complete and accurate summary of the medications that a patient has been using, together with other information which may usefully contribute to pharmaceutical care.

The patient's medication history should be obtained at the beginning of the hospital admission so as to provide any additional useful information to the prescriber that may positively influence drug therapy selection. The nature of the medication history interview will depend on the patient's condition. The pharmacist must determine the specific goals of the interview and tailor the questions accordingly. Aspects of medication use that are commonly assessed are shown in Table 13.1.

The medication history interview provides an ideal opportunity for pharmacists to apply their expertise as *'medication managers'*. It enables the pharmacist to:

- Establish a rapport with the patient
- Explain their role in patient management
- Conduct preliminary medication counselling
- Plan ongoing patient management/ pharmaceutical care

The steps involved in taking a medication history are summarised in *Appendix II*. Pharmacists should tailor their questions and discussions according to the information that is needed and the patient's ability to provide this information. Whenever possible, discussions regarding medications should be done with the patient handling the medication in question.

Table 13.1 Aspects of medication use which may be obtained from a medication history interview

History of previous allergies and/or ADRs
Indication/Purpose of each medication
Dosing regimen including dose, route, frequency and duration of therapy
Perceived efficacy of each medication
Perceived side-effects
Adherence to medication regimen
Medication administration techniques
Use of medication aids
Treatment with other systems of medicine (Ayurveda, Siddha and Unani)
Use of prescription and/or non-prescription medications
Specific problems relating to medication use
Immunisation status (if relevant)
Possibility of pregnancy in women of childbearing age
Social drug use (alcohol, tobacco, pan masala, etc.)
Evidence of drug abuse
General attitudes towards illness and medication use

The pharmacist should assess the patient's understanding and attitude towards their medications and health condition. It is important to pay special attention to the patient's concerns and tailor responses to their comments. Throughout the interview, the patient should be encouraged to speak freely, while the interviewer listens carefully and observes.

Following the interview, the data collected should be compared with the medication charts for any discrepancies (a process called *medication reconciliation*), and also to identify any drug-related problems. If appropriate, the concerned physician should be contacted to overcome those drug-related problems and amend the medication charts if needed.

Assessment of Therapeutic Goals

In order to determine the appropriateness of drug therapy, it is essential to understand the therapeutic goals for the individual patient. These may include one or more of the following:

- Cure of the disease
- Reduction/elimination of signs and symptoms
- Arresting or slowing disease progression
- Preventing disease/symptoms

These goals should be tailored to the patient's individual circumstances, and may differ from patient to patient based on their age, co-morbidities and the nature and severity of their illness. For example, for a 40-year-old patient with diabetes and hypertension, the goal may be to reduce blood pressure below 130/85 mmHg. However, in a 75-year-old patient with diabetes, hypertension and a history of postural hypotension, the goal may be to reduce blood pressure to no lower than 150/90 mmHg in order to minimise the risk of symptomatic hypotension.

Identification of Drug-related Problems

When reviewing a patient's drug therapy, one of the main objectives is to identify and resolve any drug-related problems. A drug-related problem is any event or circumstance involving drug treatment that interferes or potentially interferes with the patient achieving an optimum outcome of medical care. Eight categories of drug-related problems (DRPs) were outlined by Charles Hepler and Linda Strand in their landmark paper in 1990 (*Am J Hosp Pharm* 1990; 47:533–43), and are summarised in Table 13.2.

Table 13.2 Drug-related problems

Drug-related problems
Untreated indication
Improper drug selection
Subtherapeutic dose
Overdosage
Adverse drug reactions
Failure to receive drugs
Drug interactions
Drug use without indication

If one or more problems are identified, these should be brought to the notice of the concerned physician. Pharmacists should seek corrective measures on a priority basis, so that major problems requiring urgent action are addressed before more minor problems. While seeking corrective measures, pharmacists may suggest/ recommend suitable corrective strategies with justification.

Identification of drug-related problems involves the systematic review of each drug order on the patient's medication chart for its appropriateness. To identify drug-related problems during MOR, the pharmacist should consider the following possibilities.

Untreated indication: Does the patient have an untreated medical condition or indication which may benefit from drug therapy? When reviewing the indication for drug therapy, it is important to consider whether the indication may be an unrecognised ADR. For example, a patient who complains of diarrhoea may be taking antibiotics or other drugs which contribute to this problem. Some untreated indications may not be obvious if the patient has no associated signs or symptoms. For example, some patients with diabetes who have other cardiovascular disease risk factors may benefit from low-dose aspirin therapy as primary prevention for cardiovascular events, even though they have no current signs or symptoms.

Improper drug selection: Does the patient have a medical condition for which the wrong drug is being taken? It is important to ensure that the most appropriate drug has been chosen to treat the patient's medical condition. For example, a short course of a non-steroidal anti-inflammatory agent is the usual first-line treatment for acute gout. However, if the patient concerned also has renal impairment, a short course of prednisolone may be a more appropriate choice depending on the clinical situation. It is important to ensure that the drugs prescribed are able to achieve the therapeutic objectives (the purpose for which the drug is prescribed). However, the possibility of non-adherence to drug therapy or failure to receive drugs should be considered before deciding that a given drug is ineffective.

Subtherapeutic dose: Does the patient have a medical condition for which too little of the correct drug is being taken? The dose and dosing regimen should be individualised based on the patient's medical condition. Knowledge of clinical pharmacokinetics is useful in understanding when a maximal response is likely to occur after commencing drug treatment. For some drugs with a narrow therapeutic index and where there is an established relationship between serum concentration and therapeutic effect, therapeutic drug monitoring (TDM) can be a useful aid. Many factors need to be considered when interpreting serum drug concentrations, including co-existing diseases, concomitant drug therapy and the timing of blood sampling. For more information about this, see *Chapter 22, Therapeutic Drug Monitoring.*

Overdosage: Does the patient have a medical problem for which too much of the correct drug is being taken? Once again, TDM may be useful for some drugs. Overdosage may also occur if a patient takes a drug for a longer period than necessary. For example, if antibiotic treatment is continued after an infection has resolved, it may expose the patient to the unnecessary risk of developing ADRs and also increase the treatment cost. Overdosage can also occur if the same generic drug has been prescribed twice under different brand names. Both individual doses and the total daily dose should be assessed.

Adverse drug reactions: Does the patient have a medical condition which is the result of an ADR? The detection of an ADR is crucial in the management of any patient since failure to recognise an ADR may result in continuing patient morbidity. As a first step, the pharmacist should check that the patient is not allergic to the prescribed drug, or has had an adverse reaction to the drug in the past. Secondly, it is important to assess the patient for the presence of any new symptom, increased severity of baseline symptoms, abrupt cessation of medications or addition of anti-allergic medicines and/or steroids. All patients, especially those who are most susceptible to develop an ADR, should be monitored on a daily basis for any possible ADR. It is, therefore, essential that the clinical pharmacist has a thorough knowledge of the detection, monitoring and management of ADRs. For more information about this, see *Chapter 9, Adverse Drug Reactions and Pharmacovigilance.*

Failure to receive drugs: Does the patient have a medical condition that is the result of him or her not receiving a drug? This may be due to many factors including non-adherence, poor administration technique, missed doses due to medication errors, sub-standard drugs, non-availability of the prescribed drug or the patient's inability to pay for the medication. For example, a patient with newly diagnosed hypertension who has been prescribed an angiotensin converting enzyme inhibitor continues to have high blood pressure. On speaking to the patient, the pharmacist discovers that the patient has not been taking the drug because of its high cost. If the patient has no relevant contraindications, a low-dose thiazide or a beta blocker will be more affordable and at least equally effective.

Drug interactions: Does the patient have a medical condition that is the result of a drug–drug or drug–food interaction? Drug interactions vary in their clinical significance, and the pharmacist needs to make a professional judgement whether a change in drug therapy is necessary. For example, a patient who has been prescribed ciprofloxacin and iron tablets may not absorb ciprofloxacin if these drugs are taken at the same time. This problem can be resolved by giving the doses of these drugs several hours apart. The pharmacist should identify and resolve drug–drug interactions of clinical significance to avoid adverse consequences.

Drug use without indication: Is the patient taking a drug for which there is no valid indication? Care is needed here, as the indication for which a drug is used may not be immediately obvious. For example, tricyclic anti-depressants are often used for indications such as urinary frequency, neuropathic pain and pruritis. A pharmacist who concludes that a prescription for amitriptyline has no indication because the patient has no history of depression may be making an incorrect conclusion.

Pharmacists should prioritise any drug-related problems that are identified according to their severity and possible consequences. Using their knowledge and clinical experience, pharmacists must make a professional judgement about which problems are of greatest importance to the patient's welfare. After the drug-related problems have been assessed for severity and acuity, potential corrective action needs to be considered before deciding on the most appropriate action to resolve the problem. If a change in therapy appears necessary, the pharmacist must outline the problem to medical staff caring for the patient, and discuss the options for resolving the problem.

Individualising Medication Regimens

Once drug-related problems relating to individual drugs on the medication chart have been resolved, the next step is to consider the patient's overall medication regimen. This is particularly important for patients with chronic diseases who are on many drugs on a long-term basis. In individualising the medication regimen, the pharmacist should consider patient data including past medical history, co-morbid conditions, allergic history and concurrent disease. The aim should be to simplify the regimen as much as possible and to adjust the regimen to maximise long-term medication adherence. This may involve switching to slow-release formulations of the same drug, using a different route of administration, changing the time at which doses are taken or switching to a cheaper but effective and safe medication. Sometimes, a combination formulation can be used to replace two drugs which are being taken at similar doses as in the combination product. This should only be done after the doses for the individual drugs have been stabilised.

Monitoring of Treatment Outcome

Monitoring of treatment outcome is the key to assessing whether the therapeutic goals of drug treatment have been achieved. It is an ongoing process and involves a review of the patient's clinical status, laboratory data and other markers of drug therapy response. In hospitals, monitoring of treatment outcome is usually carried out on a daily basis by the attending doctors as part of their overall clinical review of the patient's progress and clinical status.

When evaluating a patient's response to drug therapy, the pharmacist may need to review information and data from a number of sources (Table 13.3). For example, monitoring of the effects of antibiotic treatment usually involves examining the patient's temperature chart, laboratory data (changes to indices such as white cell count and inflammatory markers such as ESR and CRP) and case note entries which describe changes in the signs and symptoms of the patient's infection. Useful information may also be obtained by speaking to patients and from evaluations undertaken by other healthcare professionals.

Some therapeutic goals require long-term follow-up. For example, a response to antidepressants may take up to 4–6 weeks to become evident. If the therapeutic goals are not achieved within the expected timeframe, pharmacists should try to identify possible causes such as medication non-adherence before considering the need for a change in therapy. This may involve dose adjustment, cessation of a drug and commencement of another drug or the addition of a second agent (see the section on clinical review later in this chapter).

Medication Chart Endorsement

Chart endorsement (annotations to the treatment chart) is one of the primary responsibilities of the pharmacist in ensuring that medication orders are unambiguous, legible and complete. It is now routine practice for pharmacists to document on the medication chart the relevant aspects of medication administration. It is essential to avoid medication errors, including those that might occur at the level of prescribing and/or administration due to incompleteness of the order, lack of adequate instructions and illegibility.

Where a chart endorsement is required, preferably with immediate notice to the concerned prescriber, all the necessary details are endorsed on the chart to avoid any confusion in drug administration and also to prevent or minimise medication errors. Some of the conditions which warrant chart endorsement include the use of unofficial abbreviations such as the abbreviation of 'unit' as 'u', incomplete documentation such as an unfilled allergy column, lack of adequate instructions such as rates of infusion for intravenous administration of vancomycin or phenytoin.

The types of annotations which may be needed are determined by considering the following:

- Is the identity of the patient (name and medical record number) on each medication chart? If not, the pharmacist should confirm the identity of the patient before completing these details on the chart.
- Is the allergy status of the patient documented on each medication chart? If not, the pharmacist should confirm these with the patient and with the patent's case notes, before annotating as needed. If no allergies are identified, then 'nil known allergies' (sometimes abbreviated as 'NKA') should be annotated on the chart.
- Is the medication name clear? Abbreviations should be avoided. For example, the abbreviation 'AZT' has been used for both azathioprine and zidovudine, which may result in the wrong drug being given unless the chart is annotated with the full generic name.
- Is the drug prescribed by the generic name? If drugs are prescribed by brand name the pharmacist should write the generic name of the drug next to the brand name.
- Is the dose clear? Both the dose and dosing frequency should be clear and unambiguous. Abbreviations such as 'u' for 'units' and 'μg' for 'mcg' should be avoided. Fractional doses should be written with a zero before the decimal point. For example, 0.5 mg should not be written as .5 mg, as the latter may result

Table 13.3 Treatment monitoring parameters and sources of information for some common diseases/conditions

Disease or Condition	*Drugs and Non-drug Treatment*	*Some Common Outcome Parameters*	*Where to Find Information*
Ischaemic heart disease /Angina	Nitrates, Beta blockers, Anti-platelet agents, Calcium antagonists	Occurrence of angina	Chest pain chart, medical or nursing notes
		Blood pressure	Observations chart
		Heart rate	Observations chart
Diabetes mellitus Type 2	Oral hypoglycaemic agents, Insulin, Diabetic diet	Blood glucose levels	Diabetes chart
		HbA1c (longterm)	Lab data
		Body weight (longterm)	Dietician reports
Acute gout	NSAIDs, colchicine, prednisolone	Uric acid level	Lab data
		Pain	Patient interview
		Redness/ tenderness	Direct observation or medical notes
Infective diarrhoea	Antibiotics Oral rehydration or IV fluids	No. and nature of bowel actions	Bowel chart
		Fluid balance	Fluid balance chart
		Skin turgor	Direct observation or medical notes
		Blood pressure	Observations chart
		Stool culture	Lab data
Major depression	Anti-depressants Psychotherapy Electroconvulsive therapy (ECT)	Appetite, mood, sleep quality, interest in activities, ability to concentrate, apathy	Can be assessed by patient interview, reading nursing/medical notes, direct observation, or reports from family members

in a ten times higher dose if the decimal point is not seen.

- Is the route of administration specified? If not, the pharmacist should endorse the chart appropriately. If there is uncertainty about the route, the pharmacist should check this with the prescriber.
- Is the date and time of drug administration clear? If the times of drug administration are inappropriate for the drug and patient concerned, then the pharmacist should annotate the chart with the recommended dosing times.
- Is a minimum dose interval stated for preparations to be taken 'as required'? Unless this is done, patients may receive more frequent doses of a medication than the doctor really intended. Also, ensure that the maximum total daily dose of a medication is stated. For example, if paracetamol is prescribed on an 'as required' basis, then the maximum dose

of 4 g per day should be stated to avoid any overdose.

- Are additional drug administration instructions given where appropriate? For example, the pharmacist may need to add directions such as 'take with food' for aspirin to avoid the risk of gastric irritation.
- Is there any over-writing which may lead to confusion? For example, has a dose been crossed out and re-written in a way which could lead to the wrong dose being administered?
- Is the cancellation of a medication order clear and unambiguous? Cancellation of medication orders should be visible and signed by the concerned prescriber.
- Is the prescription signed by a doctor? As it is a legal requirement, the pharmacist should ensure that all prescriptions are signed by the prescribing doctor.
- Has the medication chart been signed by a nurse each time a dose was due? The ideal medication chart is a combined medication order/administration record chart, where it is possible to assess drug administration at a glance. This helps in assessing medication adherence.
- Have medications been prescribed according to legal and local requirements? The pharmacist needs to ensure that the prescription meets all legal and local requirements.

Pharmacists should explain the purpose of chart endorsement to prescribers prior to commencing this service to avoid any misunderstanding. Chart endorsements, when permitted, should be initialled and dated. While reviewing medication charts to assess the need for chart endorsement, pharmacists must never try to guess the prescriber's intention from an illegible, poorly written or confusing prescription. Medication charts should be reviewed on a daily basis so that new drug orders can be annotated in a timely manner.

Documentation

The pharmaceutical care provided to a patient should be an integral part of the patient's medical record. The documentation of pharmaceutical care provided can be made either in the medication chart or in case notes with a clear title (for example, clinical pharmacy) with the pharmacist's signature. Documentation of services in the patient's medical record is then accessible to all other healthcare professionals. Computerisation of relevant information relating to pharmaceutical problems may be useful in hospitals where patients' data is accessible to healthcare providers through a networking system.

Clinical/Daily Progress Review

Clinical review is one of the integral components of medication review and should preferably be performed on a daily basis. It is the review of the patient's progress for the purpose of assessing the therapeutic outcome. The therapeutic goal for the specific disease should be clearly identified before the review as described earlier under the section on assessment of therapeutic goals.

Goals

The primary aims of the clinical review are to:

- Assess the response to drug treatment

- Evaluate the safety of the treatment regimen
- Assess the progress of the disease and the need for any change in therapy
- Assess the need for monitoring, if any
- Assess the convenience of therapy (to improve compliance)

Procedure

Ideally, clinical review should be done routinely for all patients. It is usually carried out every day by the attending doctors, while evaluating their patients, to monitor the patient outcome to drug therapy. In evaluating a patient's response to drug therapy, the pharmacist may need to review biochemical, haematological, microbiological and other investigations, as appropriate (Table 13.4). Other essential information required may be obtained from other healthcare professionals and patients.

Collection of all clinically relevant data involves the use of the following sources:

- Case notes
- Observation charts (fluid balance, blood/urine sugar, temperature and pulse)
- Medication history interview record
- Discussion with the patient and other healthcare professionals

The data should be interpreted to assess whether or not progress is being made towards the targetted objectives. These objectives should be specific to the patient's condition as mentioned earlier and could be cure of the disease, reduction in the patient's signs and symptoms, arresting/slowing the disease process, prevention of disease and improving the quality of life.

Table 13.4 Monitoring parameters to assess the patient's response to medication

Clinical parameters:
Signs Symptoms
Clinical charts:
Diabetic chart Fluid balance chart Observation chart Pain management chart Bowel chart Alcohol withdrawal chart
Laboratory parameters (if clinically indicated):
Biochemistry: *electrolytes, renal function and liver function tests* Hematological: *Total WBC, RBC indices, platelets, DC, ESR, Hb% etc.* Microbiology: *Culture results, antibiotic sensitivities* Other tests: *Echocardiogram, ECG, CT scan, MRI etc.*

The information obtained must be interpreted and evaluated with reference to:

- The clinical features of the disease being treated
- The need for an investigation
- Aspects related to drug effects (onset and duration)
- Medication history of the patient
- The desired therapeutic outcome(s)

If the therapeutic objectives are not being achieved, the clinical pharmacist should re-evaluate the appropriateness of treatment and discuss any relevant issues with the clinicians. The intervention could be of any type (change of drug, dose adjustment, cessation of drug, etc.), but the recommendations should be specific and directed towards achieving the therapeutic goals for the problem identified.

Detection and Management of Adverse Drug Reactions

Adverse drug reactions (ADRs) are one of the most important causes of morbidity and mortality. It has been estimated that approximately 10–30% of hospitalised patients will experience an ADR and 5% of hospital admissions are attributed to an ADR, of which 0.3% are fatal. It is, therefore, essential that the clinical pharmacist has knowledge of ADRs including their predictability, preventability, frequency, severity, predisposing factors and recognition, their causality assessment, management and prevention.

Definition

The World Health Organization (WHO) defines an ADR as '*any response to a drug which is noxious and unintended, and which occurs at doses normally used in man for prophylaxis, diagnosis or therapy of disease, or for the modification of physiological function*'.

Goal

The goals of ADR management include:

- Identification and monitoring of patients susceptible to ADRs
- Detection and assessment of ADRs
- Assisting in the management of ADRs
- Documentation and prevention of ADRs

Steps

In the detection and management of ADRs, pharmacists should engage in the following activities (for more information, see *Chapter 9, Adverse Drug Reactions and Pharmacovigilance*):

Identification and Monitoring of Patients Susceptible to ADRs

The patients who are most susceptible to develop an ADR should be identified and monitored on a daily basis. These patients can be identified through routine drug therapy review including MOR, clinical review and at the time of the medication history interview. Patients who are at high risk of developing an ADR include:

- Those with polypharmacy
- Those with multiple disease processes
- Geriatric and paediatric patients
- Those with inter-current diseases (renal/hepatic impairment)
- Those treated with potentially highly toxic drugs (like anti-cancer drugs)
- Those who are treated with drugs which have a narrow therapeutic index (like digoxin and amikacin)
- Those who are treated with drugs that have the potential to interact with other drugs
- Those treated with inappropriate doses and prolonged therapy

Detection and Assessment of ADRs

The detection of an ADR is crucial to the management of any patient since failure to recognise an ADR may result in continuing patient morbidity. ADRs may be identified during ward rounds with the medical team and review of the patient's chart. An ADR should always be considered as part of the broader diagnosis, and hence the differential diagnosis should include the possibility of an ADR.

In establishing the causality relationship between a suspected drug and a reaction, a temporal or possible association is sufficient for a report to be made. The assessment of a causality relationship between a drug and an ADR is often highly subjective, based on the clinician's judgement and experience. If an ADR is suspected, the assessment of ADR starts with the collection of all relevant data pertaining to patient demographics; medications including non-prescription drugs (OTC); comprehensive ADR details including a description of the reaction, time of onset and duration of the reaction, complications and or sequelae; treatment of the reaction and outcome of the treatment; and relevant investigation reports. Using all the collected data, correlation of a suspected drug with an ADR can be established and categorised by using one or more available causality assessment scales.

Assisting in the Management of ADRs

The management and prevention of ADRs is a crucial aspect in patient care activities. Rapid action is sometimes important because of the serious nature of a suspected ADR, for example, anaphylactic shock. Emergency treatment and withdrawal of all medicines may be essential. If the culprit is fairly obvious, a risk–benefit decision needs to be taken about the need for the drug (are there equally effective substitutes that are unlikely to produce the same ADR?), the severity of the reaction, and its potential for treatment. If several medicines may be causative, the non-essential medicines should be withdrawn first, probably one at a time, depending on the severity of the reaction. If the reaction is likely to be dose-related, dose reduction should be considered rather than withholding the drug. If the patient cannot manage without a medicine that has caused an adverse reaction, symptomatic relief may be given while continuing the essential treatment.

Documentation and Prevention of ADRs

Documentation of reported ADRs is essential to avoid re-exposure of the patient to the same drug or drug class. In the event of a suspected ADR, the attending pharmacist should complete appropriate documentation in the patient medical record, including attachment of alert card stickers and/or placing an alert sheet in the front of the patient's case notes. It is essential that medical staff, including the original prescriber, are notified of suspected ADRs. Also, the pharmacist should ensure completion of in-house documentation for future reference.

Conclusion

Medication review is one of the integral components of pharmaceutical care. Clinical pharmacists working in hospitals spend a considerable part of each day reviewing the drug therapy of their patients. They identify and help resolve drug-related problems and help to plan the pharmaceutical care of patients. Patient outcome can be positively affected by pharmacists identifying drug-related problems, monitoring treatment outcome, individualising medication regimens and minimising the risk of medication errors via medication chart endorsement. The role of clinical pharmacists in the healthcare system is vital in the quality use of medicines, as they are the 'medication managers'.

Exercise 1

RB, SN, PV = Initials of the nurse who has administered the medication to the patient

Medication Chart								
Patient's Name: **Mrs X**			IP No.: **130946**				Unit: Medicine	
Age: **43 years**		Sex: **Female**	Height: **159 cm**				Weight: **56 kg**	
Allergies:			Consulting Doctor:		**Dr Z**			
Regular treatment: *Date of administration*				*1st*	*2nd*	*3rd*	*4th*	*5th*
Time of administration								
Drug			8.00 AM	*RB*	*SN*	*RB*		*PV*
Levothyroxine								
Dose *25 mcg*	Route *PO*	Frequency *Twice daily*	9.00 PM	*RB*	*SN*	*RB*		*PV*
Doctor's signature								
Additional instruction								
Drug			8.00 AM	*RB*	*SN*	*RB*	*SN*	*PV*
Ferrous ascorbate								
Dose *100 mg*	Route *PO*	Frequency *Once daily*						
Doctor's signature								
Additional instruction								
Drug			8.00 AM	*RB*	*SN*	*RB*	*SN*	*PV*
Crystalline penicillin			1.00 PM	*RB*	*SN*	*RB*	*SN*	*PV*
Dose *15L U*	Route *IV*	Frequency *Q6H*	5.00 PM	*RB*	*SN*	*RB*	*SN*	*PV*
			9.00 PM	*RB*	*SN*	*RB*	*SN*	*PV*
Doctor's signature								
Additional instruction								
Drug			8.00 AM	*RB*	*SN*	*RB*	*SN*	*PV*
Amoxicillin + clavulanic acid			1.00 PM	*RB*	*SN*	*RB*	*SN*	*PV*
Dose *625 mg*	Route *IV*	Frequency *Thrice daily*	9.00 PM	*RB*	*SN*	*RB*	*SN*	*PV*
Doctor's signature								

Medication Chart								
Patient's Name: **Mrs X**				IP No.: **130946**				Unit: Medicine
Age: **43 years**		Sex: **Female**		Height: **159 cm**				Weight: **56 kg**
Allergies:				Consulting Doctor:		Dr Z		
Regular treatment: Date of administration				*1st*	*2nd*	*3rd*	*4th*	*5th*
Time of administration								
Doctor's signature								
Additional instruction								
Drug			8.00 AM	*RB*	*SN*	*RB*	*SN*	*PV*
Regular Insulin			1.00 PM	*RB*	*SN*	*RB*	*SN*	*PV*
Dose *6 units*	Route *SC*	Frequency *Thrice daily*	9.00 PM	*RB*	*SN*	*RB*	*SN*	*PV*
Doctor's signature								
Additional instruction *Give 30 minutes prior to each meal*								
Drug			8.00 AM	*RB*				
Paracetamol			1.00 PM					
Dose 650 mg	Route Oral	Frequency SOS	5.00 PM			*RB*		
			9.00 PM			*RB*		
Doctor's signature								
Additional instruction								

You are reviewing the medication chart of a patient (see previous page) who has been diagnosed during admission with primary hypothyroidism and leptospirosis associated with decreased renal function (estimated GFR: 25 ml/minute). Her past medical history reveals that she had been diagnosed with type 1 diabetes two years ago and is using regular insulin.

- Review the medication chart for potential medication errors
- List the chart annotations which may help prevent may help prevent medication errors
- Summarise potential drug-related problems in order of priority which require further investigation
- Describe how you would monitor treatment response

Discussion:

The endorsements to be made to the medication chart include:

- The Allergy column should be completed. If the patient is not allergic to any drug, then the Allergy column should be completed by writing 'NIL KNOWN ALLERGY'.

- The order for crystalline penicillin should be annotated 'Benzyl penicillin' to ensure the correct drug is administered. The dose should be written as '1.5 million units' (note that the term lakh is unknown outside of India).
- The maximum dose of paracetamol per day (4 g/day) should be annotated. This order should be cancelled and re-written on the chart used for 'When needed' medications (if available).
- SOS should be annotated 'as required' and a dosing frequency should be added.

The most important potential drug-related problems that need to be investigated further are given below:

- There is a potential risk of crystalline penicillin toxicity. Considering the patient's renal status (estimated GFR: 25 ml/minute), discuss with medical staff whether the frequency of crystalline penicillin administration should be changed from Q6H to Q8H to avoid any potential toxicity. Crystalline penicillin dose adjustment is required if GFR is $\leq$ 50 ml/minute. (DRP: Overdosage)
- The indication for amoxicillin + clavulanic acid is unclear and should be investigated. (DRP: Drug use without indication)
- Ascertain with nursing staff whether the unsigned column on Day 4 refers to non-administration of levothyroxine or administered but not initialled. If non-administered, investigate the cause for this. (DRP: Failure to receive drug)
- Concomitant administration of levothyroxine and ferrous ascorbate can lead to potential therapeutic failure due to drug–drug interaction. Iron and iron containing preparations are reported to decrease the absorption of levothyroxine. Allow an interval of 4–5 hours between the two drugs. (DRP: Drug interaction)
- Concomitant use of levothyroxine and insulin may result in reduced efficacy of insulin, and hencc an increased dose of regular insulin may be required. As thyroxine has a long half-life this effect may take some weeks to evolve. Careful monitoring of blood sugar levels should be used to guide dosage adjustment of insulin therapy. (DRP: Drug interaction)

The most important parameters that need to be monitored during therapy include:

- BSLs should be monitored carefully as insulin requirements may change during acute illness. Long-term control of diabetes should be assessed by checking the results of recent HbA1c measurements.
- Monitoring thyroid function is required to determine the patient's response to levothyroxine. Vital signs such as heart rate and blood pressure, and clinical signs of hypo or hyperthyroidism should be monitored.
- Check the complete haemogram, serum ferritin, serum iron, total iron binding capacity and percentage saturation of transferrin as the patient is receiving ferrous ascorbate.
- Monitor for temperature, inflammatory markers, WBC, culture and sensitivity tests as the patient is receiving antibiotics.

- **Renal function needs to be monitored regularly as the patient's estimated GFR is low and she is receiving crystalline penicillin and amoxicillin.**

EXERCISE 2:

Medication Chart								
Patient's Name: **Mr Y**			IP No.: **130974**					Unit: Medicine
Age: **52 years**		Sex: **Male**	Height: **162 cm**					Weight: **37 kg**
Allergies: *Hypersensitive to Penicillin*			Consulting Doctor: **Dr. Z**					
Regular treatment: Date of administration				*1st*	*2nd*	*3rd*	*4th*	*5th*
Time of administration								
Drug			8.00 AM	*RB*	*SN*	*RB*	*SN*	*PV*
Isoniazid								
Dose **300 mg**	Route **Oral**	Frequency **Once daily**						
Doctor's signature								
Additional instruction								
Drug			8.00 AM	*RB*	*SN*	*RB*	*SN*	*PV*
Rifampicin								
Dose **450 mg**	Route **Oral**	Frequency **Once daily**						
Doctor's signature								
Additional instruction								
Drug			8.00 AM	*RB*	*SN*	*RB*	*SN*	
Pyrazinamide								
Dose **1500 mg**	Route **Oral**	Frequency **Once daily**						
Doctor's signature								
Additional instruction								
Drug			8.00 AM	*RB*	*SN*	*RB*	*SN*	*PV*
Ethambutol								
Dose **800 mg**	Route **Oral**	Frequency **Once daily**						
Doctor's signature								

<table>
<tr><td colspan="10">Medication Chart</td></tr>
<tr><td colspan="4">Patient's Name: Mr Y</td><td colspan="5">IP No.: 130974</td><td>Unit: Medicine</td></tr>
<tr><td colspan="2">Age: 52 years</td><td colspan="2">Sex: Male</td><td colspan="5">Height: 162 cm</td><td>Weight: 37 kg</td></tr>
<tr><td colspan="4">Allergies: Hypersensitive to Penicillin</td><td colspan="6">Consulting Doctor: Dr. Z</td></tr>
<tr><td colspan="3">Regular treatment:
Date of administration</td><td></td><td>1st</td><td>2nd</td><td>3rd</td><td>4th</td><td>5th</td><td></td></tr>
<tr><td colspan="3">Time of administration</td><td></td><td></td><td></td><td></td><td></td><td></td><td></td></tr>
<tr><td colspan="3">Doctor's signature</td><td></td><td></td><td></td><td></td><td></td><td></td><td></td></tr>
<tr><td colspan="3">Additional instruction</td><td></td><td></td><td></td><td></td><td></td><td></td><td></td></tr>
<tr><td colspan="3">Drug
Carbidopa / Levodopa</td><td>8.00 AM</td><td>RB</td><td>SN</td><td>RB</td><td>SN</td><td>PV</td><td></td></tr>
<tr><td>Dose
25/100 mg</td><td>Route
Oral</td><td>Frequency
Twice daily</td><td>9.00 PM</td><td>RB</td><td>SN</td><td>RB</td><td>SN</td><td>PV</td><td></td></tr>
<tr><td colspan="3">Doctor's signature</td><td></td><td></td><td></td><td></td><td></td><td></td><td></td></tr>
<tr><td colspan="3">Additional instruction</td><td></td><td></td><td></td><td></td><td></td><td></td><td></td></tr>
<tr><td colspan="3" rowspan="2">Drug
Paracetamol</td><td>8.00 AM</td><td>RB</td><td>SN</td><td></td><td></td><td></td><td></td></tr>
<tr><td>1.00 PM</td><td></td><td>SN</td><td></td><td></td><td></td><td></td></tr>
<tr><td rowspan="2">Dose
650 mg</td><td rowspan="2">Route
Oral</td><td rowspan="2">Frequency
As required</td><td>5.00 PM</td><td></td><td></td><td></td><td></td><td></td><td></td></tr>
<tr><td>9.00 PM</td><td>RB</td><td></td><td></td><td></td><td></td><td></td></tr>
<tr><td colspan="3">Doctor's signature</td><td></td><td></td><td></td><td></td><td></td><td></td><td></td></tr>
<tr><td colspan="3">Additional instruction
Not to exceed 4 g/day</td><td></td><td></td><td></td><td></td><td></td><td></td><td></td></tr>
</table>

You are reviewing the medication chart of a patient who has been diagnosed during admission with culture-positive pulmonary tuberculosis. His medical history reveals that he has been suffering from Parkinson's disease for one and a half years, for which he has been taking levodopa/carbidopa.

- Review the medication chart for potential medication errors.
- List the chart annotations which may help to prevent medication errors.
- Summarise potential drug-related problems in order of priority which require further investigation.
- Describe how you would monitor treatment response

Discussion:

The endorsements to be made to the medication chart include:

- Annotate "one hour before food" on the Rifampicin order.

The most important potential drug-related problems that need to be investigated further include:

- The dose of anti-tubercular agents should be adjusted based on body weight of 37 kg. (DRP: Overdosage)
- Administration of pyridoxine 25 mg daily is required to prevent the possible development of neuropathy associated with the use of isoniazid. (DRP: Untreated indication)
- Need to ascertain with nursing staff whether unsigned pyrazinamide dose on day 5 refers to non-administration of drug or administered but not signed for. If non-administered, investigate the reason for this.(DRP: Failure to receive drugs)
- There have been reports of isoniazid reducing the therapeutic effect of levodopa with worsening of Parkinson's disease. The dose of levodopa/carbidopa may need to be adjusted if this occurs. (DRP: Drug interaction)

The most important parameters that need to be monitored during therapy include:

- The patient's sputum should be cultured monthly until sputum culture is negative.
- The patient needs to be monitored for any possible elevation in liver enzymes (hepatotoxicity) due to the use of anti-tubercular agents such as rifampicin and isoniazid.
- Baseline visual acuity (visual evoked potential) and colour discrimination should be assessed and monitored regularly as ethambutol can cause retrobulbar neuritis.
- The patient should be monitored for peripheral neuropathy due to isoniazid.
- Pyrazinamide can cause hyperuricaemia and the patient should be observed for signs and symptoms of gout.
- Monitor for any possible hypersensitivity reaction to ceftazidime, especially after the first dose.
- Monitor the patient for both clinical response and adverse effects to levodopa/carbidopa.

KEY MESSAGES

- The purpose of medication review is to maximise the effectiveness and safety of drug therapy.
- To determine the appropriateness of drug therapy, it is essential to understand the therapeutic goals for the individual patient.
- Medication review serves as a basis for identifying the patient's pharmaceutical care needs, such as medication counselling, detection and management of suspected ADRs and recommendations for therapeutic drug monitoring (TDM).
- Drug-related problems are circumstances involving a patient's drug treatment that actually, or potentially, interfere with the achievement of an optimal health outcome.
- Drug-related problems should be prioritised according to how urgently they need to be resolved.
- If the objectives of drug therapy are not being achieved, the clinical pharmacist's intervention may assist in improving the clinical outcome.
- The detection of an ADR is crucial in patient management since failure to recognise it may result in continuing patient morbidity.

Further Reading

Hepler CD and Strand LM. 1990. Opportunities and responsibilities in pharmaceutical care. *Am J Hosp Pharm* 47:533–43.

SHPA Standard of Practice for the Provision of Medication Reconciliation. 2007. *J Pharm Pract Res* 37(3):231–3 (also available on The Society of Hospital Pharmacists of Australia website: http://www.shpa.org.au)

Stebbins MR, Cutler TW and Parker PL. 2009. Assessment of therapy and medication therapy management. In: Koda-Kimble MA, Yee Young LY, Alldredge BK, Corelli RL, Guglielmo BJ, Kradjan WA and Williams BR. (ed)s. *Applied Therapeutics - The Clinical Use of Drugs*. 9th ed. Lippincott Williams & Wilkins - A Wolters Kluwer Company, Baltimore, Maryland, USA.

Wilcox C and Duguid MJ. 2001. The medication chart as an integral tool in the pharmaceutical care plan. *Aust J Hosp Pharm* 31(40): 268–274.

14 Ward Round Participation

Johnson George

Learning Objectives

Upon completion of this chapter, the reader should be able to:

- List the goals and objectives for clinical pharmacists on ward rounds
- Explain the preparation necessary to accomplish those objectives
- Understand the general guidelines for ward round participation
- Understand the types of interventions that may be made during ward rounds
- Appreciate the value of good communication skills with medical and allied health staff during ward rounds
- Understand the need for follow-up after ward rounds

In many developed countries, the pharmacy profession has undergone revolutionary changes over the past five decades. In the early 1960s, the pharmacy profession started moving away from the traditional role of a compounder preparing and selling medications to that of a pharmacy practitioner providing patient-oriented health services. In 1990, Hepler and Strand defined a new way to look at the responsibilities of the pharmacist and pharmacy services.

The 'pharmaceutical care' concept described by Hepler and Strand empowers pharmacists with greater responsibility and accountability in patient care. *Pharmaceutical care* is the process through which a pharmacist co-operates with a patient and other professionals in designing, implementing and monitoring a therapeutic plan that will produce specific health outcomes for the patient. Research has shown that multi-disciplinary healthcare teams are more effective in identifying and managing patient problems when compared with individual approaches to healthcare delivery.

The fundamental responsibility of a pharmacist is to ensure that every patient receives the most appropriate evidence-based treatment in the most convenient and cost-effective form at the right time. This involves influencing medicine use decisions not only by patients, but also by healthcare professionals. The knowledge and skills of pharmacists for combining therapeutic, pharmacological and pharmaceutical data can help ensure optimal patient outcome.

Retrospective review of medication orders by pharmacists on the wards has been shown to maximise safe prescribing. The pharmacist's impact can be substantially greater if input is provided at the time of prescribing. Clinical pharmacists are ideally placed to favourably influence prescribing and improve the quality and safety of medicine use since they have appropriate clinical knowledge and regular contact with prescribers and other members of the healthcare team.

Medical Ward Rounds

A ward round is a visit made by a medical practitioner, alone or with a team of health professionals and medical students, to hospital inpatients at their bedside to review and follow-up progress in their health. At least one ward round is conducted every day to review the progress of each inpatient, although more than one is not uncommon. In certain practice settings such as psychiatry, the so-called 'ward round' may be conducted away from the patient's bedside in a non-traditional fashion, where the team meets elsewhere to review each case.

Pharmacists' participation in medical ward rounds in the United States and United Kingdom dates back to the 1970s. The evolution was accelerated by the development of postgraduate courses in clinical pharmacy. Experience from the United States, United Kingdom, Australia and Canada has shown that the addition of a pharmacist to the healthcare team attending ward rounds in various practice settings helps ensure safe, effective and economic use of drugs. This results in decreased adverse drug events, improved patient care, reduced length of hospital stay and reduced healthcare costs. The response of the medical staff towards this relatively new role of pharmacists in those settings has been excellent.

Goals and Objectives of Clinical Pharmacists on Ward Rounds

As an important member of the healthcare team, pharmacists should attend ward rounds and clinical meetings whenever possible. This enables pharmacists to contribute prospectively to patient care by providing drug information and promoting rational drug therapy. The goals of a clinical pharmacist's participation in ward rounds are to:

- Gain an improved understanding of the patient's clinical status and progress, current planned investigations and therapeutic goals
- Provide relevant information on various aspects of the patient's drug therapy, such as pharmacology, pharmacokinetics, drug availability, cost, drug interactions and adverse reactions
- Optimise therapeutic management by influencing drug therapy selection, implementation, monitoring and follow-up
- Investigate unusual drug orders or doses
- Assimilate additional information about the patient such as co-morbidities, medication compliance or complementary and alternative medicine (for example herbal remedies) use that might be relevant to their management

- Detect adverse drug reactions and drug interactions
- Participate in patient discharge planning

Compared to doctors in non-teaching hospitals, medical practitioners in teaching hospitals have more opportunities to keep themselves up-to-date with new developments in therapeutics through continuing medical education programmes and clinical seminars. Therefore, pharmacists working in non-teaching hospitals have considerable opportunitics to promote evidence-based pharmacotherapeutics and the quality and safe use of medicines.

Ward round participation also provides many learning opportunities for pharmacists. It allows them to see first-hand how medicines are used and prescribed, and to see the effects of these medicines on patients. With time, pharmacists develop an appreciation of how the patient's own wishes and their social, cultural and economic circumstances may influence therapeutic choices.

Even for experienced clinical pharmacists in teaching hospitals, it is very rare to finish a ward round without gaining new perspectives on some aspect of therapeutics or patient care. For those involved in academia and research, ward rounds allow identification of cases for clinical teaching and publication. Finally, ward round participation strengthens the inter-professional relationship among various health professionals, leading to better healthcare practice and research.

Ward Rounds: The Indian Scenario

The Indian healthcare system is diverse, with a wide range of healthcare facilities provided in the government, private and corporate sectors. Outpatient and inpatient services are offered through these three sectors in varying capacity and scope. Inpatient services are available at primary, secondary and tertiary care hospitals. Based on their affiliation to a medical school, these hospitals are categorised as teaching or non-teaching hospitals.

An insight into the organisational aspects of hospital medical care is necessary to understand the functioning of healthcare teams. Primary care hospitals (also referred to as nursing homes in the private sector) usually undertake the early management of patients as well as treating those with minor ailments. General physicians are responsible for the management of these patients. The only difference between a primary care clinic (for example, health centre) and a primary care hospital is the availability of the inpatient service in primary care hospitals. Referral to secondary or tertiary care centres is routine for the management of more complex cases.

Secondary care hospitals have general surgical and medical teams. The general surgical team usually consists of one or more general surgeons and residents or assistants who care for patients admitted with various surgical problems. Similarly, the general medical team will have one or more physicians with specialisation in general medicine and residents or assistants, who treat most of the common medical illnesses.

Tertiary care hospitals are mainly referral centres for complex medical or surgical cases as well as for specialised treatment; however, they also offer basic health services. Each specialty may have multiple units where individual units are headed by a senior specialist and other specialists, assistants or residents make up the team. Consultants or specialists from tertiary care are sometimes invited for consultations at primary or secondary care centres. Specialty units of teaching hospitals are similar to those of non-teaching tertiary care institutions. The most senior practitioners of these units are professors or senior consultants with academic responsibilities at an affiliated medical school, and are involved in classroom teaching as well as clinical teaching at the patient's bedside.

The constitution of the healthcare team participating in a ward round varies between teaching and non-teaching hospitals, as well as between private and government hospitals. It may consist of one or more medical practitioners alone, or a team of medical practitioners and allied health professionals. Nursing staff almost invariably participate in ward rounds in all practice settings. In most primary and secondary care hospitals, one or two doctors along with a nursing staff member conduct the rounds, at least once a day. Clinical pharmacists may find it useful to join these rounds on a daily basis.

In teaching hospitals, medical and allied healthcare students may also join ward rounds for clinical learning at the patient's bedside. Allied health professionals such as pharmacists, physiotherapists, dieticians, occupational therapists or social workers may join ward rounds in selected units of some tertiary care hospitals.

Ward rounds may be classified according to the purpose of the round and composition of the participating healthcare team. The common types of ward rounds in Indian hospitals are:

- *Pre-rounds:* During these rounds, the interns or medical postgraduate students in teaching hospitals perform a daily review of patients in their unit or ward. This is largely a learning opportunity to familiarise themselves with the cases, especially new admissions or transfers, and very few management decisions are made during these rounds. Trainee clinical pharmacists may join the interns or postgraduates in their pre-rounds and complete the patient medication and clinical review at this time.
- *Registrar/Resident rounds:* In teaching hospitals, the registrars and residents, individually or as a team conduct ward rounds, at least once a day at a fixed time, usually in the morning. In the intensive care unit (ICU), rounds may be conducted several times a day. These rounds are extensive and may also involve clinical teaching to medical postgraduate students and interns. These are useful rounds for clinical pharmacists of all levels of experience to join.
- *Professor/Unit chief rounds:* In teaching hospitals, the chief of a unit or ward, or the professor in a specialty conducts rounds together with their registrars, residents, postgraduate students and interns for all patients under their care, on a daily basis or on a few days of each week. These rounds may be extensive, with time devoted to addressing more complex issues regarding diagnosis or management which the registrars or residents have encountered. These rounds may be more challenging for clinical pharmacists in terms of their clinical knowledge.

Some consultants in teaching hospitals do not get involved in regular teaching activities and may only be doing referrals on request by professors or unit chiefs. It may be difficult for clinical pharmacists to join these consultant rounds due to timing. In such instances, recommendations or advice on patient management may be conveyed verbally through other members of the medical team or written in the patient's case sheets, if permitted.

- *Teaching rounds:* In teaching hospitals, academic medical staff conduct bedside clinical teaching rounds for residents, medical postgraduate students, interns and medical undergraduate students. These are very extensive rounds and are usually conducted only a few times in a week. Although these rounds provide an opportunity for pharmacists to improve their clinical knowledge, they are generally not the best rounds for making interventions or recommendations. Some clinical pharmacists with joint academic appointments may use these rounds to teach therapeutics to medical and allied health students.

Pre-ward round preparation: Pharmacists need to prepare adequately before participating in ward rounds. Accurate and up-to-date information on the patient's health status, disease management and medical and medication history is essential for active participation in clinical decision-making. To achieve this, a review of the medication chart and case record should be completed prior to the ward round. Where necessary, further information should also be gathered from the patient or their carer. Pre-ward round preparation gives an overview of the medication and condition-related issues that may be brought up during a ward round and allows the pharmacist to be proactive during the round.

Many clinical pharmacists maintain individual patient profiles which summarise information relevant to the patient's drug therapy. This includes allergies or hypersensitivities, the reason for admission, provisional or final diagnosis, past medical history, medications on admission, relevant social history, laboratory data, other relevant investigations and reports, and other information such as medication compliance and medication administration skills.

These details are collected by reviewing the patient's case record and treatment charts as well as by interviewing the patient or carers. Information may be recorded on specific forms designed by pharmacists to suit their practice setting. An example of such a form used by a clinical pharmacist working in a general medical unit is given in Fig. 14.1. A folder with an alphabetical index is helpful for easy retrieval of patient profiles.

During pre-ward round preparation, issues may arise that need to be clarified by referring appropriate information resources. Hands-on references are useful in such circumstances. It may also be useful to make a note of the interventions or recommendations to be made during the ward rounds listed in order of priority. For all newly admitted patients, it is appropriate to collect a detailed medication history from the patient or their carers, which needs to be cross-checked with information collected by other healthcare professionals. Any relevant new information obtained during the medication history interview which may change patient management (for example, history of allergy to a medicine) should be brought to the attention of the appropriate healthcare professionals and used to update existing patient profiles. Thus, pre-ward round preparation allows the pharmacist to be well-informed and organised before discussing

Figure 14.1 Patient profile form

Name of the patient: Age/ Sex: Address:

Date of admission: *(alternatively place patient ID sticker)*

Reason for admission:

Allergies:

Past Medical History:

Past Medication History:

Complementary and alternative medicine/Over-the-counter medicines:

Social History: Smoking Alcohol

Other (e.g. recreational drugs, chewing tobacco or pan)

Drugs on admission:

Diagnosis:

Current Drugs:

Investigations:

Date					
Creatinine					
Urea					
Albumin					
RBS					
FBS					
Hb					
RBC					
WBC					
DC					
ESR					
CK					
LDH					
SGPT					
SGOT					

Other Diagnostic results:
(ECG, X-ray, CT, MRI, ECHO, USG)

Clinical Progress:
(BP, Temp, Sugar)

Other information:

patient management and contributing to the decision-making process.

Practical tips for ward round participation: Pharmacists should complete their pre-ward round preparation well ahead of commencement of the round. If there is no fixed time for a ward round, the pharmacist needs to arrange to be notified at the commencement of each round. In situations where clinical pharmacists are responsible for different wards and there is an overlap in the timing of different ward rounds, priority should be given to those rounds in which the pharmacist can contribute more.

In hospitals with a formulary or drug list, the pharmacist should ensure that all prescriptions are in accordance with the hospital formulary. This is relevant to all government hospitals and some corporate hospitals. Clinical pharmacists may wish to carry appropriate references while working in wards. British National Formulary (BNF) Drug Information Handbook and Australian Medicines Handbook (AMH) are some commonly used references. Relevant up-to-date clinical guidelines (for example, Asthma Guidelines from the British Thoracic Society, Hypertension Guidelines from the World Health Organization) are useful references for pharmacists working in specialty areas.

When identifying potential problems such as drug interactions, adverse reactions and medication errors, pharmacists should be prepared to suggest alternatives to resolve the problem. For example, if the medical team accepts the pharmacist's suggestion that amlodipine may be contributing to a patient's peripheral oedema, the pharmacist should be prepared to answer the obvious question which may follow: which alternative anti-hypertensive would you recommend for this patient? Thorough pre-ward round familiarity with the patient's medical history will allow the pharmacist to discuss the appropriate options.

Pharmacists should avoid the temptation to enter discussions concerning diagnosis. The one exception to this is where a patient's symptoms or signs are possibly drug-related. In the above scenario, for example, the pharmacist needs to consider the possibility that the patient's peripheral oedema may be due to other causes such as heart failure. The pharmacist's suggestion that the oedema may be drug-related is best offered once the more common causes of peripheral oedema have been excluded by the medical team.

Interventions during ward rounds: During ward rounds, the physician first interviews the patient or carer about the patient's symptoms, complaints and progress. This is usually followed by physical examination, then a review of laboratory data and other diagnostic tests. The attending physician in consultation with other members of the healthcare team may then make decisions regarding patient diagnosis and management. On certain occasions, the pharmacist's opinion regarding drug treatment may also be sought.

A pharmacy intervention is defined as any action by a pharmacist that directly results in a change in patient management or therapy. Opportunities for interventions arise during various clinical pharmacy activities including medication history interview, medication chart review, therapeutic drug monitoring, provision of drug information and ward round participation. Intervention by pharmacists to assist prescribing can take several forms. It can be active (the use of clinical guidelines, particularly when backed up by personal visits to influence prescribing), passive (such as drug information services) or reactive (monitoring prescriptions and seeking amendment of those that are unclear, erroneous, inadequate or inappropriate). *Practice Scenario 1* gives an example of a reactive pharmacy intervention.

Important decisions regarding inpatient management are often made during ward rounds, and clinical pharmacists participating on ward rounds may influence these decisions while they are being made. The presence of a pharmacist on ward rounds as a member of the patient care team in the 17-bed medical ICU of Massachusetts General Hospital reduced preventable adverse drug events by 72%. More than 90% of pharmacist interventions were related to medication ordering; the physician acceptance rate of these interventions was 99%. The errors identified by the pharmacist included incomplete orders, wrong dose, wrong frequency, inappropriate choice and duplicate therapy. In addition, the pharmacist provided drug use information, recommended alternative therapies that were safer or cheaper but equally effective, and identified problems relating to drug interactions, adverse drug events, drug allergies and errors in the pharmacy dispensing system (*JAMA* 1999; 282:267–270).

Pharmacist participation with the medical rounding team on a general medicine unit of a Detroit hospital was also shown to contribute to a significant reduction (by 78%) in preventable adverse drug events. Two clinical pharmacists were assigned to provide patient care services which included ward round participation, documenting pharmacotherapy history and providing patient discharge counselling. The physician acceptance rate of pharmacist interventions was 98%. The most common interventions involved recommendations for dose or frequency adjustments and for the addition of an indicated drug (*Arch Intern Med* 2003; 163:2014–2018).

The main drug-related queries that may arise during ward rounds relate to:

- dose and frequency
- choice of medication
- adverse effects
- drug interactions
- formulation
- duration of therapy
- actions and uses/pharmacology
- drug availability/supply
- identification of patient's medications on admission
- legal and administrative issues
- miscellaneous, such as storage conditions

Recommendations or interventions to be made during ward rounds need to be prioritised according to their clinical significance and likely patient benefits. Interventions are more likely to be successful when pharmacists recommend solutions/alternatives for the drug therapy problems identified. The disposition of the medical staff and time constraints should also be taken into account. The experience and communication skills of the pharmacist and their relationship with medical staff are critical factors determining the success of pharmacist interventions. *Practice Scenario 2* provides an example of how to prioritise pharmacy recommendations and interventions.

Communication during ward rounds: Clinical pharmacists must work closely with other healthcare professionals to meet the healthcare needs of patients. Effective communication skills and clinical knowledge are prerequisites for effective participation in ward rounds and clinical meetings. Pharmacists need to take an active role in patient care by conveying their views on patient management to other healthcare professionals. They need to be aware at all times that their professional duties are to the patient and should be committed to ensuring that patients receive the most appropriate drug therapy. Good inter-professional relationships are key for success. Pharmacists should try to resolve differences in opinion in a direct manner but in a way that conveys respect for others.

In most teaching hospitals in India, English is the official language of communication among healthcare professionals during ward rounds. However, on most occasions the clinicians will speak to their patients in the regional language. Knowledge of the regional language helps the pharmacist to follow the conversations between clinicians and patients. It also helps the pharmacist to interact effectively with patients. Pharmacists should be cautious while discussing drug-related issues on the ward round in the presence of patients or their carers. Interventions or recommendations should be made in a way which does not challenge the prescriber's integrity or affect the patient's faith in the prescriber.

Several barriers may exist when communicating with medical staff. Situations may arise during ward rounds where the clinical pharmacist's advice is sought on issues where they lack the appropriate knowledge or expertise. Whenever pharmacists are uncertain about an answer, they should not try to bluff or guess, but rather acknowledge this to the prescriber, and undertake to retrieve the relevant information after the ward round, and then communicate the same to the prescriber.

Health professionals and patients may underestimate the skills of the pharmacist and may question their potential role in patient care. Physicians may not accept pharmacist recommendations or may not welcome some of their suggestions. Pharmacists should not expect a 'pat on the back' from physicians even for recommendations that result in significant improvement in patient outcome.

In countries where clinical pharmacy is well established, pharmacists and physicians share responsibility for the management of the patient's drug therapy. In contrast, inter- and intra-professional hierarchy is common in most Indian clinical settings. Hence, the seniority and designation of medical staff need to be considered during the communication process. Pharmacists should always avoid open or implied criticism of other healthcare professionals. Inter-professional respect and teamwork are key factors for success. Interventions or recommendations made by the pharmacist should be made in a diplomatic way, which shows respect for the physician's clinical acumen and experience, and should not challenge a medical practitioner's integrity.

Ward round follow-up: Clinical pharmacists often encounter issues during a ward round that require some follow-up. Pharmacists should prioritise these issues according to their urgency and relevance. Some of the outstanding issues that may arise during a ward round include:

- **Responding to enquiries:** All unanswered queries raised during ward rounds should be recorded and followed-up at the earliest. Responses may be given over the telephone, by e-mail, in print or in person, as appropriate. If necessary, the information should be supported with adequate references.

- **Communicating information:** In some instances, the clinical pharmacist may need to communicate changes in drug therapy made during ward rounds to relevant healthcare personnel such as medical, nursing, pharmacy, technical or dietetics staff.
- **Completing documentation:** In some situations, recommendations or interventions made by the pharmacist during a ward round may need to be documented appropriately. ADRs identified during the round may need to be documented on an alert sheet. If the clinical pharmacist has permission to record on the patient's case sheet, relevant details should be entered with the name, contact details and signature of the pharmacist.
- **Altering the patient's care plan:** The pharmacist may need to make alterations to the patient's care plan as a result of changes in patient management (for example, monitoring of drug levels or other laboratory investigations, and recommending doses after dialysis).
- **Discussions with patients:** If appropriate, the pharmacist should discuss drug therapy issues with patients (for example, the reasons for alteration in therapy, drug administration or self-monitoring techniques and caution regarding likely adverse effects).

Getting Started

The concept of clinical pharmacy practice and the role of pharmacists in patient management may be unfamiliar for many healthcare professionals and administrators in India. Pharmacists intending to initiate clinical pharmacy services need to create awareness among key policy-makers of the importance of these services. This can be achieved through discussions with the key personnel involved in decision-making processes in various settings and formal presentations to clinical and academic meetings. In government hospitals, the official permission (Government Order) from the central or state government is the first step towards initiating clinical pharmacy services.

In both government and private teaching hospitals, the Dean, Medical Director, Resident Medical Officer, head of the Department of General Medicine and senior professors may be approached initially regarding introduction of the service. In private non-teaching hospitals, the Managing Director, Chief Medical Officer and senior physicians could be useful initial contacts. The Resident Medical Officer and senior physicians are the key personnel to be contacted in a non-teaching government hospital. In both teaching and non-teaching hospital settings, it is important to discuss the new service with the heads of the hospital pharmacy department, clinical pharmacology department and nursing services. In situations where the hospital is affiliated to a university, the heads of the pharmacy and medical schools also need to be involved.

Appropriate education and supervised training are prerequisites for pharmacists to take on clinical responsibilities. Pharmacists with a sound knowledge of therapeutics and pathophysiology and with good communication skills are suitably qualified. A postgraduate qualification in clinical pharmacy or pharmacy practice is desirable.

General medical units are usually the best areas to introduce the practice of clinical pharmacy. Experience shows that pharmacy interventions are more likely to occur with medical consultants than with surgeons. More complex drug therapy for medical patients and the availability of prescribers at the time of decision making increases the opportunities for pharmacists to contribute.

At the outset, the pharmacist could join a senior professor or physician on their ward round. Though seniority of the physicians is not a restrictive criterion, it is politically wiser to introduce the concept to one of the senior medical staff. Close observation of the physician's therapy preferences is recommended initially so that advice and suggestions are made in a way that conveys respect to the physician's current prescribing practice. The personality and co-operativeness of the pharmacist and the medical staff are critical factors in determining the success of this collaboration, especially at the beginning.

It is not possible for a single pharmacist to acquire the knowledge and expertise to advise consultants from many different specialties. Specialisation is common among clinical pharmacists, where pharmacists focus on one or more specialised areas. Though it is advantageous to gain expertise in specialised areas and focus on certain practice specialties, pharmacists should initially be prepared to take the available opportunities and acquire general skills that can be adapted in many clinical situations.

As for any novel concept, there will be both advocates and opponents of the notion of pharmacists participating in clinical decision making during ward rounds. Experience from the United States, United Kingdom, Canada and Australia shows that it may take years for this concept to gain wide acceptance by medical professionals and administrators. Pioneering practitioners and entrepreneurs of clinical pharmacy in India need to realise this and be diligent and industrious in their distinct task. Last but not least, bear in mind the words of Hippocrates, *'As to diseases, make a habit of two things - to help or at least do no harm'*.

PRACTICE SCENARIO 1

Raju, a 69-year-old retired teacher, presents to the outpatient department of a large teaching hospital with complaints of lethargy, reduced frequency of urination, swollen feet and ankles and cough. Raju has a history of congestive heart failure and has been taking ramipril and frusemide for several years. Worsening of heart failure is the provisional diagnosis made by the admitting intern. Raju is admitted to the general medical ward and intravenous frusemide is initiated.

Vidhya is the clinical pharmacist in the general medical ward. As part of her routine pre-ward round preparation, Vidhya speaks to Raju about his medication use and compliance. Raju discloses that four weeks prior to admission he had one of his wisdom teeth removed. His dentist prescribed a broad-spectrum antibiotic, and Raju was told to purchase over-the-counter ibuprofen and take it sos (when necessary) for pain relief. He developed an abscess after the extraction, requiring further dental surgery. Raju has taken ibuprofen all this time, and more at times when the abscess was causing pain. This information was not obtained by the admitting intern. The following day, Vidhya joins a consultant ward round during which Raju's progress is reviewed.

How can Vidhya contribute to the management of this patient during the ward round?

Discussion

Vidhya listens carefully to the discussion among medical staff regarding Raju's laboratory data. She calculates the estimated creatinine clearance, which is low compared to previous results for Raju at outpatient appointments. The medical team reaches the conclusion that it is a case of pre-renal acute renal failure resulting from poorly controlled congestive heart failure. The doctors question Raju about his medication compliance. At this point, Vidhya explains to the medical staff that she has interviewed Raju and discovered that he has been taking over-the-counter ibuprofen for a few weeks. She then raises the possibility of NSAID-induced acute renal failure.

The consultant agrees and thanks Vidhya for the information. He reinforces to his team the importance of taking a good medication history, including over-the-counter and complementary and alternative medicines, in all patients. Raju is advised to avoid ibuprofen and other anti-inflammatory medications in future as these may worsen his heart condition. Vidhya tells him that paracetamol is a safer alternative analgesic.

This case illustrates the importance of pre-ward round preparation. Vidhya took a complete medication history from Raju which then enabled her to make a useful contribution to the management of this case during the ward round. Clinical pharmacists should make active interventions when drug-induced conditions such as adverse reactions and drug interactions are suspected. Clinical pharmacists should also be prepared to offer solutions to the problems identified. They need to be very attentive during ward round discussions so that relevant information can be gathered to guide possible clinical pharmacy contribution.

PRACTICE SCENARIO 2

Ajith is a young and enthusiastic clinical pharmacist who has recently started working in the general medical ward of a 250-bed non-teaching hospital, where Dr Singh is the physician in-charge. Fatima is a 65-year-old woman with a history of Parkinson's disease, who was admitted to hospital following a syncopal episode. During admission, she complained of nausea and Ajith notes during his pre-ward round medication chart review that metoclopramide 10 mg three times daily has been prescribed. He is concerned that this may worsen Fatima's Parkinsonian symptoms.

Rao was admitted the previous night to the hospital with a suspected urinary tract infection. During pre-ward round preparation, Ajith noticed that gentamicin 80 mg IV twice daily had been prescribed for Rao. He remembers the advantages of once-daily dosing of aminoglycosides compared to multiple daily dosing and after calculating an estimated creatinine clearance, he decides to recommend a change in gentamicin dose to 160 mg IV once daily. He makes a note about this in his folder.

Younis is a 72-year-old diabetic patient in the same ward who has been receiving digoxin 250 mcg daily for rate control of atrial fibrillation. Younis has been complaining of nausea and vomiting since morning. Ajith thinks that these may be symptoms of digoxin toxicity and believes a serum digoxin assay would help to clarify this situation. He confirms that Younis's renal function and electrolytes are within normal limits. He feels it is appropriate to withhold the digoxin until the results of a digoxin assay are available since Younis's heart rate is well-controlled at 60–70 beats per minute.

Dr Singh had a very busy session at the outpatient this morning and does not commence the ward round until 1.00 PM. He needs to finish the round quickly before attending an important meeting with the Resident Medical Officer at 2.00 PM.

How can Ajith best prioritise the patient issues he has identified during his pre-ward round preparation?

Discussion

In these circumstances, Ajith realises that he needs to prioritise the interventions to be made. His first priority is to recommend measurement of serum digoxin concentration for Younis and withholding the drug until the result is known. Dr Singh agrees, but also expresses the view that the nausea may be due to gastroparesis. On reaching Fatima's bed, Ajith explains that due to its central dopamine blocking activity, metoclopramide may worsen her tremor and other Parkinsonian symptoms. He recommends prescribing domperidone 10 mg three times daily instead, as this drug is unlikely to worsen her symptoms as it does not pass the blood–brain barrier. Dr Singh observes that Fatima's tremor is well-controlled and metoclopramide is only a short-term therapy. He decides to continue with metoclopramide.

Ajith considers recommending a change in gentamicin dose for Rao as a lower priority as the patient is improving and it is a case of uncomplicated urinary tract infection. He plans to write a review article on the advantages of once-daily aminoglycoside dosing in the forthcoming Pharmacy Newsletter.

As a new staff member, Ajith needs to spend time observing Dr Singh's prescribing patterns and preferences so that his own recommendations can be made in a way which acknowledges the doctor's clinical judgement. He also knows that ward rounds with an experienced physician is an excellent learning opportunity, and he decides to do some background reading on gastroparesis.

Time barriers are important constraints in many hospitals where the medical staff have heavy clinical workloads. Pharmacists need to prioritise their interventions and recommendations according to their clinical significance and the potential health benefits to patients. When identifying a drug-related problem and recommending a change in therapy, pharmacists should provide a brief but clear explanation of the issue, and be ready to suggest alternative therapy, taking into account the patient's medical history. However, not all recommendations on ward rounds will be accepted, and this may be more true when the pharmacist is young and relatively inexperienced. Recommendations challenging conventional practices need to be supported by appropriate evidence from the clinical literature.

PRACTICE SCENARIO 3

During a general medical ward round in a teaching hospital, the team sees a patient admitted for an acute infective exacerbation of chronic obstructive pulmonary disease (COPD). He has been prescribed nebulised ipratropium and salbutamol, a course of high-dose prednisolone and doxycycline. He is also receiving intermittent oxygen. At home, he uses a salbutamol inhaler as needed. This is his second COPD-related hospital admission in the last 12 months. On the ward round, the team discusses options for further management of the patient at home. The pharmacist recommends pulmonary rehabilitation, influenza and pneumonia vaccination, and introduction of a regular inhaled long-acting bronchodilator (beta agonist and/or tiotropium), which will also help to reduce exacerbation frequency if used on a regular basis. The pharmacist also expresses concern about the patient's inhaler technique which he checked the previous day.

The registrar asks the pharmacist about the possible role of inhaled corticosteroids (ICS) in this patient.

How should the pharmacist respond in this situation?

Discussion

The pharmacist explains that the Global initiative for Obstructive Lung Disease (GOLD) evidence-based guidelines recommend initiation of an ICS only in patients with Stage III or IV COPD and those with repeated exacerbations. However, initiation of long-acting bronchodilators and pulmonary rehabilitation (if available) should precede the introduction of ICS. The pharmacist explains that ICS may improve the symptoms and health-related quality of life, and reduce the frequency of exacerbations, but will not modify the long-term decline in lung function. There is also evidence to suggest that ICS may increase the risk of pneumonia.

Depending on the registrar's level of interest, a copy of the GOLD guidelines could be provided to the registrar for further information. If the registrar wants further information, the pharmacist could also offer to do a comprehensive review of the topic, searching for primary research papers and other relevant references.

Pharmacists need to possess excellent clinical knowledge and communication skills to participate effectively in ward rounds in teaching hospitals. In general, treatment recommendations need to be evidence-based although when lacking, anecdotal evidence may suffice. In situations where the pharmacist is uncertain or is unable to answer a query from the practitioner, due acknowledgment of their uncertainty needs to be made. Some of the issues that arise during a ward round might remain outstanding, and require follow-up. All queries that are unanswered need to be followed-up by using appropriate references or discussing with colleagues or experts. Interventions and recommendations made by pharmacists may be supported with appropriate references, where necessary. Pharmacy interventions should be documented for performance evaluation and quality assurance purposes. In some hospitals, this is done using software written specifically for this purpose.

KEY MESSAGES

- Ward round participation is an important element of clinical pharmacy practice in the hospital setting.
- Key decisions regarding patient management are made during ward rounds and it is important for clinical pharmacists to be present at this time.
- Pre-ward round preparation and familiarity with each case is essential for active participation in the ward round.
- Recommendations during ward rounds are most likely to be adopted if pharmacists communicate these in a considered and respectful manner.
- Pharmacists may need to prioritise their recommendations during ward rounds depending on the medical staff and time constraints.
- When identifying a drug-related problem during a ward round, pharmacists should be prepared to outline solutions to the problem.
- Pharmacist interventions during ward rounds may be used as key performance indicators. Regular documentation of interventions is important for justifying the need for the service, and is also useful for quality assurance.
- Requests for drug information and other outstanding issues should be followed-up promptly after the ward round.

Further Reading

Calvert RT. 1999. Clinical pharmacy-a hospital perspective. *Br J Clin Pharmacol* 47: 231–8.

Cousins DH. 1995. Re-engineering pharmacy practice: forces for change and the evolution of clinical pharmacy practice. *Pharmaceutical Journal* 255:771–6.

Deffenbaugh JH. 1998. *Best Practices for Health System Pharmacy: Positions and Practice Standards of ASHP*. American Society of Health System Pharmacists: Bethesda.

Dooley M, Bogovic A, Carroll M, Cuell S, Galbraith K and Matthews H. 2005. SHPA Standards of Practice for Clinical Pharmacy. *J Pharm Pract Res* 35:122–46. available at: http://www.shpa.org.au/lib/pdf/practice_standards/clinical_pharm_ro.pdf

Hawkey CJ, Hodgson S, Norman A, Daneshmend TK and Garner ST. 1990. Effect of reactive pharmacy intervention on quality of hospital prescribing. *BMJ* 300:986–90.

Hepler CD and Strand LM. 1990. Opportunities and responsibilities in pharmaceutical care. *Am J Hosp Pharm* 47:533–43.

Hull JH and Eckel FM. 1973. Evaluation of the pharmacist as a drug therapy advisor on ward rounds. *Am J Hosp Pharm* 30:687–94.

Klotz R and Steffens S. 1976. Improved pharmacy services through participation in medical rounds. *Am J Hosp Pharm* 33:349–51.

Leape LL, Cullen DJ, Clapp MD, et al. 1999. Pharmacist participation on physician rounds and adverse drug reactions in the intensive care unit. *JAMA* 282:267–270.

Kucukarslan SN, Peters M, Mlynarek M and Nafziger DA. 2003. Pharmacists on Rounding Teams Reduce Preventable Adverse Drug Events in Hospital General Medicine Units. *Arch Intern Med* 163:2014–2018.

Strand LM, Morley PC, Cipolle RJ, Ramsey R and Lamsam GD. 1990. Drug-related problems: their structure and function. *DICP Ann Pharmacother* 24:1093.

Tindall WN, Beardsley RS and Kimberlin CL. 1994. *Communication Skills in Pharmacy Practice*. Lea & Febiger: Philadelphia.

15
Paediatric Pharmacy Practice

Vinita Pai and Milap C Nahata

Learning Objectives

Upon completion of this chapter, the reader should be able to:

- Understand the need for specific drugs and dose requirements for paediatric patients
- Initiate and establish a clinical pharmacy practice in paediatrics
- Collect informational resources to provide exemplary pharmacotherapy care to children
- Design tools and instruments to gather, organise and monitor clinical data with the goal of assessing and recommending changes to drug therapy
- List various factors that may alter the ability of a child to absorb drugs given by various routes of administration
- Describe the effects of age on pharmacokinetics and their significance in drug therapy
- Indicate the role of therapeutic drug monitoring in paediatric patients
- Discuss the factors affecting medication compliance in paediatric patients
- Describe methods to enhance medication safety in children and the clinical pharmacist's role in the process
- Describe the purpose and importance of medication reconciliation and the clinical pharmacist's role in this process

The paediatric population comprised only about 33% of the total world population in 2007; however, numerous acute and chronic diseases can affect this subpopulation. Premature neonates have poorly developed organ function and are at the highest risk of eliciting unexpected toxicity or poor clinical response from suboptimal dosage regimens of drugs due to altered pharmacokinetics or dose requirements in this population.

The sulfanilamide and thalidomide tragedies (deaths caused by sulfanilamide elixir and birth defects among the newborns of mothers who had used thalidomide for morning sickness) led to stricter governmental requirements for drug approval for paediatric patients. In the United States of America, the 1962 Kefauer–Harris Amendment made proof of efficacy and safety prior to drug approval in paediatric patients a requirement. This led to decreased interest within the pharmaceutical industry to seek paediatric drug approval, and infants and children became 'therapeutic orphans' in that most drugs used for them have not been adequately tested for efficacy and safety.

Numerous studies have shown that children are unique in many ways. They require different doses per kilogram of body weight than adults due to differences in pharmacokinetics, pharmacodynamics and/ or other factors. The dose requirement/kg/ day for drugs is often highest among children and lowest in premature infants, with adults in the middle. Children below the age of six years may need extemporaneously prepared dosage forms (such as oral suspensions) due to their inability to swallow tablets and capsules and the fact that doses are tailored (not fixed) based on body weight. Patients are dependent on parents or caregivers to receive optimal drug therapy. Finally, the social and economic status of parents directly influences the care they can offer to their children.

Over 80% of the drugs marketed for adults are not approved for infants and children, although many are commonly used in clinical practice. Unlabelled or off-label use of drugs is common among paediatric patients. Over 60% of children in hospitals and 90% of those in intensive care units receive unlicensed or off-label drugs. Examples of such drugs are, captopril, levofloxacin (except prophylaxis of and post-exposure treatment of anthrax inhalation), gabapentin, dexmeditomidine and morphine (oral). Often, information about the dose in milligrams per kilogram of body weight for these drugs is not available and the practitioner is left to estimate a paediatric dose based on the adult dose, using certain formulae given below.

Clark's Rule: (for infants and children)

$$\frac{\text{(Weight in pounds) x (Adult dose)}}{150}$$

Fried's Rule: (for infants and children up to 1–2 years)

$$\frac{\text{(Age in months) x (Adult dose)}}{150}$$

Young's Rule: (for children 1–12 years)

$$\frac{\text{(Age in years) x (Adult dose)}}{\text{Age + 12}}$$

These formulae are not in general use in the US because age alone is no longer considered a singularly valid criterion in determining a child's dose, and the calculated dose can easily under or overestimate the desired dose. Body surface area (BSA) may be used for calculating the doses of certain drugs such as chemotherapy agents. This is because BSA may correlate better with organ function, and thus the dose requirements for certain drugs. The Mosteller formula is most commonly used in practice.

BSA (m2) = Square root [(Body weight in kg x height in cm)/3600]

Use of unlabelled or off-label drugs may be associated with the development of adverse effects in children.

The medication use process involves appropriate drug selection, prescribing, transcribing, preparation, dispensing, administration, monitoring, assessment of clinical outcomes, and achieving patient satisfaction through improved quality of life. The purpose of this chapter is to describe the unique aspects of paediatric pharmacy practice. Information presented in this chapter will emphasise the influence of growth and maturation on drug disposition and pharmacodynamic response to drugs in children, ranging from neonates to adolescents. The role of therapeutic drug monitoring and factors affecting compliance in children will also be discussed.

Education and Training

All pharmacy students should receive didactic (classroom) lectures and clinical experience in paediatric pharmacy. Those interested in paediatric practice should complete additional courses and practical training in children's hospitals and clinics. Postgraduate residency training in paediatric pharmacy is highly recommended for additional practice and management experience to further enhance clinical skill, specifically in the area of paediatric disease management. Individuals interested in expanding their activities to paediatric research would benefit highly from completing a minimum two-year fellowship to learn skills such as identifying clinical research problems, developing objectives and hypotheses, preparing research protocols, seeking funding, conducting studies, analysing data, presenting research papers and publishing manuscripts in peer-reviewed journals to address unresolved clinical and patient care issues.

Establishing a Paediatric Clinical Pharmacy Practice

The principles of establishing a clinical practice in paediatric pharmacy are similar to those of developing a pharmacy practice in specialties. The process should be initiated by identifying the type of paediatric patients being cared for at your institution; for example, general paediatric patients seen for ailments such as gastroenteritis, respiratory infections, acute otitis media and constipation, or specialised paediatric services such as haematology and oncology or critical care.

Physicians, nurses, pharmacists and other healthcare professionals predominantly involved in the care of these patients should be identified. Drug therapy issues commonly faced by these practitioners should be recognised. A document listing the goals and clinical activities to be offered as a pharmacy practitioner to the paediatric healthcare team should be formulated.

Input from other members of the team should be sought so that these goals and activities tie in with the mission and goals of the institution, Department of Paediatrics and Department of Pharmacy to satisfy clinical needs. A close professional relationship should be fostered with the members of this team. A few chosen members of this team (for example, the Chief of Paediatrics or Chief of a specialty such as Infectious Diseases, or the Head Nurse) should be identified as primary contacts.

After the goals have been identified and approved, they should be presented to the entire department. This should be used as an opportunity to introduce the pharmacy practitioner and the value of their service to the patients. Means of easily contacting the pharmacy practitioner to provide pharmacotherapy consultation should be amply advertised. Resources needed to provide exemplary pharmaceutical care to children should be identified and sought.

These resources may include drug information resources specific to children and tools to facilitate such practice. An important component of developing an efficient clinical practice in paediatrics is the development and maintenance of a library consisting of textbooks, handbooks, primary literature and electronic and internet resources pertaining to paediatric pharmacotherapy. A list of these references is included in Table 15.1. It should be understood that this is not an exhaustive list of references, and the list can change as new publications appear.

In addition to developing an information base, clinical practitioners may also want to design tools or instruments to facilitate collection and organisation of patient-specific data while participating in multi-disciplinary patient rounds. Tables 15.2, 15.3, 15.4 and 15.5 include examples of such tools. A brief outline on how to follow a complex paediatric patient using the tools provided in these tables is given in *Case Study 8*.

Unique Aspects of Paediatric Drug Therapy

It is necessary to understand that children are not 'miniature adults'; the adult doses, scaled down based on body weight, may not be safe or effective in children. As neonates develop into infants and young adolescents, a number of physiologic events occur which change the body composition (for example, changes in body water, body fat, plasma proteins and hormonal composition); these changes influence drug disposition and dose requirements.

Certain intrinsic factors such as gender, race, heredity and inherited diseases and extrinsic factors such as acquired diseases, diet and prior exposure to drug therapy may change drug disposition in children. To provide safe and effective drug therapy to children, it is important to gain knowledge of the pharmacokinetic and pharmacodynamic properties of each drug and the effect of development on its disposition.

To understand the following sections, it is necessary to define a few terms. *Gestational age* (GA) is defined as the number of weeks from the first day of the mother's last normal menstrual period to the birth of the newborn. *Postnatal age* (PNA) is the number of weeks since birth. *Postmenstrual age* (previously known as postconceptional age [PCA]) is defined as the sum of gestational age and postnatal age.

A newborn at 38–41 weeks GA is considered a *full-term newborn*. *Neonates* are between weeks 0 and 4 weeks of postnatal age. The term neonate may also be applied to a premature newborn. Neonates born prior to 38 weeks GA are considered *premature*. A *post-term newborn* is of 42 weeks or more of gestational age. The term *infant* is used from 1 month to 1 year, *child* from 1 year to 12 years, and *adolescent* from 13 to 18 years of age (Fig. 15.1, *Case Study 1*).

Drug Delivery and Absorption

Intravenous (IV) drug delivery: Factors such as the site of injection, IV flow rate, infusion system and dose volume used can alter the predictable and complete delivery of an intravenously administered drug into systemic circulation. A site of injection distant

Table 15.1 List of print literature to be included in your clinical paediatric pharmacy programme

1.	Taketomo CK, Hodding JH and Kraus DM. 2009. *Pediatric Dosage Handbook 2010–2010*, 17th ed. Lexi-Comp, Inc: Hudson, Ohio. This is a practical, convenient and portable guide for physicians, pharmacists, residents, nurses and all medical, pharmacy and nursing students who require quick access to paediatric data concerning clinical use of medications. Also available as Pediatric Lexi-Drugs for handheld devices such as Personal Digital Assistant (PDA), Blackberry and iPhone.
2.	Buck ML and Hendrick AE. 2009. *Pediatric Medication Education Text*, 5th ed. American College of Clinical Pharmacy: Kansas City, Kansas. This book is a patient counselling aid, consisting of information on commonly prescribed paediatric medications in English and Spanish written at the 6th to 8th grade reading level. It is designed to be photocopied and distributed to patients and their families. Also available in a CD-ROM format.
3.	Bates RG and Nahata MC. 1996. *Children's Medications: A parent's guide*. Harvey Whitney Books: Cincinnati, Ohio. This book is written in laymen's language covering infants to teenagers; a profile of each drug gives information on dosage, side effects, drug–drug interactions and special precautions. Additional sections on drug administration techniques and drug use while breastfeeding are included.
4.	Nahata MC and Pai VB. 2011. *Pediatric Drug Formulations*, 6th ed. Harvey Whitney Books Company: Cincinnati Ohio. This book provides a variety of extemporaneous formulations of parenteral and oral use with documented stability data.
5.	Kliegman RM, Behram RE, Jenson HB and Stanton BF (Eds). 2007. *Nelson's Textbook of Pediatrics*, 18th ed. Elsevier Health Sciences: Philadelphia, Pennsylvania. This book provides guidance on the aetiology, epidemiology, pathology, pathophysiology, clinical manifestations, diagnosis, prevention, treatment and prognosis of virtually every medical and surgical disorder in children. It is also available as an e-dition, an online version of the textbook.
6.	Rau RE, Custer JW, Lee CK and The Johns Hopkins Hospital. 2009. *The Harriet Lane Handbook: A manual for pediatric house officers*. Elsevier Health Sciences: Philadelphia, Pennsylvania. This book provides diagnostic and management guidance, recommended tests, complete therapeutic information, comprehensive drug formulary and latest treatments in paediatric patients.
7.	American Academy of Pediatrics. *Patient Education Online: Health Care Advice for children, teens and parents*. Available at http://patiented.aap.org. (Accessed September 10, 2009). This is a comprehensive collection of AAP patient education materials in English and Spanish, which includes information on key health concerns from infancy through adolescence.
8.	*Red Book 2009: Report of the Committee of Infectious Diseases*, 29th ed. 2009. American Academy of Pediatrics: Elk Grove Village, Illinois. This provides the most current information on clinical manifestations, aetiology, epidemiology, diagnosis and treatment of childhood infectious diseases. It is also available online at http://aapredbook.aappublications.org/ (Accessed September 10, 2009).
9.	Young TE and Magnum B. 2009. *Neofax*, 22th ed. Thomson Healthcare: New York, NY. Acorn Publishing: Raleigh, North Carolina. This book is a comprehensive clinical reference providing up-to-date information on neonatal drugs and nutritional products. It also includes facts about drug use, pharmacology, adverse effects, precautions and compatibility/incompatibility guidance.
10.	Rossi S, Hurley E, Goldsworthy S, Gale S, Hanley R, Shute R, Sutcliffe A and Vitry A (eds). 2003. *Australian Medicines Handbook*, Australian Medicines Handbook Pvt Ltd.: Adelaide, South Australia. This book provides readily accessible, concise, up-to-date source of independent drug information to facilitate effective, rational, safe and economical prescribing.
11.	Kemp CA and McDowell JM (eds). *Paediatric Pharmacopoiea*, 13th ed. Royal Children's Hospital: Melbourne, Australia.
12.	Immunise Australia website at http://www.immunise.health.gov.au. (Accessed September 10, 2009).

Table 15.2 Patient demographic information sheet

<table>
<tr><td colspan="3">Patient ID:</td><td colspan="2">Name:</td></tr>
<tr><td colspan="3">Date of birth:</td><td colspan="2">Age:</td></tr>
<tr><td colspan="3">Height:</td><td>Weight:</td><td>Gender:</td></tr>
<tr><td colspan="3">Admission date:</td><td colspan="2">Date of data collection:</td></tr>
<tr><td colspan="5">Allergies:</td></tr>
<tr><td colspan="5">History of present illness:</td></tr>
<tr><td colspan="5">Past medical/Surgical history:</td></tr>
<tr><td colspan="5">Family/Social history:</td></tr>
<tr><td colspan="5">Medications prior to admission (PTA):</td></tr>
<tr><td colspan="3"></td><td colspan="2"></td></tr>
<tr><td colspan="3"></td><td colspan="2"></td></tr>
<tr><td colspan="5">Immunisations:</td></tr>
<tr><td colspan="5">Current medications:</td></tr>
<tr><td>Start date</td><td>Stop date</td><td colspan="3">Drug name, dose, route, frequency</td></tr>
<tr><td></td><td></td><td colspan="3"></td></tr>
<tr><td></td><td></td><td colspan="3"></td></tr>
<tr><td></td><td></td><td colspan="3"></td></tr>
<tr><td></td><td></td><td colspan="3"></td></tr>
<tr><td colspan="5">Relevant information from physical exam, procedures, and daily progress</td></tr>
<tr><td>Date</td><td colspan="4"></td></tr>
<tr><td></td><td colspan="4"></td></tr>
<tr><td></td><td colspan="4"></td></tr>
<tr><td></td><td colspan="4"></td></tr>
<tr><td></td><td colspan="4"></td></tr>
<tr><td></td><td colspan="4"></td></tr>
<tr><td></td><td colspan="4"></td></tr>
</table>

Table 15.3 Daily monitoring form

Date										
Date										
Weight (kg)										
T max °C										
WBC (K/mm3)										
ANC										
Hb (g/dl)										
Platelets (k/mm3)										
BUN (mg/dl)										
Cr (mg/dl)										
Na (mmol/l)										
K (mmol/l)										
Cl (mmol/l)										
CO2 (mmol/l)										
Ca (mg/dl)										
PO4 (mg/dl)										
Mg (mg/dl)										
Glucose (mg/dl)										
Triglycerides (mg/dl)										
Total protein (g/dl)										
Albumin (g/dl)										
Total bilirubin (mg/dl)										
ALT (U/L)										
In ml										
Total Output ml										
Stool Output in ml										
ALT										
AST										
Alk Phos										
Uric acid										
Cultures										
Aerobic										
Anaerobic										
Fungal										
Drug Serum Concentration										
Aminoglycoside										
Vancomycin										
Phenytoin										
Phenobarbital										
Digoxin										
Theophylline										
Cyclosproine										
Tracrolimus										

Table 15.4 Total parenteral nutrition monitoring form

Total Parenteral Nutrition										
Date										
Weight										
Duration (hours/day)										
TPN ml/day										
Intralipid g/kg										
Intralipid ml/day										
Intralipid Kcal/day										
Protein g/day										
Protein Kcal/day										
Dextrose %										
Dextrose g/day										
Dextrose kcal/day										
Total kcal/day										
Na (mEq/kg/day)										
K (mEq/kg/day)										
Cl:Acetate (ratio)										
Ca (mEq/kg/day)										
PO4 (mmol/kg/day)										
Mg (mEq/kg/day)										
Se (mg /day)										
MVI										
Insulin (units/day)										
Heparin (units/day)										
H2 antagonist (mg/day)										

Table 15.5 Monitoring pain therapy

Pain Therapy										
Drug used										
Basal rate (mg/hr)										
PCA bolus dose (mg)										
Lock out interval										
# of attempts										
# of successful attempts										
Total dose (mg)										
Pain rating										
Sedation										
Respirations										

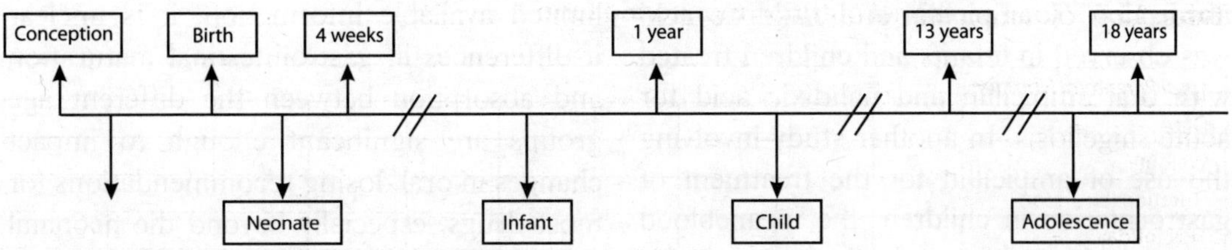

Conception | Birth | 4 weeks | 1 year | 13 years | 18 years

Neonate | Infant | Child | Adolescence

Figure 15.1 Chronological time

from the patient, slow IV flow rate and large dose volume will result in lower and delayed peak serum concentrations of the drug. This may potentially influence the therapeutic efficacy and/or safety of the drug.

A serum drug concentration, especially one different from what was predicted, should be evaluated by giving careful consideration to the abovementioned factors. Accurate drug delivery can be achieved by using syringe pumps and low-volume microbore tubings; choosing as close a site as possible to the patient; and, priming the pump and the IV tubing with sufficient volume of the drug solution to be administered. Intravenous drug admixtures may often include an amount of drug solution in excess of the amount to be administered, referred to as overfill, that is used to prime the IV tubing.

Oral absorption: Most drugs administered by the oral route are absorbed by passive diffusion. Gastric pH, gastric and intestinal motility, pancreatic enzyme activity, bacterial colonisation of the intestines, bile salt production, blood flow to the gastrointestinal tract, and the surface area of absorption affect the rate and extent of gastrointestinal absorption. These factors undergo considerable maturational changes as an infant grows into an adult.

The volume and acid concentration of the gastric juice is dependent on age and approaches the lower limit of adult values by three months of age and reaches adult values only after two years of age. The rate and extent of absorption of drugs that are weak acids or bases may depend on their partition co-efficients (Table 15.6).

Gastric pH may change with ingestion of certain foods; for example, orange juice, cranberry juice and carbonated beverages decrease gastric pH, causing acidic drugs such as itraconazole to be absorbed more readily (*Case Study* 2). Absorption of acidic drugs will decrease when given with milk or infant formula due to an increase in gastric pH.

The gastric emptying rate appears to be a function of gestational age, postnatal age as well as the nature of feeds. It is considerably delayed in neonates, reaching adult values by 6–8 months of age. Most orally administered drugs are absorbed in the small intestine; therefore, the faster the gastric emptying time, the faster the rate of absorption provided the rate of emptying from the small intestine is not faster than normal.

The rate and extent of drug absorption may be significantly altered in patients with acute changes in the gastrointestinal tract (*Case Study* 3). Decreased and delayed absorption of ampicillin and nalidixic acid was observed in infants and children treated with oral ampicillin and nalidixic acid for acute shigellosis. In another study involving the use of ampicillin for the treatment of gastroenteritis in children, the mean blood concentrations of ampicillin were lower in children with gastroenteritis than in children without the disease, possibly due to malabsorption.

Pancreatic enzymes increase the bioavailability of certain oral drugs with dosage forms requiring intraluminal (gastrointestinal) hydrolysis prior to absorption (for example, oral liquid ester formulations of clindamycin and chloramphenicol palmitate). Pancreatic enzyme activity is low at birth. Amylase activity remains low (approximately 10% of adult values) even after the first month of life. Lipase activity increases 20-fold during the first nine months after birth. Trypsin secretion in response to pancreozymin and secretin develops during the first year of life. Bile salts may influence the absorption of certain fat soluble drugs and nutrients (Table 15.6). Bile salt metabolism matures postnatally within the first few months of life and continues during the first year of life.

The composition and rate of gastrointestinal colonisation by bacterial flora depends more on diet than on age; however, its effect on intestinal motility and drug metabolism is not completely known. For example, intestinal colonisation by oral digoxin reducing anaerobic bacteria approaches adult values by two years of age; however, the degree of digoxin reduction by these bacteria observed in adults may not be achieved until adolescence. Therefore, higher digoxin bioavailability can be anticipated in infants compared to adults. Based on limited available information, it is unclear if differences in gastrointestinal maturation and absorption between the different age groups are significant enough to impact changes in oral dosing recommendations for most drugs, especially beyond the neonatal age group.

Intramuscular (IM) absorption: The surface area over which the injected drug can be distributed, blood flow to the site of injection, ease of penetration through the endothelial capillary walls and muscle activity may all influence the absorption of drugs administered intramuscularly. Absorption of drugs from an IM site of injection may be more variable in premature neonates because of decreased muscle mass and haemodynamic instability when compared to a full-term neonate. This route is more commonly used for the administration of vaccines. Drugs administered by this route are well absorbed in infants and children.

Intramuscular administration can be a painful route, especially for certain drugs such as ceftriaxone, and should be used only when oral administration is not indicated, feasible or IV access is unavailable. Pain due to IM drug administration can be minimised by applying a topical anaesthetic such as lidocaine. EMLA® is a local anaesthetic cream marketed in the US which contains a mixture of lidocaine base and prilocaine base. This cream is applied under an occlusive dressing at least an hour before the procedure to alleviate the pain caused by venipuncture.

Percutaneous absorption: Greater skin hydration, thinner and/or immature stratum corneum, and greater body surface area to weight ratio increase percutaneous drug absorption. The skin of a full-term neonate has barrier properties to drug absorption similar to those in adult skin. Premature neonates have an immature epidermal barrier and increased skin hydration compared to a full-term neonate and, therefore, exhibit increased transepidermal water loss and drug absorption.

Increased absorption of drugs may be observed in infants, compared to children and adults with equal topical drug applications (Table 15.6). Percutaneous absorption is increased through damaged skin; therefore, application of high potency corticosteroids to diaper rashes with severe perianal inflammation should be avoided.

Rectal absorption: The rectal route of administration is a useful alternative when oral administration is precluded by nausea, vomiting, seizures, or due to preparation for surgery and when the IV route is precluded either due to a lack of IV dosage form or lack of IV access. The rate and extent of absorption of certain drugs may be much improved when rectal solutions rather than suppositories are used; for example, diazepam (Table 15.6, *Case Study 4*). However, factors such as delay in onset of action and failure to reach minimal effective concentrations in plasma make the rectal route inferior to the oral and IV routes for most drugs. Suppositories should not be halved to administer a lower dose. Such administration may not guarantee delivery of the required dose since the drug may not be uniformly distributed throughout the suppository.

Drug Distribution

Volume of distribution: The apparent volume of distribution is greater for drugs that are highly distributed in tissues. Factors such as relative proportion of total body water, total body fat and differences in protein binding determine the difference in drug distribution between children and adults. Total body water as a percentage of total body weight has been estimated to be 85% in premature infants, 78% in full-term newborns and 60% in adults. Extracellular fluid volume is also markedly different in premature infants compared with older children and adults; the extracellular fluid volume may account for 50% of body weight in premature infants, 35% in 4–6-month-old infants, 25% in children of 1 year of age and 19% in adults.

Hydrophilic drugs such as aminoglycoside antibiotics are largely distributed into extracellular fluid and thus have larger volumes of distribution in neonates compared to older infants and children (Table 15.6). The larger the volume of distribution, the larger the mg/kg dose of aminoglycoside required to achieve the recommended peak serum concentration (*Case Study* 5). However, caution should be exercised in using actual body weight in calculating aminoglycoside doses in obese children (*Case Study* 6).

Total body fat increases from 1% at 29 weeks PCA to 12–16% at term and 20–25% at one year of age. It then increases between 5 and 10 years of age, followed by a decrease in boys at age 17. At puberty, there is a rapid increase in body fat in females, approaching twice the value compared to males. Lipophilic drugs will have a larger apparent volume of distribution in adults and children with a higher percentage of body fat than neonates and infants (Table 15.6).

Protein binding: The binding of drugs to circulating plasma proteins depends on multiple factors such as the total amount of proteins, the number of binding sites, binding affinity and the presence of pathophysiologic conditions (for example, change in blood pH) and/or endogenous compounds (for example, bilirubin, free fatty acids) that may alter the drug–protein interaction. Albumin, alpha-1 acid glycoprotein and lipoproteins are the important drug-binding proteins; albumin comprises 58% of all plasma proteins. Total protein concentration, including serum albumin and alpha-1 acid glycoprotein as well as their function and binding capacity, is decreased in neonates and approaches adult values by the first year of age and remains consistently stable in healthy children between 2 and 18 years of age.

Acidic and neutral drugs such as beta-lactam antibiotics, warfarin and digoxin exhibit great binding affinity for albumin; basic compounds including propranolol and alprenolol bind to alpha-1 acid glycoprotein, lipoproteins and beta-globulins. Several endogenous substances such as bilirubin and free fatty acids compete for the albumin binding sites and influence the drug–protein binding capacity. For example, bilirubin is often high in neonates and infants with increased red cell destruction and/or limited liver capacity to conjugate it. The binding capacity of bilirubin to plasma albumin is decreased in newborn infants and approaches adult values by five months of age.

Drugs highly bound to the plasma proteins, for example, sulfonamides or ceftriaxone, may displace bilirubin and contribute to high levels of displaced bilirubin in neonates and infants. Displaced bilirubin can cross the blood–brain barrier and deposit in the brain, inducing an encephalopathy termed kernicterus. The pharmacological action of a drug moiety is usually attributed to the free, unbound form of the drug. Conditions that decrease serum plasma proteins, for example, albumin, may increase the free, active fraction of highly protein-bound drugs (Table 15.6). When the toxic effects of phenytoin are manifest despite normal total phenytoin plasma concentrations, in patients with hypoalbuminemia or receiving drugs competing with phenytoin binding sites, for example, valproic acid, an unbound fraction should be measured and an adjusted total plasma concentration and therapeutic range for phenytoin should be estimated.

Drug Metabolism

Drug metabolism primarily occurs in the liver; however, the kidneys, intestine, lungs and skin may also be involved. Most drugs are metabolised to pharmacologically weaker or inactive compounds for easy excretion from the body. Some active parent compounds may be transformed into active metabolites (for example, theophylline to caffeine or codeine demethylated to morphine). Further, pharmacologically inactive compounds or prodrugs may be converted to their active moiety (for example, cyclophosphamide is hydroxylated to 4-hydroxycyclophosphamide and aldophosphamide).

Hepatic blood flow, extraction efficiencies, binding affinity and enzyme activity may affect hepatic drug metabolism. Of these, enzyme activity is greatly dependent on the age of the patient. Two primary enzymatic processes, phase I or non-synthetic reactions and phase II or synthetic reactions, are involved in drug biotransformation.

Phase I reactions include oxidation, reduction, hydrolysis and hydroxylation that introduce or reveal a functional group within the substrate that will serve as a

Table 15.6 Age-dependent differences in physiologic function and drug disposition

Physiologic Variability	*Neonate*	*Infant*	*Child*	*Pharmacokinetic Consequences*
ABSORPTION				
Gastric pH	Increased (>5)	Increased (2–4)	Normal (2–3)	Increase in bioavailability of acid lab le drugs, for example, penicillin G, ampicillin, nafcillin in neonates and infants compared to children and adults, decreased bioavailability of weak organic acids e.g phenobarbital
Gastric and intestinal emptying time	Reduced and Irregular	Increased	Increased	Increased time to achieve peak plasma acetaminophen concentration when administered with meperidine due to decreased gastrointestinal motility
Biliary function	Immature	Near adult pattern	Adult pattern	increased absorption of fat and fat soluble Vitamins D and E in infants and children
Pancreatic function	Immature	Near adult pattern	Adult pattern	increased hydrolysis and bioavailability of oral liquid ester formulations of clindamycin and chloramphenicol in infants and children
Gut microbial colonisation	Reduced	Near adult pattern	Adult pattern	Increased bioavailability of digoxin in infants compared to adults due to lack of microbial gut colonization with a oral digoxin reducing anaerobic bacteria
Intramuscular absorption	Variable	Increased	Increased to near adult pattern	Benzathine penicillin G more rapidly absorbed in children compared to adults since no measurable activity was detected in children 18 days after the injection
Skin permeability and percutaneous absorption	Increased	Increased	Near adult pattern	EMLA (eutectic mixture of local anesthetics lignocaine and prilocaine) contraindicated in patients less than 3 months of age due to risk of methemoglobinemia due to increased percutaneous absorption of prilocaine and decreased methemoglobin reductase
Rectal absorption	Increased	Increased	Near adult pattern	Increased rate and extent of diazepam absorption from rectal solution compared to suppositories, used to prevent and treat febrile seizures in infants and children [40]

Physiologic Variability	*Neonate*	*Infant*	*Child*	*Pharmacokinetic Consequences*
DISTRIBUTION				
Total body water (Extracellular water)	Increased	Increased	Near adult pattern	Increase in mean apparent volume of distribution (Vd) for hydrophilic drugs e.g gentamicin $Vd_{<34\,wk}$ 0.67 ± 0.13 L/Kg; $Vd_{34\text{-}48\,wk}$ 0.52 ± 0.10 L/Kg; $Vd_{1\text{-}4.9\,yrs}$ 0.38 ± 0.16 L/Kg; $Vd_{5\text{-}9.9\,yrs}$ 0.33 ± 0.14 L/Kg; $Vd_{10\text{-}16yrs}$ 0.31 ± 0.12 L/Kg; Vd_{adult} < 0.30 L/Kg;
Total body fat	Reduced	Reduced	Increased (age 5-10 yrs)	Increase in mean apparent Vd for lipophillic drugs e.g diazepam 1.6 – 3.2 L/Kg in adults vs 1.3 – 2.6 L/Kg in infants
Total plasma proteins	Reduced	Reduced to Near adult pattern	Adult pattern	Increase in Vd and free phenytoin concentration in neonates and children and adults with physiologic/pathologic conditions leading to altered protein concentrations
RENAL ELIMINATION				
Glomerular filtration	Reduced	Adult pattern	Adult pattern	Famotidine – 80% excreted unchanged in the urine in older children and adults; renal clearance equivalent to adults by 1 year of age
Tubular secretion	Reduced	Near adult pattern	Adult pattern	Penicillins - increased elimination half-life due to decreased excretion both by glomerular filtration and tubular secretion, therefore ↑ dosing interval in neonates and infants compared to children and adolescents
Tubular reabsorption	Reduced	Near adult pattern	Adult pattern	Specific example not available

site for a phase II conjugation reaction. In phase II reactions, the substrate may be conjugated with endogenous agents such as sulfate, acetate, glucuronic acid, glutathione and glycine, resulting in a more polar, water-soluble compound that can be easily eliminated by the renal and/or biliary system (*Case Study 7*).

The activity of the oxidizing enzymes is greatly reduced at birth, resulting in prolonged elimination of drugs such as phenytoin and diazepam. The hepatic mono-oxygenase system approaches and exceeds adult capacities by approximately six months of age. Alcohol dehydrogenase activity, detectable at ≤ 3–4% of adult activity at two months of age, approaches adult capacity after five years of age. Demethylation activity may not be seen until 14–15 months of postnatal age and may increase thereafter. Hydrolytic activity reaches adult values within the first few months of life.

Quantitatively, cytochromes P450 are the most important phase I enzymes, with the CYP1, CYP2 and CYP3 isozymes playing an important role in human drug metabolism; for example, cisapride is metabolised by the CYP 3A4 isoenzyme system and concomitant administration with CYP 3A4 inhibitors such as fluconazole can result in increased cisapride concentration, leading to prolongation of the QT interval and severe arrhythmias (Table 15.7).

The phase II enzymes consist of glucuronosyl transferases, sulfotransferases, arylamine N-acetyl tranferases, glutathione S-transferases and methyltransferases, all of which play an important role in the biotransformation of drugs (Table 15.8). Important differences exist between children and adults, and phase II enzymes do not all follow the same developmental pattern.

Drug Elimination

The kidney is an important organ for the elimination of drugs and their water-soluble metabolites. The functional capacity of the kidney increases with age. Glomerular filtration, tubular secretion and re-absorption are responsible for the renal elimination of drugs. Glomerular filtration of drugs depends on the functional capacity of the glomerulus, integrity of renal blood flow and extent of drug–protein binding. The amount of drug filtered through the glomerulus is inversely proportional to the degree of protein binding. Glomerular filtration rate (GFR) increases with increase in renal blood flow. In utero, high renal vascular resistance decreases renal blood flow, which approaches adult values by approximately 5–12 months of age.

GFR is lower for premature neonates than for full-term newborns. It dramatically increases from birth and approaches adult values by approximately 3–5 months of age. The increase in GFR is related to changes in renal blood flow; at birth, clamping of the umbilical cord increases the cardiac output and perfusion, and decreases renal vascular resistance, thus increasing renal blood flow.

The tubular secretory function does not mature at the same rate as GFR, as the proximal convoluted tubules are small relative to their corresponding glomeruli at birth. Tubular function approaches adult values by approximately 30 weeks of postnatal life, thus affecting drugs eliminated by tubular secretion in addition to glomerular filtration (Table 15.6). Tubular re-absorptive functions remain ill-defined in the paediatric population but appear to mature relative to PCA and may not be as important once the premature newborn approaches the age of a full-term infant (>36 weeks).

Table 15.7 Age-dependent differences in the activity of important drug-metabolising Phase I enzymes and drug metabolism

Enzyme	*Neonate*	*Infant*	*Child*	*Adolescent*	*Pharmacokinetic Consequences*
CYP2D6	Reduced (20% adult activity)	Reduced	Adult pattern (by age 3–5 years)	Adult pattern	O-demethylation of codeine to morphine ↓ in neonate/infants resulting in lack of efficacy and poor pain control
CYP2C19	Reduced	Adult pattern (reached by age 6 months)	Increased (peak activity at age 3–4 years)	Adult pattern (decreases to adult value at puberty)	Diazepam half-life ↑ in neonates/infants (25–100 hours) compared to children (7–37 hours) and adults (20–50 hours) due to ↓ oxidative activity
CYP2C9	Reduced	Adult pattern (reached by age 1–6 months)	Increased (peak activity at age 3–10 years)	Adult pattern (decreases to adult value at puberty)	Phenytoin half-life ↓ from 80 hours at 0–2 days, to 15 hours at 3–14 days, to 6 hours at 14–150 days of life due to slow maturation
CYP3A4	Reduced (30–40% of adult activity)	Adult pattern (by age 6 months)	Increased (at 1–4 years, then progressively ↓)	Adult pattern (at puberty)	↑ metabolism of carbamazepine to its 10, 11 epoxide in infants/children with ↑ CYP3A4 activity compared to neonates, and adults

↑ = increase ↓ = decrease

Dosing recommendations for renally excreted drugs, especially those with a narrow therapeutic index, should be based on the patient's renal function to avoid toxicity due to decreased elimination and increased accumulation. Renal function can be clinically assessed by monitoring urine output, creatinine clearance and serum creatinine. A urine output of approximately 1 ml/kg/hr in infants may be considered normal. However, urine output varies with fluid intake, hydration status, renal solute load and urine concentration capabilities, and may not accurately reflect the renal clearance of drugs primarily excreted through the kidneys, especially those eliminated by tubular secretion rather than glomerular filtration.

GFRs can be estimated by assessing creatinine clearance. This requires a 24-hour urine collection that is difficult to obtain in infants and children. Incomplete collection will lead to inaccurate results; complete collection may require catheterisation of the patients, thus, making the process more invasive. Creatinine clearance can be estimated from single serum creatinine values by using nomograms or mathematical formulas which are most convenient but less accurate. The mathematical formulas used to estimate creatinine clearance (CrCL) in adults (for example, Cockgraft and Gault, Jelliffe) cannot be used to estimate CrCL in children. The following Schwartz formula is often used to estimate CrCL in children:

$$CrCL = kL / SCr$$

Creatinine clearance (CrCL) is estimated in ml/min/1.73 m^2, where L is body length in cm, SCr is serum creatinine in mg/dL and k is a constant of proportionality based on age for all patients and also gender for those above two years of age (Table 15.9).

Table 15.8 Age-dependent differences in the activity of important drug-metabolising Phase II enzymes and drug metabolism

Enzyme	Neonate	Infant	Child	Adolescent	Pharmacokinetic consequences
N-acetyltransferase-2	Reduced (up to 2 months)	Reduced (by age 4–6 months)	Adult pattern (present by age 1–3 years)	Adult pattern	↓ acetylation of sulfapyridine (sulfasalazine metabolite) results in ↑ side effects – nausea, headache, abdominal pain in neonates and infants
Methyltransferase	Increased (50% higher than adults)	Adult pattern	Adult pattern	Adult pattern	Specific example not available
Glucuronosyl transferase	Reduced	Adult pattern (by age 6–18 months)	Adult pattern	Adult pattern	↑ ratio of glucuronide to sulfate of acetaminophen with age; newborn - 0.34; child (3–10 years) - 0.8; adolescent - 1.61 and adult - 1.8–2.3; sulfation compensates for glucuronide so no major consequences for dose adjustment in children
Sulfotransferase	Reduced (10–20% of adult activity)	Increased (for specific substrates)	Increased (for specific substrates)	Adult pattern	Specific example not available

↑ = increase ↓ = decrease

Table 15.9 Values of k for estimating creatinine clearance with the Schwartz formula

Age Group	k (mean value)
Low birth weight infants ≤ 1 year	0.33
Full term ≤ 1 year	0.45
Children 2–12 years	0.55
Females 13–21 years	0.55
Males 13–21 years	0.70

Using creatinine clearance or serum creatinine in estimating GFR has its limitations. Creatinine clearance is accurate in estimating GFR only when patients have a normal GFR. Creatinine is not completely filtered by the glomeruli. As GFR decreases, a greater proportion of creatinine is secreted, rather than being filtered, leading to an overestimation of creatinine clearance. Serum creatinine values depend on creatine metabolism in the muscles. Patients with low muscle mass (for example, premature neonates, bedridden infants and children, and cystic fibrosis patients with malnutrition) will have low serum creatinine values, and therefore creatinine clearance may not accurately reflect their renal function. Assay methodology used to determine serum creatinine concentrations should be specific and sensitive enough to detect even minor changes occurring in infants. Serum creatinine values should not be used to estimate CrCL in infants with normal renal function, but may be used in patients with renal dysfunction with elevated serum creatinine. Reproducibility of the assay method improves as serum creatinine increases. In patients on aminoglycosides, renal clearance of the aminoglycoside approximates creatinine clearance, since >90% of the dose is filtered through the glomeruli without being secreted or re-absorbed and can be used to estimate the GFR.

Therapeutic Drug Monitoring (TDM) and Treatment Outcome

TDM generally consists of serum drug concentration measurements and the use of pharmacokinetic and pharmacodynamic principles to make drug dosing recommendations. These recommendations are individualised for each patient to achieve maximum therapeutic efficacy with minimal adverse effects. Examples of maximum therapeutic efficacy include eradication of bacterial infection with aminoglycosides or control of seizures after phenytoin therapy. Prevention of adverse effects would include nephrotoxicity after aminoglycoside therapy or ataxia and nystagmus after phenytoin administration. TDM is more useful for drugs with a narrow therapeutic index and those that exhibit good correlation between serum concentration and efficacy or adverse effects.

Clinical pharmacists should develop and provide guidelines for monitoring serum drug concentration. These guidelines should include a list of drugs that need TDM, when to measure their serum concentration, which serum concentration to measure (peak, trough or both), and the therapeutic concentrations to achieve. It is essential that the nursing staff is educated to accurately document the times of drug administration and drawing of serum concentrations, respectively.

An important function of a clinical pharmacist is to obtain all the information and use appropriate pharmacokinetic equations to calculate intended serum concentrations and make appropriate dose recommendations.

The ultimate goal of drug therapy is to achieve the desired clinical outcome, with or without measuring the serum concentration of drugs. The role of TDM should not be limited to measuring serum drug concentrations but should be extended to monitoring the therapeutic outcome to drugs such as clinical response (decreased fever, normalisation of blood pressure and heart rate) and microbiological response (eradication of bacteria causing an infection). Pharmacists must ensure that expected health outcomes have been achieved and that adverse effects have been avoided or minimised.

Compliance

The term compliance has been used interchangeably with adherence. An exact definition of compliance and its distinction from non-compliance is difficult to ascertain. Often, an arbitrary percentage is deemed as compliance, such as when ≥70% of the medication is taken. Non-compliance may be observed as missing doses, delaying doses, failure to fill a prescription, wrong dose, wrong dosing interval and premature discontinuation of drug therapy. Information on non-compliance in children is limited and is complicated since parents are usually responsible for administering the medication. Non-compliance in children is comparable to that in adults and ranges from 7% to 89% for short-term acute medications and 11% to 83% for long-term chronic ones.

Non-compliance is not without consequences. It may decrease the efficacy of drug therapy and result in failure to attain the desired therapeutic goal. It may result in unnecessary modification or escalation of the drug dose. For example, non-compliance with antibiotic therapy may result in the emergence of resistant strains of organisms and greater probability of recurrent infection. Increased doses may lead to toxicity if compliance improves following an initial period of non-compliance. Thus, non-compliance may result in unnecessary morbidity and cost associated with drug therapy.

Issues unique to non-adherence in children will be addressed in this chapter. For a more global discussion on adherence, see *Chapter 7, Medication Adherence*. Family situations such as disharmony between parents or poor parental coping and problem-solving skills have been correlated with poor compliance for acute and chronic disease medication regimes. Increased family size leading to decreased parental reminders to comply, limited parental supervision, parental educational level and understanding, and developmental abilities of the child/adolescent to follow instructions may also result in poor compliance.

Adolescents may be less compliant with medication therapy. Defiance, rebellion, attention seeking, denial, confusion due to transition from parental dependency to autonomy may play an important role in non-compliance among adolescents.

Disease severity as perceived by parents rather than as assessed by the physician may affect compliance, both for acute and for chronic conditions. For example, increased compliance in children with pharyngitis compared to otitis media was due to the parents' perception that pharyngitis is a more serious disease than otitis media, leading to greater vigilance in administering and monitoring their child's therapy.

Regimen factors contributing to non-compliance include complexity, cost, type of regimen and taste of the medication. Complex drug regimens such as in paediatric transplants, requiring the administration of multiple medications, frequently decrease compliance. Bitter-tasting drugs, regimens that include only solid dosage forms such as tablets and capsules may lead to decreased compliance as the child may be reluctant or unable to swallow the medication and will fight administration of the medication.

As clinical pharmacists, we can play an important role in reviewing the medication regimens recommended for the patient. Compliance can be improved by reducing the number of doses to be taken in a day and timing the doses to fit in with the patient's daily routine (*Case Study 8*). Pharmacists can also assist in choosing a better tasting liquid product if needed. Assistance can be provided to parents in teaching them different techniques of drug administration.

The parents should be educated on how to use an oral syringe (Fig. 15.4), a medicine spoon or a medicine dropper to administer liquid medication. While using the oral syringe or medicine dropper, the parents need to squirt the liquid medicine into the side of the mouth slowly enough to allow the child to swallow the medicine naturally. The parents should be informed not to squirt the liquid at the back of the mouth since this may cause gagging. While using a medicine spoon, it should be held upright as a dose is being measured. The spoon should then be put to the child's lips and tilted slowly as the parent tells the child to pretend that she is drinking a glass of milk or juice.

With bitter-tasting medicine, the child may refuse to take any subsequent doses or spit the doses out. This could be overcome by mixing the medicine in a small volume of water or fruit juice to mask the taste. Parents should be instructed to administer the entire amount of the liquid. They should be informed that all medicines cannot be mixed with other liquids and they should consult their pharmacist or doctor before doing so. For patients who are unable to swallow tablets or capsules, the parents should be informed that the tablets can be crushed or the capsules opened and the contents sprinkled over some soft food such as ice cream, apple sauce or jelly before administration. Compliance can be improved by educating the parents and/ or the patients about their medications. This can be achieved by using patient education books and pamphlets, listed in Table 15.1. However, it is important to assess the parents' and/or patients' literacy level and their ability to read the language in which the education material is printed.

Immunisation

Pharmacists can play an essential role in immunisation programmes to demonstrate their professional role, as well as their caring. Pharmacists can participate in activities such as identifying patients needing immunisation; facilitating administration of vaccines; determining special needs for vaccines, for example those on dialysis and with immunodeficiency; monitoring efficacy, safety, contraindications of vaccines, and interactions with drugs and immunologic agents; conducting surveillance; educating parents and providers; and serving on committees to improve vaccination use. These activities can be performed in both the institutional as well as ambulatory settings.

Immunisation history should be made a part of the patient's permanent medication history and should be updated periodically. Hospitalised patients and those visiting clinics and emergency departments should be monitored and efforts made to administer the required vaccines. In pharmacies and ambulatory care settings, pharmacists can exhibit a large poster of the immunisation schedule and monitor. Brief counselling and educational brochures can be offered to parents.

Medication Safety

An estimated 6% of paediatric inpatients and 10% of children treated in the emergency room are at risk of being affected by medication errors. Children offer a unique challenge in the prevention of medication errors and adverse drug events. A common definition of medication error is '*an error in prescribing, dispensing or administering a medication*'.

A medication error can occur at any stage of the use of a drug to treat a disease state. Errors that occur during prescription of a medication may include those in drug selection, dose calculation, frequency of administration or use of incorrect dosage form or route of administration. Since most drugs require weight-based dosing, more dose calculations are required in children than in adults. Some IV drugs may need to be diluted before dispensing, thus requiring more calculations.

Common errors made during dispensing intravenous medications may include using a wrong solvent or diluting to an incorrect concentration. Errors involved in drug administration may include incorrect administration technique, administration at incorrect times or missed doses. When patients with similar names are admitted to the same unit, medications prepared for one could be inadvertently administered to the other.

Nearly 25% of medication errors are preventable. Children, especially neonates, have limited ability to buffer the effects of erroneous drug administration. Aspirin, metoclopramide and tetracycline are examples of drugs where children are more susceptible to their adverse effects than adults. The most common drugs associated with medication errors are antibiotics, analgesics, anti-neoplasties, anti-convulsants, sedatives and fluids and electrolytes. Aspirin can cause Reye's syndrome with fatal results in children when used during viral illnesses such as influenza A or B, or varicella. Children are particularly susceptible to the toxic effects of metoclopramide such as agitation, irritability, neck pain and rigidity and extrapyramidal symptoms. Tetracycline can cause discolouration of the teeth during the first eight years of life.

Prescribing errors can be avoided if clinical pharmacists participate in physician rounds, doctors use a computerised physician order entry system or with bar coding or point of care use, and pharmacists provide readily usable drug information to physicians. A systems approach should be used to address medication errors – the medication use system must have checks and balances.

Doses, drug concentration and administration procedures should be standardised for all patients within an institution. Pharmacists must prepare all high-risk drug doses to prevent errors on the medical wards by individual nurses or compounders. Pharmacists should routinely perform certain steps to detect any errors in paediatric prescriptions. All dose calculations should be checked. Patient weight and height must be recorded; the pharmacist should evaluate whether they seem reasonable for the patient's age. The indication for the drug and the dosage regimen should be verified by referring to a standard paediatric reference. Look-alike packages and sound-alike names should be avoided by manufacturers. The Institute for Safe Medication Practices (http://www.ismp.org) in the US collects and disseminates information about medication errors.

Medication Reconciliation

Medication reconciliation as defined by the Institute for Healthcare Improvement, an independent not-for-profit organisation helping to lead the improvement of healthcare throughout the world, as 'comparing a complete list of a patient's current home medications, dose, dosage form and frequency to the medication orders written by the physician upon admission to the hospital and during each subsequent transition point in order to identify and reconcile the discrepancies'. The Joint Commission, an institution that evaluates and accredits more than 16,000 healthcare organisations and programmes in the US, has designated medication reconciliation as a national patient safety goal, specifically Goal 8, since 2004.

Goal 8 is to 'accurately and completely reconcile medications across the continuum of care'. The rationale behind this goal is to prevent harm to the patient from adverse drug events due to miscommunications regarding their medications. The incidence of such adverse events increases when multiple healthcare professionals and care givers are involved in providing care to patients. Accurately maintaining a current list of medications whenever new medications are ordered, current medications are discontinued or adjusted, whenever a patient is transferred from one service to another or discharged and re-admitted is essential to reduce such transition-related adverse drug events.

Clinical pharmacists are uniquely positioned to help hospitals achieve these goals. Most often, they are the consistent participant in the healthcare team. Attending physicians, medical residents, medical students and nurses taking care of the patient may change and rotate out depending on the length of the patient's hospitalisation. However, a clinical pharmacist assigned to a service is always available. Pharmacists can assist by obtaining patient medication histories that are often more complete and accurate than those obtained by physicians or nurses.

Medication reconciliation should consist of four main steps. The *first step* is to develop a complete list of the medications the patient is currently taking at home (including drug, dose, route, dosage form and frequency). This can be achieved by conducting a thorough medication history, and family members may also be involved in this process. The *second step* is to compare the medications ordered for the patient while admitted to the hospital to the list created under Step One. Any discrepancy (additions, deletions, duplications or omissions for drugs, changes in doses, dosage forms, routes, frequencies) are reconciled and documented while the patient is still in the hospital; this is *Step Three*.

Step Four consists of transmission of this information when and if the patient is transferred to another provider/service/unit or discharged. At this point, the current provider should transmit this up-to-date reconciled medication list and documents to the receiving provider/patient/care giver. Pharmacists can be involved in performing all four steps.

CASE STUDY 1

YZ is a 14-day-old premature neonate, born at 28 weeks of gestation.

Calculate his GA, PNA and postmenstrual age.

His gestational age is 28 weeks, postnatal age is 14 days or 2 weeks, and his postmenstrual age is 30 weeks (28 weeks + 2 weeks).

CASE STUDY 2

AB, a seven-year-old girl weighing 20 kg, is diagnosed with an immunocompromising disease. She is currently neutropaenic. Her absolute neutrophil count (ANC) is 150/mm^3. She has just completed a three-week therapy of liposomal amphotericin B (Ambisone®) 100 mg IV every day at 5 mg/kg/day. She has been afebrile since amphotericin B was administered. In addition, she is also on ceftazidime 1 g IV every 8 hours (150 mg/kg/day) and vancomycin 400 mg IV every 8 hours (60 mg/kg/day). A decision to stop amphotericin B and to start itraconazole 50 mg PO every 12 hours (5 mg/kg/day) was made in consultation with a paediatric infectious diseases specialist. The specialist also recommended measuring peak serum concentration for itraconazole two hours after the dose, 3–5 days after starting therapy. The level was low at 150 ng/ml (therapeutic range: >250 ng/ml). A list of other drugs includes:

- Cotrimoxazole 5 cc (40 mg trimethoprim) in the morning and 7.5 cc (60 mg trimethoprim) in the evening on Saturday and Sunday
- Chlorhexidine mouthwash 5 ml swish and spit four times a day
- Filgrastim 100 mcg SC daily (5 mcg/kg/day)
- Paracetamol 200 mg PO every 4–6 hours prn
- Total parenteral nutrition over 24 hours
- Ranitidine 50 mg PO twice a day (5 mg/kg/day)

What would be your recommendation for the lower itraconazole level?

Itraconazole needs an acidic gastric pH for complete absorption. The decreased concentration of itraconazole in this child can be explained by concurrent ranitidine therapy. Administering it with carbonated beverages or orange juice, which would temporarily decrease gastric pH and probably enhance absorption, can increase the absorption of itraconazole. Another option would be to increase the itraconazole dose until the required therapeutic drug concentration is obtained.

CASE STUDY 3

CD is a 9-year-old girl (weight 25 kg) with a severe seizure disorder due to hypoxic ischaemic insult to the brain during birth. She is on phenobarbitone and phenytoin for seizure control. She is admitted for symptoms of drug toxicity such as increased lethargy and nystagmus. Her phenobarbital serum concentration is 74 mcg/ml (normal: 10–40 mcg/ml) and phenytoin serum concentration is 38 mcg/ml (normal: 10–20 mcg/ml). All other laboratory values including liver function tests were within normal limits. She has normal respiration without need for intubation. Patient has had surgery for Nissen fundoplication with placement of a gastrostomy tube. Her only medication other than the anti-epileptics is metoclopramide at 2.5 mg PO four times a day.

She has a urine output of 2.5 ml/kg/hour indicating normal renal function. The mother reports that CD has had no bowel movement for the past four days despite a typical adequate diet. She also denies administering any extra doses of any drug.

What do you think is causing the increased serum concentrations of phenobarbital and phenytoin?

The lack of bowel movement indicates slowing of gastrointestinal emptying; this increases gastrointestinal absorption of the drugs administered, even at normal doses. Both phenytoin and phenobarbitone are weak acids. Decreased gastrointestinal transit time results in prolonged exposure to the stomach acid, both drugs remain unionised and hence there is increased absorption. This has resulted in increased serum drug concentrations. The administration of both drugs should be stopped until the serum concentrations return to normal. Monitor phenytoin serum concentration daily until it reaches 10–20 mcg/ml and then resume her normal dose. Monitor phenobarbitone serum concentration every 2–3 days until it reaches 20–40 mcg/ml and then resume her normal dose. Constipation should be relieved by administering drugs such as lactulose, sennosides, magnesium salts such as magnesium hydroxide or magnesium citrate until the patient has a bowel movement and returns to a normal bowel movement schedule.

CASE STUDY 4

EF is an 18-month-old baby weighing 10 kg, receiving carbamazepine to control her seizure disorder. Her dose is 75 mg three times a day (22.5 mg/kg/day) (3.75 ml three times a day) administered as an oral suspension 100 mg/5 ml. EF is scheduled for Nissen fundoplication with placement of a gastrostomy tube and is NPO (nothing per os, nothing by mouth) for 8 hours before surgery, including her oral medications. The seizure disorder is well controlled on her current dose. The neurologist as well as the general surgeon do not want the carbamazepine serum concentration to drop while she is NPO or during surgery.

What would be your recommendations?

An oral suspension of carbamazepine can be administered rectally in patients who are orally restricted. Total absorption, maximum serum concentration and time to achieve maximum serum concentration were comparable between patients receiving carbamazepine tablets orally and suspension rectally. The only drawback with rectal administration is the strong defecatory urge. This can be reduced by mixing the oral suspension with water in a 1:1 proportion before administration.

CASE STUDY 5

GH is a three-day-old, postnatal age neonate, born at 39 weeks of gestation. He weighs 3 kg and is admitted to the general paediatrics floor with fever of unknown origin. He is started on ampicillin 150 mg IV every 8 hours (150 mg/kg/day) and gentamicin 6 mg (2.5 mg/kg/dose) IV every 12 hours. His blood urea nitrogen (BUN) and serum creatinine (SCr) are 5 mg/dL and 0.6 mg/dL, respectively, with a urine output of 2.5 ml/kg/h. The gentamicin peak and trough serum concentrations were 5 mcg/ml and 1.0 mcg/ml, respectively. The calculated Vd was 0.57 L/kg.

IJ is a 10-year-old girl weighing 30 kg and being treated with gentamicin 60 mg IV every 8 hours (2.5 mg/kg/dose) for Gram-negative *Escherichia coli* pyelonephritis. Her BUN and SCr are 15 mg/dL and 0.8 mg/dl, respectively. The gentamicin peak and trough serum concentrations were 7 mcg/ml and 0.5 mcg/ml, respectively. The calculated Vd was 0.31 L/kg.

Explain why different serum peak concentrations are obtained in the two patients despite using the same dose (2.5 mg/kg/dose).

Extracellular fluid volume is markedly different in premature infants compared with older children and adults; the extracellular fluid volume may account for 50% of body weight in premature infants, 35% in 4–6-month-old infants, 25% in children 1 year of age and 19% in adults. Hydrophilic drugs such as aminoglycoside antibiotics largely distribute into the extracellular fluid and thus have larger volumes of distribution in neonates on a per kg basis compared to older infants and children (gentamicin distribution volumes $Vd_{< 34\ wk}$ 0.67 ± 0.13 L/kg; $Vd_{34–48\ wk}$ 0.52 ± 0.10 L/kg; $Vd_{1–4.9\ yrs}$ 0.38 ± 0.16 L/kg; $Vd_{5–9.9\ yrs}$ 0.33 ± 0.14 L/kg; $Vd_{10–16\ yrs}$ 0.31 ± 0.12 L/kg; Vd_{adult} < 0.30 L/kg). The larger the volume of distribution, the larger the mg/kg dose of aminoglycoside required to achieve the recommended peak serum concentration. GH is a neonate with larger Vd compared to IJ and therefore will need a higher individual mg/kg dose to achieve identical serum concentrations. However, because the clearance is lower in neonates, the dose would be given at an extended interval so that the daily maintenance dose will be smaller in neonates than in the older population.

CASE STUDY 6

MN is a 16-year-old girl weighing 80 kg and is 165 cm tall. She is admitted for a urinary tract infection. Gentamicin 160 mg IV every 8 hours is prescribed for her.

What would be your reaction to this dose?

Although the dose is correct at 2 mg/kg/dose, the patient is overweight for her age. The dose of 160 mg is based on her actual body weight that includes adipose tissue. Gentamicin is a hydrophilic drug and will distribute only in the non-adipose tissue. Dosing based on actual weight may lead to toxicity. A paediatric patient may be considered obese if actual body weight (ABW) is >120% weight for height on the US National Center for Health Statistics growth chart. To calculate weight for height, plot the patient's height on the growth chart. Note the percentile it corresponds to for the patient's age (MN's height falls between the 50th and 75th percentiles for her age). Find the weight corresponding to that percentile for that age (MN's 75th percentile weight for her age is 62 kg). If patient's actual weight is >120% of this weight, calculate dosing weight:

Dosing weight (DW) = IBW + 0.4 (ABW – IBW)

IBW is the weight corresponding to the patient's height on the growth chart.

MN's actual body weight is 80 kg which is about 129% of her weight for height. Therefore, her dosing weight is = 62 + 0.4 (80 – 62) = 69.2 kg

Her gentamicin dose should be 138 mg IV Q 8 hours instead of 160 mg IV every 8 hours. Recommend the measurement of peak and trough serum concentrations around the second dose to make sure that dosing recommendations are appropriate.

CASE STUDY 7

KL is a 39-week, postconceptional age neonate born at 28 weeks' gestational age weighing 2 kg. He is admitted to a paediatric intensive care unit with the diagnosis of 'gasping syndrome', with metabolic acidosis, respiratory distress needing intubation, hypotension needing fluids and vasopressors, lethargy and with decreased urine output (<1 ml/kg/hour). Among other significant laboratory values, the following have been included: urine benzoate levels of 10.1 mg/mg creatinine, hippurate levels of 8 mg/mg creatinine (normal values = 0–trace); serum benzoic acid levels were 20 mEq/l (normal = 0).

History of Present Illness: KL demonstrated an increase in the number of apnoeic episodes requiring increased oxygen, body temperature of 38.3 °C, decreased oral intake, and lethargy. He was taken to the nearest emergency department. Among other things, a fluid bolus was ordered to resuscitate his decreasing blood pressure. He received two 30 milliliter boluses of 0.9% sodium chloride (normal saline). However, the normal saline administered was obtained from multidose vials of bacteriostatic 0.9% sodium chloride containing 0.9% benzyl alcohol.

Past Medical History: KL was a 28-week premature baby discharged from the hospital at PCA of 38 weeks with a diagnosis of bronchopulmonary dysplasia, apnoea of prematurity and retinopathy of prematurity. During the hospital stay, he had acute respiratory distress syndrome needing surfactant therapy, prolonged intubation to provide oxygen, corticosteroids and diuretics. He was sent home on 0.1 l of oxygen by nasal canula and an apnoea monitor.

The medical student wonders why serum benzoic acid concentrations were measured. How would you explain it to him?

Benzyl alcohol is normally oxidised rapidly to benzoic acid, which is conjugated with glycine in the liver and excreted as hippuric acid. However, this metabolic pathway may not be well developed in KL. Benzyl alcohol was metabolised to benzoic acid, which could not be conjugated by the immature liver but accumulated, causing increased serum levels and metabolic acidosis. Benzyl alcohol was inadvertently administered to the premature neonate with of bacteriostatic 0.9% sodium chloride for resuscitation. In 1982, the USFDA issued a warning against the use of agents or reconstituted solutions containing benzyl alcohol in newborn infants. A dose greater than 90 mg/kg/day was considered toxic. KL received two 30 ml boluses = 60 ml containing 0.9% benzyl alcohol. Therefore, KL received 540 mg of benzyl alcohol or 270 mg/kg of benzyl alcohol.

The administration of preservative-free (benzyl alcohol–free) parenteral drugs is ideal in neonates, especially premature ones, to avoid the risk of accumulation of benzoic acid. Not all parenteral drugs are manufactured benzyl alcohol–free; as a result, these need to be diluted with other benzyl alcohol–free diluents to decrease the amount of benzyl alcohol that may be administered.

CASE STUDY 8: HOW TO FOLLOW A COMPLEX PAEDIATRIC PATIENT

Patient ID: 1234567		Name: John Doe	
Date of Birth: 1/1/1995		Age: 14 years	
Height: 168 cm	Weight: 63.5 kg		Gender: Male
Admission date: 2/1/2009		Date of data collection: 2/1//2009	
Allergies: Penicillin, Cephalosporin, Sulfa			
History of Present Illness: Seen in bone marrow transplant clinic on 2/1/09 due to increased stool output and skin rash due to suspected acute graft host disease (aGVHD), a complication of the bone marrow transplantation. Diarrhoea started 2 days ago and the rash has now spread to 75% of body surface area. Admitted for intravenous medications and treatment of aGVHD.			
Past Medical/Surgical History: Acute lymphocytic leukaemia diagnosed Jan 2000 with multiple relapses and status post-allogeneic matched unrelated bone marrow transplantation in Jan 2009. Epilepsy diagnosed at one year of age on levetiracetam, last seizure 2005. Delayed development and learning disability with writing and reading skills at kindergarten or 1st grade level.			
Family/Social History Lives with maternal grandparents; grandmother is the primary care giver.			

Medications Prior to Admission (PTA):	
Levetiracetam 750 mg capsule: 750 mg orally twice a day	Voriconazole 250 mg orally two time daily (using 200 mg and 50 mg tablets)
Lansoprazole 30 mg capsule: 30 mg orally once a day	Levafloxacin 500 mg capsule: 500 mg orally once daily
Mycophenolate 250 mg capsule: 1000 mg orally three times a day	Acyclovir 200 mg capsule: 400 mg orally two times daily
Tacrolimus 0.5 mg/ml oral suspension: 0.8 mg orally two times a day	
Immunisations: Up-to-date prior to transplant	

Current Medications: (after admission to the hospital)		
Start Date	Stop Date	Drug name, dose, route, frequency
2/1/09		Levetiracetam 750 mg IV every 12 hours
2/1/09		Levofloxacin 500 mg IV daily
2/1/09		Lansoprazole (delayed release capsule) 30 mg orally daily
2/1/09		Mycophenolate 1000 mg IV every 8 hours
2/1/09		Paracetamol 650 mg orally every 6 hours as needed for fevers > 38 °C
2/1/09		Tacrolimus 0.3 mg IV every 12 hours
2/1/09		Fentanyl Patient Controlled Analgesia (PCA) order
2/1/09		Acyclovir 400 mg IV twice daily
2/1/09		Voriconazole 250 mg IV twice daily
2/6/09		Pentamidine 260 mg IV every 4 weeks (last dose 1/9/09)
2/7/09		Immune globulin 32.5 g IV every 2 weeks (last dose 1/10/09)
2/1/09		Methylprednisolone 60 mg IV every 12 hours

Relevant information from physical exam, procedures, and daily progress
2/1/09 JD admitted for aGVHD symptoms of diarrhoea and full body rash; stool cultures sent; methylpredinisolone started; all oral drugs changed to intravenous; JD started on fentanyl patient controlled analgesia for abdominal pain; also made NPO for gut rest and total parenteral nutrition started
2/2/09 JD afebrile; pain worsening requiring increase in PCA; tacrolimus level normal after change from oral to IV; stool cultures negative for infectious cause of diarrhea; TPN adjusted for electrolytes; blood glucose high due to steroids may need insulin; stool out put still high
2/3/09 Afebrile; labs stable; still hyperglycemic; increased PCA; stool output stable; skin rash resolved
2/4/09 Afebrile; labs stable; still hyperglycemic; pain under control; stool output stable
2/5/09 Afebrile; labs stable; still hyperglycemic; pain under control; stool output stable
2/8/09 Afebrile; labs stable; still hyperglycemic; pain under control, weaning PCA; stool output decreasing
2/10/09 Afebrile; labs stable; still hyperglycemic; pain under control, weaning PCA; no liquid stool gut aGVHD resolving; anticipate discharge home in the next week on oral prednisone

Daily Monitoring Form

Date	2/1	2/2	2/3	2/4	2/5	2/6	2/7	2/8	2/9	2/10
Weight (kg)	63.5	63.2	64	63.7	64.2	64.9	65.5	65.3	65.1	65.2
T max °C	37.7	37	37.1	37.5	36.9	37.2	37.2	37.1	37.5	37.8
WBC (K/mm3)	8.6	10.2	9.1	13.5	18.4	19.8	17.3	17.5	12.8	11.3
ANC	6708	7854	8654	12420	17112	18216	15224	15575	11776	10057
Hb (g/dl)	12.9	12.0	9.9	12.1	11.4	10.2	12.7	11.5	10.4	11.9
Platelets (K/mm3)	184	181	138	141	145	131	129	124	112	104
BUN (mg/dl)	14	12	10	12	12	14	14	15	14	13
Cr (mg/dl)	0.42	0.41	0.38	0.37	0.34	0.32	0.34	0.33	0.35	0.31
Na (mmol/l)	132	132	133	136	137	136	135	134	137	137
K (mmol/l)	4.4	4.4	4.2	4.1	4.3	4.3	4.6	4.4	4.7	4.0
Cl (mmol/l)	101	103	104	105	107	105	105	104	105	105
CO2 (mmol/l)	27	28	27	28	26	26	28	27	29	27
Ca (mg/dl)	8.2	8.2	8.1	8.3	8.5	8.3	8.1	8.0	8.3	8.3
PO4 (mg/dl)	2.5	3.1	2.6	3.0	3.1	3.1	3.0	3.4	3.4	3.4
Mg (mg/dl)	1.7	1.7	1.5	1.7	1.6	1.6	1.5	1.4	1.3	1.5
Glucose (mg/dl)	177	137	158	200	182	188	191	190	179	200
Triglycerides (mg/dl)					241					
Total protein (g/dl)	5.1		5.1			5.2			5.2	
Albumin (g/dl)	3.1		3.0			3.5			2.9	
Total bilirubin (mg/dl)	0.6		0.3			1.0			1.0	
ALT (U/L)	67		60			135			49	
In ml	6646	7052	6889	6422	6402	7004	6504	6662	7586	6541
Total Output ml	7100	7543	7110	7130	6640	7500	6795	5920	8945	7445
Stool Output in ml	4775	4660	3136	3275	2515	2000	1480	845	300	No liq stool
Microbiology Cultures										
Stool 2/1/2009	Clostridium difficile toxin negative; Adenovirus negative; Rotavirus negative									
	Culture negative									
Drug Serum Concentration										
Tacrolimus (5-15 ng/ml)	7			9			10			10

Total Parenteral Nutrition										
Date	2/1	2/2	2/3	2/4	2/5	2/6	2/7	2/8	2/9	2/10
Weight	63.5	63.2	64	63.7	64.2	64.9	65.5	65.3	65.1	65.2
Duration (hours/day)	24	24	24	24	24	24	24	24	24	24
TPN ml/day	2040	2040	2040	2040	2040	2040	2040	2040	2040	2040
Intralipid g/kg										
Intralipid ml/day	360	360	360	360	360	360	360	360	360	360
Intralipid kcal/day	720	720	720	720	720	720	720	720	720	720

Protein g/day	90	90	90	90	90	90	90	90	90	90
Protein kcal/day	360	360	360	360	360	360	360	360	360	360
Dextrose %	15	15	15	15	15	15	15	15	15	15
Dextrose g/day	306	306	306	306	306	306	306	306	306	306
Dextrose kcal/day	1040	1040	1040	1040	1040	1040	1040	1040	1040	1040
Total kcal/day	2120	2120	2120	2120	2120	2120	2120	2120	2120	2120
Na (mEq/kg/day)	4	4	4	4	4	4	4	4	4	4
K (mEq/kg/day)	1	1	1	1	1	1	1	1	1	1
Cl:Acetate (ratio)	75:25	75:25	75:25	75:25	75:25	75:25	75:25	75:25	75:25	75:25
Ca (mEq/kg/day)	0.2	0.2	0.2	0.2	0.2	0.2	0.2	0.2	0.2	0.2
PO4 (mmol/kg/day)	1	1	1.5	1.5	1.5	1.5	1.8	1.8	1.8	1.8
Mg (mEq/kg/day)	0.25	0.25	0.25	0.25	0.25	0.25	0.25	0.25	0.25	0.25
Se (mg /day)	40	40	40	40	40	40	40	40	40	40
MVI	10 mL	10 mL	10 mL	10 mL	10 mL	10 mL	10 mL	10 mL	10 mL	10 mL
Insulin (units/day)	0	0	0	0	0	0	0	0	0	0
Heparin (units/day)	0	0	0	0	0	0	0	0	0	0
H2 antagonist (mg/day)	0	0	0	0	0	0	0	0	0	0

PAIN THERAPY										
Drug used	Fentanyl									
Date	2/1	2/2	2/3	2/4	2/5	2/6	2/7	2/8	2/9	2/10
Basal rate (mcg/hr)	35	45	50	50	50	45	40	35	30	25
PCA bolus dose (mcg)	35	45	50	50	50	45	40	35	30	25
Lock out interval (minutes)	15	15	15	15	15	15	15	15	15	15
# of attempts	37	15	10	8	9	9	0	0	0	0
# of doses	18	15	10	8	9	9	0	0	0	0
Total daily dose (mcg)	1470	1755	1700	1600	1650	1485	960	840	720	600
Pain rating out of 10	10	8	6	4	4	3	3	3	2	1
Sedation	alert	alert	alert	alert	alert	alert	alert	alert	alert	alert
Respiratory rate breaths/minute	16-24	16-24	16-20	16-25	15-23	14-22	12-22	16-25	16-24	16-20

How to follow a complex paediatric patient?

As part of a multi-disciplinary healthcare team, clinical pharmacists can play an important role in making valuable pharmacotherapeutic recommendations and facilitate the care of the patient during rounds. To be effective during rounds, the clinical pharmacist should engage in an activity that could be labelled pre-rounding. This involves:

1. Preparing a list of all the patients on your healthcare team's ward.
2. Reviewing their health information and gathering pertinent data before rounds using the tables shown above.

3. Prioritising the patients you would review based on their acuity of care. This is not necessarily medical acuity but pharmacy acuity. Examples of patients with high pharmacy acuity of care would include those on drugs which require therapeutic drug monitoring, those with worsening renal and/or hepatic function which impacts drug dosing or those with infectious diseases who require multiple antibiotics.
4. Determine the patient's medications prior to admission (medications they use at home) and ensure those are ordered for them upon admission, if necessary.
5. Check each medication to ensure it is indeed indicated in your patient.
6. Check the accuracy of the doses being administered (mg/kg/day or mg/kg/dose).
7. Make a list of the patient's medical issues/problems.
8. Check to ensure that each medical problem is being treated, when appropriate.
9. List all the parameters to monitor in each patient to assure efficacy and safety of the administered drug therapy.
10. Observe for resolution of the patient's medical problems.

Areas where a clinical pharmacist would be involved in making recommendations/interventions for JD include:

1. Infectious diseases – to recommend appropriate antibiotics based on culture results.
2. Pain control – to recommend the starting dose and titration of the PCA based on JD's pain.
3. Total parenteral nutrition – to make an initial recommendation on the amount of carbohydrates, proteins and lipids and on further titration of the TPN to achieve adequate nutrition.
4. Total parenteral nutrition – to make an initial recommendation and on further titration of electrolyte supplementation to obtain stable, normal laboratory values.
5. Therapeutic drug monitoring – to monitor tacrolimus serum concentrations and recommend dose changes based on the results.
6. Management of hyperglycemia – to recommend insulin dose and titration, and patient education if insulin is needed on a long-term basis.
7. To assist the healthcare team to switch to oral medications once JD is ready to go home.

CASE STUDY 9

JD from **Case Study 8** is ready to go home on the following oral medications:

Prednisone (10 mg oral tablet): Take one tablet (10 mg) by mouth twice daily

Levofloxacin (Levaquin™) 50 mg/ml oral liquid: Take 10 ml (500 mg) by mouth once daily

Mycophenolate (Cellcept™) 250 mg oral capsule: Take 4 capsules (1000 mg) by mouth three times daily

Tacrolimus 0.5 mg/ml oral suspension (extemporaneously compounded): Take 1.4 ml (0.7 mg) by mouth twice daily

Voriconazole (VFend™) 200 mg and 50 mg tablet: Take one 200 mg and one 50 mg tablet (250 mg) by mouth twice daily

Acyclovir (Zovirax™) 200 mg/5 ml oral suspension: Take 10 ml (400 mg) by mouth twice daily

Lansoprazole (Prevacid™) 30 mg delayed-release oral capsule: Take 1 capsule (30 mg) by mouth once daily

Levetiracetam (Keppra™) 750 mg tablet: Take 1 tablet (750 mg) by mouth twice daily

Although JD is 14 years old, he is not able to adhere to his daily medications on his own without forgetting or missing a dose; this is because of his developmental delay. His grandmother expresses some frustration due to the number of medications that need to be administered.

How would you help JD and his grandmother improve their adherence to his complicated therapy?

Inquire about JD's ability to swallow tablets and capsules. He may not be able to swallow large tablets or capsules, and hence those may need to be substituted with a liquid formulation. The pharmacist can help the grandmother understand the complicated drug administration schedule by preparing a medication plan for JD (Fig. 15.2) and also by writing clear instructions for each drug (Fig. 15. 3). All daily medications should be administered at the same time. An attempt should be made to match the frequencies and administration times for most of the drugs administered during the day. For example, prednisone, tacrolimus, voriconazole, acyclovir and levetiracetam are all scheduled twice daily and should be administered at 9 AM and at 9 PM. Levofloxacin and lansoprazole are scheduled once daily and should be administered either at 9 AM or at 9 PM, based on JD's preference, and with other medications. This would prevent JD and his grandmother from forgetting to administer them. Mycophenolate is scheduled three times daily; two of the three doses should be scheduled with other medications at 9 AM and at 9 PM. The third dose should be scheduled for early afternoon with some regular activity that JD participates in, such as return from school or with an afternoon snack. Review information about each drug with the grandmother using patient education materials. You may ask JD's grandmother to fill any new prescriptions and bring her home medications to the hospital room.

As you review the instructions with her, you can identify each medication by opening the bottle. You may also ask her to demonstrate how she would administer liquid medications using the oral syringes (Fig. 15.4). Review the storage conditions, number of refills available and when to call for a refill or new prescription. Review the following information with the grandmother: the drug, the dose, frequency, the reason for using a particular drug, what to expect for efficacy and for side effects. Ask the grandmother to repeat the information in response to your open-ended questions, such as 'What did the doctor say this medicine is being used for?', 'What did the doctor tell you to expect?' and 'What did the doctor say the side effects would be from taking this medicine?'. This information may need to be reviewed again on subsequent visits. The clinical pharmacist should let the grandmother know about their availability to answer any questions or provide more information if needed. You may also offer the grandmother a medication administration schedule form (Fig. 15.5) which she can use to mark off the drugs each day as she administers it. You may also ask her to bring in the completed schedule form.

MEDACTIONPLAN™

My Daily Schedule

8/29/2009 4:13:00 PM
Revised by: Vinita Pai

Doe, John DOB: **01-01-1995** MRN: **1234567**
Allergies: **Cephalosporins, Penicillins, Sulfa**

Take These Medications	At These Times			Purpose
	9am	4pm	9pm	
GENERIC **Prednisone** 10mg Tablet(s) By mouth	1 Tablet(s)		1 Tablet(s)	Prevents and treats acute graft versus host disease.
Levofloxacin Suspension (Levofloxacin) 50 mg/mL By mouth	10 mL(s) (500mg)			Treats/prevents bacterial infections
Cellcept® (Mycophenolate mofetil) 250mg Capsule(s) By mouth	4 Capsule(s)	4 Capsule(s)	4 Capsule(s)	Prevents and treats acute graft versus host disease.
Tacrolimus Suspension (Tacrolimus) 0.5 mg/mL By mouth	1.4 mL(s) (0.7mg)		1.4 mL(s) (0.7mg)	Prevents and treats acute graft versus host disease.
VFend® (Voriconazole) 200mg Tablet(s) By mouth	1 Tablet(s)		1 Tablet(s)	Prevents/treats fungal infections
VFend® (Voriconazole) 50mg Tablet(s) By mouth	1 Tablet(s)		1 Tablet(s)	Prevents/treats fungal infections
Zovirax® (Acyclovir) 200 mg/5 mL By mouth	10 mL(s) (400mg)		10 mL(s) (400mg)	Treats/prevents viral infections
Prevacid SoluTab® (Lansoprazole) 30 mg Delayed release tablet(s) By mouth	1 Delayed release tablet(s)			Treats/prevents stomach ulcer/heartburn
Keppra® (Levetiracetam) 750mg Tablet(s) By mouth	1 Tablet(s)		1 Tablet(s)	Treats epilepsy

❑ Only take the medications listed in your Daily Schedule. Check the date of your last schedule to make sure you have the most current medication list. The pharmacist may make a generic substitution for the medication shown in your Daily Schedule. The medication name, dosage strength, shape, color, and size may change as a result of this substitution. Please check dosage strength on your prescription bottle against the dosage strength shown on your daily schedule. Call your healthcare professional's office immediately if you receive medication that is different from what was prescribed or if you have questions about your medication.
1 teaspoon = 5mL, 1 tablespoon = 15mL

Patient verbalized understanding of instructions/explanations regarding medications? ___No ___Yes

Healthcare Provider/Title: ______________________ Date:__________

[I, the patient][We, the family] understand these medications and have received specific instructions for taking them from this healthcare professional.

Patient/Family Member: ______________________ Date:__________

Keep your med schedule updated on ***www.MyMedSchedule.com.*** Ask your healthcare facility to send your schedule to you so you can keep your schedule current.

Figure 15.2 Case Study 9, example of medication schedule to improve adherence

MEDACTIONPLAN™
Special Instructions

8/29/2009 4:13:00 PM
Revised by: Vinita Pai

Doe, John DOB: **01-01-1995** MRN: **1234567**
Allergies: **Cephalosporins, Penicillins, Sulfa**

Please follow these instructions to help you get the best results from your medication. Call your transplant coordinator immediately if you have any questions or experience any problems with your medication. Do not stop taking your medication without your physician's approval.

Take These Medications	Instructions
GENERIC **Prednisone** 10mg Tablet(s) By mouth	Take with food to reduce nausea or stomach upset. Take 1 tablet twice daily Edit Instructions
Levofloxacin Suspension (Levofloxacin) 50 mg/mL mL(s) By mouth	Take 10 mL once daily. Take as directed by your doctor. Take on an empty stomach, 1 hour before or 2 hours after meals. Do not skip doses. Finish full course of therapy unless advised by your doctor. Edit Instructions
Cellcept® (Mycophenolate mofetil) 250mg Capsule(s) By mouth	Take 4 capsules three times daily. Do not break, crush or chew capsules. May take with food to reduce nausea or stomach upset. Edit Instructions
Tacrolimus Suspension (Tacrolimus) 0.5 mg/mL mL(s) By mouth	Take 1.4 mL twice daily. Take as directed by your doctor. Tell your doctor if you have any signs or symptoms of an infection. Report any unusual bleeding or bruising. Take medication at the same time each day on an empty stomach. Protect from light. Edit Instructions
VFend® (Voriconazole) 200mg Tablet(s) By mouth	Take 1 capsule twice daily. Combine with 50 mg tablet. Take at least one hour before or one hour after a meal. Edit Instructions
VFend® (Voriconazole) 50mg Tablet(s) By mouth	Take 1 capsule twice daily. Combine with 200 mg tablet.Take at least one hour before or one hour after a meal. Edit Instructions
Zovirax® (Acyclovir) 200 mg/5 mL mL(s) By mouth	Take 10 mL twice daily. Shake well before use. Drink plenty of fluids while taking this medication. Edit Instructions
Prevacid SoluTab® (Lansoprazole) 30 mg Delayed release tablet(s) By mouth	Take one tablet daily. Do not chew or crush tablets. Edit Instructions
Keppra® (Levetiracetam) 750mg Tablet(s) By mouth	Take one tablet twice daily. Take with or without food. Edit Instructions

☐ Only take the medications listed in your Daily Schedule. Check the date of your last schedule to make sure you have the most current medication list. The pharmacist may make a generic substitution for the medication shown in your Daily Schedule. The medication name, dosage strength, shape, color, and size may change as a result of this substitution. Please check dosage strength on your prescription bottle against the dosage strength shown on your daily schedule. Call your healthcare professional's office immediately if you receive medication that is different from what was prescribed or if you have questions about your medication.
1 teaspoon = 5mL, 1 tablespoon = 15mL

References: 1. Full Prescribing Information for respective products and brands. **2.** FDA/Center for Drug Evaluation and Research, Division of Library and Information Services. [FDA Web site]. Available at http://www.fda.gov/cder/consumerinfo/default.htm.

Keep your med schedule updated on ***www.MyMedSchedule.com.*** Ask your healthcare facility to send your schedule to you so you can keep your schedule current.

Figure 15.3 Case Study 9, example of medication instructions for patients

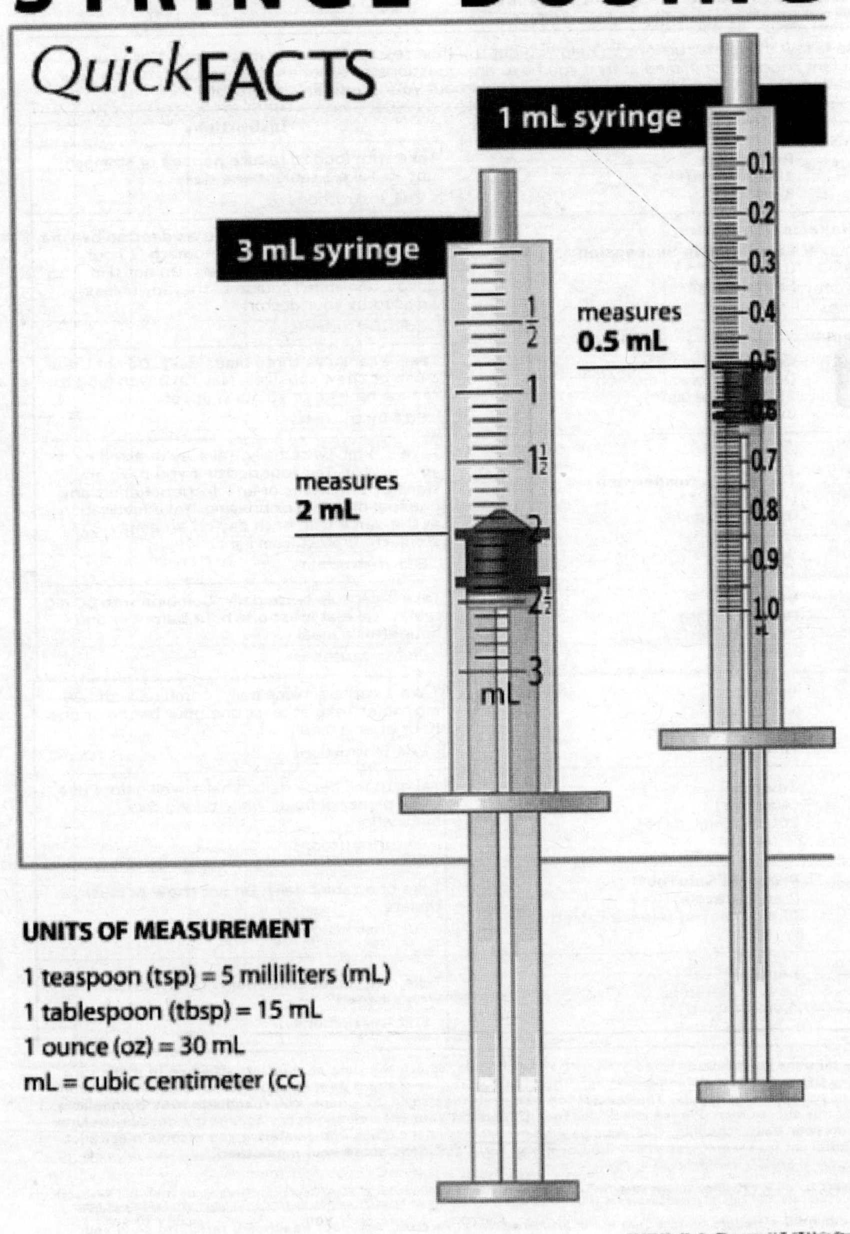

Figure 15.4 Case Study 9, measuring liquids in oral syringes

MEDACTIONPLAN™

Weekly Med Checklist

8/29/2009 4:13:00 PM
Revised by: Vinita Pai

It is important to bring this completed list with you to each healthcare or dental visit.

Doe, John DOB: **01-01-1995** MRN: **1234567**
Allergies: **Cephalosporins, Penicillins, Sulfa**

Medication	Dose	Time	SUN	MON	TUES	WED	THUR	FRI	SAT
		Date:	/	/	/	/	/	/	/
Prednisone 10mg *Prevents and treats acute graft versus host disease.*	1 Tablet(s)	9am							
	1 Tablet(s)	9pm							
Levofloxacin Suspension (Levofloxacin) 50 mg/mL *Treats/prevents bacterial infections*	**10mL(s)** (500mg)	9am							
Cellcept® (Mycophenolate mofetil) 250mg *Prevents and treats acute graft versus host disease.*	4 Capsule(s)	9am							
	4 Capsule(s)	4pm							
	4 Capsule(s)	9pm							
Tacrolimus Suspension (Tacrolimus) 0.5 mg/mL *Prevents and treats acute graft versus host disease.*	**1.4mL(s)** (0.7mg)	9am							
	1.4mL(s) (0.7mg)	9pm							
VFend® (Voriconazole) 200mg *Prevents/treats fungal infections*	1 Tablet(s)	9am							
	1 Tablet(s)	9pm							
VFend® (Voriconazole) 50mg *Prevents/treats fungal infections*	1 Tablet(s)	9am							
	1 Tablet(s)	9pm							
Zovirax® (Acyclovir) 200 mg/5 mL *Treats/prevents viral infections*	**10mL(s)** (400mg)	9am							
	10mL(s) (400mg)	9pm							
Prevacid SoluTab® (Lansoprazole) 30 mg *Treats/prevents stomach ulcer/heartburn*	1 Delayed release tablet(s)	9am							
Keppra® (Levetiracetam) 750mg *Treats epilepsy*	1 Tablet(s)	9am							
	1 Tablet(s)	9pm							

☐ **Only take the medications listed in your Daily Schedule. Check the date of your last schedule to make sure you have the most current medication list. The pharmacist may make a generic substitution for the medication shown in your Daily Schedule. The medication name, dosage strength, shape, color, and size may change as a result of this substitution. Please check dosage strength on your prescription bottle against the dosage strength shown on your daily schedule. Call your healthcare professional's office immediately if you receive medication that is different from what was prescribed or if you have questions about your medication.**
1 teaspoon = 5mL, 1 tablespoon = 15mL

Keep your med schedule updated on *www.MyMedSchedule.com.* Ask your healthcare facility to send your schedule to you so you can keep your schedule current.

Figure 15.5 Case Study 9, example of a weekly medication administration schedule

KEY MESSAGES

- Developing and maintaining a library consisting of textbooks, handbooks, primary literature and electronic/internet sources pertaining to paediatric pharmacotherapy is an important component of developing an efficient clinical practice in paediatrics.
- Knowledge of the pharmacokinetic and pharmacodynamic properties of each drug and the effect of development on its disposition is necessary to provide safe and effective drug therapy to children.
- The goals of therapeutic drug monitoring should be to maximise the potential for positive therapeutic outcome while minimising toxicity.
- Accurate information on non-compliance in children is difficult to obtain since parents are usually responsible for administering the medication.
- Prescribing errors can be minimised by the use of a clinical pharmacist, computer order entry, bar coding or point of care use and readily usable drug information for physicians and other healthcare personnel.
- Clinical pharmacists are uniquely positioned to achieve medication reconciliation, a process to accurately and completely reconcile medications across the continuum of care.

16 Clinical Pharmacy for Geriatric Patients

Rohan A Elliott

Learning Objectives

Upon completion of this chapter, the reader should be able to:

- Describe the health problems that commonly affect elderly patients
- Explain why elderly patients are at increased risk of adverse drug outcomes
- Understand the physiological changes that occur with ageing and how these impact on drug therapy
- Identify drugs that commonly cause adverse effects in the elderly and therefore need to be used with extra caution
- Understand that some diseases and adverse drug reactions may not present with typical symptoms in older patients
- Contribute to the prevention of drug-related problems in elderly patients by recommending avoidance of high-risk drugs and suggesting modified dose-regimens where appropriate
- Recognise and overcome communication barriers in elderly patients
- Understand the role clinical pharmacists can play in relation to common geriatric health problems

Geriatrics is the branch of medicine that is concerned with the medical and social aspects of health and illness in the elderly. The term 'elderly' generally refers to people aged 65 years and above. However, the physiological changes associated with ageing occur gradually over a lifetime, with significant patient-to-patient variability; so the choice of '65 years' is arbitrary, and sometimes the definition is extended to include people aged 60 years and above.

The Ageing Population

The proportion of elderly people within the populations of developed countries grew dramatically in the 20th century. For example, in the US, only 2% of the population was 65 years or older in 1900, but by 2000 it had risen to 13%. These increases were primarily due to declining infant and child mortality (due to improved standards of housing, hygiene and nutrition) and falling birth rates, and to a lesser extent to advances in curative and preventative medicine. By the year 2050, it is expected that 20% of the US population will be 65 years or older.

In developing countries, this demographic change has been slower. For example, in India in 2006 only 8% of the population was aged 60 years or older. However, this figure is likely to rise dramatically during this century, primarily due to falling birth rates, with the proportion of the population aged 60 years and above expected to reach 21% in 2050.

Currently, there are 90 million people in India aged over 60 years, and as this number grows it will become increasingly important for pharmacists to contribute to rational and safe medication use in the elderly.

Reasons for Caution When Using Medications in the Elderly

The incidence of adverse drug reactions (ADRs) and other adverse outcomes such as medication errors and drug-related hospital admissions increases with age. Data from cross-sectional studies suggest that about one in six elderly people taking multiple medications experience an ADR. Drug-related problems contribute to 10–20% of hospital admissions among older people.

However, old age as such is not an independent risk factor for ADRs and other adverse drug outcomes. The main reasons for increased risk are:

- Use of multiple medications (polypharmacy)
- Altered drug response
- Inappropriate prescribing
- Medication non-compliance

Polypharmacy: The prevalence of many diseases increases with age. Therefore, elderly people often suffer from multiple co-existing health problems (Table 16.1). Many of these are chronic problems which require long-term drug therapy, and sometimes combination drug therapy; so older people are frequently prescribed multiple medications ('polypharmacy').

Table 16.1 Common diseases and health problems affecting the elderly

Osteoarthritis
Visual and hearing impairment
Cardiovascular diseases (hypertension, ischaemic heart disease, heart failure)
Cerebrovascular diseases (like stroke)
Impaired mobility and falls
Constipation
Urinary and/or faecal incontinence
Chronic bronchitis, chronic obstructive airways disease
Depression
Osteoporosis
Cancer
Dementia
Malnutrition and related problems
Infectious diseases (especially respiratory and urinary tract infections)

Studies have consistently reported a positive association between the number of medications and the risk of ADRs, drug interactions, unplanned hospital admissions and medication non-compliance. Therefore, although the use of multiple medications may be unavoidable in patients with multiple co-existing medical conditions, care must be taken to avoid *unnecessary* polypharmacy.

Altered drug response: Elderly patients, especially the very old (over 75 years) and the frail, tend to be more sensitive to the effects of medications compared to younger adults. This is a result of physiological changes that occur with ageing, resulting in altered pharmacokinetics and pharmacodynamics. Older patients are therefore more prone to adverse effects and often require lower doses.

ADRs may present insidiously, without typical symptoms, in the elderly, and therefore they can be difficult to distinguish from new onset of illness. This can result in misdiagnosis and the introduction of an additional drug to treat the symptoms, thereby contributing to polypharmacy.

Inappropriate prescribing: Inappropriate prescribing for elderly patients is common. Studies from many different countries have consistently reported that around 20–40% of elderly people take at least one inappropriate medication.

As well as over-prescribing or inappropriate drug choice, under-prescribing is also common. For example, angiotensin converting enzyme (ACE) inhibitors decrease the morbidity and mortality associated with heart failure, but these drugs are commonly under-prescribed in the elderly.

Non-compliance: Poor compliance with prescribed drugs is common. Between 30% and 50% of elderly people do not take their medications as prescribed. Contributing factors include polypharmacy, complex dosing regimens, cognitive impairment, visual impairment, impaired dexterity (such as difficulty in getting tablets out of containers), ADRs, inadequate patient counselling, illiteracy and poverty.

Pharmacokinetic Changes with Ageing

Renal elimination: There are a number of pharmacokinctic changes that occur with ageing, but perhaps the most important is reduced renal function. Glomerular filtration rate and renal drug clearance decrease by 30–50% on average between the ages of 40 and 90 years, although there is variability among patients, and fit, healthy older people may retain near-normal renal function.

Elderly patients, especially those with pre-existing chronic renal impairment, are also at increased risk of acute renal failure as a result of dehydration, heart failure and hypotension (due to decreased kidney perfusion). Drugs that are extensively excreted unchanged by the kidneys and have a low therapeutic index usually require dosage reduction in the elderly. Dose adjustment is also required for drugs that are not themselves renally cleared, but which have an active or toxic metabolite that is renally excreted (Table 16.2).

Serum creatinine levels are often used as an indicator of renal function, but it is important to be aware that in older people this may not be reliable. Reduced muscle mass associated with ageing results in less creatinine production, which may offset any decrease in creatinine excretion via the kidneys. Therefore, an older person may have a 'normal' serum creatinine level, but still have markedly reduced kidney function.

Table 16.2 Pharmacokinetic changes associated with ageing

Pharmocokinetic Parameter	*Change*	*Cause*	*Effect*	*Examples of Drugs Affected*
Absorption	Rate reduced; extent usually unchanged (some exceptions, as listed)	Decreased acid secretion, delayed gastric emptying, decreased motility and decreased intestinal blood flow	Generally no significant effect. Potentially reduced absorption of a limited number of drugs and nutrients	Calcium, iron compounds, ketoconazole, vitamin B_{12}
First-pass metabolism	Reduced	Reduced liver blood flow, liver mass and intrinsic metabolic capacity	Greater bioavailability of some drugs	Chlorpromazine, labetolol, levodopa, metoprolol, nortriptyline, propranolol, prazosin, verapamil
Distribution – body composition	Altered	Decreased muscle mass and total body water, increased body fat	Fat-soluble drugs – increased volume of distribution, resulting in prolonged half-life and accumulation	Diazepam, lignocaine, thiopentone, tricyclic anti-depressants
			Water-soluble drugs – reduced volume of distribution, resulting in higher serum levels following acute dosing	Cimetidine, digoxin, ethanol, gentamicin, paracetamol
Distribution – protein binding	Reduced	Lower serum albumin	Decreased total plasma concentration (but unchanged unbound [active] concentration) of highly albumin-bound drugs	Phenytoin, diazepam, NSAIDs, tolbutamide, valproate, warfarin
Renal excretion	Reduced	Reduced glomerular filtration rate	Prolonged elimination half-life, accumulation and greater steady-state concentrations of some drugs or their metabolites	Digoxin, lithium, aminoglycosides, metformin, glibenclamide, vancomycin, fluoroquinolones, allopurinol,* pethidine,* dextropropoxyphene,* metoprolol*
Metabolism	Reduced oxidative (Phase I) metabolism	Decreased liver blood flow and mass. Reduced oxidative microsomal enzymes	Prolonged elimination half-life, accumulation and greater steady-state concentrations of some drugs	Diazepam, imipramine, fentanyl, metoprolol, nitrazepam, phenytoin, labetolol, propranolol, levodopa, theophylline verapamil, warfarin
	Unchanged conjugative (Phase II) metabolism	Preserved conjugative enzymes	Drugs which are conjugated are largely unaffected	Lorazepam, oxazepam, temazepam, isoniazid, rifampicin, paracetamol, most NSAIDs

* Parent drug not renally excreted, but metabolite is renally excreted.

To accurately determine renal function in the elderly, creatinine clearance needs to be determined either by direct measure (24-hour urine collection and assay) or by estimation using a formula such as the Cockroft and Gault equation (see *Case Study 1*).

Metabolism: There is great inter-individual variability in the decline in liver function with age, possibly due to the many factors that affect liver function (such as nutritional status, genetics, disease states, concurrent drug use and environmental factors such as smoking). There is generally a decrease in liver blood flow and mass with age, and a reduction in function of some hepatic enzyme systems. In general, drugs metabolised by oxidative (phase I) pathways by mixed-function oxidase enzymes are most affected. The rate of clearance of drugs metabolised by these systems may be decreased by 20–40% with ageing. The clearance of drugs metabolised solely by conjugation (phase II) pathways is typically unaffected (Table 16.2). Drugs that are not dependent on the mixed-function oxidase system for removal from the body should be used preferentially in elderly patients (see *Case Study 2*).

Absorption and first-pass metabolism: A number of physiological changes occur within the gastrointestinal (GI) tract with ageing, but clinically significant alterations in drug absorption are uncommon. The rate of absorption may be reduced but, with a few exceptions, the extent of absorption is usually unchanged (Table 16.2).

First-pass metabolism (pre-systemic metabolism after oral absorption) may be decreased, primarily due to a reduction in liver blood flow rate, and to a lesser extent due to the reduced intrinsic metabolic capacity of the liver. This results in increased bioavailability of some drugs after oral administration, particularly those that have high first-pass extraction (Table 16.2).

Drug distribution: Body composition changes with ageing. Lean body mass and total body water decrease, and fat mass increases as a proportion of total body weight. This affects the disposition of drugs in different ways (Table 16.2). The most important effect is that lipid-soluble drugs are taken up into the tissues to a greater extent, and therefore have increased volume of distribution and prolonged duration of action.

Levels of plasma albumin (the main plasma protein) may decline with age, and therefore protein binding of highly bound drugs tends to be reduced (Table 16.2). In contrast to albumin, alpha1-glycoprotein, which primarily binds basic drugs (such as propranolol) may be increased so that binding of highly bound drugs tends to be increased. However, the clinical significance of altered protein binding is usually minimal because compensatory changes in volume of distribution and/or drug clearance prevent the unbound (active) drug concentration from changing significantly. It does become important, however, when interpreting measured serum drug levels for highly protein-bound drugs (like phenytoin), because measured levels are usually *total* concentrations (*bound* plus *unbound*); so the altered proportion of unbound drug needs to be considered.

Pharmacodynamic Changes with Ageing

Pharmacodynamic changes (altered responsiveness to a given serum drug level) may be due to alterations in receptor and/

or tissue responsiveness, or changes in homeostatic responses.

Altered receptor or tissue sensitivity: The central nervous system (CNS) is particularly vulnerable to alterations in drug response. For example, adverse effects of benzodiazepines occur at lower drug concentrations in the elderly than in young patients. The ageing brain loses a significant number of active cells, and some brain atrophy is common.

There is also reduction in cerebral blood flow, and a selective decline in some nerve pathways. For example, the number of cholinergic neurons in some parts of the brain decreases with age. Loss of large numbers of cholinergic neurons results in memory loss, confusion and other cognitive impairments. Elderly patients are, therefore, more sensitive to the effects of drugs with anti-cholinergic properties, since these exacerbate the cholinergic deficit (see *Case Study* 3).

Monoamine oxidase activity increases with normal ageing, resulting in a decline in noroadrenaline and dopamine levels in the brain. The decline in dopamine is associated with increased sensitivity to dopamine blocking agents (for example, anti-psychotic drugs). Increased sensitivity to drug effects in the CNS may be displayed as excessive sedation, confusion or behavioural disturbances (such as agitation and aggression), which can easily be misdiagnosed as dementia or psychosis.

Iatrogenic confusion and behavioural disturbances are relatively common in older adults. In one study, 11% of patients above 65 years experienced cognitive impairment as a result of an ADR, and the risk increased nine-fold when patients were taking four or more medications.

The elderly also exhibit increased sensitivity to the effects of warfarin, and may require doses 30–40% lower than that given to younger patients. This may be due to a combination of pharmacokinetic and pharmcodynamic changes – increased pharmacodynamic sensitivity may be due to an age-related decline in the hepatic synthesis of the vitamin K–dependent clotting factors.

Altered homeostasis: The adverse effects of medications in the elderly often result from impaired secondary compensatory mechanisms (homeostasis). For example, postural hypotension is common in older patients and results from impaired baroreceptor function, reduced compensatory tachycardia and vasoconstriction in response to hypotension, and failure of cerebral blood flow autoregulation.

Postural hypotension is often aggravated by drugs with sympatholytic activity (like alpha receptor blockers, phenothiazines), volume depleting drugs (like diuretics) and vasodilating agents (such as nitrates). Patients with impaired cardiac output who are on diuretics are especially vulnerable (see *Case Study 2*).

Ageing impairs balance and posture maintenance, and some drugs (such as benzodiazepines) may adversely affect balance and contribute to falls. The homeostatic and autonomic mechanisms involved in renal function, blood glucose control and bladder function may also be impaired in old age and be associated with greater sensitivity to drug effects. The efficiency of thermoregulation may be reduced in old age and the consumption of drugs such as phenothiazines or alcohol may result in hypo or hyperthermia.

Appropriate Prescribing for the Elderly

Appropriate prescribing for the elderly requires a balanced and cautious approach. Polypharmacy should be avoided where possible; however, under-prescribing of essential drugs should also be avoided.

A drug should only be prescribed when there is good evidence to support its use (that is, it has been proven to reduce morbidity or mortality associated with the condition being treated). Drugs should be avoided when the risks associated with their use in an elderly patient outweigh the potential benefits.

Dose selection and adjustment is important. A good general rule is to 'start low and go slow', especially when using drugs to which the elderly are known to be more sensitive (Tables 16.2 and 16.3). For example, a general guideline for CNS-active drugs is to start with one-third to one-half of the usual starting dose for younger patients and slowly titrate the dose against the clinical response. Where possible, dose selection and adjustment should be guided not just by age, but also by knowledge of the patient's weight, renal function, hepatic function and other medications.

Principles of appropriate prescribing for elderly patients are summarised in Table 16.4.

Role of the Clinical Pharmacist in Geriatrics

The overall goal of the clinical pharmacist in geriatrics, as in other medical disciplines, is to promote the rational and safe use of drugs. When dealing with the elderly, however, extra attention needs to be paid to dose adjustment, minimising unnecessary polypharmacy, identifying and preventing ADRs and enhancing compliance. The clinical pharmacist needs to have an understanding of the common health problems affecting the elderly (Table 16.1), and also be aware of drugs that need to be used with extra caution in older people (Table 16.3). An appreciation of the fact that disease and ADR presentation may be altered in the elderly is also important. Roles for the clinical pharmacist in geriatrics are summarised in Table 16.5.

In recognition of the specialised knowledge needed by pharmacists working with elderly patients, the Commission for Certification in Geriatric Pharmacy (www.ccgp.org) was established in the USA. It provides a competency-based examination that can be taken by pharmacists in any country who wish to have their geriatric pharmacy expertise recognised by obtaining the 'Certified Geriatric Pharmacist' (CGP) credential.

Communicating with the Elderly Patient

Effective communication with older patients can be challenging due to additional communication barriers that may not exist in younger patients. Common barriers include impaired hearing, vision and cognition. Polypharmacy also makes communication more challenging because of the increased volume and complexity of information that needs to be delivered, understood and remembered. Illiteracy may also complicate the communication process.

Most of these problems can be overcome with some forethought and planning. Hearing impairment may be overcome by talking more loudly and/or moving closer to the patient. In the hospital setting, it is

Table 16.3 Drugs that need to be used with caution in the elderly because of increased risk of toxicity

Drug	Significant Adverse Effects	Special Consideration
ANALGESICS		
Non-steroidal anti-inflammatory drugs (NSAIDs), including COX-2 inhibitors	GI ulceration and bleeding, renal impairment, fluid retention, hypertension and confusion	Try paracetamol first. Monitor renal function, cardiac status, blood pressure. Avoid indomethacin and phenylbutazone because of increased incidence of adverse effects (CNS and haematological, respectively).
Opioid analgesics	Sedation, respiratory depression, constipation, hypotension, confusion	Start with lower doses and increase gradually. Monitor for adverse effects. Prevent constipation with dietary measures and/or laxatives.
Propoxyphene (dextropropoxyphene)	Confusion, dizziness, cardiotoxicity, dependence	Not recommended because of long half-life and dependence potential, and because efficacy is not significantly better than paracetamol.
ANTIBIOTICS		
Aminoglycosides (for example, gentamicin)	Renal impairment, hearing loss	Use lower doses. Avoid in the presence of significant renal impairment unless TDM available.
Flucloxacillin	Increased risk of hepatitis in people >55 years	Use alternative antibiotic if possible. Dicloxacillin is also associated with increased hepatitis risk in older people, but may be safer than flucloxacillin.
Nitrofurantoin	Peripheral neuropathy (more common in renal impairment), pulmonary fibrosis, and hepatitis with long-term use	Not recommended in the elderly, especially those with moderate-to-severe renal impairment. Monitor renal, liver and respiratory function during long-term use.
Sulphamethoxasole-Trimethoprim (cotrimoxazole)	Serious hypersensitivity reactions (Stevens–Johnson syndrome, blood dyscrasias)	Trimethoprim alone is equally effective (and safer) for most urinary tract infections.
ANTI-DIABETIC AGENTS		
Long-acting oral sulphonylureas (chlorpropamide, glibenclamide, glimepiride)	Increased risk of hypoglycaemia. Risk of SIADH with chlorpropamide	Shorter-acting agents are preferred (for example, gliclazide, glipizide). Chlorpropamide should never be used because of its very long half-life.
Phenformin, Metformin	Lactic acidosis (especially in the presence of renal impairment, hepatic impairment or heart disease) (may be fatal)	Metformin is the preferred agent (lower incidence of lactic acidosis). Reduce dose in renal impairment. Avoid in severe renal failure (creatinine clearance < 30 ml/min).
ANTI-GOUT AGENTS		
Allopurinol	Rash, renal failure	Reduce dose to 100–200 mg per day
Colchicine	Diarrhoea, dehydration	Not recommended for chronic therapy

Drug	Significant Adverse Effects	Special Consideration
ANTI-PARKINSONIAN AGENTS		
Amantadine	Confusion, peripheral oedema, rash	Not recommended. If given, use low dose.
Anti-cholinergics (benztropine, trihexyphenidyl)	Confusion, urinary retention, postural hypotension	Generally not recommended – sometimes useful if tremor refractory to other treatment
Levodopa	Confusion, hallucinations, postural hypotension, nausea, involuntary movements	Use lowest effective dose
Dopamine agonists (for example, bromocriptine, cabergoline, pergolide)	As for levodopa, especially confusion and nausea	
CARDIOVASCULAR DRUGS		
ACE inhibitors	Hyperkalaemia, renal impairment, hypotension, cough	Start with small doses and increase gradually to target dose. Monitor blood pressure, renal function and potassium level.
Amiodarone	Hyper or hypothyroidism, taste disturbance, headache, dizziness, fatigue, neurotoxicity (tremor, ataxia, paraesthesia, peripheral neuropathy, limb weakness), sleep disturbances. GI adverse effects (nausea, vomiting, constipation) more frequent in the elderly usually dose-related	Use with caution and close monitoring for toxicity. Use lower doses. Adverse effects are slow to resolve after drug is stopped due to very long half-life.
Beta-blockers	Depression, lethargy, bronchospasm, bradycardia, hypotension, exacerbation of peripheral vascular disease, insomnia, vivid dreams	Avoid in reversible airways disease and peripheral vascular disease. Propranolol and timolol not recommended because of higher incidence of adverse effects.
Digoxin	Confusion, bradycardia, arrhythmias, nausea	Use lower doses. Avoid hypokalaemia. Not first-line therapy for heart failure (ACE inhibitor preferred). Monitor serum levels if available.
Disopyramide	Strong anti-muscarinic and negative inotropic effects	Use other anti-arrhythmic agents if possible. Use reduced dose.
Methyldopa	Depression, postural hypotension, bradycardia	Not recommended - safer agents available.
Nitrates and nicorandil	Postural hypotension, dizziness, headache	Start with lower doses. Monitor BP.
Pentoxifylline	Hypotension, dizziness, flushing. May potentiate the effects of anti-hypertensives.	Limited efficacy in peripheral vascular disease. Doubtful efficacy in cerebrovascular disease. Monitor BP.
Prazosin	Stress incontinence, postural hypotension	Not recommended – safer agents available
Reserpine	Depression, sedation, postural hypotension	Not recommended – safer agents available
Verapamil	Constipation, bradycardia, dizziness, heart failure	Avoid in heart failure. Monitor for constipation.

Drug	*Significant Adverse Effects*	*Special Consideration*
DIURETICS		
Loop and thiazide (for example, frusemide, hydrochlorothiazide)	Dehydration, hypotension, hyponatraemia, hypokalaemia, hyperglycaemia, hyperuricaemia, incontinence, confusion	Use lowest dose possible. Monitor electrolytes and glucose.
Potassium-sparing (for example, amiloride)	Hyperkalaemia (especially if used in conjunction with an ACE inhibitor)	Monitor potassium
PSYCHOTROPIC AGENTS		
Barbiturates (for example, phenobarbitone, primidone)	Sedation, confusion, osteoporosis, dependence	Generally not recommended because of long half-life and toxicity. Safer agents available for insomnia and epilepsy.
Benzodiazepines (for example, diazepam, oxazepam, temazepam, nitrazepam)	Confusion, drowsiness, memory impairment, falls, dependence	Use for short periods only (up to 2 weeks) or use intermittently. Try non-drug measures for insomnia and anxiety. Avoid long half-life agents (diazepam, flunitrazepam, chlordiazepoxide, nitrazepam).
Butyrophenones (for example, haloperidol)	Confusion, drowsiness, extrapyramidal effects, tardive dyskinesia, akathisia. May increase risk of stroke and death.	Ensure appropriate indication for treatment exists. Use lowest effective dose. Avoid long-term use if possible.
Phenothiazines (for example, chlorpromazine, thioridazine, prochlorperazine)	Confusion, drowsiness, anti-cholinergic effects, extrapyramidal effects, tardive dyskinesia, akathisia. May increase risk of stroke and death.	As above
Atypical anti-psychotics (for example, risperidone, olanzapine, quetiapine)	Drowsiness, weight gain, anti-cholinergic effects, impaired glucose tolerance (especially olanzapine). Postural hypotension and extrapyramidal effects at higher doses (especially risperidone). May increase risk of stroke and death.	Generally preferred over typical anti-psychotics (phenothiazines and butyrophenones). Use lowest effective dose. Avoid long-term use if possible.
Tricyclic anti-depressants (for example, amitriptyline, imipramine, doxepin, dothiepin)	Anti-cholinergic effects, hypotension, falls	Start with low dose and gradually increase. Give as a single night-time dose. Selective serotonin reuptake inhibitors (SSRI) are generally preferred because they are better tolerated, but they are more expensive.
MISCELLANEOUS		
Anti-histamines (for example, diphenhydramine, chlorpheniramine, promethazine)	Anti-cholinergic effects (blurred vision, urinary retention, constipation, confusion), sedation	Use smallest dose and shortest duration possible.
Anti-spasmodics (for example, dicyclomine, propantheline, belladonna alkaloids)	Anti-cholinergic effects (as above), sedation	Risk of side effects often outweighs minimal benefits. Avoid long-term use.
Cimetidine	Confusion, gynaecomastia, significant drug interactions	Other histamine-2 receptor blockers preferred (for example, ranitidine).

Drug	Significant Adverse Effects	Special Consideration
Corticosteroids (systemic)	Hyperglycaemia, osteoporosis, peptic ulceration, depression, skin atrophy, slowed wound healing, confusion	Use smallest dose and shortest duration possible. Prefer inhaled steroid for airways disease
Theophylline	Confusion, nausea, arrhythmias	Low therapeutic index, increased risk of toxicity due to altered pharmacokinetics and reduced clearance in heart failure. Generally not considered first-line therapy – inhaled beta-agonists and inhaled corticosteroids preferred.
Warfarin	Increased anti-coagulant response and risk of bleeding. Drug interactions.	Start with lower dose. Monitor INR regularly. Avoid concurrent drugs which significantly interact with warfarin.

COX-2: Cyclo-oxygenase-2; INR: International normalised ratio; NSAID = Non-steroidal anti-inflammatory drug; SIADH: Syndrome of inappropriate anti-diuretic hormone; TDM = Therapeutic drug monitoring

best not to talk to the patient from the end of the bed, especially in a shared ward where there is likely to be a lot of background noise. Instead, move closer and preferably sit down next to the patient. Facing the patient and projecting the voice towards the patient is also important.

Visual impairment may be overcome by ensuring that written information is presented in large writing. Colour-coding of medication packaging may also be helpful if the patient cannot read the name on the package.

Cognitive impairment may make it necessary to spend more time with the patient to elicit a medication history or to provide medication counselling. Information presented to the patient will need to be kept simple and it may be necessary to go through the information more slowly. Memory impairment may be overcome by going through the information on more than one occasion, and providing written information to prompt the patient's memory. A written medication list, which outlines the name, strength, dose and duration of each medication is helpful, especially if the patient is on multiple medications.

Since elderly patients are more likely to be dependent on others to help them with their medications, it is often necessary to involve other people in the communication process. The patient's carer (often a family member) may be able to provide a more complete medication history, and may need to receive medication counselling if they will be assisting with medication administration.

Common Problems in the Elderly and the Role of the Clinical Pharmacist

Osteoarthritis: Osteoarthritis, a disease of weight-bearing joints (especially the knees, hips, feet, ankles and lower back), is one of the most common health problems affecting the elderly (prevalence approximately 60%). Pain secondary to osteoarthritis can have a significant impact on a patient's function and quality of life. However, it is often under-diagnosed and under-treated, partly because older patients tend to under-report pain.

The clinical pharmacist can help guide prescribers in the selection of appropriate

Table 16.4 Prescribing principles for elderly patients

Consider whether drug therapy is indicated
• Clearly define the disease to be treated; do not just treat symptoms.
• Put the problem in context. Is it affecting the patient's quality of life or causing functional decline? Is there evidence that drug therapy will reduce the symptoms or mortality?
• Consider non-drug alternatives (like physical therapy, counselling, relaxation techniques) for symptoms such as chronic pain, insomnia, anxiety.
• Avoid prescribing drugs to treat the adverse effects of other drugs. A new symptom following the recent introduction of any medication should be suspected as being due to that medication (be aware of atypical presentations of ADRs in the elderly).
• Avoid under-treating diseases for which there is strong evidence for the benefits of drug therapy (atrial fibrillation, heart failure, osteoporosis).
Select drug, dosage and duration
• Where possible, avoid (or use with extra care) drugs that commonly cause problems in the elderly (refer to Table 16.3).
• Modify drug doses to allow for age-related physiological changes and pathological processes (such as renal impairment). A good general rule is to 'start low and go slow' – adjust doses according to the patient's response.
• Keep the drug regimen as simple as possible by minimising the number of drugs prescribed and minimising dose frequency.
• Where possible, predetermine the duration of treatment and communicate this to the patient.
Monitor drug therapy
• Carefully monitor for adverse reactions, including atypical ones such as confusion and postural hypotension.
• Regularly review the patient's medications, and stop those that are no longer required.
• Regularly review the patient's compliance to therapy.

drugs and non-drug therapy. Analgesics and non-steroidal anti-inflammatory drugs (NSAIDs) can help control pain and disability, but should not be the first-line of therapy.

Non-pharmacological strategies can reduce pain and increase function, and may slow disease progression. These include exercise (to increase and maintain strength and flexibility), massage, hot or cold packs, weight reduction if obese, and functional aids (such as a walking stick). If drug therapy is required, a trial of paracetamol should be recommended before moving on to more expensive and potentially toxic agents such as NSAIDs (see *Case Study 2*).

Immobility and falls: Over 50% of patients over the age of 75 years have impaired mobility, and around 20% are house-bound because of it. Causes include:

- Pain and stiffness in the joints, muscles, and bones (for example, arthritis, gout, polymyalgia rheumatica, Paget's disease)
- Weakness (for example, peripheral neuropathy, myopathy, hypokalaemia, anaemia, dyspnoea, disuse)

Table 16.5 Roles of the clinical pharmacist in geriatrics

Roles
• Inform medical and nursing staff of the potential hazards of polypharmacy, altered pharmacokinetics and pharmacodynamics, and poor compliance.
• Recommend avoidance of (or extra caution with) drugs that have a high risk of problems in the elderly (Table 16.3).
• Ensure doses are adjusted to account for age-related pharmacokinetic and pharmacodynamic changes and pathological processes (such as renal impairment).
• Identify adverse drug reactions, including atypical reactions.
• Educate patients about their medications, and involve their family so that they are able to assist with managing the medications and enhancing compliance.
• Minimise unnecessary polypharmacy by regularly reviewing patients' chronic medications:
– Ensure there is an indication for each medication (recommend ceasing unnecessary drugs)
– Ensure there is no significant contraindication to any prescribed medication (suggest safer alternatives)
– Identify ADRs (which may have gone undetected and/or have resulted in the addition of another medication)
– Simplify complex dosing regimens (change from multiple daily to once- or twice-daily dosing where possible)
– Simplify the drug regimen by replacing multiple drugs with one drug where possible (see *Case Study 2*)
• Recommend strategies to prevent complications of hospitalisation, for example:
– Avoid sudden withdrawal of sedating medications (like benzodiazepines) on admission
– Recommend low-dose unfractionated heparin (or low molecular weight heparin) for deep vein thrombosis prophylaxis if the patient is unable to mobilise or has had major orthopaedic or abdominal surgery
– Recommend the short-term use of laxatives in immobile patients, especially if they are on opioid analgesics

- Orthopaedic handicaps (for example, previous road accident trauma)
- Foot disorders (such as painful corns and calluses, severe ischaemia, infection)
- Psychological causes (for example, anxiety and fear of falling, especially following previous falls)
- Psychiatric causes (such as depression and apathy, dementia)
- Neurological causes (such as Parkinson's disease, poliomyelitis, hemiplegia secondary to stroke)
- Drug-related causes (such as sedation, dizziness, falls, extrapyramidal effects, myopathy; Table 16.6)

The complications of impaired mobility can be serious, and therefore potentially reversible causes should be identified and treated. Physical complications may include muscle wasting, osteoporosis, pressure sores, constipation, incontinence, deep vein thrombosis (DVT) and falls. Psychological complications may also occur, including loss of confidence and depression or anxiety (due to loss of independence, social isolation and fear of falling).

Falls in old age are common and can cause significant injury (fractures, bruising, head injuries) and disability. Principal causes of recurrent falls include:

- Age-related changes (such as increased postural sway, impaired compensatory mechanisms)
- Impaired sensory input (for example, visual and hearing impairment, vertigo, dizziness, peripheral neuropathy)
- Joint and muscle disorders (such as arthritis, myopathy)
- Neurological impairment (such as Parkinson's disease, hemiplegia)
- Epilepsy
- Decreased cerebral perfusion (for example, hypotension, low cardiac output, dehydration, transient ischaemic attacks)
- Environmental effects (such as sub-standard accommodation, environmental hazards such as objects on the floor or poor lighting, unfamiliar environments such as hospitals)
- Drug effects (such as sedation, postural hypotension, cardiac arrhythmias; Table 16.6)

Table 16.6 Drugs which are known to affect mobility and/or increase the risk of falls

Drug Effect	***Examples of Drugs***
Postural hypotension, dizziness	Anti-depressants Anti-psychotics Anti-Parkinsonian agents Anti-hypertensives Benzodiazepines Diuretics Nitrates
Impaired balance and postural control	Benzodiazepines
Extrapyramidal effects (dopamine antagonism)	Anti-psychotics Prochlorperazine
Vestibular system effects/Eighth cranial nerve damage	Aminoglycosides Loop diuretics Aspirin (high dose)
Muscle weakness or pain (muscle wasting, myopathy)	Corticosteroids HMG CoA reductase inhibitors (for example, simvastatin)
Blurred vision	Drugs with anti-cholinergic effects NSAIDs Eye ointments (transient effect) Pilocarpine eye drops

The clinical pharmacist should be alert for instances where a patient's medications may be contributing to poor mobility or falls (see *Case Study 2*), and should recommend alternative safer medications in these situations.

Fractures and osteoporosis: Fractures are a common cause of disability in the elderly, and are usually due to bone disease (such as osteoporosis) and/or falls. Common sites of fracture are the thoracic and lumbar spine (vertebral crush fractures), forearm or wrist (usually due to reflex extension of the arm during a fall) and neck of femur (hip).

Around one in four elderly patients who suffer an injurious fall die within one year of their injury. Fracture of the hip is a serious injury and is associated with significant morbidity and mortality. It may result in a prolonged period of hospitalisation, immobility and secondary complications such as pressure sores, DVT and infections.

Osteoporosis, a disease characterised by decreased bone density, increases the risk of fracture. The prevalence of osteoporosis increases with age, and is more common in women than in men. There is gradual and progressive loss of bone after the age of 35 years, normally at a rate of 0.2% of total bone mass per year, increasing to 1% per year in postmenopausal women (due to decreased oestrogen production). By the age of 80 years, women will have lost about 30% of their original bone mass, and men 10%.

Additional factors contributing to reduced bone mineral density and osteoporosis include:

- Calcium or vitamin D deficiency
- Inactivity/Immobilisation
- Chronic use of systemic corticosteroids
- Excess glucocorticoid production
- Oestrogen or androgen deficiency
- Smoking
- Alcohol excess
- Hyperthyroidism
- Renal failure

The clinical pharmacist should be able to provide advice to doctors and patients about the prevention and treatment of osteoporosis. Prevention strategies include regular weight-bearing exercise, maintenance of adequate calcium intake and regular exposure to sunlight (15–30 minutes/day) to increase vitamin D production in the skin. Drug treatment is recommended following a low-trauma fracture (for example, fracture following a fall from standing height or less) or non-traumatic vertebral fracture, when bone mineral density is low (T-score < –2.5), and in patients on long-term oral corticosteroids.

Confusion, delirium and dementia: The term 'confusion' refers to a disturbance of higher mental function. There are four syndromes associated with confusion: delirium, dementia, focal neurological syndromes (for example, stroke, transient ischaemic attack, Korsakoff's syndrome) and some psychiatric disorders (for example, depression, schizophrenia). Only the first two syndromes are discussed in this chapter.

Delirium occurs in 20–50% of all hospitalised elderly patients, and has a mortality rate in the order of 15–20%. Also referred to as 'acute brain syndrome', delirium is a reversible syndrome with rapid onset, occurring over a period of hours to days. It is characterised by impaired cognitive function in association with altered consciousness, awareness and attention. This is in contrast to dementia, which is of gradual onset, occurring over years, and characterised by irreversible cognitive impairment with normal consciousness. The prevalence of dementia increases exponentially with age, affecting about 2% of people aged between 65 and 75 years, rising to more than 20% of those aged over 80 years.

There is almost always an identifiable (potentially reversible) underlying cause for delirium (such as infection, fluid or electrolyte disturbance, urinary retention, faecal impaction, pain, stroke, myocardial infarction, renal failure, alcohol withdrawal or medications). Often there is more than one contributing factor. Medications are implicated in 20–40% of cases, with anti-cholinergic and sedative drugs being the most frequent offenders. Polypharmacy is also a strong risk factor. Abrupt withdrawal of chronic sedative or anxiolytic drugs may also trigger delirium.

The major causes of dementia are Alzheimer's disease (70%) and vascular ('multi-infarct') dementia (20%). Other common forms of dementia include Lewy body dementia, dementia associated with Parkinson's disease and alcohol-related dementia. Less common causes include cerebral neoplasm, neuro-syphilis, AIDS, hypothyroidism, vitamin B_{12} deficiency, hydrocephalus and subdural haematoma. Patients with dementia are at increased risk of developing delirium, often triggered by seemingly trivial insults (such as urinary tract infection).

Since confusion is common in the elderly, clinical pharmacists need to be aware of drugs that may precipitate or exacerbate confusion (Table 16.3, *Case Study* 3). Pharmacists should ensure that such drugs are only used when an appropriate indication exists and no suitable alternatives are available, and that doses are minimised.

Symptomatic treatment is sometimes required for behavioural disturbances (agitation, aggression) associated with delirium and dementia, and the clinical pharmacist can help guide appropriate drug selection. Drug therapy should only be used where environmental and behavioural strategies, such as correction of sensory impairment (sight and hearing) and removal of trigger factors (pain, infection, medication, excessive stimulation) have failed. Anti-psychotic drugs (such as haloperidol, risperidone) are the first choice, although their efficacy is modest and they may themselves worsen cognitive function (see *Case Study* 3).

Adverse effects are common (for example, Parkinsonism with butyrophenones; sedation, anti-cholinergic effects and postural hypotension with phenothiazines). There is emerging evidence that anti-psychotics are associated with increased risk of stroke and death, so treatment should be limited to the lowest dose and shortest duration possible. Other drugs for disturbed behaviour have not been subjected to well-designed controlled trials and should be considered second-line therapy. These include benzodiazepines, beta-adrenergic antagonists and anti-convulsants. They are all associated with significant side effects in the elderly such as sedation, worsening of cognitive function and falls.

Anaemia: Anaemia is common in the elderly, but it does not occur as a natural consequence of ageing. A pathological or nutritional cause is always responsible, and should be sought. Anaemia may aggravate underlying ischaemic heart disease or heart failure because of the decreased oxygen-carrying capacity of the blood. The commonest types of anaemia in elderly people are iron-deficiency anaemia, anaemia of chronic disease and megaloblastic anaemia. Multiple causes of anaemia may co-exist in one patient.

Iron-deficiency anaemia: This may be caused by poor dietary intake of iron or chronic blood loss (commonly from the gastrointestinal tract or, less often, the genitourinary tract or elsewhere). Defective absorption may be a contributory factor if chronic gastritis, gastrectomy or small bowel disease is present. Pure nutritional deficiency of iron is uncommon in well-nourished persons, so unless there is reason to suspect nutritional deficit, a source of blood loss should be investigated. The clinical pharmacist should be alert to possible drug-related causes of blood loss, such as NSAIDs or warfarin. NSAIDs (including low-dose aspirin) should be stopped if gastrointestinal bleeding is suspected or proven.

Treatment of iron-deficiency anaemia generally requires only oral iron replacement in addition to the treatment of any underlying lesion. Selection of an appropriate iron supplement is important because many multivitamin preparations and tonics do not contain sufficient amounts of elemental iron. The dose of elemental iron required is 2–3 mg/kg/day (about 120–200 mg) initially, reduced to about 65–100 mg/day once the haemoglobin level has started to rise (see *Case Study 2*).

Anaemia of chronic disease: This type of anaemia is caused by chronic diseases including infections, inflammatory disorders (such as rheumatoid arthritis) and cancers. It often co-exists with other types of anaemia. The anaemia is usually mild and there is no specific therapy other than treatment of the underlying disease.

Megaloblastic anaemia: This is caused by the deficiency of vitamin B_{12} or folic acid. This type is less common, but if untreated can cause irreversible neurologic damage.

Folate deficiency is more common than vitamin B_{12} deficiency and is usually due to poor diet with or without malabsorption. Other factors are increased demand (infection, cancer, haemolysis), anti-convulsants (phenytoin, carbamazepine) and chronic alcoholism. Treatment requires correction of the underlying cause plus oral folate supplementation. Folate should not be given until vitamin B_{12} deficiency has been excluded, because doing so may mask pernicious anaemia while allowing neurologic damage to progress.

Vitamin B_{12} deficiency is usually caused by pernicious anaemia (an autoimmune disease that results in gastric atrophy and failure of intrinsic factor secretion). Other causes are gastrectomy, some bowel disorders and nutritional deficiency (especially in vegans and vegetarians). Oral vitamin B_{12} is ineffective in pernicious anaemia and regular intramuscular injections are required.

Urinary incontinence: Urinary incontinence is the involuntary or inappropriate loss of urine. It is an unpleasant, distressing and embarrassing condition which affects 10–15% of older people. Causes of incontinence in the elderly are summarised in Table 16.7.

Clinical pharmacists need to be aware of the many drugs that can cause or exacerbate urinary incontinence (Table 16.7), and should understand the limited role that drug therapy plays in its treatment. Before introducing a drug to treat incontinence,

Table 16.7 Causes of urinary incontinence in older people

Primary causes:

Urinary tract infection

Pelvic floor muscle weakness

Outflow obstruction (such as prostatic hyperplasia, urethral stricture)

Atrophic vaginitis or urethritis secondary to oestrogen deficiency

Detrusor instability (unstable bladder)

Impaired bladder contractility

Secondary causes:

Polyuria (for example, diabetes, diuretic therapy)

Impaired mobility (for example, arthritis, Parkinson's disease, stroke)

Constipation and faecal impaction (as a result of pressure on the bladder exerted by faecal mass)

Neurological causes (for example, stroke, neuropathy)

Psychiatric causes (for example, delirium, dementia, depression)

Drugs:

Class	***Examples***	***Mechanism***
Analgesics	Codeine, morphine	Constipation
Antacids	Aluminium hydroxide	Constipation
Anti-cholinergics	Propantheline, disopyramide, anti-histamines, tricyclic anti-depressants	Inhibition of detrusor contractility (promotion of incomplete bladder emptying), confusion, constipation
Anti-hypertensives	Alpha adrenergic blockers (for example, prazosin, phenoxybenzamine, labetolol, doxazosin)	Urethral sphincter relaxation, decreased urethral pressure
	Verapamil	Constipation
Diuretics	Frusemide, thiazides	Increase bladder filling rate, urinary frequency
Sedatives	Benzodiazepines, anti-psychotics, anti-histamines	Clouded consciousness, reduced awareness of bladder sensation

all current drugs that might contribute to incontinence should be reviewed. Some drugs may be discontinued, reduced in dosage or exchanged for a drug less likely to cause incontinence.

Drug therapy is rarely effective in curing urinary incontinence, but may reduce the severity of symptoms in some patients with urge incontinence due to detrusor muscle instability. There is a high placebo response rate (30–40%). Anti-cholinergic drugs such as propantheline, imipramine and oxybutinin are sometimes useful; however, these can cause serious side effects in the elderly (Table 16.3) and should not be used as first-line therapy. Treatment of underlying causes should occur first (antibiotics for UTI, laxatives for constipation), and non-drug measures should be considered (for example, bladder retraining, pelvic muscle exercises, absorbent pads, catheters). Local oestrogen replacement (by oestrogen vaginal cream or pessaries) may be beneficial in women with atrophic changes.

Constipation and faecal incontinence: Constipation is a common complaint in the elderly. Colonic transit time increases with age, and is especially prolonged in immobile patients. Inadequate fluid intake is also a frequent contributor. Acute constipation is especially common in hospitalised patients. Some medications can cause or exacerbate constipation, including opiates, verapamil, iron, aluminium-containing antacids and drugs with anti-cholinergic activity (like the tricyclic anti-depressants, phenothiazine anti-psychotics, anti-spasmodics, some anti-Parkinsonian medications).

Severe constipation can result in faecal impaction which can then lead to faecal incontinence. This occurs because of the continued presence of a faecal mass in the rectum which causes reflex anal sphincter relaxation and irritation of the rectal mucosa, leading to mucus and fluid production and involuntary passage of usually liquid stools. Faecal incontinence affects about 15% of older hospitalised patients but is less common in the community.

Prevention of constipation in ambulatory patients can usually be achieved with adequate fluid and fibre intake and exercise. An oral laxative may be used prophylactically for short periods when constipation is likely to occur; for example, during periods of immobilisation or hospitalisation or when opioid analgesics are being used. In frail elderly patients, especially if fluid intake is poor, increasing the fibre intake is inappropriate and long-term use of a stimulant laxative may be required.

Management of acute constipation may require a short course of oral and/or rectal laxatives. In chronic constipation, the cause needs to be identified and treated (for example, poor diet, inadequate fluid intake, constipating drugs, obstructing lesions of the bowel). If there is faecal loading or impaction, manual disimpaction may be required, followed by enaemas and oral laxatives until the bowel is clear.

The clinical pharmacist needs to be aware of the drug and non-drug causes of constipation, and should have a good understanding of the role and adverse effects of the various types of laxatives (stimulant, bulking, softening and osmotic). Laxatives are commonly used inappropriately, and the pharmacist can play a role in improving their use by educating doctors, nurses and patients. Awareness that faecal incontinence and diarrhoea may be secondary to constipation is also important so that the inappropriate use of anti-diarrhoeal drugs is avoided.

Infections: Certain infections occur more frequently in the elderly, for example pneumonia and urinary tract infection (UTI). This is probably a result of factors such as impaired immunity, physiological changes (such as decreased cough reflex, incomplete bladder emptying, hormonal changes affecting mucous membranes in women) and predisposing illnesses (diabetes increases the risk of UTI, stroke may increase the risk of aspiration pneumonia because of impaired swallowing reflex).

Morbidity and mortality from infections is greater in the elderly, particularly if treatment is delayed. Although patients may sometimes present with typical symptoms, often the usual diagnostic features (such as fever) are absent. Onset of illness may be insidious, and the patient may present with delirium, drowsiness, dehydration, deterioration of pre-existing conditions (such as CCF, diabetes), incontinence (with UTIs) or unexplained change in functional capacity.

As well as appropriate antibiotic therapy, attention to supportive measures is critical because the risk of developing complications such as hypoxaemia, fluid and electrolyte disturbances and worsening of underlying conditions is greater.

The clinical pharmacist should be alert to the atypical symptoms of infection in the elderly, and play a role in recommending appropriate antibiotic and supportive therapy (see *Case Study 3*).

Complications of Hospitalisation

Hospitalisation of patients of any age can result in complications, but the elderly are at greatest risk. This is because of the combined effects of the ageing process, pre-existing chronic diseases and disabilities, and exposure to multiple drugs.

It is common, especially during the early phase of hospitalisation, for older patients to experience episodes of confusion and disturbed behaviour even in the absence of underlying dementia. This may be because of the underlying illness, exposure to (or rapid withdrawal of) drugs affecting mental function, or being in a foreign environment. Immobility during hospitalisation can lead to muscle wasting, joint stiffness, contractures, pressure sores, constipation and DVT. Hospital-acquired infections, especially pneumonia, are more common in the elderly. Adverse drug reactions are also common in the hospitalised elderly patient, and the clinical pharmacist has a major role in preventing and identifying these. Some strategies the clinical pharmacist can recommend to help prevent complications of hospitalisation are included in Table 16.5.

CASE STUDY 1

Mrs UP is a 73-year-old woman with a history of atrial fibrillation (AF) and type 2 diabetes mellitus. She presents to the hospital outpatient clinic with complaints of weight loss, headache and dizziness. Her son, who has accompanied her to the clinic, reports that she has recently had very poor appetite and episodes of confusion. Current medications include digoxin 250 mcg once a day six days per week, perindopril 5 mg daily aspirin 150 mg daily, and glibenclamide 5 mg bd.

On presentation, her weight is 50 kg, BP 140/80 and pulse 50 beats/min. A blood test is ordered, and the results are as follows:

Sodium 136 mmol/L (135–145)

Potassium 4.2 mmol/L (3.5–5.0)

Creatinine 96 micromol/L (30–110)

Haemoglobin 115 g/L (120–160)

Random blood glucose level (BGL) is 2.7 mmol/L (4.0–8.0)

Consider whether any of Mrs UP's symptoms could be drug-related.

Discussion

Decreased appetite, dizziness and bradycardia could be symptoms of digoxin toxicity. Digoxin is 50–70% eliminated by the kidneys and has a low therapeutic index. Although Mrs UP's serum creatinine is within the normal range, it can be a misleading indicator of renal function in older people, as outlined previously. An estimated creatinine clearance needs to be calculated using the Cockroft and Gault equation, which takes into account age and weight as well as serum creatinine:

$$\frac{(140 - \text{Age in years}) \times \text{Weight (kg)} \; (\times 0.85 \text{ for women})}{0.814 \times \text{Serum creatinine (micromol/L)}}$$

Mrs UP's estimated creatinine clearance is calculated to be 36 ml/minute, indicating mild to moderate renal impairment. Dosage reduction of digoxin is recommended when creatinine clearance is less than 50 ml/min. In this case, a 50% reduction, to 125 mcg, would be appropriate. Serum digoxin level, if available, could be measured to guide dosage adjustment, but it is possible to manage the patient without measuring this. Dose reduction can be based on creatinine clearance, combined with clinical observation to determine efficacy (in the case of AF, by monitoring pulse rate) and identify early signs of toxicity (for example, nausea, loss of appetite). The drug should be withheld for two or three days before commencing the new dose to enable the digoxin level to decrease. Patient counselling is also crucial to make the patient aware of the early signs of toxicity and the need to report these signs as soon as possible. Given that the patient is confused, and the son is present, including the son in the medication counselling would be useful.

Confusion, headaches and dizziness could be caused by hypoglycaemia. Glibenclamide is an oral hypoglycaemic agent with a relatively long duration of action (16–24 hours). It is not recommended for elderly patients, especially those with renal impairment, because of increased risk of hypoglycaemia. The likelihood of hypoglycaemia is further increased by the fact that Mrs UP has not been eating much lately. Hypoglycaemia is confirmed by her BGL measurement of 2.7. In this case, glibenclamide should be stopped and if the BGL rises again above acceptable levels, a shorter-acting, non-renally eliminated, oral hypoglycaemic agent should be substituted (like gliclazide or glipizide). Education regarding diet and signs of hypoglycaemia would be useful.

Outcome

Digoxin was withheld for three days, then recommenced at 125 mcg daily six days per week. Mrs UP's heart rate increased to 65 bpm, she felt less nauseous and her appetite improved. Glibenclamide was changed to gliclazide 80 mg mane, and she had no further hypoglycaemic episodes.

CASE STUDY 2

Mrs AN is a 69-year-old woman with a history of hypertension, heart failure, angina, osteoarthritis, iron-deficiency anaemia and anxiety. She is in hospital for the treatment of a fractured wrist following a fall. When questioned, she reports feeling light-headed when she stands up. She has daytime drowsiness and poor short-term memory. Current medications include frusemide 40 mg daily, potassium chloride 600 mg tds, digoxin 125 mcg daily, prazosin 5 mg tds, metoprolol 50 mg bd, diclofenac 50 mg bd, diazepam 5 mg bd, Globac® 10 ml daily, and aspirin 150 mg daily.

Her weight is 55 kg, BP 120/70 and pulse 70 beats/min. A blood test is ordered, and the results are as follows:

Sodium 132 mmol/l (135–145)

Potassium 4.5 mmol/l (3.5–5.0)

Creatinine 80 micromol/l (30–110)

Haemoglobin 105 g/l (120–160)

Mrs AN is taking nine medications. Consider whether this level of polypharmacy is appropriate by reviewing the indication for each agent. Could the number of medications be reduced? Also consider whether there are any potential drug-related problems.

Discussion

There is an indication for each of Mrs AN's medications (see the table on the next page), so at face value the medications seem reasonable. However, it may still be possible to reduce the number of medications. Mrs AN is taking digoxin and frusemide for heart failure, and she is not taking an ACE inhibitor. It may be possible to replace digoxin and/or frusemide (and potassium) with an ACE inhibitor. These drugs decrease morbidity and mortality in heart failure, and their inclusion may also help control Mrs AN's hypertension, enabling prazosin to be reduced or stopped. This could reduce the number of medications by up to three.

In any older patient who has had a fall, possible drug-related causes need to be considered, and in this case there are several medications that could be contributory. Mrs AN reports feeling dizzy upon standing, so postural hypotension should be considered. Her current BP is slightly low, but to find out whether she has postural hypotension, BP needs to be measured in both the lying and standing positions (standing BP should be taken at least 3 minutes after rising because BP may not drop immediately). Mrs AN's lying BP was 130/70, and 5 minutes after standing it decreased to 100/60, confirming the presence of postural hypotension. Prazosin (and other alpha adrenergic receptor antagonists) are a common cause of postural hypotension in elderly patients, and are best avoided. Frusemide and metoprolol could also be contributing to postural hypotension, so if the problem persists despite dose reduction or cessation of prazosin, these could also be reviewed.

Another possible cause of Mrs AN's dizziness, and also her drowsiness and memory impairment, could be the benzodiazepine. Diazepam is metabolised by oxidative pathways to active metabolites that are also eliminated by hepatic metabolism and have very long half-lives in older people (up to 220 hours). Because of its long duration of action, it is more likely to cause adverse effects compared with shorter-acting agents. Shorter-acting benzodiazepines (such as oxazepam, lorazepam and temazepam) primarily undergo conjugation, which is less affected by ageing, and are without active metabolites, meaning that accumulation and prolonged sedation is less likely. Long-term use of any benzodiazepine is best avoided, but if a benzodiazepine is indicated, diazepam could be gradually weaned (to avoid withdrawal), and oxazepam substituted.

Drug	***Indication***
Digoxin 125 mcg daily	**Heart failure**
Frusemide 40 mg daily	**Heart failure**
Potassium chloride 600 mg tds	**Hypokalaemia secondary to diuretic therapy**
Prazosin 5 mg tds	**Hypertension**
Metoprolol 50 mg bd	**Ischaemia heart disease (angina) and heart failure**
Diclofenac 50 mg bd	**Osteoarthritis**
Diazepam 5 mg bd	**Anxiety**
Globac® 10 ml daily	**Iron-deficiency anaemia**
Aspirin 150 mg daily	**Thromboprophylaxis for ischaemic heart disease**

Another potential problem with Mrs AN's medications is the NSAID diclofenac. NSAIDs are a common cause of adverse effects in the elderly, and should be avoided whenever possible. Adverse effects may include GI bleeding (and iron-deficiency anaemia), renal impairment, fluid retention and antagonism of the effects of diuretics and anti-hypertensives. Paracetamol is recommended as first-line drug therapy for osteoarthritis because it is safer and less expensive. Therefore, it would be worth recommending a trial of paracetamol (taken regularly, three to four times a day) instead of diclofenac.

Finally, Mrs AN's iron dose is very low (Globac® contains only about 18 mg elemental iron per 10 ml). If she is still iron-deficient, she would require a dose in the order of 60–150 mg per day. A product containing a greater amount of iron could be recommended (for example, Orofer® which has 100 mg elemental iron per capsule).

Outcome

Prazosin was stopped, and Mrs AN was started on ramipril 1.25 mg daily. This low dose was selected because patients on diuretics have increased risk of first-dose hypotension due to activation of the renin–angiotensin system. Her BP was monitored for a few days, and then the dose increased to 2.5 mg daily. The frusemide dose was decreased to 20 mg daily (and potassium to 600 mg bd). Digoxin was discontinued. The diazepam dose was decreased to 5 mg nocte, and naproxen changed to paracetamol 1 g tds. Globac® was changed to Orofer®. A few days later, Mrs AN was discharged from hospital.

Ten days after discharge, Mrs AN was reviewed in the outpatient clinic. Her CCF remained well-controlled, so the frusemide and potassium were stopped, and the ramipril dose increased to 5 mg daily (in CCF, the ACE inhibitor should be increased to the maximum tolerated dose, to achieve maximum long-term benefit). Since stopping prazosin, she reported feeling less dizzy, and her drop in systolic BP when standing was now only 15 mmHg. Her osteoarthritis pain was well controlled using paracetamol so this was continued. The diazepam dose was further reduced to 2.5 mg nocte, and then changed to oxazepam. She is now on six medications.

CASE STUDY 3

Mr SK is a 76-year-old man who presents to the emergency department with confusion, hallucinations and aggressive behaviour. He has a history of hypertension and tuberculosis, but no history of psychiatric illness or dementia. According to his wife, his aggressive behaviour is very out of character and has developed rapidly over the past few days.

Current medications listed in Mr SK's medical notes are propranolol 40 mg bd and Becosules® one capsule daily. Upon questioning his wife about recent medication use, you find out that he has recently had a non-specific gastric complaint and has been taking Spasmindon® tablets three times a day.

On presentation, Mr SK is afebrile, weighs 65 kg, has a BP of 140/80 and pulse of 75 beats/min. A blood test is ordered, and the results are as follows:

Sodium 140 mmol/l (135–145)

Potassium 4.3 mmol/l (3.5–5.0)

Creatinine 79 micromol/l (30–110)

Haemoglobin 125 g/l (140–180)

White cell count 13.8 (4–11)

A diagnosis of delirium (acute brain syndrome) is made, and Mr SK is started on chlorpromazine 50 mg bd to control his hallucinations and aggressive behaviour. Over the next 24 hours, there is little improvement in Mr SK's condition – he remains confused and disorientated, although he appears to be having fewer hallucinations and is quite sedated.

What could be the possible drug and non-drug causes of Mr SK's symptoms? Is chlorpromazine appropriate therapy for his symptoms?

Discussion

Delirium in older people may be precipitated by a range of drug and non-drug factors. Anti-cholinergic medications, such as dicyclomine (contained in Spasmindon®), are one of the more common drug-related causes of delirium, and this may be one explanation for Mr SK's symptoms. However, Mr SK has a raised white cell count, suggesting the possibility of infection. Although he is afebrile and has no specific symptoms suggestive of infection, it should be considered as a potential cause of his delirium. Infections may present without the classic signs and symptoms in older patients, and patients may present with deteriorating mental and/or physical function.

Management of delirium requires removal or treatment of precipitating factors; however, symptomatic treatment may also be required for psychiatric symptoms if these are a danger to the patient or to other people. For this indication, an anti-psychotic is usually given. Butyrophenones are generally preferred because they cause less anti-cholinergic side effects and postural hypotension compared with phenothiazines. Low doses should be utilised (for example, haloperidol 0.5–2.0 mg per day until symptoms resolve). The newer 'atypical' anti-psychotics (risperidone, olanzapine) appear to have similar efficacy to the older anti-psychotics, and offer the advantage of a lower incidence of Parkinsonian side effects; however, they are also more expensive.

Outcome

Urine examination, using a urinary reagent strip ('dipstick test') revealed the presence of leukocytes and nitrites in urine. This is indicative of urinary tract infection (UTI). Intravenous antibiotic therapy was commenced. Upon recommendation of the clinical pharmacist, chlorpromazine 50 mg bd was changed to haloperidol 0.5 mg bd and Spasmindon® was discontinued. These interventions were made to minimise the potential for adverse anti-cholinergic effects, which could be contributing to his ongoing delirium.

Three days later, Mr SK was less confused and aggressive. His white cell count was 9.6. The haloperidol dose was reduced to 0.25 mg bd, and the antibiotic was switched from intravenous to oral. After a week, Mr SK's mental function had returned to normal, so haloperidol was stopped, and he was discharged with three more days of oral antibiotics to complete the treatment for his UTI.

Exercise: Medication Review

If you have access to patients in a teaching hospital, identify three in-patients over the age of 65 years. For each patient, complete the following tasks:

- Take a detailed medication history from the patient and/or family member. Remember to ask about over-the-counter medications which the patient may be taking. (Only one student should interview each patient).
- Identify the indication for each drug by referring to the patient's medical history and by asking the patient if needed. Is the patient taking medications for which there is no apparent indication? Have any drugs been prescribed to treat the potential side effects of other drugs?
- Calculate the patient's estimated creatinine clearance using the Cockcroft–Gault equation. Check whether the dose of any renally cleared drugs is appropriate.
- Identify whether the patient is taking any drugs listed in Tables 16.3, 16.6 and 16.7. Are these medications causing adverse effects? If so, what recommendations would you make to address these?
- Does the patient have any medical conditions for which they are not receiving treatment? If so, can you identify any contraindications to treatment? Remember also to consider the overall context of the patient's medical condition.

KEY MESSAGES

- The prevalence of chronic disease increases with advancing age, and therefore elderly patients tend to use more medications than younger patients.
- The incidence of adverse drug reactions increases with advancing age.
- Polypharmacy (use of multiple medications) is an independent risk factor for adverse drug reactions and drug interactions.
- Physiological changes occur with increasing age and may result in altered pharmacokinetics and pharmacodynamics for many drugs.
- Some drugs are associated with greatly increased risk of adverse effects in the elderly and should be avoided or used with extra caution.
- Dose reduction is required for many drugs in the elderly.
- Poor compliance with medications is common in elderly patients.
- The clinical pharmacist can play an important role in promoting rational and safe medication use in elderly patients.

Further Reading

Aronow WS, Frishman WH and Cheng-Lai A. 2007. Cardiovascular drug therapy in the elderly. *Cardiology in Review* 15(4):195–215.

Hilmer SN, McLachlan AJ and Le Couteur DG. 2007. Clinical pharmacology in the geriatric patient. *Fundamental & Clinical Pharmacology* 21:217–30.

Hilmer SN. 2008. ADME-Tox issues for the elderly. *Expert Opin Drug Metab Toxicol* 4(10):1321–31.

George J, Elliott RA and Stewart DC. 2008. A systematic review of interventions to improve medication taking in elderly patients prescribed multiple medications. *Drugs & Aging* 25(4):307–24.

Kane RL, Ouslander JG, Abrass IB and Resnick B. 2008. *Essentials of clinical geriatrics*, 6th ed. New York: McGraw-Hill.

Mintzer J and Burns A. 2000. Anticholinergic side-effects of drugs in elderly people. *J Royal Soc Med* 93(Sep):457–62.

Nicholl C, Wilson J and Webster S. 2007. *Lecture notes: Elderly Care Medicine*, 7th ed. Blackwell Publishing: Oxford.

Woodward MC. 2003. Deprescribing: Achieving better health outcomes for older people through reducing medications. *J Pharm Pract Res* 33:323–8. Free full-text available at http://jppr.shpa.org.au/lib/pdf/gt/Dec2003.pdf

Websites of Interest

American Geriatrics Society

http://www.americangeriatrics.org

British Geriatrics Society

http://www.bgs.org.uk

Commission for Certification in Geriatric Pharmacy

http://www.ccgp.org

Geriatrics

http://www.geri.com/geriatrics

Journal of Pharmacy Practice and Research, Geriatric Therapeutics

http://jppr.shpa.org.au

Veterans' Medicines Advice and Therapeutics Education Services (Veterans' MATES)

https://www.veteransmates.net.au

17 MEDICATION USE IN PREGNANCY AND LACTATION

Katy E Trinkley and Milap C Nahata

Learning Objectives

Upon completion of this chapter, the reader should be able to:

- Understand the need for close monitoring of medication use during pregnancy and breastfeeding
- Describe the properties of medications that increase their likelihood of crossing the placenta or excretion into breast milk
- Identify limitations of the informational resources used to determine the risks of medication use in pregnancy and lactation
- Utilise published information to determine the risk of medication use during pregnancy and lactation
- Design and implement a therapeutic plan to treat pregnant and lactating women

Many pregnant and breastfeeding women may experience chronic and acute diseases, which often require treatment with medications. Studies involving the use of medications in pregnant and breastfeeding women are, however, limited, making it difficult to determine the risks of medication use in these populations. Often, decisions rely on less convincing evidence, such as animal studies or case reports. While some general guidelines and recommendations regarding the risks of medication use during pregnancy and lactation are available, all pregnant and breastfeeding women are advised to be cautious whenever they take a medication. Pharmacists, with expertise in pharmacology and therapeutics, can play a pivotal role in advising other clinicians and patients on the selection of medications and on the risks of medication use during pregnant and breastfeeding.

An important lesson was learned from a tragedy of birth defects associated with the use of thalidomide by pregnant women. In the 1950s, thalidomide was widely used in Europe by pregnant women as a sleep aid and to treat morning sickness. Some American women travelling to Europe also found relief with the use of thalidomide. Animal studies of thalidomide did not reveal any potential congenital harm; however, after a decade of use, scientists discovered the foetal toxicity of thalidomide. Thousands of congenital birth defects occurred, including shortened or absent limbs in the newborns of mothers who took thalidomide during pregnancy. This led the US Food and Drug Administration (FDA) to mandate that the manufacturers of new drugs prove both the safety and the efficacy of drugs for their labelled indication and in the intended population prior to approval. A consequence of this regulation is that few drugs are approved for safe use in pregnant women.

Pharmacokinetics/ Pharmacodynamics

When recommending a medication for use in pregnant or lactating women, it is important to know that most medications ingested have the potential to cross the placenta or be excreted into breast milk, and hence affect the foetus or newborn, respectively. The likelihood of crossing the placenta or being excreted into breast milk is influenced by the physiologic characteristics and physicochemical properties of the drug.

Agents of low molecular weight, high lipophilicity, that have low plasma protein binding and are non-ionised at physiologic pH are more likely to cross the placenta or be excreted into breast milk. Drugs with shorter half-lives are eliminated from maternal circulation faster, minimising the time of exposure for the foetus or newborn and thus decreasing the risk of harm.

The application of many of these principles is demonstrated with the use of warfarin during pregnancy. Commonly used to prevent thrombotic complications, warfarin is a known teratogen and is contraindicated for use during pregnancy. Although it is 99% bound to plasma proteins and ionised at physiologic pH, this is in equilibrium with thc 1% that is unbound and non-ionised at physiologic pH. Because of warfarin's long elimination half-life of approximately 40 hours, there is ample time for the unbound and non-ionised warfarin to cross the placenta, thus exposing the foetus to warfarin and its teratogenicity. Even after warfarin therapy is discontinued, its teratogenic potential continues to be a threat to the foetus until it is eliminated from maternal circulation.

If warfarin is not stopped far enough in advance of the time of conception to allow for its elimination from maternal circulation, the foetus is at risk. Therefore, it is important for pregnant women to avoid warfarin; in addition, all women of childbearing age should avoid becoming pregnant while taking warfarin and allow adequate time to elapse between discontinuation and conception to prevent congenital harm.

Weighing the Risks Against the Benefits

As with any medication, the benefit of use must outweigh the risk of use. In the case of pregnant or lactating women, there is the added complexity of weighing the benefit to the mother against the risk to the foetus or newborn. For example, it is well known that anti-depressants can pose some risk to the foetus or newborn, yet physicians still prescribe them to pregnant and breastfeeding women. This is because the significant and known risk of suicide in untreated, severely depressed, pregnant and breastfeeding women may potentially pose a greater risk to the foetus or newborn than anti-depressants.

Under-treating a medical condition due to concerns of exposing the foetus to potentially harmful medications can sometimes be more harmful to the foetus than the medications themselves, as is the case with diabetes. Hyperglycaemia associated with uncontrolled diabetes significantly complicates pregnancy, and can result in birth trauma, pre-eclampsia, miscarriage and long-term complications in infants including diabetes and cognitive deficits. Hence, it is especially important to adequately control glycaemia during pregnancy with appropriate management, including medication and lifestyle changes.

An important factor in treating pregnant or breastfeeding women is choosing the medication with the least risk to the foetus; this depends on many factors, including how extensively it has been studied and the quality of those studies. While manufacturers of newly approved medications are required to report on the potential risks of use during pregnancy and lactation, the safety statement may be limited to findings of case reports or animal studies. The latter are helpful in identifying potential risks to the foetus or nursing child, but are not indicative of how a drug will affect humans.

There are significant interspecies differences in the effects of drugs ingested, which was illustrated with the use of thalidomide. Although thalidomide was found to result in no harm to the offspring of pregnant and lactating animals, its use during human pregnancy resulted in significant harm to the foetuses. For ethical reasons, however, human safety studies in pregnant and lactating women are often not conducted and clinicians are sometimes forced to rely on case reports or animal studies to aid in the decision of a medication's risk of harm. Thus, medications which have safely been used in patients over extended durations should be preferred over newer medications with limited clinical data. This is because, over time, as more patients use a medication, the likelihood of uncovering adverse drug events increases, as does the possibility of identifying delayed adverse drug events, which are more common than those discovered at the time of birth.

At birth, the prevalence of birth defects is 2–3%, which increases to 5–6% at one year of age, when previously hidden defects are discovered. This was exemplified with the use of diethylstilbestrol (DES) in the late 1930s through 1971. DES was used during pregnancy to prevent miscarriage and other pregnancy complications. Although DES resulted in no apparent harm to the foetus at birth, it was later discovered that DES had harmed the foetus, but these effects were not apparent until the child reached puberty. After 30 years of use in pregnant women, it was realised that female foetuses exposed to DES are at a significantly increased risk of vaginal adenocarcinoma, infertility, miscarriage and preterm birth in their own pregnancy following puberty.

Estimating Risk during Pregnancy

After determining that a medication is safe and effective and that the benefits outweigh the risk, the primary safety concern is to the foetus. When determining the risks of medication use during pregnancy, many additional factors are considered, the foremost being the time of use in relation to the foetus's stage of development, the dose and duration of use, and the extent to which it crosses the placenta.

Nearly all medications cross the placenta to some degree; the amount that crosses is, however, the concern. As the pregnancy progresses, the foetus undergoes different stages of development, during which it is more or less vulnerable to certain medications. As such, it is important to realise that exposure of the foetus to certain medications at specific developmental time points can have drastically different effects. During approximately the 5th week of gestation, placental transport between the mother and foetus begins, allowing for potential transfer of medications from the mother to the placenta. Although there is a risk of congenital harm any time during pregnancy, generally, the first 12 weeks of gestation are considered the stage during which the foetus is most susceptible. This is the time when critical organs, including the heart, brain, spinal cord and limbs are developing.

Non-steroidal anti-inflammatory drugs (NSAIDs) are examples of medications where the safety profile changes depending on the stage of pregnancy. NSAIDs are associated with inhibition of prostaglandins and the risk of premature closure of the ductus arteriosus, as well as inhibition of uterine contractions; these should be avoided in the later stages of pregnancy, particularly during the last eight weeks, when the ductus is most sensitive to their effects. In addition, NSAIDs may cause foetal harm, including spontaneous abortions when used during the earlier stages of pregnancy and should thus be used with caution throughout pregnancy.

In addition to foetal development, physiological changes also occur in the mother as a result of the pregnancy, including cardiovascular, haemodynamic and renal changes. These changes vary with the stage of pregnancy, and are not necessarily consistent across all pregnant women. For example, in pregnant women, cardiac output increases by 30–50%, plasma volume begins to increase around the 4th week of gestation, and renal clearance may increase by as much as 50%. Therefore, medications may need to be monitored more closely and doses may need to be adjusted, especially those with narrow therapeutic windows. The serum concentrations of certain medications (such as lamotrigine, levetiracetam) may also need more frequent monitoring.

Following the FDA requirement of proven safety and efficacy, the FDA created a system to categorise the safety of drug use during pregnancy; this is known as the *Pregnancy Risk Categories*. Although some countries, including Australia and Germany have developed their own unique rating systems, the US Risk Category system is used most commonly in the US and in most other countries.

Under this system, drugs are categorised as Category A, B, C, D or X, based on the evidence for foetal risk, where Category A designates a medication that is thought to pose the least risk to the foetus and Category X designates a drug that has a known risk of harming the foetus. Due to ethical issues of studying medication use in pregnant women, only a limited number of safety studies have been conducted. Therefore, the categories consider safety studies in both humans and animals and are defined

Table 17.1 Definitions of FDA Pregnancy Categories assigned to medications used during pregnancy

Category	***Definition***
A	Controlled studies in women fail to demonstrate a risk to the foetus in the first trimester (and there is no evidence of a risk in a later trimester), and the possibility of foetal harm appears remote.
B	Either animal reproduction studies have not demonstrated a foetal risk but there are no controlled studies in pregnant women or animal reproduction studies have shown an adverse effect (other than a decrease in fertility) that was not confirmed in controlled studies in women in the first trimester (and there is no evidence of a risk in later trimesters).
C	Either studies in animals have revealed adverse effects on the foetus (teratogenic or embryocidal or other) and there are no controlled studies in women, or studies in women and animals are not available. Drugs should be given only if the potential benefit justifies the potential risk to the foetus.
D	There is positive evidence of human foetal risk, but the benefits from use in pregnant women may be acceptable despite the risk (for example, if the drug is needed in a life-threatening situation or for a serious disease for which safer drugs cannot be used or are ineffective).
X	Studies in animals or humans have demonstrated foetal abnormalities or there is evidence of foetal risk based on human experience or both, and the risk of the use of the drug in pregnant women clearly outweighs any possible benefit. The drug is contraindicated in women who are or may become pregnant.

in Table 17.1. Categorical assignments are made by the manufacturers, although some older drugs, available before the FDA created the Pregnancy Categories, have not been assigned categories and do not reflect new information made available following the initial categorical assignment.

Given the limitations of the Pregnancy Categories in determining the safety of medication use during pregnancy, it is important to not rely solely on the Pregnancy Category assignment. Classification of a drug into Category A does not necessarily mean it is safe for use in pregnant women. Assignment of Category A simply means that a medication has not been shown in animal and human studies to cause harm to the foetus. Although few drugs (such as levothyroxine, liothyronine, folic acid) are assigned to Category A, practising physicians do consider other medications appropriate for use during pregnancy. The drugs considered contraindicated for use during pregnancy and given a rating of Category X are listed in Table 17.2.

Despite the best efforts of the FDA, the Pregnancy Categories have not been enough to prevent foetal harm, which was illustrated with the use of isotretinoin. Since it was first marketed in the US in 1982, isotretinoin has been assigned a Pregnancy Category of X. Despite this warning, isotretinoin was used for the treatment of severe acne in pregnant women. One year after the availability of isotretinoin in the US, birth defects including hydrocephalus and spontaneous abortions were reported, which totaled 78 in 1989.

Another lesson was learned following the use of etretinate, an analogue of isotretinate, used for the treatment of psoriasis. Etretinate,

Table 17.2 Category X drugs: Contraindicated for use during pregnancy

Abarelix	Fluorouracil	Miglustat
Acetohydroxamic acid	Fluoxymesterone	Misoprostol
Acitretin	Fluvastatin	Nafarelin
Ambrisentan	Follicle stimulating hormone/ Lutenizing hormone	Nandrolone
Anastrozole		Norethindrone
Anisindione	Follitropin alfa	Oxandrolone
Atorvastatin	Follitropin beta	Oxymetholone
Benzphetamine	Ganirelix	Plicamycin
Bexarotene	Goserelin	Pravastatin
Bicalutamide	Histrelin	Progestin
Bosentan	Iodinated glycerol	Quazepam
Cerivastatin	Isoflurophate	Quinestrol
Cetrorelix	Isotretinoin	Raloxifene
Chlorotrianisene	Leflunomide	Ribavirin
Chorionic gonadotropin	Lenalidomide	Rosuvastatin
Clomiphene	Leuprolide	Simvastatin
Danazol	Levonorgestrel	Sitaxsentan
Degarelix	Lorazepam	Sodium iodide
Demecarium	Lovastatin	Stanozolol
Dienestrol	Lutropin alfa	Tazarotene
Diethystilbestrol	Medroxyprogesterone	Temazepam
Dutasteride	Megestrol	Testosterone
Ergotamine	Menadiol	Thalidomide
Estazolam	Mequinol/tretinoin	Tositumomab
Estradiol	Methotrexate	Triazolam
Estrogen	Methyltestosterone	Triptorelin
Estropipate	Methysergide	Urofollitropin
Etretinate	Mifepristone	Vitamin A, high dose
Finasteride		Warfarin

also contraindicated for use during pregnancy, has resulted in similar birth defects to isotretinoin. The lesson learned was that drugs can cause foetal harm even if discontinued prior to pregnancy. One of the many reports of congenital defects resulting from the use of etretinate was a child born with cardiac and CNS malformations, despite the mother discontinuing etretinate 11 months prior to conception. Because of etretinate's high lipophilicity, storage in maternal adipose tissues and long elimination half-life of approximately 120 days, insufficient time was allowed for its elimination from maternal circulation prior to conception.

The isotretinoin and etretinate incidents heightened awareness of the uncertainty and potential risks of medication use during pregnancy. As an added measure to prevent foetal harm, isotretinoin, thalidomide and other drugs with similar potential risks are now available only through restricted access programmes, which require a woman to use two forms of contraception during treatment and for one month after discontinuation.

Estimating Risk during Lactation

Determining whether to recommend a medication for use during lactation depends on the available literature, physiologic characteristics and a drug's physicochemical properties, as well as consideration of the potential adverse reactions observed in adults and children. Although some cytotoxic drugs have not been studied for use in lactation, their mechanism of action and extensive adverse effect profile in adults deter their use during lactation. Factors to consider, such as the available studies, duration of the child's exposure, age of the nursing child and the milk–plasma drug concentration ratio, are helpful in determining the risks. Nursing children of younger age are at greater risk of harm because they tend to eliminate drugs more slowly, allowing for greater amount and duration of drug exposure.

Although a higher medication milk–plasma concentration ratio is thought to expose nursing children to greater amounts of the drug and thus increase the risk, there has been little correlation between this concentration ratio in the mother and the concentration in the nursing child's blood or urine. To minimise the potential exposure of the nursing infant, dosing schedules should not overlap with breastfeeding times. Ideally, breastfeeding should be completed immediately prior to the time of the nursing mother's next dose, because the concentration of the drug in breast milk should be lowest at this time. In reality, timing breastfeeding around maternal drug schedules is difficult due to the frequency of feeds, especially with newborns who often require feeding as frequently as every two hours. To further decrease the medication concentration in breast milk, medications with shorter half-lives are preferred.

While women should be encouraged to breastfeed, because of its many advantages over formula, some women do not. It may also not be an option due to maternal use of high-risk medication, insufficient milk supply, inability to tolerate feeds or lifestyles that are not conducive to breastfeeding. Women who work or who are outside the privacy of their homes during times of breastfeeding, may find breastfeeding a challenge. These women should be educated on alternatives to traditional breastfeeding, including the use of formulas for newborns and infants, the option of supplementing breast milk with formula, and the use of breast milk pumps to store the milk for future feeds.

Unlike drug use during pregnancy, no formal rating system has been developed for lactation, but the American Academy of Pediatrics (AAP) offers direction in choosing a medication for use during lactation with lists that categorise medications as Maternal Medication Usually Compatible With Breastfeeding, Cytotoxic Drugs That May Interfere With Cellular Metabolism of the Nursing Infant, Drugs for Which the Effect on Nursing Infants Is Unknown but May Be of Concern and Drugs That Have Been Associated With Significant Effects on Some Nursing Infants and Should Be Given to Nursing Mothers With Caution.

These lists are updated periodically, with the most recent update in 2001 and are found in Tables 17.3 to 17.6. Although a medication may be categorised as Compatible with Breastfeeding, the child may still ingest small amounts, and hence be at risk; however, when given at the recommended dose, the

Table 17.3 Drugs that have been associated with significant effects on some nursing infants and should be given to nursing mothers with caution

Acebutolol	Aspirin	Phenindione
5-Aminosalicylic acid	Clemastine	Phenobarbital
Atenolol	Ergostamine	Primidone
Bromocriptine	Lithium	Sulfasalazine

Table 17.4 Drugs for which the effect on nursing infants is unknown but may be of concern

Alprazolam	Diazepam	Tinidazole
Amitriptyline	Doxepin	Trazadone
Amoxapine	Fluoxetine	Trifluoperazine
Amiodarone	Fluvoxamine	Lorazepam
Buproprion	Haloperidol	Midazolam
Chloramphenicol	Imipramine	Perphenazine
Clofazimine	Lamotrigine	Prazepam
Clomipramine	Mesoridazine	Quazepam
Desipramine	Metoclopramide	Temazepam
Paroxetine	Metronidazole	
Sertraline	Nortriptyline	

Table 17.5 Cytotoxic drugs that may interfere with the cellular metabolism of the nursing infant

Cyclophosphamide	Doxorubicin
Cyclosporine	Methotrexate

medication breast milk concentration may be lower than that shown to harm the nursing child. As with pregnancy, most medications are excreted into breast milk, but the extent and effect of the nursing child's exposure are uncertain.

Discontinuation of Medications Associated with Withdrawal

Medications that require tapering or monitoring when discontinued in adults to prevent withdrawal may also require the same measures in the newborn. Medications used during pregnancy or lactation that affect the foetus or child can continue to have effects on the newborn following delivery and cessation of breastfeeding. At childbirth and upon discontinuation of breastfeeding, the maternal transfer of medication stops abruptly and could thus precipitate withdrawal in the newborn or child. Examples of medications that may necessitate tapering or close monitoring include opioids, anti-depressants and corticosteroids.

Screening all Women of Childbearing Age

When making a medication recommendation for any woman of childbearing age, it is important to screen for those who are

Table 17.6 Maternal medication usually compatible with breastfeeding*

Acetaminophen	Dyphylline	Moxalactam
Acetazolamide	Enalapril	Nadolol
Acitretin	Erythromycin	Nalidixic acid
Alcohol	Estradiol	Naproxen
Acyclovir	Ethambutol	Nefopam
Allopurinol	Ethanol	Nifedipine
Amoxicillin	Ethosuximibe	Nitrofurantoin
Antimony	Fentanyl	Norethynodrel
Atropine	Fexofenadine	Norsteroids
Azapropazone	Flecainide	Noscapine
Aztreonam	Fleroxacin	Ofloxacin
B1	Fluconazole	Oxprenolol
B12	Flufenamic acid	Phenylbutazone
Baclofen	Fluorescein	Phenytoin
Barbiturate	Folic acid	Piroxicam
Bendroflumethiazide	Gadopentetic	Prednisolone
Bishydroxycoumarin	Gentamicin	Prednisone
Bromide	Gold salts	Procainamide
Butorphanol	Halothane	Progesterone
Caffeine	Hydralazine	Propoxyphene
Captopril	Hydrochlorothiazide	Propranolol
Carbamazepine	Hydroxychloroquine	Propylthiouracil
Carbetocin	Ibuprofen	Pseudoephedrine
Carbimazole	Indomethacin	Pyridostigmine
Cascara	Iodides	Pyrimethamine
Cefadroxio	Iodine	Quinidine
Cefazolin	Iodine	Quinine
Cefotaxime	Iohexol	Riboflavin
Cefoxitin	Iopenaoic acid	Rifampin
Cefprozil	Isoniazide	Scopolamine
Ceftazidime	Interferon alpha	Secobarbital
Ceftriaxone	Ivermectin	Senna
Chloral hydrate	Vitamin K1	Sotalol
Chloroform	Kanamycin	Spironolactone
Chloroquine	Ketoconazole	Streptomycin
Chlorothiazide	Ketorolac	Sulbactam
Chlorthalidone	Labetolol	Sulfapyridine
Cimetidine	Levonorgestrol	Sulfisoxazole
Ciprofloxacin	Levothyroxine	Sumatriptan
Cisapride	Lidocaine	Suprofen
Cisplatin	Loperamide	Terbutaline
Clindamycin	Loratadine	Terfenadine

Clogestone	Magnesium sulfate	Tetracycline
Codeine	Medroxyprogesterone	Theophylline
Colchicine	Mefenamic acid	Thiopental
Contraceptive pill with estrogen/ progesterone	Meperidine	Thiouracil
Cycloserine	Methadone	Ticarcillin
Vitamin D	Methimazole	Timolol
Danthron	Methohexital	Tolbutamide
Dapsone	Methydopa	Tolmetin
Dexbrompheniramine maleate with d-isoephedrine	Methyprylon	Trimethoprim/ sulfamethoxazole
Diatrizoate	Metoprolol	Triprolidine
Digoxin	Metrizamide	Valproic acid
Diltiazem	Metrizoate	Verapamil
Dipyrone	Mexiletine	Warfarin
Disopyramide	Minoxidil	Zolpidem
Domperidone	Morphine	

*These drugs are considered safe for use in pregnancy by the AAP at the recommended doses. Inclusion in this category does not mean a medication is not excreted in breast milk.

currently pregnant or breastfeeding, wanting to become pregnant, and for those at risk of becoming pregnant. For all women of childbearing age, recommendations should include use of a medication that is proven to be safe in pregnancy or a recommendation for contraceptive methods. In addition, all women should be educated aboout the potential risks associated with medication use on the foetus should they become pregnant, as well as the risks of medication use when breastfeeding.

Further, women identified as trying to become pregnant should, at the minimum, be instructed to take a folic acid supplement beginning a month prior to conception and continue it for the first 12 weeks of gestation to prevent neural tube defects. Women may also be instructed to continue folic acid supplementation throughout pregnancy, and to take mineral and vitamin supplements to meet the recommended daily dietary allowances for pregnancy.

Conclusion

When determining the risks of medication use during pregnancy and lactation, it is important to realise that nearly all medications have the potential to cross the placenta and be excreted in breast milk, thus harming the foetus or nursing child. Weighing the risks against the benefits of medication use depends on many factors, including consideration of all available safety studies, physiologic changes and the physicochemical and pharmacokinetic properties of the drug. Extensive consideration of all factors is imperative before beginning any medication in pregnant or breastfeeding women. There are many resources available to assist in risk assessment, but ultimately, the decision process must involve a review of the latest primary literature and be individualised to the patient.

CASE STUDY 1

MS is a 45-year-old Indian woman who presents to her primary care physician 18 days after starting hydrochlorothiazide 25 mg to treat a blood pressure of 167/106 mmHg. Today her blood pressure is 164/105 mmHg and her pulse is 65 beats/min. Her target blood pressure is <130/80. Other than hypertension and type 2 diabetes, she has no significant medical problems or family history. She currently takes hydrochlorothiazide 25 mg daily, metformin XR 2000 mg daily, atorvastatin 40 mg at bedtime and aspirin 81 mg daily. Pertinent lab investigation values as of yesterday are serum creatinine 0.89 mg/dl and serum potassium 3.8 mmol/l. The physician asks for your recommendation to control blood pressure in this patient who is trying to get pregnant.

Discussion

According to JNC 7, MS's diabetes is a compelling indication for an ACE inhibitor or angiotensin receptor blocker (ARB); however, she is trying to become pregnant and ACEs are Pregnancy Category X and ARBs are Category D. Thus, another agent, such as methyldopa, a beta blocker with intrinsic sympathomimetic activity (ISA) or amlodipine is a better option for MS. Methyldopa is Pregnancy Category B, beta blockers with ISA and long-acting nifedipine are Category C. Methyldopa, although a weak anti-hypertensive agent, is most commonly used in pregnant women, followed by the beta blocker labetalol. Some experts consider beta blockers with ISA to be Pregnancy Category D in the second and third trimesters of pregnancy, and beta blockers without ISA should not be used during pregnancy because they may cause intrauterine growth restriction. Reasonable recommendations for adjunctive anti-hypertensive therapy include methyldopa 250 mg twice daily, labetalol 100 mg twice daily, or long-acting nifedipine 30 mg daily. Part of the recommendation should include starting daily prenatal vitamin with folic acid, as well as stopping atorvastatin which is Pregnancy Category X and aspirin, which is Category C. For MS, aspirin is being used for cardioprotection, meaning the benefit to the mother does not outweigh the potential risk to the foetus; further, MS no longer meets the criteria for using aspirin as primary prevention based on the updated recommendations from the American Diabetes Association.

Should MS become pregnant, consideration should be given to adding or switching to an ACE inhibitor following delivery. MS has a compelling indication for an ACE inhibitor, and ACEs are considered safe for use during lactation. It is important to ensure, prior to beginning an ACE, that MS is not trying to become pregnant and is using appropriate contraceptive measures because it is contraindicated for use in pregnant women.

CASE STUDY 2

JT is a 29-year-old African-American woman with a chief complaint of feeling depressed. She gave birth to her first child one month ago and is currently breastfeeding. A nine-point depression assessment survey (PHQ9) was administered today and she scored 23, which is considered 'severe depression.' She has no history of depression or other co-morbidities. Today her BP is 138/85 mmHg. What would you recommend to JT's physician for the treatment of her depression?

Discussion

Although all anti-depressants are excreted in breast milk, hence posing a risk to the nursing child, the benefit to the mother appears to outweigh the risk to the child. Prior to starting any medication, the mother should be informed of the risk to the child and presented the option of using formula as an alternative to breastfeeding. If the mother chooses to continue breastfeeding, selective serotonin receptor inhibitors (SSRIs), trazodone, buproprion and tricyclic anti-depressants (TCAs) are considered to be Drugs for Which the Effect on Nursing Infants Is Unknown but May Be of Concern by the AAP. Other anti-depressants, such as the selective serotonin and norepinephrine reuptake inhibitors (SNRIs), have not been categorised by the AAP. Therefore, recommending an agent considered 'of concern' would be preferred over an agent such as an SNRI which has been studied less extensively for its safety during lactation and which could be more harmful. First-line agents for treating depression are SSRIs, of which fluoxetine is commonly used during lactation and which could be more harmful because of their shorter half-life, but may not be preferred due to its long half-life. Thus, other SSRIs such as citalopram or sertraline may be recommended for this patient because of their shorter half-life. Alternatives to an SSRI may be trazodone, buproprion or a TCA.

KEY MESSAGES

- Nearly all medications can cross the placenta or be excreted in breast milk.
- Factors such as the time, amount and duration of medication exposure can significantly influence the risk of harm to the foetus or nursing infant.
- All women of childbearing age, regardless of pregnancy status, should be educated about the risks of medication use during pregnancy.
- Nursing mothers should be educated about the risks of medication use and ways to minimise the extent of the child's exposure.
- It is important to thoroughly review all sources of information to help determine the risks of medication use during pregnancy and lactation.
- No reference, including the FDAs Pregnancy Categories, should be solely relied upon to determine the risk of medication use during pregnancy or lactation.
- The benefit of medication use during pregnancy or lactation must outweigh the risk of use to the foetus or child and include a consideration of both the available literature and other factors, such as the time, amount and duration of medication exposure.

Further Reading

American Academy of Pediatrics Committee on Drugs. 2001. Transfer of drugs and other chemicals into human milk. *Pediatrics* 108:776–789.

American College of Obstetricians and Gynecologists. 2007. *Guidelines for Perinatal Care*, 6th ed., ACOG: Washington, DC.

Briggs GG and Nageotte MP (eds). 2009. *Diseases, Complications, and Drug Therapy in Obstetrics - A Guide for Clinicians*. ASHP: Bethesda, MD.

Briggs GG, Freeman RK and Yaffe SJ. 2011. *Drugs in Pregnancy and Lactation. A Reference Guide to Foetal and Neonatal Risk*, 9th ed. Philadelphia: Lippincott, Williams & Wilkins.

DRUGDEX® System [Internet database]. Thomson Reuters (Healthcare) Inc: Greenwood Village, Colorado: Thomson Reuters (Healthcare) Inc. Updated periodically.

Federal Register. 1980. 44:37434–37467.

Folic acid for the prevention of neural tube defects: U.S. Preventive Services Task Force recommendation statement. 2009. *Ann Intern Med*150:626–631.

Hale TW. 2010. *Medications and Mother's Milk: A Manual of Lactational Pharmacology*, 11th ed. Pharmasoft Publishing L.P: Amarillo.

Herbst AL, Ulfelder H and Poskanzer DC. 1971. Adenocarcinoma of the vagina. Association of maternal stilbestrol therapy with tumor appearance in young women. *N Engl J Med* 284:878–881

Kaufman RH, Adam E, Hatch EE, Noller K, Herbst AL, Palmer JR and Hoover RN. 2000. Continued follow-up of pregnancy outcomes in diethylstilbestrol-exposed offspring. *Obstet Gynecol* 96:483–489.

Kitzmiller JL, Gavin LA, et al. 1991. Preconception care of diabetes. Glycemic control prevents congenital anomalies. *JAMA*13; 265:731–736.

Lammer EJ. 1988. Embryopathy in infant conceived one year after termination of maternal etretinate. *Lancet* 2:1080–1081.

Li DK, Liu L and Odouli R. 2003. Exposure to non-steroidal anti-inflammatory drugs during pregnancy and risk of miscarriage: population based cohort study. *BMJ* 327:368–372.

Public Affairs Committee of the Teratology Society. 2000. Teratology Society Public Affairs Committee Position Paper: Thalidomide. *Teratology* 62:172–173.

Rosa FW. 1983. Teratogenicity of isotretinoin. *Lancet* 2:513.

van Oppen ACC, Stigter RH and Bruinse HW. 1996. Cardiac output in normal pregnancy: a critical review. *Obstet Gynecol* 87:310–318.

Website of Interest

REPRORISK system; commercially-available CD-ROM that contains electronic versions of REPROTEXT, REPROTOX, Shepard's Catalog and TERIS. The system is available from Micromedex, Inc.

http://www.micromedex.com/products/reprorisk/

18
CRITICAL APPRAISAL: HOW TO READ A RESEARCH PAPER

Karin Nyfort-Hansen

Learning Objectives

Upon completion of this chapter, the reader should be able to:

- Define the terms research literature, critical appraisal and evidence-based medicine
- Summarise the types of research literature which are most relevant to clinical pharmacists
- Explain why critical appraisal is an important skill for clinical pharmacists
- Summarise the factors to be considered when choosing a paper for critical appraisal
- Explain the difference between absolute risk reduction and relative risk reduction
- Critically appraise a paper reporting a drug trial
- Critically appraise a paper describing a systematic review/meta analysis
- Critically appraise a paper presenting therapeutic guidelines

For health and science professionals, the term 'literature' refers to the body of articles published in biomedical and scientific journals. It is this literature we turn to when we need to answer questions such as 'Which is the best drug for this disease?' or 'Is this new drug better than the old one?'. Many of the articles in biomedical journals describe research studies investigating various aspects of disease causation, diagnosis, screening, prognosis and management. Research papers on management often report on the effects of drugs, but non-drug therapy such as surgery and lifestyle interventions may also be the topic of investigation.

Types of Drug Therapy Research Papers

Drug therapy research ranges from laboratory and animal investigations to studies in healthy volunteers, individual patients, patient cohorts or entire populations. The studies of greatest interest to clinical pharmacists include those that focus on clinical efficacy, short- and/or long-term drug toxicity, drug pharmacokinetics, dose–response relationships and drug therapy monitoring. Trials of drug efficacy compare a drug treatment with either placebo or other treatments commonly used for that disease, and those of greatest relevance study the drug in patients who are similar to our own. Other types of research papers that may be of interest include systematic reviews/meta analyses, therapeutic guidelines, population studies, economic analyses, qualitative research, drug utilisation evaluations and case series.

What is Critical Appraisal?

Critical appraisal is the ability to read original research papers in a way that allows us to judge their scientific value and to consider how the results can be applied in practice. Skills in critical appraisal are essential for clinical pharmacy practice as they allow us to independently evaluate the significance of research findings for our patients. Without this ability, we are much more likely to be persuaded by the advertising and promotional claims of the pharmaceutical industry, which often use highly selective data from research papers to support the use of their products.

The main aim of critical appraisal can be summarised as: *Should this paper, in conjunction with other relevant literature and clinical experience, change clinical practice?* This implies that while it is possible to judge the scientific value of a paper as it stands, the true purpose of critical appraisal is the consideration of whether the results should be applied in practice. To do this, it is necessary to have an understanding of the background to the study, knowledge of relevant previous studies, relevant clinical experience and an understanding of the needs of individual patients.

Choosing a Paper for Critical Appraisal

Every year, hundreds of biomedical journals publish thousands of research papers on drug therapy. However, only a few of these are likely to, or should, change prescribing practice. Many studies have methodological problems, which put the results in some doubt, and most clinicians, usually very wisely, wait to see if the results are replicated in subsequent studies.

So how do clinical pharmacists decide which research papers are important to read? Most pharmacists 'filter' articles to select those that are most likely to be of greatest clinical relevance and significance. In order to judge the relative importance of a paper, consideration needs to be given to factors such as:

- Is this paper addressing an important or controversial therapeutic issue which is of relevance to my patients?
- Is this study the first evidence for the efficacy of a new drug class or treatment?
- Does this study involve more patients or is it continued for longer than previous studies?

- Is the studied population different in any way from previous studies?
- Does the methodology address the methodological problems identified in previous studies of this drug?

If the answer to any of these questions is 'Yes', then it is likely that the paper may be worthy of critical appraisal. Consideration also needs to be given to the type of study that is described. Some studies may be more important to read because they use a study design (the way the study was conducted) which provides stronger evidence than other types of study design. A ranking or hierarchy of evidence is presented in Table 18.1.

Table 18.1 Hierarchy of evidence. The relative weight carried by different types of primary study in descending order of quality. Well-conducted systematic reviews and meta analyses provide stronger evidence than an RCT, which is stronger than other types of study design. Methodological flaws in individual studies may affect ranking in any given situation.

1	Systematic reviews and meta analyses
2	Randomised controlled trials
3	Non-randomised trials
4	Cohort studies
5	Case-control studies
6	Cross-sectional surveys
7	Case reports

Critical Appraisal of Primary Research Papers

Research papers appearing in the biomedical literature usually conform to a standard format known as IMRAD: **I**ntroduction (background details and the research question), **M**ethods (how the study was conducted and details of statistical analysis), **R**esults and **D**iscussion (authors present their study findings and interpret the results in light of other research findings, and possible implications for current clinical practice).

When reading a paper, people often start with the abstract and then proceed to the paper as presented, finishing with the discussion and conclusion. Abstracts can be misleading, however; for example, they are more likely to include significant results than non-significant ones. A more questioning or critical approach examines particular aspects of the paper and study design. When reading a paper, the aims of the study should be identified first. This should be followed by a reading of the methods and results sections, which enables you to draw your own conclusions about whether the study design and the results met the stated aims.

Evaluating the Methods Section

The methods section tells you whether the study design chosen by the investigators was sound and likely to answer the research question. If you are trying to decide whether a paper is worth reading, you should do so on your evaluation of the study design, rather than on whether the results are 'statistically significant' or study outcomes changed in the direction which you would like them to. You may have noticed that drug advertising and promotional material often contain quotations from the results section of research papers, but little, if any information about study methods.

When reading the methods section, you should find descriptions of the study design, specific interventions to be studied, the outcomes to be measured, how subjects were recruited and who was included or excluded, how bias was avoided or minimised, the duration and completeness of follow-up and the statistical methods which were used. All these should be described in detail and each needs to be considered carefully during the appraisal process. In the following discussion, these ideas are explained further. Some common terms used to describe the design features of clinical trials are summarised in Table 18.2.

The best choice of study design depends on the research question, but in general, when testing the efficacy of drug treatments,

Table 18.2 Terms used to describe the design of drug trials

Term	*Meaning*
Double-blind	Neither subjects nor investigators know treatment allocation
Single-blind	Subjects do not know which treatment they are receiving, but investigators are aware of treatment allocation
Placebo-controlled	Control subjects receive inactive (placebo) treatment, which should be identical in appearance and method of administration to active medication
Open-label study	Subjects and investigators are aware of treatment allocation
Prospective study	A study using data to be gathered in the future
Retrospective study	A study using data available from the past
Multi-centre	Used to describe trials which are conducted in more than one institution
Case-control study	A study which identifies a group of patients having the outcome of interest, and compares them to a matched group of patients who do not have the outcome of interest
Cross-over	Each subject receives both the intervention and the control treatments (in random order), usually separated by a wash-out period during which subjects receive no treatment (to minimise interference between treatments)
Cross-sectional survey	A study which surveys a population about a condition or exposure, or both, at one point in time
Cohort study	A non-experimental study design which follows a group of people (cohort) prospectively and then examines how events differ among people within the group
Factorial design	Allows investigation of the separate and combined effects of more than one independent variable (drugs) on a given outcome
Parallel group comparison	Each group receives a different treatment, with both groups being entered into the study at the same time. Results are analysed by comparing groups
Paired comparison	Subjects receiving different treatments are matched to balance potential confounding factors. Results are analysed in terms of differences between subject pairs
Within subject comparison	Subjects are assessed before and after an intervention. Results are analysed in terms of subject changes

the *randomised controlled trial (RCT)* is considered the preferred study design. In an RCT, subjects are randomly allocated to either an intervention group (such as drug treatment) or a control group (such as placebo treatment). Both groups are then followed up for a specified time period and analysed in terms of specific outcomes, which are defined at the outset of the study. The method of randomisation should be stated. The randomisation process aims to ensure that the two groups are very similar, so that any known or unknown variables (confounding factors) which may affect outcomes are evenly distributed between the groups. Any differences in outcome can then more confidently be attributed to drug treatment.

All studies and trials are subject to bias or confounding. It can be difficult to understand the difference between these two terms. *Confounding* relates to the possibility of alternative explanations of the study results, whereas *bias* relates to problems with the study design. Good study designs aim to minimise bias. While the randomisation process aims to minimise bias between the intervention and control groups by ensuring that similar subjects are in each group, biases may still be present.

These include selection bias (such as failure to randomise all eligible patients), performance bias (such as differences in the care provided apart from drug treatment), exclusion bias (for example, differences in withdrawal from the study) and detection bias (such as failure to blind assessors). When reading a paper, it is important to look for potential biases that may be present because this can influence our interpretation of the study results.

All studies usually have some type of inclusion and exclusion criteria, which define the characteristics of the patients who were recruited into the study. Typical selection criteria may relate to age, sex, severity of disease and co-morbid conditions; exclusion criteria are often used to ensure patient safety. When reading the methods section, you should pay attention to these criteria, as they will help you decide how similar the study subjects are to the patients you encounter in your daily practice, and whether the results can be generalised to your patients.

Check whether the criteria have introduced any bias, for example, selection bias may have occurred if the study has excluded patients who may not respond as well to treatment. Always check the settings and locations in which the study was carried out. These can also affect the generalisability of results, as outcomes in some trials may be affected by factors such as patient ethnicity, climate and local dietary patterns.

The term '*placebo effect*' is used to describe the positive (and sometimes negative) clinical response which subjects may have when given a placebo ('dummy') medication. Doctors and other assessors can also make assessments, quite unintentionally, which are influenced by their preconceptions of how effective the study treatment is likely to be. The gold standard for RCTs is a trial where patients, doctors and other assessors are unaware of a subject's randomisation status. The term '*double-blind*' implies that neither the caregiver nor the patient knows which treatment was received. The term, however, is ambiguous with regard to blinding of other persons, including those assessing patient outcomes. Authors should therefore state clearly who was blinded. Look for this when you are reading the methods section.

Drug trials without any blinding are known as *'open label'* and have greater potential for bias than blinded studies.

When reading the methods section, the drug treatment or any other intervention should be fully described. This includes the drug(s) names and formulations, the doses used, administration details and the duration of treatment. Details of the placebo treatment should also be included; for example, that it looked identical to the intervention medication. If a comparator drug has been administered rather than a placebo, consider whether subtherapeutic doses of the comparator drug have been used to enhance differences in outcome between the two treatments. Also check whether the comparator was formulated or packed to look identical to the intervention medication, and administered in the same way. A well-conducted trial will also include measures of compliance, such as tablet counts, and these should also be described.

RCT investigators will study a variety of outcomes or *'end points'* to evaluate the effects of the study treatment. The outcome considered by the investigators to be of greatest importance is the 'primary outcome'. Other outcomes of interest are called 'secondary outcomes.' Sometimes the primary or secondary outcome may be a 'composite' end point, in which a number of different outcomes are combined. This is usually done for rare events to minimise the follow-up time and the number of patients required to be recruited.

For example, a trial of an anti-hypertensive may have a composite end point of cardiovascular death, myocardial infarction and stroke. The components of a composite end point should be expected to have similar relative risk reductions, and each component should be of similar importance to the patient. In a paper, all outcomes should be identified and completely defined, including who assessed the outcome and by what method.

Some outcomes may be objective (for example, blood pressure measurements, mortality rates), others may be subjective in nature (such as entries in a patient diary) and others may be partly both (for example, interpretation of a chest x-ray, quality of life measurements). Good study designs will use previously validated scales or instruments where they are available.

When reading a paper, you need to decide how relevant or important each outcome is for patient prognosis. Direct real-life outcomes of efficacy, such as changes in disease progression or mortality rates, are the preferred outcome measures. However, these are often difficult to measure and may require long periods of follow-up, and surrogate end points may be used in their place. A *surrogate end point* is relatively easily measured and is assumed to predict a rare or distant outcome of an intervention, but is not in itself a direct measure of either harm or clinical benefit. Examples include blood pressure measurements, sputum smears or the minimum inhibitory concentration of an anti-microbial. Data on surrogate end points are less persuasive evidence than clinical data relating to morbidity, mortality or hospitalisation.

For example, a study that reports on the effects of a new hypoglycaemic agent is much more persuasive if micro and macrovascular outcomes are studied in addition to surrogate end points such as blood glucose or HbA1c measurements. This is because the drug may have other effects in the body (for example, hyperlipidemia or other unknown negative effects) which may offset the clinical benefits of a reduction in blood glucose.

When reading the methods section, you should consider whether the duration of treatment and follow-up is sufficient to draw meaningful conclusions for each of the outcomes assessed. For example, asthma medications are often assessed using a variety of outcomes, such as changes in beta agonist use or lung function tests, or the number of night-time awakenings due to asthma symptoms. However, some outcomes, such as the number of asthma exacerbations, may require months or years of follow up because these events occur much less frequently. Studies of insufficient duration will not provide reliable results about such outcomes.

Statistics: The types of statistical tests used in the study are also described in the methods section. Research papers use statistics for both descriptive and inferential purposes. In the former situation, they are used to summarise data, commonly through the use of means, medians or ranges. For inferential purposes, statistics are used to draw a conclusion from the results.

Statistics can be a complex and sometimes intimidating subject, and as a result many clinicians rely on the statistical expertise of the investigators and the journal's independent reviewers. A basic knowledge of biostatistics can help you independently evaluate whether the statistical tests used in a paper are appropriate. However, even without this expertise, you should try to develop a 'feel' for the results data to identify the key information that leads to the study's conclusions.

The most important question to ask yourself when reading about the statistical analysis is 'Are the authors using a statistical test which is appropriate for their data?'. All statistical tests are either parametric (they assume that the data was sampled from a particular type of distribution, such as a normal distribution) or non-parametric (no such assumption is made). In general, parametric tests are more powerful than non-parametric tests and so should be used if possible. The term *'tail'* refers to the extremes of data distribution, and the term *'outliers'* refers to individual unusually high or low results. Generally, we wish to know whether extreme high or low values could have occurred by chance, and to do this we need a statistical test which is 'two-tailed' rather than 'one-tailed'.

A two-tailed test should always be performed if there is uncertainty about whether the effect of an intervention (drug) is positive or negative. A one-tailed test can be used if the investigators are sure that the outcome will be either positive or negative. Paired (or matched) statistical tests should be used if the data we wish to analyse are paired, that is, measured on two occasions such as before and after treatment. A summary of some commonly used statistical tests and the type of data for which they should be used is presented in Table 18.3. For a detailed discussion of these tests, readers should refer to texts on biostatistics.

For clinical trials with two randomised treatment groups with equal numbers and an event outcome, a quick and simple statistical test can be used to assess the evidence for a treatment difference (Fig. 18.1). This test ignores the number of subjects randomised and the follow-up time by assuming these are virtually equal. It is therefore unreliable if there is a considerable difference in treatment group size. Also, if event rates are high, the

Table 18.3 Some appropriate statistical tests of significance according to data type and study design

	Two Comparison Groups		***More than Two Comparison Groups***	
Type of Data[1]	Unpaired Data	Paired Data	Unpaired Data	Paired Data
Nominal	Chi square[2]	McNemar	Chi square	Cochran Q test
Ordinal	Mann–Witney U test	Wilcoxon	Kruskal–Wallis	Friedman
Parametric	Student t-test	Paired student t-test	Analysis of variance (ANOVA)	ANOVA

[1] For further information on these terms, readers should consult a text on biostatistics

[2] If the number of patients in groups is less than or equal to 20, or if the number of observations in at least one cell is less than five, use Fisher's exact test

For a clinical trial with equal randomisation, the number of events (outcome of interest) in the two treatment groups is a and b, respectively. Calculate z using the following equation:

$$Z = \frac{(a-b)}{\sqrt{(a+b)}}$$

The P values in the table should approximate the conventional tests used in research papers, such as a log rank test.

Value of Z	*P Value*
1.28	0.2
1.64	0.1
1.96	0.05
2.05	0.04
2.17	0.03
2.32	0.02
2.58	0.01
3.29	0.001
3.89	0.0001

Fig. 18.1 A simple statistical test for a significant difference between treatments (Reproduced from BMJ 2006; 332:1256–8 with permission from the BMJ Publishing Group)

test becomes conservative, and p values are larger than they should be.

Evaluating the Results Section

When examining the results section, the first thing you should look for is that the randomisation process did indeed produce similar groups. Papers which report RCTs should include a table in which important patient characteristics (such as age, sex and any potential confounding factors such as disease severity) for both groups at study commencement (baseline) are summarised. This table should be examined carefully to identify any variables which may be dissimilar and which may be important to consider when interpreting the results. At this point, you should also think about whether there are potential confounding factors which have not been documented. For example, a study that is investigating the effects of a new anti-hypertensive agent should provide details on how many patients in each group were receiving other medications which may raise or lower the blood pressure.

Another factor to consider when interpreting the results is the subjects who withdraw from a study (sometimes called drop-outs). These may include those who do not respond adequately to treatment or who experience adverse effects. Studies involving drug treatments should generally undergo 'intention to treat' analysis. This means keeping patients in their original groups for statistical analysis, whether or not they complete or even receive the treatment to which they were allocated. Unless this is done, the original balance of variables resulting from randomisation will be lost, and treatment efficacy may be over-estimated.

The results of intention to treat analysis usually also reflect more closely what may happen in actual clinical practice. When reading a paper, check that the analysis included intention to treat and that all subjects enrolled in the trial were accounted for. A flow diagram indicating the numbers of patients moving through different stages of the study, and the numbers withdrawn or lost to follow-up is often useful. Check that the numbers on the diagram account for all patients entered into the study, and that the authors provide a full explanation why patients were excluded or lost to follow-up.

The authors should present results for all the outcomes listed in the methods section and provide reasons for any missing results. For each outcome, results should be reported as a summary of the outcome for each group together with the contrast between groups, known as the *'effect size'*. Clearly labelled tables or graphs should be used to summarise the data.

Investigators are often interested in whether a subgroup of patients (for example, younger vs older patients, patients with mild disease vs severe disease) may achieve greater or less benefit from drug treatment. If the results around primary and secondary outcomes are modest or inconclusive, investigators may perform multiple subgroup analyses in an attempt to find a subgroup of patients who appear to gain greater benefit from treatment. The results of subgroup analyses should be judged cautiously, and are best viewed as hypothesis-generating.

Many reports of RCTs provide inadequate information on adverse effects. We need information about the risks as well as the benefits of drug treatment, as these can have a major impact on whether a drug treatment is clinically acceptable and useful. This is particularly important when a drug is being used in essentially healthy patients to modify the risk of some future adverse event. At a minimum, authors should summarise the frequency of the most commonly reported adverse effects for each group, and the reasons for treatment discontinuation. Given the limited size and duration of most trials, adverse effects occurring less often than 1 in 1000 subjects, or which may be delayed, will generally remain undetected.

In any study, there is the possibility that any differences we observe between groups of patients may simply have occurred by chance. The concept of statistical significance helps us decide whether it is reasonable to attribute such differences to chance or whether it is more likely that there is a real difference between the two groups. The p value, the probability that any particular outcome has arisen by chance, is commonly used to describe the level of significance. Conventionally, a p value of less than 1 in 20 (expressed as $p < 0.05$) is considered to be 'statistically significant'. A p value above 0.05 tells us that either there is no difference between the groups, or there were too few subjects to demonstrate such a difference if it existed (the study is described as 'under-powered' in the latter situation). When examining the results of a paper, check to see if the results reported for the intervention group are statistically significant from those reported for the control group.

Confidence intervals (CI) are another measure often reported in study results. A *confidence interval* is the range within which the true size of effect lies with a given degree of assurance. It is used because the same study carried out with different samples of patients would not give identical results, but would be spread around the true difference for the whole population. By noting the 95% CI around a result when reading a paper, you will be able to say that there is a 95% chance that the real difference lies between these two limits. The larger the number of subjects, the narrower the CI, which means that the result is more likely to reflect the true difference between the groups. A wide confidence interval means the true size of effect is less certain.

Sometimes we want to know the relationship between two variables. The statistical methods used to define the relationship between two variables are termed correlation and regression analysis. *Correlation analysis* provides a measure of the strength of a relationship. It is important to remember that correlation does not imply causation, that is, that one variable causes the other. *Regression analysis* is a way of mathematically describing the relationship between variables. It aims to allow one dependent variable (for example, heart disease) to be predicted from one or more independent predictor variables (for example, hypertension or smoking). If there is more than one predictor variable, the technique is described as multiple regression.

Remember that a statistically significant result may not be clinically significant. Increasingly, pharmaceutical companies are conducting very large trials which detect small treatment effects. To make conclusions about the clinical significance of these effects, the results should be expressed in terms of the likely benefit an individual patient could expect. *Absolute risk* is the probability that an individual will experience a specified outcome during a specified time period. The change in absolute risk, or *absolute risk reduction* (ARR), is the difference between how often an outcome occurs in the treatment group compared to the control group. However, it can still be difficult to imagine what figures for ARR actually mean for an individual patient.

The 'number needed to be treated' (NNT) is often used to overcome this problem. This refers to how many patients would need to be treated with the study treatment over a stated period of time for one person to benefit in the outcome of interest. If the NNT is not stated, an easy way to calculate this is by inversing the absolute risk reduction (Example 1).

Evaluating the Discussion

Inferences, opinions and hypotheses about the results appear in the discussion section. Here the authors may compare their results with other studies, discuss the significance of their findings and summarise the limitations of their study. After going through the discussion, readers need to judge whether the authors' conclusions are justified, taking into consideration the design and conduct of the study, the statistical analysis employed and the study's limitations (Fig. 18.2).

Evaluating Other Parts of the Paper

The introduction provides background information about the topic and should explain why current research is needed. Other

Example 1: Absolute Risk vs Relative Risk

In an RCT comparing amodiaquine with the comparator drug chloroquine for the treatment of uncomplicated *Plasmodium falciparum* malaria, the relapse rate after 21 days is found to be 15% for chloroquine and 5% for amodiaquine. These figures represent the absolute risk of relapse in these two groups. The change in absolute risk is the difference in absolute risk (AR) between the two groups. Here, it is 15% minus 5%, that is 10% or 0.1, and this is referred to as the absolute risk reduction (ARR). This means that the probability of relapse is reduced by 10% in patients taking amodiaquine for 21 days compared to chloroquine. The number needed to treat (NNT) is the inverse of ARR; that is, 1 divided by 0.1, or 10. This means that ten patients would need to be treated with amodiaquine for 21 days in order to prevent one more case of relapse relative to treatment with chloroquine.

Relative risk (RR) is the ratio of how often an outcome (relapse) occurs in the treatment group (amodiaquine) compared with the control group (chloroquine). A relative risk of 1.0 indicates there is no difference in the risk of relapse between the two groups. Relative risk is calculated by dividing the incidence of relapse in the amodiaquine group by the incidence of relapse in the control (chloroquine) group. In this example, the relative risk is 5% divided by 15%, or 0.33. This means that patients in the amodiaquine group are one-third as likely to relapse compared to the chloroquine group. The relative risk reduction (RRR) is 1.0 minus 0.33, or 0.66 or 66%. The problem with relative risk is that it does not tell us anything about the size of the underlying risk of relapse in the two groups and therefore how many people are likely to benefit. For example, if the absolute risks of relapse in another similar study (Study 2) happened to be 3% for the chloroquine group and 1% for the amodiaquine group, the ARR would be 2% (0.02) and the NNT would be 1 divided by 0.02 or 50. However, the RRR would still be 66%.

	Absolute Risk of Relapse in Amodiaquine Group	*Absolute Risk of Relapse in Chloroquine Group*	*Absolute Risk Reduction (ARR)*	*Number Needed to Treat (NNT)*	*Relative Risk (RR)*	*Relative Risk Reduction (RRR)*
Study 1	5%	15%	10%	10	33%	66%
Study 2	1%	3%	2%	50	33%	66%

A relative risk reduction of 66% sounds much more impressive than an absolute risk reduction of 10% or 2%. You can see from this example why pharmaceutical company advertising often uses misleading graphical illustrations of relative risk reduction.

parts worthy of examination include the title, author affiliations, acknowledgments and references.

Author affiliations and acknowledgments should be examined to rule out potential conflicts of interest such as consultancy work for the sponsoring company or share ownership. Many journals now require authors to state their potential conflicts of interest, so that readers can consider if these may have influenced the authors to conduct research or present their results in a way which is favourable to their own interests.

Reference citations should be examined if these are of central importance to the research question or conclusions. Caution should be adopted if references are from obscure journals or unpublished such as conference papers or academic theses. This is because these references are unlikely to have undergone the close scrutiny of peer review.

Reaching a Conclusion

At the end of the critical appraisal process, you should ask yourself: *Should this paper, in conjunction with other relevant literature and clinical experience, change clinical practice?* Whether the results of a study can be applied to patients in the real world (external validity) is a matter of judgement. It can be helpful at this point to discuss your conclusions about the paper with others, particularly colleagues who have relevant clinical experience.

Secondary journals (ACP Journal Club, Evidence-Based Medicine) publish independent abstracts of trials which contain valuable information about the research methods which may be omitted from the original papers. Journal clubs, where a group of pharmacists and/or other practitioners meet regularly to discuss new research papers, are a useful way of sharing your views and developing your critical appraisal skills. It is also a very good way of keeping up-to-date with new therapeutic developments.

Critical Appraisal of a Systematic Review or Meta Analysis

For any research question, results of individual RCTs may vary, with some studies studying the same intervention producing large effects, others smaller effects and others perhaps even negative effects. A systematic review applies a rigorous and usually replicable method to summarise research findings from different primary studies relating to the same research question. Its method includes a specified aim, a comprehensive strategy for searching for primary studies, criteria for inclusion or exclusion of any study and an explicit process for grading the quality of studies. Sometimes, the results of a systematic review are combined numerically, and this is called meta analysis.

Systematic reviews and meta analyses have become popular because they help clinicians consolidate evidence and draw conclusions from a large number of studies in a rigorous way. Systematic review or meta analysis aims to minimise bias (for example, by including published and unpublished reports in every language) and random error (by amassing very large numbers of subjects). Many of the factors we need to consider when reading a systematic review are the same as those outlined for the appraisal of an individual study report. However, there are a few additional points which need to be considered.

The question examined by a systematic review or meta analysis needs to be defined very precisely so that the search for relevant

- Use of faulty comparators
- Use of surrogate end points
- Use of composite end points
- Use of post-hoc or multiple subgroup analyses
- Reporting of small treatment effects
- Reporting and discussion of relative risk reduction rather than absolute risk reduction
- Lack of safety and toxicity data

Fig. 18.2 Clinical trial characteristics which increase the risk of being misled

Example 2: Forest Plot for a Meta Analysis

Meta analysis of unscheduled intravenous infusion among children randomised to reduced osmolarity and standard WHO rehydration solutions. (Reproduced from *BMJ* 2001; 323:81–5 with permission from the BMJ Publishing Group)

Study	Intervention n/N	Control n/N	Odds ratio (95% CI fixed)	Weight %	Odds ratio (95% CI fixed)
Bangladesh 1995a[11]	4/19	5/19		3.0	0.75 (0.17 to 3.36)
Bangladesh 1996a[13*]	0/18	0/18		0.0	Not estimable
CHOICE 2001[14]	34/341	50/334		34.5	0.63 (0.40 to 1.00)
Colombia 2000[15]	7/71	16/69		11.1	0.36 (0.14 to 0.95)
Egypt 1996a[17]	6/45	5/44		3.3	1.20 (0.34 to 4.26)
Egypt 1996b[18]	1/94	8/96		5.9	0.12 (0.01 to 0.97)
India 1984a[19*]	0/22	0/22		0.0	Not estimable
India 2000b[21]	11/88	12/82		8.2	0.83 (0.35 to 2.01)
Mexico 1990a[22]	2/82	7/84		5.1	0.28 (0.06 to 1.37)
Panama 1982[23*]	0/33	0/30		0.0	Not estimable
USA 1982[23]	0/15	1/20		1.0	0.42 (0.02 to 11.03)
WHO 1995a[24]	33/221	43/218		27.9	1.20 (0.43 to 1.18)
Total (95% CI)	98/1049	147/1036		100.0	0.61 (0.47 to 0.81)

x^2=6.52, (df=8), z=3.50

0.01 0.1 1 10 100

Favours treatment Favours control

*No patients required intravenous infusion

Reprinted with permission from BMJ Publishing Group (BMJ, 2001, 323: 81–5)

This systematic review aimed to compare the effectiveness of two rehydration solutions in children admitted to hospital with dehydration and acute diarrhoea. The primary outcome studied was the subsequent need for unscheduled IV infusion. Twelve studies were included and are listed in the left-hand column. The 'squares' indicate the estimated mean odds ratio for each trial, with a pooled result at the bottom. The relative size of the 'square' indicates the relative number of patients in each study (also indicated by the Weight column). The 95% confidence interval (CI) for each study is indicated by the horizontal line extending from either side of the 'square'. Note that the two largest studies have narrow CIs. The vertical line indicates an odds ratio (OR) of 1 which indicates there is no difference between treatments. A value less than 1.0 indicates that the reduced osmolarity solution is better than the WHO rehydration (control) solution in preventing unscheduled IV infusions following admission to hospital. Where the horizontal lines intersect the unity OR line, the observed effect is not significant at the usual 0.05 significance level. This type of figure allows readers to quickly visualise the results of the meta analysis. The pooled results show that reduced osmolarity solutions were associated with fewer unscheduled infusions than the WHO rehydration solution (OR 0.61, 95% CI 0.47–0.81).

articles can be thorough and objective. The search methods should be described in detail so that readers can be assured that the search has been as complete as possible. Apart from searching standard databases such as Medline and Embase, a rigorous search would include hand-searching of journals, conference proceedings, theses and the databanks of pharmaceutical companies.

This is important because negative trials are less likely to be submitted and selected for publication, the so-called '*publication bias*'. The criteria used to include and reject trials must also be explicit. Independent evaluations by more than one individual may be used to confirm study validity and eligibility for inclusion in the systematic review. This gives additional reassurance that the studies that have been included meet the selection criteria.

We then need to look at the results of the systematic review. Are the effects of treatment consistent from study to study? The results of a systematic review are more convincing if the treatment effect in each study is at least in the same direction, even though the degree of efficacy may vary. If there is inconsistency (heterogeneity), the authors should explain why this may have happened (for example, differences in doses or patient characteristics). The results are also strengthened if the authors have used individual patient data rather than summary tables or published reports for their analysis. Most reviews use odds ratios (ORs) or relative risks (RRs) to present their results. These are respectively the odds (chance) and relative risk of an event in a patient in the treatment group relative to that of a patient in the control group. These results are often presented graphically (Example 2).

Critical Appraisal of Cohort Studies

As with RCTs, cohort studies compare outcomes in groups that did and did not receive a drug intervention. Unlike RCTs, they measure outcomes in the real world and can be used to assess whether the efficacy observed in an RCT also occurs in a broader population. They often study large groups of subjects for long periods of time, and are useful for the study of long-term outcomes and rare adverse events.

In cohort studies, allocation to receive a drug intervention is not random as in an RCT, but depends on prescribing patterns, local policy and individual physician choice. This means that these studies are subject to selection bias, where a range of known and unknown factors (confounders) may influence the outcome under study, apart from the intervention itself. A well-conducted cohort study will attempt to minimise this by careful selection of appropriate comparison groups, identification of potential confounders and the use of certain statistical techniques.

When reading a cohort study paper, look for a clear justification for why the two groups were selected and how they were defined. One way of minimising selection bias is to limit inclusion to those with a specific clinical characteristic. However, this restriction will limit the generalisability of the results.

In RCTs, known and unknown confounders can be expected to be evenly distributed between the comparison groups. Cohort studies do not have this safeguard and it is therefore important that investigators identify potential confounders through a detailed literature review, and determine their distribution in the intervention and comparison groups. This is usually presented in the first table of the paper.

Certain confounders (such as exercise, diet, medication adherence) may be difficult to measure, particularly if the study is retrospective and relies on administrative or clinical databases. For example, cohort studies may use records of prescription filling as a surrogate measure of medication adherence. Significance tests such as χ^2 (for dichotomous variables) or *t* tests (for continuous variables) are used to identify imbalances in the distribution of confounders between the groups. However, these tests are sensitive to sample size, and may not be meaningful when used in very large cohort studies.

Regression analysis and stratification are two techniques which are used in cohort studies to reduce confounding. In regression analysis, the outcome of interest is the dependent variable and the potential confounders and intervention are independent variables. Regression analysis estimates the association of each independent variable with the dependent variable after adjusting for the effects of all the other variables. If the outcome is binary (for example, the occurrence of a stroke), a logistic regression model is appropriate, whereas a proportional hazards model would be used if the outcome is timed to an event (such as the time before a stroke occurs).

When assessing the results of regression analysis, you should compare the adjusted and unadjusted estimates of effect. If these differ greatly, it suggests that differences in baseline characteristics have had a substantial effect on the outcome.

Most regression techniques assume a constant relationship between the outcome and intervention in all subjects. In stratification, the study population is divided into subgroups based on characteristics which may be confounders. These groups are more similar with respect to that characteristic and this may give less biased estimates of the intervention outcome. However, the groups may still be imbalanced in other ways and smaller groups mean that the power of the study is reduced.

In cohort studies, a sensitivity analysis may be done to estimate how sensitive the results are to bias due to unmeasured confounders. As with any study, the results of a cohort study need to be considered in the context of other evidence, and the biological plausibility of the results.

Critical Appraisal of Therapeutic Guidelines

Therapeutic guidelines are statements that are formulated to help clinicians choose the most appropriate treatment in specific clinical circumstances. Guidelines may be based on a systematic evaluation of current evidence or may be a statement of recommendations from a panel of selected experts. In the latter case, they are referred to as 'consensus' guidelines. Therapeutic guidelines generally have two distinct parts. The first is a *summary of the evidence* relating to the subject area, and the second is a set of *recommendations and protocols* for applying the evidence to patients.

If you are evaluating therapeutic guidelines, the following are some of the factors to consider when assessing their validity and reliability. Guidelines should be based on high-quality research studies. These should be identified during a comprehensive literature review conducted within the recent past. This may be 12 months for areas where the evidence has changed quickly, but longer periods, say 24–36 months, may be acceptable where new evidence is produced more slowly.

Unlike systematic reviews which tend to be undertaken on topics where there is high-quality evidence (that is, randomised controlled trials), therapeutic guidelines tend to be 'necessity-driven' and use the best available evidence that can be found. This means that they may combine high-quality evidence with evidence of a more uncertain quality. These different 'levels' of evidence should be acknowledged by tagging each recommendation to indicate the strength of evidence upon which it is based. This means that we can identify which recommendations are based on solid evidence and which are more uncertain. In addition, each recommendation should be linked to a specific reference, so readers can track the evidence back to its source.

Having decided that the therapeutic guidelines are valid, you then need to decide how applicable the guidelines are to your patients. Many guidelines are written by groups in the USA or UK, and the majority of included studies will be from non-Indian settings. There may be cultural, economic, legal, geographic, organisational, authoritarian or behavioural barriers to implementing the recommendations in your practice setting. For example, guidelines from Western countries may recommend certain types of drug therapy and monitoring which may place a considerable financial burden on many Indian patients.

What is Evidence-based Medicine?

Health professionals have traditionally used various approaches for making clinical decisions. These include decision-making by anecdote (for example, using a drug to treat a condition because it worked well for a similar patient), by 'press cutting' (for example, using a drug based on the results section of a single published study), based on pharmaceutical company advertising, and based on cost minimisation. These approaches to clinical decision-making are still very common, even though they are not based on sound scientific evidence.

In recent years, evidence-based medicine (EBM) has stimulated interest among health professionals as an alternative approach for clinical decision-making. According to one definition, it is the *"conscientious, explicit and judicious use of current best evidence in making decisions about the care of individual patients"*. This involves several essential steps: converting your information needs into an answerable question, tracking down the best evidence, appraising this evidence critically both for its validity and its usefulness, and integrating the results of your appraisal with your clinical expertise and the needs of your individual patient. From this definition, it can be seen that skills in critical appraisal are essential for the practice of EBM.

A number of developments have made it easier to adopt an EBM approach to clinical practice. These include the publication of systematic reviews and electronic evidence-based journals, and the availability of information technology which has vastly improved our ability to track down available evidence. The Cochrane Library is one of the leading EBM databases. Published articles are entered into the Cochrane databases by members of the Cochrane Collaboration, an international network of researchers who use strict methodological criteria to classify each article.

In many countries, the EBM approach to clinical practice has in turn been accompanied by a gradual change from an authoritarian healthcare culture to one where there is increased emphasis on the ability to access, interpret and apply knowledge. As a result, many pharmacists with critical appraisal skills have been able to participate more fully in clinical decision-making.

Conclusion

Skills in critical appraisal are essential for clinical pharmacy practice. Although initially the concepts and terms may be difficult to understand, perseverance will be rewarded by a greatly enhanced ability to provide high-quality therapeutic advice and drug information. This in turn will lead to greater respect for the pharmacist's advice and opinion on drug therapy. Once skills in critical appraisal have been acquired, they will be used routinely whenever reference is made to the biomedical literature.

Group Exercise: Journal Club

Select a recently published primary research paper that describes an RCT of relevance to your patients. Distribute a copy to each group member, then read the paper individually using the critical appraisal approach described in this chapter. Within a few days, discuss the paper as a group, with the aim of sharing opinions and ideas about each section of the paper. During your discussion, consider the following questions:

Objectives

1. Are the aims of the study summarised clearly and unambiguously?
2. Why do the authors think this study needs to be done?

Methods

3. What type of study design have the investigators chosen? Discuss the important features of this design.
4. Do you think the study design was appropriate for the research question?
5. How relevant are the outcomes for patient prognosis? Do they include measures of morbidity and mortality, or only surrogate outcomes?
6. How were the subjects recruited? Discuss possible bias that may be present as a result.
7. Examine the reasons why some people were excluded from the study. Why was this done?
8. What information was collected about each subject?
9. Is the intervention treatment clearly described and in sufficient detail?
10. Where was the study conducted? Do you think the subjects enrolled in the study are likely to be similar to Indian patients?
11. Who was blinded during the study? Did this include all assessors?
12. Was the study continued for long enough to reliably assess each of the outcomes?

Statistical analysis

13. Was the study done on an intention to treat basis? What does this mean?
14. What types of statistical tests were used? Depending on your knowledge in this area, are these appropriate?
15. If the two groups are of similar size, estimate the p value using the method shown in Fig. 18.1. Is this similar to the p value in the paper?

Results

16. Are there any important baseline differences between the intervention and control groups?
17. Are there any confounding factors which may have influenced the results but which are not accounted for?
18. Are the results for each outcome statistically significant?
19. If the results are statistically significant, do you think they are clinically significant? Have the authors expressed their results in terms of absolute risk reduction or number needed to treat? If this has not been done, try to calculate this.
20. Have the authors presented data on the adverse effects of drug treatment?

Discussion

21. Discuss the limitations of the study.
22. Do you agree with the authors' conclusions about their results?

Other parts of the paper

23. Discuss possible conflicts of interest. Did a drug company sponsor this study? Are the authors connected with this company in any way?

Reaching a conclusion

24. What factors do you need to consider when applying the results of the paper to your own patients?
25. Does the trial have any of the characteristics of potentially misleading trials listed in Fig. 18.2?
26. Do you think this paper should change clinical practice, taking into consideration other relevant literature and clinical experience?

Exercises

Test your understanding: Number needed to treat

1. A six-month randomised trial comparing a new oral anti-inflammatory with inhaled beclomethasone for the prevention of asthma exacerbations found a 50% relative risk reduction with the new drug. There were 145 patients in the beclomethasone group and 165 patients in the new drug group.

   How many patients need to be treated with the new drug for six months to prevent one additional asthma exacerbation?

   a. Cannot be calculated because the p value is not stated
   b. 2 patients for six months
   c. 10 patients for six months
   d. Cannot be calculated because absolute risk reduction is not stated

Answer: The number of patients who need to be treated with the new drug for six months in order to prevent one additional asthma exacerbation is the number needed to treat (NNT). Figures for relative risk reduction alone do not allow us to calculate NNT as the underlying rate of exacerbations in the two groups is not known. Therefore, answers b and c are incorrect. NNT is the inverse of absolute risk reduction but in this example, the absolute number of asthma exacerbations in two groups is unknown, and so NNT cannot be calculated. P values are not used to calculate NNT.

2. In a 12-month study comparing a new drug with placebo for the prevention of myocardial infarction (MI) in patients with a history of coronary heart disease, the incidence of MI was 15% in the placebo group and 10% in the group receiving the new drug.

   Based on these results, how many patients need to be treated with the new drug to prevent one additional MI over 12 months?

   a. 5
   b. 10
   c. 20
   d. 25

Answer: The number of patients who need to be treated with the new drug for 12 months in order to prevent one additional MI is termed the number needed to treat (NNT). A drug with a low NNT is more effective than one with a higher NNT. In this example, the absolute risk reduction (ARR) is 5% or 0.05 (15% minus 10%). The NNT is the inverse of the ARR (1/0.05), which is 20. This means 20 patients with coronary heart disease would need to be treated with the new drug for 12 months in order to prevent one additional MI. Note that the NNT should always specify for how long a drug needs to be taken to achieve the specified benefit.

KEY MESSAGES

- Skills in critical appraisal are essential for clinical pharmacists.
- The main aim of critical appraisal is to assess whether a research paper, in conjunction with other literature and clinical experience, should change clinical practice.
- Many papers published in medical journals have potentially serious methodological flaws.
- The randomised controlled trial is the preferred study design to investigate the efficacy of drug treatment.
- The efficacy of a drug should ideally be measured in terms of clinical end points that are relevant to patients, rather than surrogate end points.
- Statistical significance is not the same as clinical significance.
- Results of drug trials should be expressed in terms of absolute risk reduction or 'number needed to treat'.

Further Reading

Dans AL et al. 1998. How to Decide on the Applicability of Clinical Trial Results to Your Patient *JAMA* 279:545–549.

Glasziou P, Del Mar C and Salisbury J. 2007. *Evidence-Based Practice Workbook*, 2nd ed. Blackwell Publishing.

Greenhalgh T. 2006. *How to Read a Paper: The Basics of Evidence Based Medicine*, 3rd ed. Wiley-Blackwell. *(Highly recommended. Relevant chapters in this book were published as a series of articles in the BMJ in 1997, and may be easier to access.)*

Hollis S and Campbell F. 1999. What is meant by intention to treat analysis? Survey of published randomised controlled trials. *BMJ* 19:670–4.

Gaddis ML and Gaddis GM. 1990. Introduction to biostatistics: Parts 1–6. *Annals of Emergency Medicine* 19:86–89,309–315,591–597,820–825, 1054–1059, 1462–1468.

Scott IA and Greenberg PB. 2005. Cautionary tales in the clinical interpretation of therapeutic trial reports. *Internal Medicine Journal* 35:611–621.

Strauss SE et al. 2005. *Evidence-based Medicine: How to Practice and Teach EBM*, 3rd ed. Churchill Livingstone.

Websites of Interest

University of Sheffield (provides online courses in critical appraisal)
(http://www.shef.ac.uk/scharr/ir/units/critapp)

Centre for Evidence-Based Medicine in Toronto, Canada (useful information on practising and teaching EBM, also has statistics calculators).
(http://www.cebm.utoronto.ca)

Supercourse, WHO Collaborating Centre University, Pittsburgh (An excellent library of lectures from around the world on many areas of epidemiology, including study design and critical appraisal)
(http://www.pitt.edu/~super1)

An online revised version of **Statistics at Square One**, a best-selling statistical textbook in the UK.
(http://bmj.com/collections/statsbk/index.shtml)

The Cochrane Collaboration
(http://www.cochrane.org)

American College of Physicians Journal Club
(http://www.acponline.org/search)

Turning Research into Practice
(http://www.tripdatabase.com)

19
Drug Information

M Ramesh and Graeme M Vernon

Learning Objectives

Upon completion of this chapter, the reader should be able to:

- Describe the scope of drug information practice and its contribution to patient care
- List the skills required to provide drug information advice to healthcare professionals
- Explain the nature of drug information resources
- State the basic principles of indexing and searching computerised databases
- Describe a systematic approach to answering drug information enquiries
- Understand the importance of identifying and interpreting evidence to support clinical decisions

Introduction

Providing drug information is a fundamental responsibility of all pharmacists irrespective of the practice setting. The pharmacy profession has traditionally been seen as suppliers of medicines, but this function will be of limited benefit and can cause adverse outcomes in the absence of appropriate information support. Drug information means providing clinically relevant information on any aspect of drug use relating to individual patients, or general information on how best to use drugs for populations.

Pharmacists have a unique range of knowledge and skills which are required for drug information practice. These include knowledge of pharmaceutics, pharmacology, pharmacokinetics and pharmacotherapy. All of these are required to optimise the use of drugs in the treatment and prevention of disease. Drug information can be challenging but also exciting. It requires much of the knowledge that pharmacists acquire as students and allows them to apply these skills to improve health outcomes.

Pharmacists provide information across the spectrum of clinical practice. Providing concise information to patients during counselling is an important aspect of pharmaceutical care. Pharmacists also often provide basic drug information to other health professionals in the course of their clinical activities. Pharmacists who specialise in drug information perform similar functions but they have access to more resources and have greater opportunities to refine their skills. Hence, they can provide greater depth to the analysis, interpretation and response, and they can do this more efficiently.

They should also understand the quality of the evidence base used to support a conclusion and be aware of information resources which may be relevant but not accessible at the time a recommendation is required in clinical practice. Providing a drug information service is a professional activity which carries the same responsibilities as direct patient care. Information provided to support policy decisions can affect many people (hospital, regional or national populations) and poor-quality information can cause as much damage to public health as inadequate quality control in pharmaceutical manufacturing.

The term '*drug information service*' can be applied to any activity where information about drug use is transferred, and includes patient-related aspects of pharmaceutical care. A '*drug information centre*' is an area where pharmacists (or other health professionals) specialise in providing information to health professionals or the public. The unique aspect of the drug information centre is that it draws together a range of information resources and makes these accessible to people who know how to make the best use of them.

Drug information centres vary in size according to the volume of requests. A centre can be large (national or regional) and focus solely on providing information, or be incorporated into clinical service units with patient care functions. Most are operated by pharmacists but some also use the services of librarians and medical specialists (usually clinical pharmacologists). What makes it a 'centre' is the concentration of resources and trained professionals which together have a greater potential value than if the same resources were disseminated and used by individuals in multiple locations.

The term '*medicines information*' can be used to avoid confusion with services which are limited to problems relating to drugs of abuse. Medicines information has been adopted as the preferred description in the United Kingdom but is used less frequently in other countries where English is a major language. In some languages, 'drugs' and 'medicines' are not distinguished with specific words, so the potential difference in meaning can be lost in translation.

Drug information centres were first established in the USA in the early 1960s and developed in parallel with clinical pharmacy services. Centres are usually located in hospitals or support clinical training programmes, and exist in most countries which have well developed clinical pharmacy services. There has been limited momentum in establishing drug information centres in developing countries in conjunction with patient care services.

Drug information centres can limit their services to health professionals but some also offer a service to the public. There are also centres which specialise in information for the public. The training and skills required for a public-focused service differ from those for health professionals, and can be more challenging. A drug information centre can also contribute to pharmacovigilance (adverse drug reaction reporting), drug use reviews, health education programmes and clinical research. Poison information services can be co-located with drug information services, but specific training and resources are required to provide poison information to health professionals and the public.

The internet has created a means of remote access for reference sources and provides additional means of interacting with drug information services. Although individual clinicians (and the public) can now access a wider variety of drug information sources, this information may not be of high quality and requires careful interpretation. Drug information centres are more likely to be able to afford the cost of high-quality resources. Using their knowledge of drugs, pharmacists can help place the available information within the context of all relevant information prior to drawing conclusions.

At the most basic level, a drug information service can consist of a small selection of textbooks, access to the internet and a selection of the most relevant medical and pharmaceutical journals. Usually, one pharmacist will be responsible for maintaining the resources, recording requests and responses, and for quality assurance. This person will require specific training in literature searching and critical analysis, and will have sufficient clinical experience to interpret information for patient care. The most valuable resources will depend on the range of patient care provided but could include those listed in Table 19.1.

Drug Information Resources

Information about drugs is available in a wide range of formats, media types and levels of quality. The internet has enlarged the scope of information available to much of the world's population and has vastly

Table 19.1 Suggested resources for a basic drug information service

AHFS Drug Information (American Society of Health-System Pharmacists, USA)
Martindale: The Complete Drug Reference (Pharmaceutical Press, UK)
Goodman and Gilman's The Pharmacological Basis of Therapeutics (McGraw-Hill, USA)
British National Formulary (Pharmaceutical Press, UK) or Australian Medicines Handbook (AMH, Australia)
Meyler's Side Effects of Drugs (Elsevier, The Netherlands)
Drug Prescribing in Renal Failure (American College of Physicians, USA)
British National Formulary for Children (Pharmaceutical Press, UK)
Drugs in Pregnancy and Lactation, (Lippincott, USA)
Handbook of Injectable Drugs (American Society of Health-System Pharmacists, USA)
Iowa Drug Information Service (The University of Iowa, USA)
Drugdex (included in Micromedex Healthcare Series, Thomson Reuters, USA)

improved access to information for health professionals. However, the range of quality is as varied as the volume of information available. Medical research is often reported in the media before there is an opportunity for critical analysis and before the new information can be placed in a clinical perspective. Information on drugs approved and marketed in one country is now available globally, and this provides a means of indirect advertising and pressure for public access to new drugs.

There is often a tendency to seek information which is available without charge on the internet. While it is important for drug information pharmacists to be aware of the nature of free drug information, they should have access to sources which have acceptable standards of quality and reliability. They should also respect the intellectual property rights of the authors and publishers. There are provisions within the copyright laws which allow access to material required for research or private study, but this does not allow further distribution without permission.

Information sources have traditionally been categorised as primary, secondary or tertiary, according to the nature of the content and speed of publication. However, the most important point is to distinguish primary sources (original reports) from all other sources (reviews). Electronic formats, and ready access to updates, have blurred the divisions previously applied to secondary and tertiary sources.

Primary Resources

Primary literature describes unique experiences which change the world in terms of available knowledge. Primary reports include the results of research at all levels (from molecular science to controlled clinical trials) and also clinical experience in the form of individual responses to drugs and small case series. Primary literature is published principally in scientific journals in the form of research results, concise reports and letters to the editor. Adverse drug reaction reports are an example of primary literature and these can be published in journals or contributed to pharmacovigilance centres.

Primary literature can be seen as the building block on which medical science (and therefore clinical practice) is based. It is essential to understand its nature and to be able to critically analyse its content using the full text of reports. It is important to understand that clinical research needs to be replicated at different sites and in relevant populations before it is accepted as the basis for changes in standards of care. Initial reports of adverse reactions may (or may not) be a signal for serious concern and potentially for withdrawal of a drug from use on safety grounds. Primary literature provides a 'first look' at how clinical practice may evolve but it must be constantly monitored and interpreted carefully.

Secondary Resources

Secondary sources consist of reviews of primary reports. Journals often publish a mixture of primary and secondary reports but there are also journals which are devoted to reviews of previously published material. Reviews can be informal, often by a single author recognised as a specialist in the field. These provide a personal perspective of the literature and can include comments on how the author might apply the information in practice. This type of report is sometimes called a 'narrative review' and this term may appear in the title to distinguish it from a more formal analysis, referred to as a 'systematic review'.

In a *systematic review*, the authors (usually a team) use a rigorous (and defined) method to search for all relevant information (including unpublished studies) and select those studies which meet criteria for scientific quality. The selected studies are then analysed and conclusions drawn. In many cases, the results of a number of studies are merged using a process called '*meta-analysis*'. This process aims to create the equivalent of one large study with greater statistical power than the separate studies.

There are a number of electronic knowledge systems which can be considered as secondary sources of information. These include Drugdex (Micromedex, USA) and International Pharmaceutical Abstracts (American Society of Health-System Pharmacists, USA). These systems are electronic, include summaries of the primary reports and are updated regularly.

Secondary sources provide a condensed and refined view of primary data and are often used in drug information practice to provide rapid responses to clinical questions. However, published reviews may not include recent primary reports, and narrative reviews may reflect the authors' clinical perspective and limited access to the relevant information.

Tertiary Resources

Tertiary resources are summaries of the primary and secondary published literature. Printed textbooks are the main example and these are characterised by a slow rate of revision compared to secondary sources. Although they are revised less frequently, these texts tend to be more comprehensive and should undergo a more thorough review and editing process than secondary sources. Many major textbooks are now published electronically as well as in print, so sections can be updated progressively rather than waiting for a complete revision at the time of printing (usually every 3–5 years).

In drug information practice, a tertiary text will usually be consulted first as a quick reference and, if necessary, secondary and primary sources are then checked for a more complete response.

Journals

Most of the important research and clinical experience is published in scientific journals (or 'periodicals'). Because of the large volume of information, there is continuing effort to improve our ability to locate the most relevant information and access the full text of the documents. Most journals have to rely on subscriptions or advertising to support the cost of accurately transmitting information to readers. However, there is growing awareness of the need to improve access to information where it is most needed. This includes an increasing number of open-access journals which are usually only published electronically (to minimise costs).

Most of the research and review articles published in reputable journals have undergone peer review. This process helps the journal editors select material which is of an acceptable standard and to improve the quality of how the information is presented to readers. This usually involves anonymous reviews from experts in the field who advise on whether the material warrants publication and how it could be improved with additional details, mode of presentation or interpretation of the results. Peer review is generally accepted as the best approach to maintaining the quality of scientific publications but it can only provide a limited perspective (usually from a few individuals). Sometimes, incorrect information is published (and later corrected) or incorrect information is deliberately submitted for publication (scientific fraud) and it is not detected by the editors or the peer review process.

All clinical trials are performed at a particular time and under specific conditions so we cannot necessarily extrapolate the results to our patient population. Even the best research is subject to random variation and therefore a single study is not sufficient to prove a point. We should look for more than one source of research and opinion before implementing changes in practice.

Bibliographic Databases

These services are sometimes called *indexing and abstracting services* because they provide a copy of the published abstract of primary and secondary reports, together with an indexed database to help locate relevant reports. The Iowa Drug Information Service (IDIS) also includes the full text of articles from around 200 medical and pharmaceutical journals. Medline and Embase are the largest and most frequently used bibliographic databases.

Medline is produced by the US National Library of Medicine and uses US conventions for indexing and journal coverage. It is available free of charge in the form of PubMed and has traditionally been used in medical and educational institutions. Embase has a European perspective and has more comprehensive indexing (including drug terms) than Medline. However, Embase is only available by subscription. These databases are used to locate published literature (primary and secondary) and the indexing allows searches to be broad or focused. The databases can directly link to the full text of journal articles but only some full-text articles will be available free of charge.

Searching Computerised Databases

Journal articles within databases are labelled with a range of information which characterises each article and allows users to locate relevant articles. Some of the indexing relates to publishing details and is highly predictable. This includes the title (and authors' abstract, if available), the authors' names, their institution, the journal name and specifics about how and where it was published. In addition to these basic details, indexing terms are usually added by the database publisher to help users locate useful material. In general, these terms can be called '*keywords*' but they are most useful when they are selected from a controlled and structured list. In Medline, these are called Medical Subject Headings (MeSH). The main advantage of having a controlled list of headings is that there should be only one term for each concept. This creates a standard term for each disease and drug (regardless of variations in spelling) but means that new or less important concepts may not have a subject heading. In this case, the indexer will select the closest term (usually a more general term) to describe a concept.

Searches for groups of related terms are linked together in '*trees*'. The tree structure lists general terms at the top with '*branches*' for groups of related terms, with the most specific terms at the end of the branch. We can search for specific terms or groups of terms at any level of the tree. Searching for related terms within a hierarchical list of headings is called an '*explosion*', and the process provides considerable power and flexibility for the user.

In some databases (including Medline and Embase), subheadings can be applied by the indexer to modify the meaning of the selected headings. For example, the subheading of 'adverse effects' can be applied to a drug name heading to indicate that, in that article, the drug has been associated with an adverse outcome. Similarly, a disease heading given a subheading of 'drug therapy' helps users locate articles that deal with the use of drugs to treat that disease. Limits can also be applied to a search so that the output can be restricted to the subjects (for example, human), language (for example, English) or type of publication (for example, review, letter).

It is usually necessary to combine two or more concepts to provide a focused search. This can be done with the Boolean operators 'AND', 'OR' and 'NOT'. We use OR to expand the scope of our search; for example, 'liver diseases' OR 'bile duct diseases' if we are interested in all aspects of hepato-biliary disease. We could then combine this broad concept with a group of drugs that may be associated with those diseases. That is:

liver diseases OR bile duct diseases
AND
non-steroidal anti-inflammatory drugs

This will create a much smaller set of articles which have been indexed with a drug term within our definition of non-steroidal anti-inflammatory drugs (NSAIDs) and any one disease term from either the 'liver' or 'bile duct' group. In practice, these three terms would be exploded to include all the specific drugs and diseases within the three groups. We could also apply subheadings to refine the search; for example, a subheading of 'adverse effects' could be applied to the NSAID terms to specify that we are interested in articles where the NSAID may have caused liver disease. However, in this case, the subheading will not have a great effect as NSAIDs are not used to *treat* liver disease. The 'NOT' operator is rarely used as it can exclude articles which have relevant headings as well as the heading that we exclude. In our example above, we could exclude articles about aspirin-induced Reye's syndrome by applying the heading for this specific disease as a 'NOT' within our definition of the diseases of interest, or after combining the disease and drug terms.

Medline is available in many formats including the open-access version called PubMed. This format defaults to a simplified search process which creates reasonable quality searches based on simple words or phrases provided by the user. A similar approach is used by other vendors of the Medline database. These automatic searches can produce impressive results in a short period of time; however, it is best to understand the structure and potential of the database rather than rely on the 'autopilot' approach. Both have their place in practice but it is necessary to understand how automated search works and appreciate its limitations.

Other Sources of Drug Information

The internet has enhaced our access to information from reputable organisations.

National libraries offer reliable information and links to useful sites, including open-access journals. Many clinical guidelines and drug assessments are not indexed in bibliographical databases but can be located on recognised sites or using search engines which focus on reputable sources of information. Examples of specific sites include:

- National Institute for Health and Clinical Excellence, UK (www.nice.org.uk)
- National Prescribing Centre, UK (www.npc.co.uk)
- National Prescribing Service, Australia (www.nps.org.au)
- Canadian Agency for Drugs and Technologies in Health (www.cadth.ca)

Search tools for clinical guidelines include:

- National Guideline Clearinghouse, USA (www.guidelines.gov)
- National Library for Health, UK (www.library.nhs.uk).

Product information is available for approved drugs in many countries including:

- DailyMed, USA (dailymed.nlm.nih.gov/dailymed)
- European Medicines Agency (www.emea.europa.eu)
- Medicines.org.uk, UK (www.medicines.org.uk).

Clinical questions often arise as media reports or news items on internet services. This means that the questions are publicly raised before there is an opportunity to consider all the data and determine whether the new information warrants a change to clinical practice. Retrospective analysis of patients' health records is becoming increasingly easier due to improvements in technology and many questions arise from the exploration of large populations rather than prospective controlled trials. Analysing databases for outcomes can identify potential problems with a low incidence but it does not provide direct evidence of cause and effect, and this can make it difficult to interpret and apply these data for individual patients.

Drug information is about understanding all available information resources, selecting and using the most useful, and being able to retrieve and interpret that information in a clinical or public health context.

Answering Drug Information Questions

Drug information enquiries in clinical practice often reflect circumstances which are unusual in some way, and beyond the scope of average patients and situations. Prescribers will be familiar with established drugs but may ask about new drugs, new or unusual adverse effects, or how to manage therapy in a patient with interacting drugs or complications such as renal or liver disease.

In many cases, these questions are beyond the scope of the product information. However, this is not surprising because the product information summarises the experience of small populations in clinical trials. In clinical practice, we encounter more complicated patients (who would have been excluded from clinical trials) and may need to use drugs beyond the approved indications and dosage. The product information is also unlikely to include recent research into how a drug can be used or recent adverse effects which may preclude its use.

The nature of enquiries will depend on the scope of the drug information service.

However, a general clinical service is likely to be asked about efficacy, therapeutic strategies, dosage and administration, adverse reactions, interactions, use in paediatrics and the elderly, and safety during pregnancy and breastfeeding. It is often necessary to seek further details from the enquirer in order to provide a meaningful response. However, systematic questioning for unnecessary detail will not be appreciated.

Adopting a stepwise approach may reduce literature search time, avoid overlooking significant information and help the enquirer understand the search strategy. The basic steps to approaching drug information enquiries are summarised below. A model recording form is shown in Fig. 19.1.

Requester's details: Identify the enquirer and obtain sufficient contact details. For regular clients, these details should be recorded in a database to facilitate future enquiries.Gauge the depth of response required. Experienced clinicians are likely to prefer concise factual information whereas junior staff may also seek guidance on clinical management. A deadline for a response should always be established. For clinical questions, this often relates to imperatives for patient movement, timing of procedures and staff rosters. If a specific deadline is not offered then an expected response time should be provided. This can be extended later to adequately address the issue; however, the enquirer can be advised and a revised deadline negotiated.

Background information: Further details can be sought from the enquirer but this should focus on the question at hand and not attempt to cover all the clinical details. This is a difficult step and clinical pharmacy experience is needed to maximise the outcome of this initial exchange of information. It may be necessary to obtain additional information such as age, other medical conditions, renal and liver function, other relevant drugs (including traditional medicines), history of allergic reactions and stage of pregnancy.

Refine and categorise the question: Having accepted the enquiry, it may be necessary to understand some aspects of the question before seeking an answer. For pharmacists, this applies particularly to medical terminology and aspects of disease and pathology. This information may help to refine the question and to estimate the time required to achieve an acceptable response.

This is important because all searches must be conducted within the constraints of available resources and the required deadline. It is rarely possible to create a perfect answer, and beyond a reasonable point, there is a diminishing return in terms of increased quality or confidence in the response. For clinical purposes, a concise and rapid response will be preferred to one which is protracted and delayed. Of course, the reverse is true for research projects.

Almost all drug information requests can be categorised by their nature and this will dictate the most efficient and rewarding strategy. Selecting the resources most likely to contain the required information can save time and also increase the accuracy of the response. Search patterns can be used as a guide to the best approach for different types of questions. This is particularly helpful in training new drug information pharmacists. Experienced staff are less likely to apply a formal search pattern but will automatically follow an established process for specific types of questions.

Develop a strategy and conduct a search: Consider all the available information

Figure 19.1 Model recording form

DRUG INFORMATION REQUEST | Enquiry number:

Enquirer (name): | Phone/fax:

Address: | Email:

Profession:

Pharmacist: ☐ Hospital ☐ Community ☐ Other

Doctor: ☐ Hospital ☐ Community ☐ Other

Nurse: ☐ Hospital ☐ Community ☐ Other

Other HCP:____________

Received by

☐ Telephone ☐ Email ☐ Mail

☐ In person ☐ Other

Received by (name): | Date/time received:

Reply required by (date/time): | Patient related?: yes/no

Purpose of enquiry: Individual patient care / update knowledge /others | Gender: male/female

Renal / hepatic status: | Age: Weight:

Enquiry details:

Enquiry type:

☐ Adverse reaction / toxicity

☐ Availability/identity/cost

☐ Dose/administration

☐ Evaluation

☐ Interaction

☐ Pharmacokinetic

☐ Pharmaceutical

☐ Pregnancy/lactation

☐ Therapeutic strategy

☐ Other

Background (other drugs and/or medical conditions, stage of pregnancy, breastfeeding): | Relevant laboratory results

Resources used:

☐ AHFS Drug Information	☐ Drug Interaction Facts	☐ Product information
☐ British National Formulary (BNF)	☐ Goodman and Gilman	☐ Meyler's Side Effects of Drugs
☐ BNF for Children	☐ Handbook of Injectable Drugs	☐ Reference texts (other)
☐ Clinical advice	☐ Iowa Drug Information Service	☐ Stockley's Drug Interactions
☐ Drug Prescribing in Renal Failure	☐ Martindale	☐ Therapeutic Guidelines
☐ Drugdex	☐ Medline	☐ Websites
☐ Drugs in Pregnancy and Lactation	☐ Pharmaceutical manufacturer	☐ Other

Reply given by (name):	Form of reply: ☐ Written ☐ Verbal ☐ Phone ☐ Email ☐ Fax ☐ Mail
Date/time:	Time spent: (min.) Deadline met? yes/no

Keywords (for indexing):

Reply (referenced)

Outcomes

Enquirer's feedback:

Patient outcome:

Quality assurance:

resources and prioritise them based on the probability of locating the required information. In many cases, beginning the search with tertiary sources (textbooks) and then progressing to secondary literature will provide an adequate answer, and there will be no need to attempt a literature search.

In addition to electronic and printed resources, it may be possible to seek an opinion from a more experienced colleague or specialist. It may also be necessary to apply first principles; for example, the kinetics of a drug in renal impairment may not have been studied but can be predicted based on its chemistry and the nature of the renal replacement therapy (dialysis or haemofiltration).

Record the resources used and a summary of the information derived. However, only the most relevant references need be documented in the actual reply.

Interpret data: The information retrieved must be critically evaluated within the context of the enquiry. It is important to consider consistency of information between various references and whether clinical research is relevant to your population or a specific patient. Where possible, the full text of published reports should be consulted as it is often the details, such as how the patients were selected for a trial, how the drug was given, and limitations of the study (noted in the discussion), which will help with interpretation for specific enquiries.

Absolute answers are rare in drug information, and as a drug information pharmacist you may be the last resort for a person seeking an answer. Often there is limited data and conflicting research or opinions and this lack of certainty must be summarised and included in a response. However, clinical decisions still have to be made and you may be required to advise on patient care in an environment with limited evidence.

Formulate and provide a response: Answers should be derived only after critically analysing the available information obtained from a comprehensive search. It is also important to provide a formulated response to the enquirer in a timely manner. All responses should be documented with the minimum detail necessary to justify the response. Even rapid verbal responses should include the resources used as well as the question and response. The question should be restated to confirm that it has been correctly interpreted. Clinicians prefer direct and concise replies but this does not mean that all the necessary detail should not be recorded and referenced within the drug information service. Often, additional (sometimes predictable) questions are raised when providing a response, so extra detail is handy if this occurs.

If a written response is provided, state the answer first and then justify it with the details. Do not write a paper which arrives at a well-reasoned conclusion at the end. All written responses should be based on a template which includes the contact details of your service as well as the question (as you have interpreted it).

If responding by telephone, document the main points you need to state before making the call. For urgent responses, a detailed record can get completed later but it is easy to be sidetracked during telephone conversations and you must remember to convey all of your essential points during the discussion. Restate the question at the beginning of the conversation as this allows the enquirer to focus on the subject and to confirm that you have correctly interpreted it.

Follow-up and document the outcome: Try to determine the consequences of your advice and any patient outcomes. This may only be possible in a hospital or clinic but it is critical to developing skills in drug information. Advice provided should be recorded in at least one mode of documentation (log book, paper worksheet, computer programme). While drug information pharmacists have access to many skills and information resources, they often lack feedback and the opportunity to learn from clinical experience. Practising clinical pharmacists have the advantage that they receive continuous education based on the response of their patients to interventions. Drug information services which are located within patient care areas are more likely to receive this important type of feedback through clients and colleagues. Feedback can also be sought by email, written requests or by the telephone. Where possible, include outcomes as a part of the enquiry record. If enquiry records are indexed, this information can be retrieved to help with future responses.

Quality assurance: Establishing a process for quality assurance in drug information is difficult because the service may be considered as the highest authority to those seeking guidance. However, there is no reason why drug information pharmacists cannot learn to improve their techniques and efficiency, and it is important to demonstrate that the service endeavours to maintain and improve its quality. The quality assurance programme is an integral part of a drug information service as it provides opportunities to improve and to provide guidelines for future development.

Quality assurance can be assessed in terms of resources and operating procedures. It is necessary to maintain up-to-date references and search strategies. This is best done by regular comparison to similar services and accepted standards.

Output is best assessed within the service and by external peer review. Within the service, there will be time for many responses to be checked by a colleague prior to making the final response. It will generally not be possible to arrange for peer review of all responses but routine random samples of enquiries can be assessed in this way. It may be possible to have a sample of enquiries considered by drug information pharmacists or clinical pharmacists from another site, and where possible, medical staff can contribute to the assessment. Although only a proportion of the workload can be considered in this way (due to time constraints), it is important that all enquiries are subject to random selection for review. General assessment of the service can also be sought from users through periodic circulation of feedback questionnaires.

Conclusion

Drug information is a specialty within the field of clinical pharmacy. A drug information pharmacist has access to the resources and skills required to make the best use of available knowledge. A drug information service draws together a wide range of information resources, and the knowledge and experience of a specialist pharmacist makes the overall service more valuable than its individual components. The value of drug therapy can be optimised only if we base our practice on all the available evidence and translate this knowledge into patient care.

Practice Scenario 1

You are a clinical pharmacist responsible for the drug information service in your hospital. One of the resident doctors asks you for advice regarding a 34-year-old male who has developed thrombocytopaenia. The patient has been taking ranitidine as maintenance treatment of gastro-oesophageal reflux and was admitted to hospital with severe pain in his left leg. He was diagnosed with deep vein thrombosis (DVT) and started on subcutaneous heparin 15,000 units every 12 hours. Six days after starting heparin, his platelet count was noted to be below the normal range of 150–450 x 10^3/mcl (150–450 x 10^9/l). Daily platelet counts were ordered and now, after three days, showed a substantial decline to 76.

Step 1: Requester's details

The first step is to understand the nature of the enquirer and the urgency of the enquiry. In this case, the doctor is the vascular surgery resident and has been asked to investigate possible drug causes by her consultant who is keen to continue therapy for the leg thrombosis. You agree to provide a response by telephone by the end of that afternoon.

Step 2: Background information

You arrange for a clinical pharmacist to obtain further details from the medical records on the ward. You are informed that the patient's only other medical problem is the reflux disease (which was diagnosed six months ago), but he has a family history of thrombosis and his father died from a 'clot in the lung'. His reflux was initially treated with 4 weeks of omeprazole 20 mg daily and has been well controlled with his current ranitidine dose, and he does not take any other medication. On admission, his platelet count was 410 and heparin was started immediately after the diagnosis of DVT (by ultrasonography). Subsequent platelet counts on Days 3–9 were 293, 287, 305, 292, 175, 138 and 76 x 10^3/mcl. There is no evidence of bleeding and no further symptoms of thrombosis. A blood sample has been sent to an external laboratory to test for heparin-induced thrombocytopaenia (HIT) but the result may take up to a week.

Step 3: Refine and categorise the question

Assuming this is drug-induced, there are two questions: Has ranitidine or heparin caused the thrombocytopaenia, and should there be a change in therapy? Therefore, the enquiry can be classified as an adverse drug reaction question and a therapeutic strategy question. Given the timing of the drug exposure, your clinical experience suggests that heparin would be more likely to be the cause, and if so, a change of anti-coagulant may be required. Therefore, you decide to check both drugs for evidence of causing thrombocytopaenia and prepare to offer advice on subsequent therapy if heparin needs to be replaced.

Step 4: Develop a strategy and conduct a search

The product information for both ranitidine and heparin confirms that both drugs can cause thrombocytopaenia but does not provide details of severity or time to onset. The text, *AHFS Drug Information*, confirms that ranitidine can cause thrombocytopaenia and that it is usually reversible. AHFS also indicates that heparin-induced thrombocytopaenia can be mild and transient, or more severe with an average onset of 5–9 days. It quotes recommendations for monitoring and management based on guidelines published by the American College of Chest Physicians.

You conduct a PubMed search using the appropriate headings for ranitidine and thrombocytopaenia, and a more focused search for reviews of the management of HIT. There are a number of case reports implicating ranitidine with thrombocytopaenia but apparently no evidence for a late-onset effect. Recent reviews of HIT include one by local authors (*J Assoc Physicians India* 2008; 56:622–7) and the US guidelines cited in *AHFS Drug Information*. The full text of these recommendations is located on National Guideline Clearinghouse, and a search of the NHS Evidence locates the full text of a review of management (*Br J Haematol* 2006; 133:259–69).

Step 5: Interpret data

Ranitidine is unlikely to have caused the thrombocytopaenia, given the duration of exposure and the rapid and substantial decline in platelets. Although it is not possible to access all the case reports, the widespread use of ranitidine suggests that acquiring this information will probably not change our view and may delay appropriate management of HIT. Current reviews of HIT emphasise the high risk of venous and arterial thrombosis associated with this condition and recommend an immediate change from heparin to a non-heparin anti-thrombotic. Low–molecular weight heparins have an unacceptable risk of cross-reactivity with heparin and warfarin should only be reinstated when platelets have returned to normal because it can increase the risk of venous ischaemia. The best option is likely to be danaparoid (a heparinoid), preferably given as an intravenous infusion with monitoring of its effects. Other options include the direct thrombin inhibitors lepirudin and argatroban, but these are less likely to be readily available.

Step 6: Formulate and provide a response

By mid-afternoon, you have collected enough information to advise the doctor that HIT is most likely and that the thrombotic consequences could be severe especially given this patient's family history of thrombotic disease. Urgent advice should be sought from a haematology specialist. Danaparoid is likely to be the best therapeutic option.

You provide copies of the two guidelines, together with a copy of the product information for danaparoid, and offer to provide details of other anti-coagulants if required.

Step 7: Follow-up and document the outcome

After providing your response, you document the details for an adverse drug reaction report. A supply of danaparoid was obtained and an infusion started that evening. The patient's platelets gradually returned to normal over the course of one week and he had no further thrombotic events, although there were some minor bleeding episodes. He was transferred to warfarin and the danaparoid stopped after his INR was stable (after three days).

The patient's outcome is documented in your drug information record and added to the adverse reaction report. Prior to discharge, the patient is provided with an alert card so that he can inform future health carers of this problem.

Practice Scenario 2

You are responsible for a drug information service in a major hospital and you receive a telephone call from a cardiologist who is concerned that proton pump inhibitors reduce the anti-thrombotic effects of clopidogrel. He read this in a news report on the internet and is concerned because clopidogrel is given to reduce the chance of a subsequent myocardial infarction.

Step 1: Requester's details

In this case, the enquirer is a cardiac specialist and the question does not relate to a specific patient but he is keen to resolve the issue as it may affect the outcomes of his patients in general. You agree to respond by telephone before he leaves for a conference in three days. He also provides an email address for you to forward any additional information.

Step 2: Background information

The enquirer often prescribes omeprazole to reduce the risk of gastric bleeding in patients who need both aspirin and clopidogrel for 12 months after coronary stents. He consulted the product information for clopidogrel but there were no warnings about concurrent use with inhibitors of gastric acid.

Step 3: Refine and categorise the question

This is an interaction question. Given that these drugs have been used for many years, there may be recent evidence to indicate adverse outcomes or a pharmacological basis for an interaction. If there is a clinically significant interaction, the enquirer will probably want to know how it occurs and if it would be the same for proton pump inhibitors other than omeprazole. He may also be interested in other anti-thrombotics with the same efficacy as clopidogrel which could avoid such problems.

Step 4: Develop a strategy and conduct a search

Your drug interaction search strategy includes product information, Medscape Drug Interaction Checker and a literature search. Given that this was encountered as a news item, you also decide to check the US Food and Drug Administration website for recent alerts.

There is no interaction listed in the clopidogrel product information (August 2008); however, the omeprazole product information indicates that it is mainly metabolised via the hepatic cytochrome P450 system (CYP2C19) and may be expected to interact with the metabolism of other drugs metabolised by this enzyme; it does not specify if this would increase or decrease the metabolism of the other drugs. The product information for clopidogrel indicates that it is extensively converted to an 'inactive' metabolite but provides no useful details.

The Medscape Drug Interaction Checker reports a moderate interaction between clopidogrel and 'selected proton pump inhibitors' and the risk to the patient should be assessed and action taken as needed. This assessment was based on a number of published reports. In healthy subjects, omeprazole and lansoprazole decreased the effects of clopidogrel on platelets. A retrospective review of patients who had received coronary stents indicated that a proton pump inhibitor may have increased the risk of a major cardiovascular event; however, this was not apparent in another retrospective review. In another study, esomeprazole and pantoprazole had no effects on platelet response to clopidogrel. This was supported by a further retrospective review which indicated that a proton pump inhibitor other than pantoprazole could have increased the risk of a subsequent myocardial infarction. The Medscape review also quoted an FDA early communication about an ongoing safety review of clopidogrel (26 January 2009) which notes a pharmacological basis for an interaction and a recommendation that healthcare providers 're-evaluate the need for starting or continuing' a proton pump inhibitor in patients taking clopidogrel. No further updates from the FDA were located at the time of the enquiry.

A search of PubMed (using the MeSH heading for proton pump inhibitors combined with 'clopidogrel') located a more recently published retrospective study which indicated the possibility that clopidogrel's efficacy could be reduced if taken with proton pump inhibitors (Ho et al. 2009. *JAMA* 301:937–44). A further study comparing the platelet aggregation of clopidogrel after omeprazole, pantoprazole or esomeprazole was also located. This confirmed the effect of omeprazole in attenuating platelet aggregation but not pantoprazole or esomeprazole (Sibbing D et al. 2009. *Thromb Haemost* 101:714–9).

Within Medline, clopidogrel has a pharmacological action heading of 'platelet aggregation inhibitor' and a search for this as a major heading (linked to a subheading of 'therapeutic use') located several reports of a new drug (prasugrel) which could have similar uses to clopidogrel but be less likely to be affected by metabolic interactions. Prasugrel has been approved for use in Europe and the product information indicates that its conversion to an active form does not depend on a single enzyme (as is the case with clopidogrel).

Step 5: Interpret data

Clopidogrel is a 'prodrug' which requires conversion to its active form in the liver by the action of several enzymes including CYP2C19. This pharmacological profile is not well described in the product information because the data was not available at the time of registration. Subsequent studies have shown that drugs which inhibit this enzyme can reduce the amount of the active form available to inhibit platelet aggregation and therefore to reduce the risk of arterial thrombosis. These concerns led to retrospective reviews of data from large groups of patients who had taken clopidogrel, and some of these studies indicated that taking a proton pump inhibitor was associated with a higher risk of thrombosis. These studies are indirect evidence and it is difficult to determine whether these apparent decreases in efficacy would be clinically significant for an individual patient, bearing in mind that not taking a proton pump inhibitor is likely to increase the risk of serious gastric bleeding (particularly if aspirin is also required). The retrospective studies do not differentiate between proton pump inhibitors but there is limited evidence that pantoprazole and esomeprazole may not cause this interaction.

Step 6: Formulate and provide a response

Based on the available data, there is concern that clopidogrel may be less effective if taken concurrently with omeprazole and other proton pump inhibitors, with the possible exceptions of pantoprazole and esomeprazole. Current data may lead to changes in recommendations for patient management. Until the information is fully assessed, pantoprazole or esomeprazole could be used if a proton pump inhibitor is clearly indicated. Histamine H2 antagonists could be used in high doses but the efficacy of this approach with aspirin and clopidogrel is not established. Prasugrel is available as an alternative to clopidogrel but further assessment of its relative benefits and risks are required, as well as further investigation of its interaction potential with proton pump inhibitors.

Step 7: Follow-up and document the outcome

After providing your summary and recommendations to the cardiologist, you alert the clinical pharmacists in your hospital and prepare an update for the hospital drug bulletin.

To follow developments, you create an automatic search strategy in PubMed for articles with clopidogrel or prasugrel in their titles, and register your email address with the FDA so you can be alerted to further information about their continuing assessment. This will enable you to respond to the cardiologist's request for further information as it becomes available.

KEY MESSAGES

- Information is an essential component to optimise the use of drugs for individuals and populations.
- A drug information service must be integrated with the clinicians it supports.
- Clinical decisions must be based on objective evidence and this requires access to published research and clinical reports.
- A drug information pharmacist should make the best use of available information resources and his or her skills, and provide a critical assessment of the available data.
- Providing a drug information service is a professional activity which carries the same responsibilities as direct patient care.

Further Reading

Bernknopf AC, Karpinski JP, McKeever AL, Peak AS, Smith KM, Smith WD et al. 2009. Drug information: from education to practice. *Pharmacotherapy* 29 (3):331–46.

Websites of Interest

United Kingdom Medicines Information (UKMi)

(www.ukmi.nhs.uk)

20 POISON INFORMATION

M Ramesh and Shobha Churi

Learning Objectives

Upon completion of this chapter, the reader should be able to:

- Explain the importance and usefulness of a poison information service in patient care
- List the differences between a poison information centre and a drug information centre
- Describe the functions of a poison information centre
- Explain the organisation of a poison information centre
- List important poison information resources
- Describe the systematic approach in answering a poison information query

Introduction

The number of chemicals, poisonous household products and medicines on the Indian market is increasing day by day, which consequently increases the risk of misuse of these products and leads to greater incidence of intentional and unintentional poisoning. The impact of poison information services on the quality of healthcare is very significant, and hence there is an increased need for poison information services to prevent and manage the morbidity and mortality caused by poisoning. Such services are designed to provide immediate, round-the-clock toxicity assessment and treatment recommendations for the effective management of poisoning cases.

Poison information (PI) is a specialised area of drug information which includes information about the toxic effects of chemicals and pesticides, hazardous material spills, household products, overdose of therapeutic medicines, plants including mushrooms, animal toxins from the bites of snakes, spiders and other venomous creatures, and stings.

A poison information service deals with the risk assessment, diagnosis, management and prevention of exposure to any poison, in patients of any age irrespective of type (intentional or accidental) and route of exposure. The goal of poison information services is to reduce the morbidity and mortality caused by poisoning and improve the patients' health-related quality of life.

These services are mainly provided to the general public as well as to healthcare professionals. As the patient load is ever increasing, physicians may not be able to search and interpret the information from a vast literature in a short period. Poison information services are of great help to physicians in the immediate management of all types of poisoning cases.

Specialist pharmacists with knowledge of clinical toxicology and with the skills required for provision of drug and poison information can contribute to the management of poisoning cases. Pharmacists can acquire the required knowledge and skills through appropriate training in the area of poison information which enables them to evaluate poisoning cases with in-depth understanding, and thereby provide valuable information.

The pharmacist's knowledge of pharmacology, drug products, pharmacokinetics, drug interactions, adverse drug reactions and clinical use of drugs with skills in information retrieval, drug information evaluation, patient history-taking and communication are strong assets to pharmacists working as poison information specialists in the area of clinical toxicology practice.

Poison information services are provided by a specialised centre known as a poison information centre (PIC) or poison control centre (PCC). It provides immediate information on poisoning management through well-trained poison information specialists. A PIC functions 24 hours a day, round the year with the objective of continually improving health outcomes by providing a timely, safe information service appropriate to the needs of the enquirer related to poisoning, suspected poisoning and prevention of poisoning. It also aims to prevent unnecessary visits to doctors and hospitals and to ensure that patients who are poisoned receive the most effective treatment promptly. The size of the PIC may vary depending on call volumes and should ideally be located adjacent to the emergency department. A PIC may operate locally, providing services to populations of a specific geographical location, or may extend its service to the regional/national level.

Evolution

After the Second World War, a large number of medicines and chemicals were introduced into the market. Consequent to this, globally there was a higher incidence of intentional and unintentional poisoning, especially in children. Healthcare professionals had little knowledge about the ingredients present in the new products. In view of the increasing incidence of poisoning and lack of awareness among the public about the effects of poisoning, the first poison information services were established.

In Europe in the late 1940s, special toxicity wards for treating poisoning cases were established in Copenhagen and Budapest, and in 1949, the Netherlands started a poison information centre. Subsequently, Dr Roy Goulding started a PIC at Guy's Hospital, London, and around the same time, a service was also developed by Dr Henry Mathew in Edinburgh. In the USA, pharmacist Louis Gdalman initiated a poison information service at St Luke's Hospital in the 1930s and the service was widely recognised by physicians throughout the country. In the late 1940s, he started recording information on small cards and later developed a data collection form. In the 1950s, he established an extensive library on the management of acute and chronic poisoning, and in 1953 the poison information centre at Presbyterian St Luke's Hospital, Chicago was formally recognised. Subsequently, similar centres began in different parts of the world. All the centres provide an invaluable service by creating public awareness of poisoning and providing toxicological, diagnostic and therapeutic assistance to healthcare professionals.

In India, poison information services are essential as poisoning is common and is one of the main causes of death. The World Health Organization (WHO) reported that in 2000, unintentional poisoning was the ninth most common cause of death globally and the sixth most common cause of death in India in the age group of 15–29 years.

In India, management of acute poisoning cases is difficult for physicians working in emergency departments because typically very little information is available regarding the nature and amount of the substance ingested at the time of presentation. Also, toxicology analysis services are not readily available. Increased mortality and morbidity may result from lack of access to information (for the physician treating the poisoned patients) and lack of awareness about prevention, first aid measures and management of different poisoning cases.

Poison information centres can play a vital role in the prevention and management of poisoning cases through the provision of information to the general public and to healthcare professionals. As of 2010, there were only four WHO-recognised centres in India. In addition, a few other centers offer a poison information service as part of a comprehensive patient care programme. The first National Poison Information Centre was established in December 1994 at the All-India Institute of Medical Sciences (AIIMS), New Delhi. The other centres were subsequently established at the National Institute of Occupational Health, Ahmedabad, Government General Hospital, Chennai and Amrita Institute of Medical Sciences and Research, Cochin.

Considering the incidence rate of poisoning cases in India, these centres may not be able to meet the demand for poison information. Since a limited number of PICs provide the vital service of poison management in India, the need for establishing several such centres with well-equipped and well-trained personnel is greater.

Role of the Poison Information Centre

Although there are several reasons for establishing a poison information centre, minimising poisoning deaths due to accidental or intentional poisoning or overdose among the general public is the ultimate goal. Providing the general public and healthcare professionals with information on poisoning prevention and management (identification/assessment and management) by providing rapid access to poisoning information is another key goal.

The PIC also conducts educational programmes for healthcare professionals of the hospital where the PIC is located, and outreach programmes at smaller hospitals may also be developed. These highlight the services of the poison information centre, especially the identification of the poisoning substance, first aid measures and the treatment and prevention of poisoning cases. PIC staff can also assist with rationalisation of antidote stocks.

There are direct benefits to the public and healthcare professionals from the services provided by the PIC. It provides public health benefits by reducing morbidity and mortality from poisoning. Healthcare professionals have access to up-to-date and relevant information about poisoning management. The PIC achieves its goals and benefits by performing several functions (Table 20.1). It can also be involved in developing contingency plans and responding to chemical disasters in association with other responsible organisations.

Table 20.1 Functions of a poison information centre

Functions
Patient management
Toxicological analytical services
Toxicovigilance
Education and training of healthcare professionals and public
Prevention of poisoning
Research in poisoning
Development of therapeutic guidelines/protocols for poison management

Organisation

PICs can operate effectively with various types of organisational structures. However, the organisation pattern of a PIC should be based on the anticipated *'ideal human exposure call volume'* (average number of queries that the poison information centre receives regarding the management of poisoning cases in humans). The majority of PICs are connected with hospitals and to some extent to universities and with the public health service of the country at national or regional level. Networking with all other existing PICs at a regional, state or national level in a systematic way is essential not only for maintaining uniformity of services but also to ensure better utilisation of available resources.

This also allows the development of a national database on poisoning and the formulation of expert management advice. It is important to liaise with hospitals and analytical laboratories in the management of poisoned patients. A reliable source of financial support is needed to ensure the stability and effective functioning of a PIC. Although the centre can remain independent and autonomous through self-finance, in most countries, PICs rely on government funding as part of a public health service.

Personnel: An adequate number of staff is essential for effective and round-the-clock functioning of the centre. The PIC is usually staffed by a physician (medical director), a pharmacist (technical director), an administrator, at least one clinical toxicologist and a poison information specialist with the required secretarial assistance. Personnel working in PICs should have unique qualifications and distinct responsibilities. Moreover, training of staff in the area of clinical toxicology and communication skills makes them more confident and prepares them well in providing such services. The responsibility of medical and technical directors is to promote research, raise funds, ensure quality service and undertake further development of the information service.

The medical functions of the centre must be the responsibility of a clinical toxicologist, who is a qualified physician with several years of experience in the treatment of poisoning cases and with experience and understanding of other areas such as emergency medicine, paediatrics, public health, internal medicine, intensive care and forensic medicine. The clinical toxicologist may provide expert advice to national decision-making bodies, and is often responsible for training at hospitals and medical faculties, and takes part in the multi-disciplinary teaching of toxicology.

The poison information specialists should be trained properly to carry out the basic functions of the centre. The responsibilities of the poison information specialist include:

- Provide poison information
- Prepare standard protocols
- Maintain an accurate record of all queries
- Participate in continuing education
- Update and maintain information resources
- Carry out research activities

A public education coordinator can liaise with the public and reduce the incidence of accidental poisoning by developing and distributing educational materials and also by conducting public education programmes. It is also desirable to have an administrative director, who is responsible for the financial, administrative and other non-medical aspects of the centre.

Facilities

- *Location:* A feasible location for the PIC is within a hospital or an area closely associated with a hospital providing emergency and intensive care services. Ideally, the PIC should be co-located with a hospital clinical toxicology service which is concerned with the identification, treatment and prevention of the harmful effects of chemicals, including natural substances, on humans. This type of setup will provide ready access to a network of medical disciplines that will support and enhance the work of the centre. Other locations include a medical library, medical university, pharmacy department and medical or pharmacy college. Regardless of the location, it is wise to have a liaison with a hospital/ university medical library.
- *Space:* The PIC should be placed in a spacious facility to accommodate the service's staff and needs. A work area of 200 square feet per workstation is recommended, with a separate office for the medical director and manager/ supervisor. The working area should have adequate lighting and ventilation.
- *Equipment:* The PIC should be well equipped with the necessary basic facilities, including furniture, to allow it to function effectively. Communication equipment is vital for the centre. As most communication with the enquirer is over the phone, at least two telephones with sufficient incoming lines with toll-free numbers should be reserved to receive the queries. It is essential to have other fast and reliable communication options such as fax and e-mail. It is also important to be equipped adequately with computers, printers, a photocopying machine and uninterrupted power supply (UPS). Book shelves and filing cabinets for storage of case records and documentation files for systematic storage and easy retrieval of data are also essential. A lockable cabinet should also be available to store confidential data. For toxicological screening purposes, either the required

facilities need to be created or the centre can liaise with a well-equipped laboratory which carries out toxicological analysis.

- *Information resources:* Information pertaining to the management of poisoning cases is available from a wide range of information sources including primary, secondary and tertiary resources and the internet (Table 20.2). Although the amount and quality of information available in these resources vary, it is essential to have all types of information resources to provide poison information. Among tertiary resources, the standard textbooks of medicine (general and paediatric), chemistry, pharmacology, analytical toxicology and animal and plant toxins of the region and standard

Table 20.2 Minimum resources required for a poison information centre

Tertiary Resources:
Medical and general toxicology:
Murray L, Dary F, Little M and Cadogan M (eds). 2007. *Toxicology Handbook*. Churchill Livingstone, Elsevier: Australia.
Drat RC, Hurlbut KM, Kuffur EK and Yip (eds.) *The five-minute toxicology consult*, current edition. Lippincott Williams and Wilkins: Philadelphia.
Bates N, Edwards N, Roper J and Volans G (eds). *Paediatric Toxicology: Handbook of Poisoning in Children*, current edition. Macmillian Reference Ltd: London.
Erickson TB, Ahrens MR, Aks S, Baum C and Ling L (eds). 2005. *Pediatric toxicology: Diagnosis and Management of the Poisoned Child*. McGraw-Hill: USA.
Olson KR (ed). 2004. *Poisoning and Drug Overdose*. McGraw-Hill.
Goldfrank LR, Flomenjbaum NE and Lewin NA (eds).2006. *Goldfrank's Toxicologic Emergencies*, 6th ed. Appleton and Lange: Norwalk.
Osterhoudt K, Perrone J and DeRoos F (eds). 2004. *Toxicology Pearls*. Hanley & Belfus Medical Publishers: Philadelphia.
Ellenhorn MJ, Schonwald S, Ordog G and Wasserberger J (eds). 2006. *Ellenhorn's Medical Toxicology: Diagnosis and Treatment of Human Poisoning*, current edition. Williams and Wilkins: Baltimore.
Occupational and industrial toxicology:
Budavari S (ed). 1996. *Merck index: An Encyclopedia of Chemicals, Drugs and Biologicals*, 12th ed. Merck & Co: Rahway, NJ.
Hayes WJ and Laws ER (eds). 1991. *Handbook of Pesticide Toxicology*, (3 volumes). Academic Press: San Diego, USA.
Analytical toxicology:
Baselt RC and Cravey RH. 1995. *Disposition of toxic Drugs and Chemicals in Man*, 4th ed. Chemical Toxicology Institute: Foster City, CA.
Formulary manuals:
American Hospital Formulary Service Drug Information (annual publication). American Society of Hospital Pharmacists: Bethesda, MD.
Indian Pharmacopoeia
United States Pharmacopeia
British National Formulary

Medical dictionaries:
Stedman's medical dictionary
Dorland's medical dictionary
Oxford medical dictionary
Secondary resources:
POISINDEX
WikiTox http://curriculum.toxicology.wikispaces.net/
Toxbase
Intox
MEDLINE
Toxicology abstracts
Toxline
Excerpta medica
Index medicus
Primary resources
Human and experimental toxicology. Published by Macmillan, Basingstoke, England.
On-line journal scanning services, for example, AMEDEO, Current Awareness in Clinical Toxicology
Clinical toxicology. Published by Informa Healthcare.
Neurotoxicology. Published by Raven Press, New York, USA
Pharmacology and toxicology. Published by Munksgaard, Copenhagen, Denmark
Toxicology. Published by Elsevier, Limerick, Ireland.
Toxicology and applied pharmacology. Published by Academic Press, San Diego, CA, USA.
Journal of Medical Toxicology.
Indian Journal of Environment & Toxicology
Indian Journal of Toxicology
Journal of Indian Society of Toxicology

medical dictionaries are essential. A list of medicines, agricultural and other chemical products with their ingredients available in the local market, and the local pharmacopoeia are also useful. Secondary sources such as POISINDEX, TOXINZ, HyperTox and Intox are a must for the quick retrieval of updated information. Several countries have their own databases for products available in their region. However, the countries which do not have such databases can select the specific and relevant database which fulfills their needs. Many databases are available both online and on CD-ROM. Primary resources include journals of medicine and toxicology, and the use of these is essential for updated and recent advances in a particular area. The internet provides a vast amount of information but the quality and reliability of this information must be ensured prior to use. Apart from these information resources, it is important to develop treatment protocols for the management of the most common types of poisoning for use by clinicians. Also, developing education material such as posters on the safe use of pesticides and chemicals, and booklets and leaflets on the safe storage of medicines and household products at home are of great importance in educating the public and in the prevention of poisoning.

Legal and ethical prerequisites: It is recommended that the PIC be officially recognised either by government authorities or the WHO. To carry out the functions effectively, the centre should have independent status, stability and neutrality. Ideally, the centre should have a governing body incorporating experts to provide policy guidance and assist in fund-raising but the body should not involve itself in the daily activities of the centre. In addition, the centre should maintain confidentiality of the data it handles. Usually the centre is required to provide the information free of cost to enquirers. But, occasionally, the centre may charge for the services being offered for its own viability. In such instances, it should be on a 'no loss–no profit' basis.

Policies and procedures: For the effective functioning of the centre, it should have well-defined policies and procedures. The policies and procedures may vary from one centre to another depending on the scope of service, financial support and the centre's requirements. The PIC should develop policies for personnel, methods of operation, documentation of services and quality assurance programmes, staff training, confidentiality, and ethical and legal aspects. Policies pertaining to personnel should indicate the mode of recruitment of personnel, qualifications and training required if any, and the position of staff with distinct responsibilities. The method of operation should detail the handling of poisoning cases starting from receipt of the query until final documentation. There should be clear escalation protocols which specify the circumstances when an enquirer should be referred on to the toxicology registrar or consultant clinical toxicologist. Detailed policies and procedures are to be established with respect to a quality assurance programme and quality improvement strategies. Similarly, the guidelines for staff training and confidentiality are crucial.

Training of staff: Adequate training to site personnel is essential especially for newly recruited and inexperienced staff. The PIC should provide either internal or external training to the staff in the various areas of poison information. The PIC should develop and implement a needs-based staff training manual. This would assist in training new and inexperienced staff in various areas and ensure that uniformity in training is maintained. Training components may include updating of knowledge in clinical toxicology, communication skills, handling of databases, retrieval of information, interpretation and analytical skills, and handling of equipment such as computers, telephones and other instruments.

Systematic Approach in Handling Poison Information Queries

Handling a poison information query is the ultimate responsibility of the poison information specialist. To handle the query, the specialist should have good skills in communicating clearly and concisely to elicit and/or present explanatory or interpretive information. It is necessary to establish and maintain effective working relationships with other employees of relevant organisations. The poison information specialist should adopt the skill of reacting calmly and effectively in emergency and stressful situations.

Identifying the exposures that are potentially serious and which require immediate medical assessment and those that represent a minimal risk of toxicity can greatly aid in the effective management of poisoning. By identifying exposures that represent a minimal risk of toxicity, unnecessary presentations to doctors and hospital emergency departments can be avoided. The poison information specialist must assess each call carefully by listening to the caller and asking open-ended questions.

Often the information provided by the caller is insufficient to give an accurate answer; in such cases, further targetted questions should be asked. The poison information specialist taking the call must make a decision based on the information given by the caller, an assessment of the reliability of the history, their own clinical judgment and the information retrieved from available sources.

For a complicated query for which information is not available, or when the enquirer is not satisfied with the information provided, the poison information specialist should contact/transfer the call either to the manager/director or the consultant clinical toxicologist and seek their expert advice. The following steps should be adopted to systematically approach a poison information query.

Step 1: Obtain the Requester's Demographics

Receive and accept the query related to the service either over the phone or in person. Establish the identity of the enquirer by gathering contact details. Also obtain all required information from the requester that will allow you to reply to the query. If the enquirer is a healthcare professional, the position and anticipated knowledge of the enquirer should be determined. If it takes time to obtain information, ask the enquirer to call back or note their contact number. Queries relating to potentially serious poisoning cases need to be answered immediately, and for a query with minimal toxicity an appropriate deadline for a response should be established.

Step 2: Collect Background Information

It is important to collect all the required background information to provide appropriate information. Obtaining relevant information often requires targetted questioning, and additional care is required to accurately identify the poisoning substance. However, all critical information should be obtained in a short time to maximise the patient outcome as otherwise it may be counter-productive.

Basic information that is required includes the age and/or weight of the victim, substance/product name, route of contact (ingestion, inhalation, dermal, ocular), quantity and/or strength involved, time elapsed since exposure, patient's condition (signs, symptoms, etc.), treatment received and the health status of the patient including medication history, allergies and relevant pre-existing conditions.

Step 3: Assess the Patient's Condition

Appropriate background information about the patient's condition allows for better understanding of the actual query to be answered. Firstly, the urgency of the situation should be assessed in terms of whether it is an emergency, serious, not serious or no problem. Assess the likelihood of toxicity associated with the exposed toxins based on the nature of the substance, type of exposure and quantity consumed. Assessment of signs and symptoms of toxicity and analytical testing of the compound may greatly aid in determining appropriate patient management and whether first aid, observation, medical treatment, home treatment or no treatment is appropriate.

Step 4: Develop and Conduct a Search Strategy

Select and prioritise the information resources based on the probability of locating the desired information. It is ideal to locate the information based on the probable efficiency of information sources in the literature hierarchy. Although in many instances the information can be provided with the use of tertiary resources, it is worthwhile to consider other information sources, as appropriate.

Searching for information in databases like POISINDEX may enable the poison information specialist to retrieve comprehensive information in a short time. In addition, the use of developed poison management protocols may serve as a ready-to-use resource, especially in emergency situations. The information resources used should be documented on the basis of their usefulness in responding to the query.

Step 5: Evaluate and Provide Information

The retrieved information should be thoroughly and critically evaluated. Comprehensive information needs to be provided to ensure the recommended line of management is based on all of the current evidence available. The response should be generated only after critically evaluating all the information available. However, consistency of information among the resources used should be ensured.

Interpretation of the information available in various resources should be patient specific and made considering all relevant factors. In case of lack of information or conflict of information in the available sources, a decision may be taken based on professional knowledge and previous experience. Information may be provided verbally/written/printed form/through fax or e-mail, as appropriate. However, timely or immediate delivery of the response is critical. If more time is required to evaluate and formulate the response, minimum vital information is to be provided at the earliest possible time.

Step 6: Conduct Follow-up and Document

Follow-up of the case is vital to assess the patient outcome and also to ascertain whether provision of any additional information is useful in the management of the poisoning. A personal visit may be more useful and is possible only when the victim is admitted to a hospital where the poison information centre is co-located. In other cases, follow-up can be made through other modes including telephone enquiry and e-mail. Documenting the details of enquirer, query and response (Fig. 20.1) in at least one mode of documentation (paper, computer, log book, etc.) is essential for several reasons. It not only helps for future reference for similar

Poison information (PI) request and documentation form					**PI request number:**
Date:		**Time:**			
Type of population	**Type of poisoning Agent(s)**	**Reason**			
		Intentional	**Accidental**	**Adverse reaction**	**Unknown**
1. Children 2. Adult 3. Elderly 4. Pregnant	1. Pesticides 2. Household products 3. Bites/stings 4. Medicines 5. Others	1. Suicidal 2. Misuse 3. Abuse	1. General 2. Occupational 3. Environmental 4. Others	1. Drug(s) 2. Food 3. Vaccine(s) 4. Device(s) 5. Others	1.Unknown reason

Patient Details	**Enquirer Details**
Name: Age: Sex: ☐ Male ☐ Female Weight: Pertinent Medical History: Tel. No: Address:	Name: Enquirer back ground: ☐ General Public ☐ Doctor ☐ Pharmacist ☐ Other healthcare professional Tel. No: Address: **Call site:** Residence ☐ Work place ☐ Health care facility ☐ Other ☐

Substance Details:
Substance 1: ---------------------------- Substance 2:----------------------------
Quantity consumed: ---------------------- Quantity consumed: -------------------------
Ingredients:
Time since exposure:
Route of exposure:
☐Ingestion ☐Inhalation ☐Ocular ☐Dermal ☐Bite/sting ☐Parenteral
☐Other ☐Unknown
First Aid measures (If any):

Symptoms present ☐Yes ☐No
If yes symptoms present (specify) ....
Is symptoms related to substance: ☐Yes ☐No
If yes symptoms related to: ☐Substance 1 ☐Substance 2
The urgency of the situation: ☐Emergency ☐Serious ☐Not serious ☐No problem
What action to be taken: *☐First aid* *☐Medical assessment* *☐Observation*
☐Home treatment *☐No treatment*

Information provided:

Mode of provision: ☐ Verbal ☐ Written ☐ Printed ☐ Other

Time taken to provide information:

References consulted (specify): ☐ Tertiary resources
☐ Secondary resources
☐Primary resources
☐Others

Follow up details (Outcome):

Received and completed by:
(Name & Signature)

Reviewed by:
(Name & Signature)

Figure 20.1 Model documentation form

queries, but also justifies the professional value and acts as a protective measure against legal liability.

Step 7: Maintain Confidentiality

All issues relating to the query are to be kept confidential by the centre for socio-legal reasons. The details of the enquirer should not be disclosed to anyone, including family members and healthcare professionals, without the consent of the enquirer.

Comparison of PIC and Drug Information Centre

Drug information centre (DIC) refers to the specialised activity of provision of information related to drug use. Both DIC and PIC have a common goal: to provide comprehensive, accurate and timely information to enhance the medical care of patients. Despite the similar organisational and operational modalities including the procedure for retrieval of information, there are several differences between a DIC and PIC (Table 20.3).

Quality Assurance

Quality assurance (QA) activities should be an integral part of the poison information service for several reasons. A formalised quality assurance programme must be developed and implemented continually in the PIC for the services provided. The aim is to improve the quality of service provided and thereby improve patient health outcomes. Assessment of the performance level of the centre in meeting the needs of the public and healthcare professionals is the key factor to consider in a quality improvement programme. It should include performance indicators and evaluation methods for monitoring the quality, appropriateness, timeliness of management or treatment recommendation and effectiveness of service. Performance evaluation of staff regarding knowledge, skills in retrieval and communication may be evaluated periodically to assess their ability to effectively handle queries. Other options

Table 20.3 Differences between a drug information centre and a poison information centre

Parameter	*Drug Information Centre*	*Poison Information Centre*
Clientele of service	Mainly healthcare professionals	Mainly general public
Expected call volume	Minimal	Maximum
Call complexity	High	Low
Reply time	More	Less (immediate)
Information resources required	Less	More
Working hours	Regular working hours on week days	Round the clock and round the year
Staff requirement	Fewer numbers	Greater numbers
Operation cost	Less expensive	More expensive
Financial support	Sponsoring institution	Government/Non-government organisation/Public

for quality assessment include feedback from users through questionnaires, reviewing and evaluation of services against predefined standards/checklist and peer review of answered queries.

The QA can be applied to different areas of practice, which may be divided into the levels of inputs, processes and outputs. The *inputs level* in poison information service refers to the areas of staff, resources, facilities and organisation. The *processes level* includes the areas of receiving queries, search strategy, data collection, literature evaluation, formulation of reply, documentation and storage. *Outputs level* refers to the areas of user satisfaction and patient outcome. All these help in resolving identified problems to improve patient care in a timely manner. If the quality of service is not up to the expected level and demands are not met, the centre should develop appropriate policies and strategies and implement them and then re-assess in order to promote or increase the level of performance.

In addition, clinical governance of the PIC should include meetings at regular intervals to discuss quality improvement strategies regarding complicated enquires/cases, to review any complaints to the PIC, to maintain statistics of hospitalised poison cases, to review management protocols and to plan educational activities and prevention programmes. As part of the quality improvement programme, the PIC staff should receive feedback from the consultant clinical toxicologists or registrar regarding all cases that have been referred to them as per escalation protocols.

Conclusion

Skilled pharmacists can play an important role as poison information specialists. This role is most effective when the PIC is co-located with a clinical toxicology service within a hospital treating poisoning cases. Experienced pharmacists may also serve as advisors to analytical toxicology laboratories, as expert witnesses in legal proceedings, and may also work in the safety offices of the pharmaceutical industry.

Pharmacists in India are already providing pharmaceutical care in many hospitals. Now it is a challenge for the profession to extend their role in healthcare as poison information specialists in clinical toxicology practice. There is a need for a centralised database and expert advice on toxicological cases to assist physicians, and to educate the public in the prevention and the overall management of poisoning in India.

Practice Scenario 1: (Query from the Public)

You are working as a poison information specialist in an independent poison information centre located in a university hospital. You receive a call from an anxious father who is seeking advice regarding treatment measures for his daughter who consumed kerosene.

The poison information specialist should follow the steps given below to provide the information.

Step 1: Obtain the requester's demographics

First, receive the query politely over the phone and establish the identity of the caller. While collecting the demographic details of the caller, understand the depth of the problem and the urgency of the query. In this case, since the caller is in an anxious state, provide counselling to help him remain calm. You should provide advice on first-aid measures immediately if the child's condition is serious, and define the appropriate timeline for further delivery of complete information.

Step 2: Collect background information

You are required to collect relevant background information to provide appropriate information. Ask for the enquirer's occupation, qualification and assess his knowledge regarding this situation. The enquirer says he is a farmer and does not know about first aid for this type of poisoning. Ask the caller to provide details of the patient and collect information on the patient's age and weight, route of exposure, quantity of kerosene consumed and time elapsed since exposure. Confirm the quantity of kerosene consumed by asking how much kerosene was originally in the container and how much is left after consuming. Also ask about the patient's condition, whether the patient has any signs and symptoms of poisoning (coughing, choking, tachypnoea, dyspnoea, cyanosis, rales, haemoptysis, pulmonary oedema, pneumatocoeles, lipoid pneumonia or respiratory arrest) and if any first aid was given. The enquirer tells you that his daughter is five years old, weighs approximately 14 kg and that she consumed two or three mouthfuls of kerosene 30 minutes back. She does not have any signs or symptoms. The enquirer is sure about the consumption of kerosene which was stored in an unlabelled water bottle and kept in the kitchen within reach of the child. You also understand that first aid was not given to the child. Collect the contact details of the enquirer for the purpose of follow-up.

Step 3: Assess the condition

Considering all the background information provided, there appears to be no evidence of any serious toxicity associated with kerosene consumption, as the victim did not develop any signs and symptoms thirty minutes after consumption. Observing the type of exposure (oral) and the time elapsed since consumption (30 minutes), it is unlikely that the patient would develop any further complication thereafter. Hence you decide that except for observation and first-aid measures, this patient does not require any treatment or hospitalisation. Also, analytical testing for the level of toxic substance in plasma would not be helpful. Although the case is non-serious and the urgency of this query is low, the information needs to be provided at the earliest possible opportunity.

Step 4: Develop and conduct a search strategy

The identification of appropriate resources is important in this step and the search for information should be carried out immediately. In this case, information about first-aid measures and the required treatment need to be provided. You must make a note that the information is available in tertiary resources including Ellenhorn's Medical Toxicology and Poisoning and Drug Overdose by Kent R Olson, and secondary resources like POISINDEX. In addition, referring to a treatment protocol (if developed and used by the PIC) is also useful to obtain immediate information. The information available in POISINDEX suggests that kerosene is unlikely to produce systemic symptoms following accidental ingestion. Also, it is difficult to estimate the amount of hydrocarbons capable of producing severe symptoms. Emesis is not recommended following hydrocarbon ingestion because of the risk of aspiration. An asymptomatic patient can be observed for 4–6 hours and discharged if they remain asymptomatic and do not have an abnormal chest x-ray. Results of a study of poison centre calls involving hydrocarbon ingestion indicated that accidental ingestion of a small quantity of hydrocarbons can be handled at home, provided the patient is asymptomatic, there is access to follow-up and there is no indication of child abuse or attempted suicide.

According to information available in Ellenhorn's Medical Toxicology, a chest x-ray should be obtained for all patients clinically suspected of aspiration regardless of whether symptoms are present. Asymptomatic children with a normal chest x-ray need not be admitted to the hospital. Ingestion of most petroleum distillate concentrations below 1–2 ml/kg does not cause systemic toxicity. Substantially larger quantities may be necessary to produce central nervous system depression. Gastrointestinal decontamination in accidental petroleum distillate ingestion is not recommended because of the severe aspiration hazard.

Upon referring to Poisoning and Drug Overdose by Kent R Olson, you note that aliphatic hydrocarbons and simple petroleum distillates such as lighter fluid, kerosene, furniture polish and gasoline are poorly absorbed from the GI tract and do not pose a significant risk of systemic toxicity after ingestion, as long as they are not aspirated. And the toxic dose is variable, depending on the agent involved and whether it is aspirated, ingested, injected or inhaled. Pulmonary aspiration of as little as a few milliliters may produce chemical pneumonitis. Pulmonary aspiration usually causes immediate onset of coughing or choking, tachypnoea and wheezing. For agents with no known systemic toxicity, gut decontamination is neither necessary nor desirable because any gut-emptying procedure increases the risk of aspiration.

Step 5: Evaluate and provide information

After evaluating this data, the information is to be provided over the phone to the enquirer with reassurance about the patient's condition. In this case, considering the substance ingested, quantity consumed and absence of toxicity symptoms, you would advise that the victim does not require hospital admission as she is asymptomatic, and also because kerosene is unlikely to cause toxic symptoms at the dose consumed by the victim. Management is largely supportive and no specific antidotes are available. You would inform the caller that inducing vomiting is contraindicated in the case of kerosene poisoning due to possible aspiration and hence advise him not to try to make the child vomit. As the patient was asymptomatic at the time of ingestion and did not have any coughing, gagging, choking or vomiting at the time of ingestion and thirty minutes after, there is no need to seek medical attention. If persistent cough, fever or respiratory distress does not appear within six hours of ingestion, it is unlikely that aspiration pneumonitis will occur. However, the child should be closely monitored at home for six hours, with the recommendation that immediate medical assessment at a hospital is required if persistent cough, fever or respiratory distress develops. Ask the enquirer to call back if any further information is needed or if the patient develops any signs or symptoms.

Step 6: Conduct follow-up and document

Follow-up is necessary in this case to ensure that the victim is asymptomatic up to six hours after ingestion. Using the contact details obtained, you may call the father to learn about the condition of his daughter. It may be necessary to develop further strategies depending on the information obtained at follow up. Document the information provided and the follow-up details in the appropriate records.

Step 7: Maintain confidentiality

You should not disclose details pertaining to the victim and the enquirer so as to maintain confidentiality.

Practice Scenario 2: (Query from a Physician)

A physician working in the emergency department of a hospital walks into the PIC located adjacent to the emergency ward and seeks information on how to manage a patient poisoned with the substance 'Laxmanrekhaa' (Cypermethrine 1% w/w with adjuvant 99% w/w). The physician asks you to provide information on the constituents of 'Laxmanrekhaa' and the relevant treatment for the patient who has been admitted to the emergency ward.

As a poison information specialist, you use a systematic approach to provide the requested information:

Step 1: Obtain the requester's demographics

In this case, you receive the query in person, which assists you to understand the depth of the problem and urgency of the situation. Collect and record the demographic details of the doctor. You need to provide the required information in a timely manner after establishing the timeline with the physician to answer the query.

Step 2: Collect background information

Collect the relevant background information to provide appropriate information. Since the enquirer is a physician, determine his position and experience and confirm the anticipated knowledge or level of information required. The physician says that he has been working in the hospital for two years since obtaining his MD qualification in general medicine. Now you need to collect other background details including patient-specific details such as the age and weight, route of exposure, quantity of poison consumed and time elapsed since exposure. You also need to obtain information pertaining to the patient's condition such as whether the signs and symptoms can be observed and if any first aid was given.

The enquirer tells you that the patient is seven years old, weighs approximately 18 kg, and accidentally consumed around 10 g of Laxmanrekhaa an hour ago. The victim is complaining of an oily taste and burning sensation in the mouth, nausea and vomiting. After hospital admission, gastric lavage was started to prevent further absorption. After obtaining background information from the enquirer, you understand that he does not know the ingredients of Laxmanrekhaa and also requires written information about the relevant treatment or specific antidote for poisoning by it. Also you note that no treatment measures have been given except for gastric lavage. Finally, you need to collect the contact details of the enquirer for the purpose of provision of information and follow-up.

Step 3: Assess the patient's condition

Although the patient shows signs and symptoms, his condition is not serious as he is conscious and stable. Considering the presenting symptoms, substance and quantity consumed, you decide that he may require treatment for his presenting condition. You also understand that gastric lavage may be of little help in this case as pyrethroids are generally absorbed rapidly from the gastrointestinal tract. However, the patient should be monitored carefully in the emergency department for 4–6 hours for any signs of CNS depression, seizure or the development of delayed pulmonary symptoms.

Step 4: Develop and conduct a search strategy

In this case, immediate identification of useful resources and retrieval of appropriate information is important. You are confident that the ingredients of Laxmanrekhaa have to be identified first, followed by management information. Specific resources with information regarding the ingredients of insecticides, fungicides, rodenticides and household products available in the Indian market are lacking. Hence, the use of a developed protocol that contains the details of ingredients present in the various toxic compounds may be of great assistance in identifying the ingredients present in Laxmanrekhaa. After searching for the ingredients of this poison, the next step is to retrieve information on the treatment or management of the patient by referring to useful tertiary sources and secondary databases like POISINDEX, Intox and HyperTox. According to the list of products and their ingredients, Laxmanrekhaa contains cypermethrin, which is a type II pyrethroid. The available information sources suggest that there is no specific antidote for pyrethroid poisoning and the treatment is symptomatic and supportive (gastric lavage and activated charcoal). Although ingestion of pyrethroids poses the greatest risk for systemic toxicity, the signs and symptoms of acute intoxication appear to be reversible. Initial symptoms after ingestion are usually gastrointestinal, with abdominal pain, vomiting and diarrhoea beginning within 10 minutes to an hour. Only the ingestion of a large volume (200–500 ml) of concentrated formulations may cause coma and seizures within 20 minutes.

Step 5: Evaluate and provide the information

According to POISINDEX and the treatment protocol, treatment is mainly basic life support and there is no specific antidote for cypermethrin poisoning. As per the request of the physician, you provide the information on management in a printed or written format. Your information in this case relates to cypermethrin, a pyrethroid compound which is the ingredient of Laxmanrekhaa. Inform the enquirer that although nausea and vomiting commonly occurs within 10–60 minutes of ingestion, oily taste and burning sensation in the mouth and laryngitis have also been reported. There is no specific antidote for pyrethroid poisoning and management is symptomatic and supportive. However, advise the enquirer to monitor fluid status and serum electrolytes if there is severe vomiting. Also, it is necessary to monitor the patient carefully in the emergency department for 4–6 hours for any signs of CNS depression, seizure or the development of delayed pulmonary symptoms.

Step 6: Conduct follow-up and document

You may follow up the case and provide further information if required. In this case, it is necessary to ensure that there are no further complications over the next 4–6 hours. Information on the patient's condition may be gathered either by making a direct visit to the patient's bedside or by calling the enquirer. Document the information provided and the follow-up details in the appropriate records.

Step 7: Maintain confidentiality

You should not disclose the details pertaining to the victim and the enquirer so as to maintain confidentiality.

KEY MESSAGES

- Provision of poison information helps in reducing the morbidity and mortality associated with poisoning.
- Knowledge of clinical toxicology and good analytical and communication skills are essential for the effective provision of poison information.
- Clinical management decisions should be taken only after critically evaluating all currently available evidence.
- A poison information specialist should apply all his/her skills while adopting a systematic approach in handling poison information queries.
- Educating healthcare professionals and the public regarding the implications and management of various poisoning compounds is the key element in preventing/minimising poisoning cases.
- A quality assurance programme should be considered as one of the integral components of a poison information service to improve the quality of service offered and thereby improve patient health outcomes.

Further Reading

Anthony MB, CSPI and Natlie MB. 1997. The nation's first control centre: Taking a stand against accidental childhood poisoning in Chicago. *Vet Human Toxicol* 39(2):115–119.

Laborde A. 2004. New roles of poison control centres in the developing countries. *Toxicology* 198:273–277.

Peter AC. 2007. Pharmacist as clinical toxicologist: Reflection on evolution, challenges and opportunities. *Ann Pharmacother* 41:1708–1711.

Ponampalan R and Anatharaman V. 2003. The need for drug and poison information – The Singapore physicians' perspective. *Singapore Med J* 44(5):231–242.

Roberts RW and Russell WL. 2007. Pharmacist-based toxicology service. *Ann Pharmacother* 41:1719–1724.

Tong TG, Becker CE, Foliart D et al. 1982. A model poison control system. *West J Med* 137:346–350.

Website of Interest

World Health Organization Guidelines for Poison Control

http://www.who.int/ipcs/publications/training_poisons/guidelines_poison_control/en/index.html

21 CLINICAL PHARMACOKINETICS

Roger L Nation and Craig R Rayner

Learning Objectives

Upon completion of this chapter, the reader should be able to:

- Define the term clinical pharmacokinetics
- Define the main pharmacokinetic parameters
- Describe how each pharmacokinetic parameter may be determined
- Explain the clinical significance and use of each pharmacokinetic parameter
- Calculate the main pharmacokinetic parameters from a patient scenario
- Appreciate how using pharmacokinetic principles, a dosing regimen may be determined to achieve a target concentration in a patient

What is Clinical Pharmacokinetics and Why is it Important?

Clinical pharmacokinetics is concerned with the process of using pharmacokinetic principles and pharmacodynamic criteria to assist in the selection of appropriate drug dose regimens for individual patients.

In essence, pharmacokinetics (*what the body does to the drug*) is the study and knowledge of the factors that determine the time-course of the drug within the body, including the absorption, distribution, metabolism and excretion of the drug. Most commonly, we are interested in the factors that determine the time-course of drug concentration in blood (or, more typically, plasma) because it is reasonably easy to collect samples of blood for the measurement of plasma concentrations. In addition, in many cases, the concentration of the drug in plasma will provide a reflection of those in the tissues of the body, including the sites where the desired and undesired effects are elicited. This does not mean that the actual concentration in plasma will be the same as that in tissues; indeed, this is usually not the case.

Whereas pharmacokinetics is concerned with the time-course of the drug within the body, pharmacodynamics (*what the drug does to the body*) is the study of the

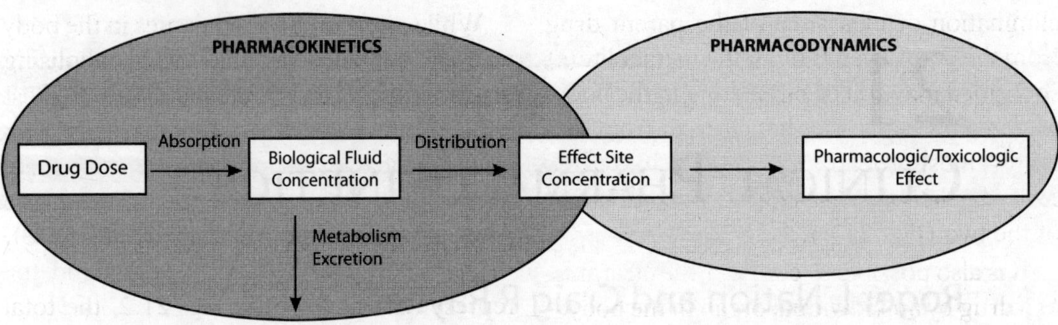

Figure 21.1 Clinical pharmacokinetics is concerned with the process of using pharmacokinetic principles and pharmacodynamic criteria to assist in the selection of appropriate drug dose regimens for individual patients.

relationship between drug concentration and pharmacological and toxicological response (Fig. 21.1). For many drugs, there is a relationship between these responses and the plasma drug concentration. For drugs where the plasma concentration most commonly associated with toxic effects overlaps with that required for the desired clinical effect, intra- and inter-individual variability in pharmacokinetics is particularly important. Variability in pharmacokinetics may arise as a result of the impact of genetic influences, disease states, environmental factors (such as cigarette smoking), ageing, drug interactions, etc.

In this chapter, we define the main pharmacokinetic parameters, describe briefly how they are determined and, most importantly, explain the clinical significance and use of each parameter. Usually, poor ability to use pharmacokinetics in the clinic arises from an inadequate understanding of the important parameters. Therefore, we have chosen to take a descriptive approach to each parameter, from simple first principles. Where necessary, we have used equations; the reader who is prepared to work their way through these will be rewarded with an enhanced understanding of the material and an increased ability to apply clinical pharmacokinetic principles to individualise and improve drug therapy. The principles discussed in this chapter will provide a sound foundation that will be developed further in *Chapter 22, Therapeutic Drug Monitoring*.

PHARMACOKINETIC PARAMETERS OF CLINICAL IMPORTANCE

Clearance

What is clearance? Clearance is the pharmacokinetic parameter that describes the efficiency of elimination (or clearance) of a drug from the body. When the term clearance is used, we usually refer to the elimination of a drug from the body – this is sometimes described as 'total body clearance' or 'systemic clearance'. Thus, clearance describes the *irreversible* elimination of a drug from the body in the form of unchanged drug (for example, excretion of the parent or unchanged drug in urine) and by biotransformation to other chemical entities (metabolites of the drug). It should be noted that metabolism contributes to the elimination or clearance of the parent drug from the body, even though the metabolite(s) so formed may still be circulating in the body. Metabolites will also be cleared from the body – most probably by excretion into urine or by further metabolism, or a combination of the two (Fig. 21.2).

It is also possible to consider the clearance of a drug by an individual organ in the body – this is done most commonly for the kidneys, where we can refer to the renal clearance (CL_R) of the unchanged drug. Renal drug clearance provides a measure of the efficiency of elimination of the (unchanged) drug by the kidneys. As one might expect, the renal clearance of a drug is likely to be decreased in patients with impaired kidney function (for example, in renal disease and in the elderly). It is convenient to describe the clearance by all other pathways as non-renal clearance (CL_{NR}); the most common form of non-renal clearance is biotransformation (or metabolism) of the drug to form metabolites.

While many organs and tissues in the body possess enzymes capable of metabolising drugs, the liver contains the highest concentration of these enzymes. Therefore, it is reasonable, in most cases, to assume that the non-renal clearance of a drug occurs predominantly in the liver (hepatic clearance). In accordance with these concepts and the representation shown in Fig. 21.2, the total body clearance (CL) of a drug can therefore be considered as the sum of renal clearance and non-renal clearance. Thus:

$$CL = CL_R + CL_{NR} \quad (1)$$

It can be appreciated that the efficiency of drug elimination will be dependent on the efficiencies of clearance by the renal and/or non-renal routes, and the relative importance of these clearance pathways in the overall clearance of the drug from the body.

It is very important and useful to recognise that total body clearance is the *proportionality constant* between the rate of drug elimination from the body at a particular point in time

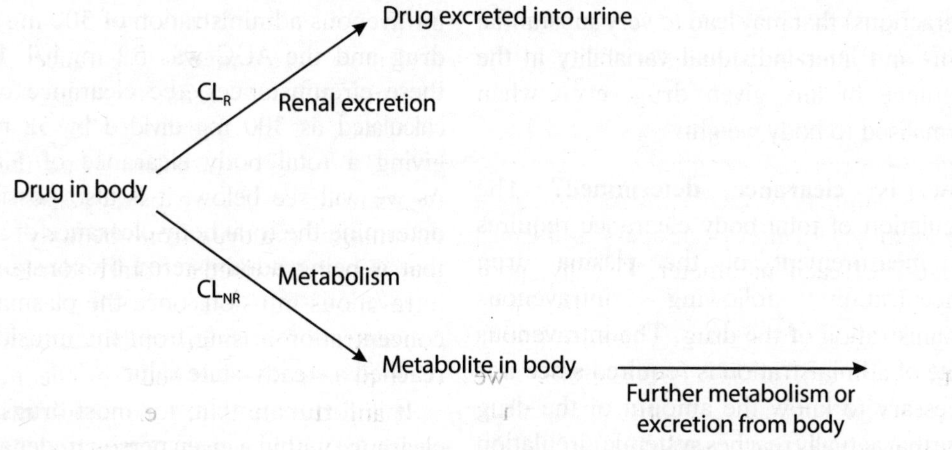

Figure 21.2 Diagrammatic representation of the pathways most commonly involved in the clearance of a drug from the body, where CL_R and CL_{NR} represent the renal and non-renal clearance components, respectively, of total clearance.

and the concomitant concentration of the drug in plasma. That is:

$$\text{Rate of elimination from the body} = CL \times C \qquad (2)$$

where C is the plasma concentration of the drug. In keeping with the above proportionality, because the rate of elimination has units of mass per unit time (such as mg/min) and plasma concentration has units of mass per volume (such as mg/l), it follows that clearance has units of volume per unit time or flow (l/min). Thus, if the total body clearance of a drug is 500 ml/min, the rate of elimination of the drug from the body when the plasma drug concentration is 2 mg/l will be 1 mg/min (0.5 l/min x 2 mg/l = 1 mg/min); under these circumstances, when the plasma concentration is 1 mg/l, the rate of elimination will be 0.5 mg/min, and so on.

Sometimes clearance is normalised to body weight (l/min/kg). It must be noted, however, that there are many factors (such as kidney or liver disease, ageing and drug interactions) that may lead to very substantial intra- and inter-individual variability in the clearance of any given drug, even when normalised to body weight.

How is clearance determined? The calculation of total body clearance requires the measurement of the plasma drug concentration following intravenous administration of the drug. The intravenous route of administration is required since it is necessary to know the amount of the drug dose that actually reaches systemic circulation intact. Following the intravenous injection of a dose, the plasma drug concentration will decline as a function of time as the drug is cleared (eliminated) from the body, as shown for a hypothetical drug in Fig. 21.3.

Using appropriate techniques (that will not be discussed in this chapter), it is possible to calculate the area under the plasma drug concentration versus time curve (AUC), from zero time (that is, immediately after administration of the dose) to infinite time (a time sufficient for virtually all the administered dose to have been eliminated from the body). Note that, in accordance with the units for the plasma concentration and time axes in Fig. 21.3, the units of the AUC are the product of concentration and time. Thus, the unit of AUC for the example shown in Fig. 21.3 is mg.h/l. The total body clearance (CL) can then be calculated as the dose (D) administered intravenously divided by AUC. That is:

$$CL = D / AUC \qquad (3)$$

In accordance with the earlier discussion, the clearance term will have units of flow D (mg) divided by AUC (mg.h/l), giving a clearance value with units of l/h. The data in Fig. 21.3 was obtained following the intravenous administration of 300 mg of the drug and the AUC was 52 mg.h/l. Under these circumstances, the clearance can be calculated as 300 mg divided by 52 mg.h/l, giving a total body clearance of 5.8 l/h. As we will see below, it is also possible to determine the total body clearance of a drug that is being administered by constant-rate intravenous infusion, once the plasma drug concentration arising from the infusion has reached a steady-state value.

It is fortunate that, for most drugs, total clearance within a given person under a given set of conditions remains relatively constant across the range of clinically relevant plasma concentrations. That is, doubling of the dose

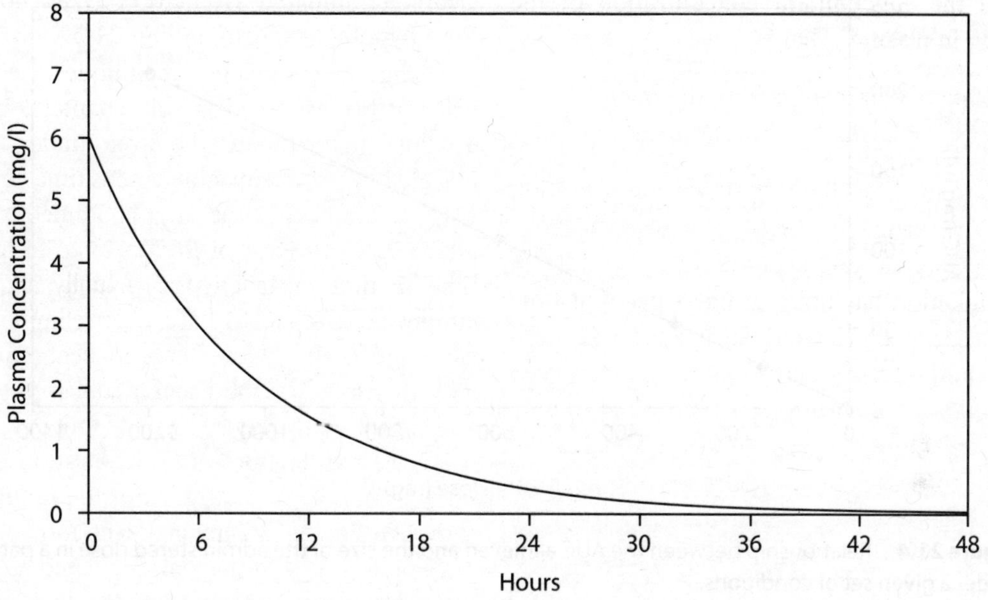

Figure 21.3 Plasma concentrations of a drug as a function of time following the administration of an intravenous dose of 300 mg at zero time. The data is shown on linear–linear axes. Note that is this data is also shown in Fig. 21.8.

administered will lead to doubling of the plasma concentration and AUC, and so on (Fig. 21.4). Note that the slope of the line in Fig. 21.4 is the reciprocal of clearance (see equation (3)) and, because there is a straight line relationship, it is evident that CL must be independent of the plasma concentration. In this circumstance, clearance is said to be 'linear'. 'Non-linear' pharmacokinetics occurs when there is a non-linear relationship between the plasma concentration achieved and the dose administered. Fortunately, this is an uncommon occurrence with most drugs in the clinical setting. One clinically important example of non-linear pharmacokinetics occurs with phenytoin, where doubling of the dose may lead to a much greater than doubling of the plasma concentration, because of saturation of the enzymes responsible for the metabolism of this drug. The readings at the end of the chapter may be consulted by those interested in obtaining further information on non-linear pharmacokinetics.

Why is clearance important clinically? Consideration of the material immediately preceding this section gives an indication of why clearance is so important. Rearrangement of equation (3) gives:

$$AUC = D / CL \quad (4)$$

Thus, it can be seen that the magnitude of the plasma concentrations achieved after a single intravenous dose of a drug (the level of exposure of the body to the drug, expressed as AUC) is directly proportional to the size of the dose administered and inversely proportional to the clearance of the drug in the patient concerned. Using the hypothetical drug example above, if the total body clearance of the drug is decreased

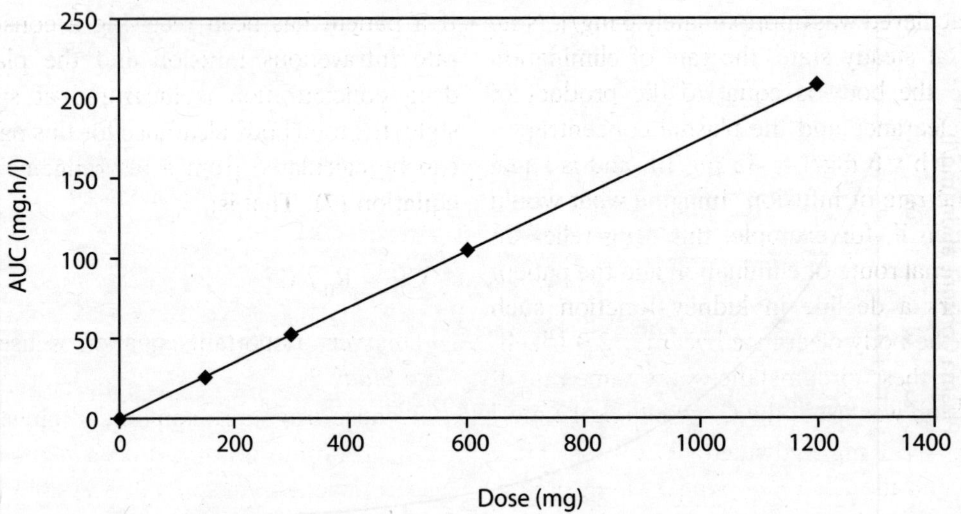

Figure 21.4 Relationship between the AUC achieved and the size of the administered dose in a patient under a given set of conditions.

to 2.9 l/h (for example, as a result of kidney or liver disease, or as a result of a drug interaction), administration of a 300-mg intravenous dose would result in doubling of the plasma concentration at each time point, and the AUC would be about 104 mg.h/l (twice that observed above). This very important issue of variability in clearance is explored in the *Case Studies*.

Perhaps a better way to understand the importance of clearance in the clinical setting is to consider the events that occur after a constant-rate intravenous infusion is started in a patient. As shown in Fig. 21.5, after commencing the infusion, the plasma concentration will increase with time and approach a plateau or steady-state concentration. By definition, at steady-state, the rate at which the drug is entering systemic circulation (the infusion rate) must equal the rate at which the drug is being eliminated from the body. That is, at steady state:

Rate of infusion = Rate of elimination (5)

Because by definition the rate of elimination is equal to the product of clearance and plasma concentration (see equation (2)), it follows that at steady state:

$$R_0 = CL \times C^{ss} \quad (6)$$

where R_0 is the rate of infusion and C^{ss} is the steady-state plasma drug concentration. Rearrangement of equation (6) gives:

$$C^{ss} = R_0 / CL \quad (7)$$

This equation, derived from very simple and straightforward first principles, *is very important in the clinical setting*. It demonstrates that the steady-state plasma drug concentration is directly proportional to the rate of infusion and inversely proportional to the clearance in a particular patient. The hypothetical drug shown in Fig. 21.5 was infused at 35 mg/h into a patient who had a clearance for this drug of 5.8 l/h. In accordance with equation (7), the

C^{ss} achieved was approximately 6 mg/l. Note that at steady state, the rate of elimination from the body is equal to the product of the clearance and the plasma concentration (5.8 l/h x 6 mg/l = 35 mg/h), and is equal to the rate of infusion. Imagine what would happen if, for example, this drug relies on the renal route of elimination and the patient suffers a decline in kidney function such that the body clearance becomes 2.9 l/h. If, under these circumstances, the same rate of infusion was used, the C^{ss} would be 12 mg/l (C^{ss} = 35 mg/h divided by 2.9 l/h). If a concentration of about 6 mg/l was desired in these circumstances (as in the original case), it would be necessary to use an infusion rate of 17.5 mg/h, which is half of that used previously.

These considerations point to another method for the determination of clearance. If a patient has been receiving a constant-rate intravenous infusion and the plasma drug concentration is measured at steady state, the total body clearance for this patient can be calculated from a rearrangement of equation (7). That is:

$$CL = R_0 / C^{ss} \quad (8)$$

This very important equation is used in *Case Study 2*.

Because drugs are commonly administered orally according to a fixed dose regimen (a certain dose administered at a certain dose interval), it is highly instructive to consider what determines the magnitude of the steady-state plasma drug concentration with this type of regimen. As shown in Fig. 21.6, after commencing the regular administration of a dose at a set dose interval, the plasma

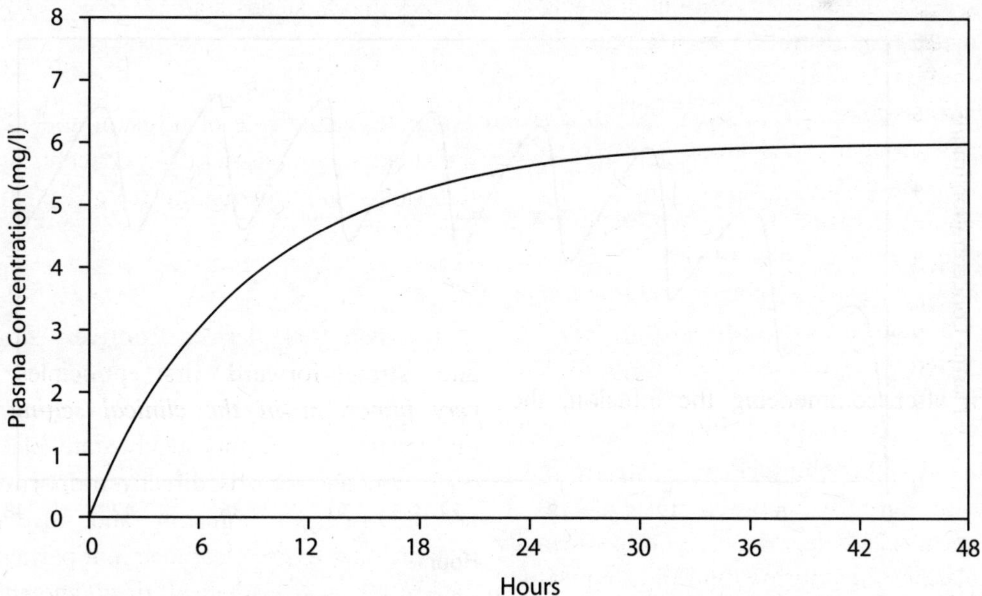

Figure 21.5 Plasma concentration time profile for a drug administered to a patient by constant-rate intravenous infusion at a rate of 35 mg/h. The total body clearance for this drug in this patient was 5.8 l/h; the half-life was 6 h.

drug concentration rises to a plateau. In contrast to the situation that occurs with a constant-rate intravenous infusion (Fig. 21.5), the profile is characterised by 'peaks' and 'troughs' that result from the absorption and elimination of each dose (Fig. 21.6). It is convenient and useful to define the average plasma drug concentration at steady state (C_{av}^{ss}) which approximates the average of the 'peak' and 'trough' concentrations at steady state.

In an analogous manner to that described for the intravenous-infusion scenario described above, at steady state the following condition must apply:

Rate of delivery to systemic circulation = Rate of elimination (9)

The term on the left-hand side of the equation is the average rate of delivery of the drug to systemic circulation. This rate is equal to the time-averaged rate at which the drug is administered orally (the size of each individual dose (D) divided by the dosage interval (τ) multiplied by the fraction of each orally administered dose that reaches systemic circulation intact (f); the latter term is the bioavailability, which will be discussed in more detail later. Therefore,

Rate of delivery to systemic circulation

$$= \frac{f \times D}{\tau} \qquad (10)$$

Because by definition the rate of elimination is equal to the product of clearance and plasma concentration (see equation (2)), it follows that at steady state:

$$\frac{f \times D}{\tau} = CL \times C_{av}^{ss} \qquad (11)$$

Rearrangement of equation (11) gives:

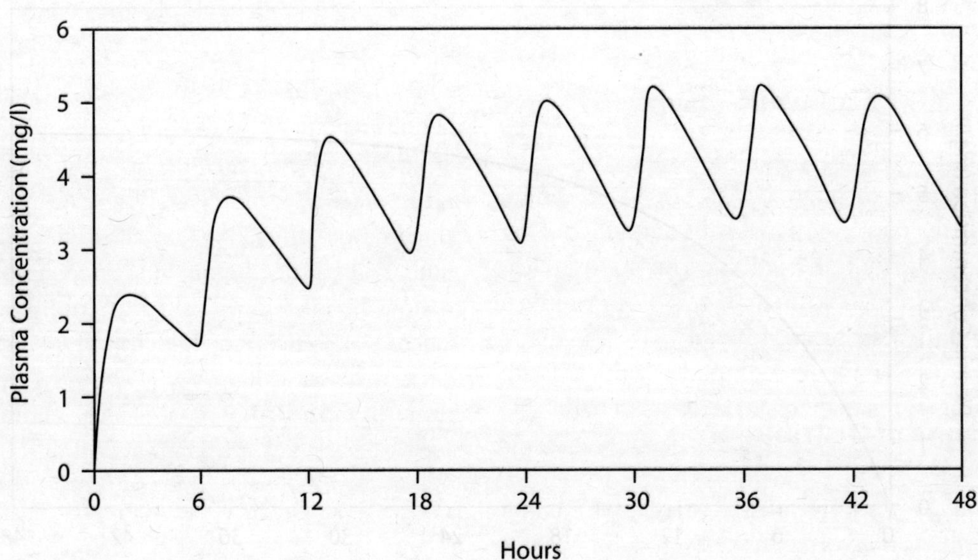

Figure 21.6 Plasma concentration time profile for a drug administered to a patient as a 300 mg oral dose given every 6 hours. The total body clearance, half-life and bioavailability for this drug in this patient were 5.8 l/h, 6h and 0.5, respectively.

$$C_{av}^{ss} = \frac{f(D/\tau)}{CL} \quad (12)$$

Once again, this is *a very important and useful equation in the clinical setting*. It demonstrates that the magnitude of the average steady-state plasma concentration achieved is determined by the dose regimen (the size of each dose (D) and how often it is given (τ)) and the pharmacokinetic parameters bioavailability (f) and clearance (CL).

The hypothetical drug represented in Fig. 21.6 had a clearance of 5.8 l/h and an oral bioavailability of 0.5 (only 50% of each orally administered dose reached systemic circulation intact) in the patient in question. Under these circumstances, when 300 mg is administered orally every 6 hours, the average steady-state plasma drug concentration will be approximately 4.3 mg/l (C_{av}^{ss} = (0.5 × 300 mg / 6 h) divided by 5.8 l/h), as shown in Fig. 21.6. If the clearance were to decrease to 2.9 l/h and the dose regimen and bioavailability remained the same, the average steady-state plasma concentration achieved would be about 8.6 mg/l.

These considerations above show why *clearance* is such *a very important pharmacokinetic parameter*. The reader will have an opportunity to apply these important concepts in the *Case Studies*.

Volume of Distribution

What is volume of distribution? Drug distribution involves the *reversible* movement of drug molecules between blood (plasma) and the various tissues in the body. Drugs may bind to proteins and other macromolecules present in plasma and tissues, but it is only the unbound drug that is capable of moving across cell membranes to enter and leave the tissues (Fig. 21.7). It is important to appreciate that drug distribution is a dynamic process and that drug molecules will move down concentration gradients for the unbound drug in the various regions of the body. Thus, just after the intravenous administration of a dose of drug, most of the drug molecules in the body will reside in plasma; drug molecules will move down a concentration gradient into tissues until an 'equilibrium' is reached between the unbound concentration of the drug in plasma and that in tissue fluid (Fig. 21.7). Therefore, the concentration of drug in plasma will decline with time as a result of drug elimination (an irreversible process) and distribution of the drug into tissues. A while after administration, drug molecules will move back from tissue sites into plasma as the concentration of unbound drug in plasma decreases as a result of ongoing clearance.

The volume of distribution of a drug provides a measure of its extent of distribution within the body. It is very important to recognise that the volume of distribution of a drug usually bears no relationship to the actual (or physical volume) of the body; for this reason, it is quite often referred to as an *apparent* volume of distribution. Thus, whereas the actual volume of an adult human body may be about 50 l, the volumes of distribution of drugs range from as little as about 5 l (warfarin) through to approximately 20,000 l (chloroquine). This can be appreciated readily when it is understood that the volume of distribution of a drug (V) is really nothing more than the proportionality constant that relates the total amount of drug in the body at a particular

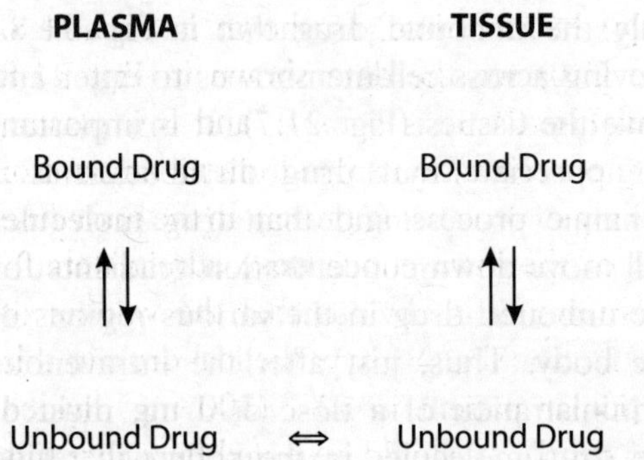

Figure 21.7 Diagrammatic representation of drug distribution within the body, showing the plasma and tissue regions of the body. For simplicity, the schema shows distribution processes only; elimination would be occurring simultaneously, but is not shown.

point in time with the simultaneously occurring concentration of the drug in plasma (the latter being a circulating body fluid that is relatively easily accessed for the measurement of drug concentration). That is:

$$A = V \times C \qquad (13)$$

where A is the total amount of drug in the body. Because it is technically difficult (but not impossible) to measure the unbound concentration of a drug in plasma, the concentration of the drug (C) in equation (13) refers to the total concentration of the drug in plasma (the sum of the concentrations of the unbound and bound drug in plasma; Fig. 21.7). It is the total concentration in plasma that is most commonly measured in pharmacokinetic studies and when undertaking therapeutic drug monitoring to optimise drug therapy in the clinical setting.

Thus, for a drug with an apparent volume of distribution of 10,000 l, the total amount of drug in the body when the plasma drug concentration is 5 μg/l must be 50,000 μg or 50 mg. When the plasma drug concentration is 1 μg/l, the amount in the body is 10,000 μg or 10 mg, and so on. As is evident from Fig. 21.7, the magnitude of the (apparent) volume of distribution of a drug depends mainly on the relative extent of binding of the drug to plasma proteins and tissue components (the latter may include partitioning of the drug molecules into adipose tissues and other lipid environments outside plasma). A drug that has high (reversible) affinity for tissue 'binding' sites relative to plasma protein binding sites will have a large volume of distribution, and vice versa. A large volume of distribution for a drug relative to the physical volume of plasma (~ 3 l) simply indicates that at any particular point in time, the majority of the drug in the body is in tissues.

As with clearance, volume of distribution may be normalised to body weight (l/kg). Fortunately, for many drugs, the body weight normalised volume of distribution is relatively constant across the population. For example, the volume of distribution of theophylline is about 0.5 l/kg for most patients, a value that is used in *Case Study 1*.

How is volume of distribution determined? As with the determination of clearance, the calculation of volume of distribution requires the measurement of the plasma drug concentration following intravenous administration of a drug. It is evident from equation (13) that knowledge of the total amount of drug in the body at a given time together with the plasma drug concentration at this same point in time permits calculation of the volume of distribution. That is:

$$V=\frac{A}{C} \qquad (14)$$

where A and C are the total amounts of drug in the body and the plasma drug concentration, respectively, at the same point in time. Immediately following an intravenous injection of the drug, the amount of drug in the body is known – it is equal to the dose administered. Knowledge of the initial plasma drug concentration (C(0)) achieved just after administration of the intravenous dose (D) therefore allows calculation of volume of distribution according to:

$$V=\frac{D}{C(0)} \qquad (15)$$

An estimate of C(0) may be obtained by back-extrapolating the plasma drug concentration profile (on a semilogarithmic scale) to zero time, as shown in Fig. 21.8. The C(0) for the data shown in Fig. 21.8 (and Fig. 21.3) is 6 mg/l, and this plasma drug concentration arose from an amount of 300 mg of drug being present in the body (the size of the intravenous dose administered). Therefore, it is obvious that the volume of distribution for this hypothetical drug in this particular patient is 50 l (300 mg divided by 6 mg/l). It should be noted here that this method of estimation of V is acceptable for the circumstances that prevail for the example shown in Figs 21.3 and 21.8 (administration of the drug by intravenous injection and where the resultant plasma drug concentrations decline according to a straight line on semilogarithmic coordinates). The use of this method in other circumstances (where a prominent 'distribution phase' occurs after intravenous injection (see below) or where

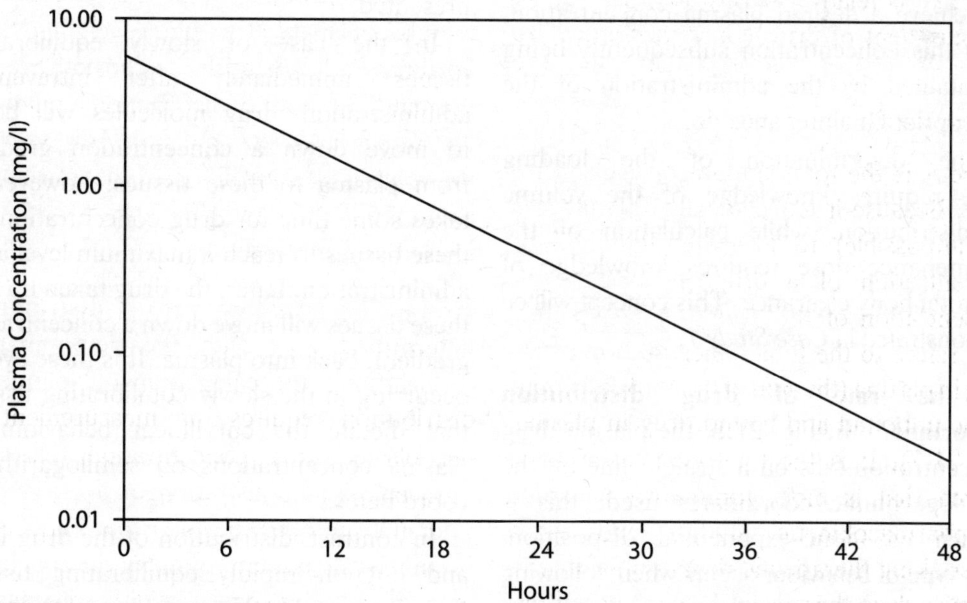

Figure 21.8 Plasma concentration of a drug as a function of time following the administration of an intravenous dose of 300 mg at zero time. The data is shown on semilogarithmic axes (logarithmic y-axis and linear x-axis). The data is the same as that shown in Fig. 21.3.

the drug is infused intravenously over a certain period) may be inappropriate, and alternative methods for determination of volume of distribution may be required.

Why is volume of distribution important clinically? The principal application of the volume of a distribution of drug is in determining the size of the dose necessary to achieve a desired initial plasma drug concentration. By rearranging equation (15), we obtain:

$$D = V \times C(0) \tag{16}$$

If, for example, it is desired to achieve an initial plasma drug concentration of 6 mg/l for a drug with a volume of distribution of 50 l, it will be necessary to administer an intravenous dose of 300 mg (50 l multiplied by 6 mg/l). Most commonly, this approach is used to calculate the loading dose needed to achieve a desired plasma concentration, with this concentration subsequently being maintained by the administration of the appropriate maintenance dose.

The determination of the loading dose requires knowledge of the volume of distribution, while calculation of the maintenance dose requires knowledge of the total body clearance. This concept will be demonstrated in *Case Study 1*.

Is the rate of drug distribution important? In Fig. 21.8, the plasma drug concentration falls on a straight line on the semilogarithmic coordinates used; this is known as mono-exponential disposition. This type of behaviour occurs when, following intravenous injection, the drug distributes rapidly into (and, later, out of) the various tissues in the body into which it distributes. Mono-exponential drug disposition is perhaps the exception rather than the rule. If samples of blood are collected early enough after intravenous administration, for many drugs the plasma concentrations, when plotted on semilogarithmic coordinates, will be seen to decline rapidly at first before entering a slower (log-linear) decline (Fig. 21.9).

The period over which the early, more rapid, decline in plasma concentrations occurs is often referred to as the 'distribution phase'. The type of plasma concentration versus time profile shown in Fig. 21.9 may often be described mathematically by a bi-exponential equation. This type of behaviour occurs when the drug does not distribute rapidly into, and out of, at least some of the tissues of the body. This is shown diagrammatically in Fig. 21.9, where the time-courses of drug concentrations in rapidly and slowly equilibrating tissues are presented.

In the case of slowly equilibrating tissues, immediately after intravenous administration, drug molecules will begin to move down a concentration gradient from plasma to these tissues; however, it takes some time for drug concentrations in these tissues to reach a maximum level after administration. Later, the drug taken up into these tissues will move down a concentration gradient, back into plasma. It is these events occurring in the slowly-equilibrating tissues that dictate the curvilinear behaviour of plasma concentrations on semilogarithmic coordinates.

In contrast, distribution of the drug into, and out of, rapidly equilibrating tissues occurs so quickly that the shape of the time-course of concentrations in these tissues mimics that seen for plasma. It should be noted that the factors that determine

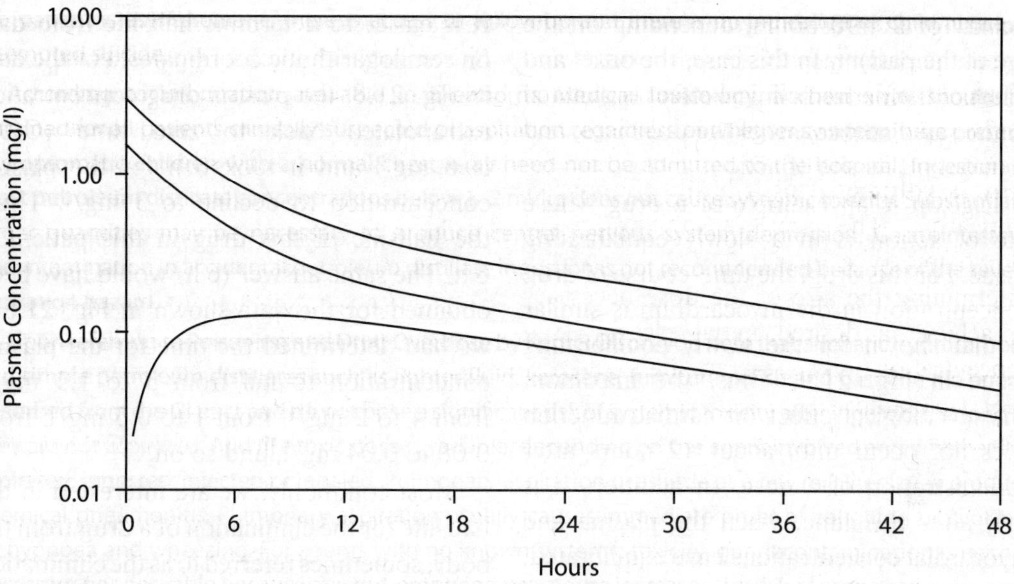

Figure 21.9 Concentration of a drug in plasma and two different tissues as a function of time following the administration of an intravenous dose at zero time. The data is shown on semilogarithmic axes. The top line shows the concentration in plasma, while the middle and bottom lines show the time-courses of the drug in rapidly and slowly equilibrating tissues, respectively.

whether or not a drug distributes rapidly or slowly into a particular type of tissue include the physicochemical properties of the drug (such as molecular size, lipohilicity) and the physiological properties of the tissue (such as mass of tissue, tissue blood flow and physicochemical nature of the tissue).

Can the rate of distribution be important clinically? Yes! Depending on whether the site of action of the drug is in a rapidly or slowly equilibrating tissue, the rate of onset and offset of pharmacological effect may be determined by distribution events. This may be demonstrated using two examples.

Diazepam administered intravenously is used for the treatment of status epilepticus. The plasma concentration time-course for this drug is similar to that for the hypothetical drug shown in Fig. 21.9. Such curvilinear behaviour for plasma concentrations on semilogarithmic coordinates arises because there are some tissues in the body that behave as slowly equilibrating sites for this drug. However, the brain, which is the site of action for diazepam, behaves as a rapidly equilibrating tissue; this is because the blood flow per gram of brain tissue is relatively high, and diazepam, being a lipophilic molecule, is able to readily diffuse across the blood–brain barrier, initially into and later out of the brain. As a consequence, the concentration time-course for diazepam in the brain is similar to that in plasma. Thus, the intravenous administration of diazepam is usually rapidly effective in halting seizure activity, but the duration of effect may be only 30 minutes or so, despite the fact that the terminal half-life of diazepam is in the vicinity of 20–90 hours, depending on the age of the patient. In this case, the onset and offset of the desired clinical effect is dictated by the rapid movement of the drug into, and then out of, its site of action.

Digoxin is an example of a drug whose site of action is in a slowly equilibrating tissue. For this drug, the time-course of drug concentration in the myocardium is similar to that shown for the slowly equilibrating tissue in Fig. 21.9. Thus, the maximum pharmacological effect on cardiac function does not occur until about 12 hours after administration of a dose. In addition, it is only after this time, when the plasma and myocardial concentrations have equilibrated, that the concentrations in plasma and myocardial tissue decline in parallel. This explains why it is important, when performing therapeutic drug monitoring in patients receiving digoxin, to wait at least 12 hours after the most recent dose (at steady state) before collecting a blood sample for estimation of plasma concentration (see *Case Study 4*). It is important to note that while the heart is a slowly equilibrating tissue for digoxin, for many other drugs, this well-perfused organ is a rapidly equilibrating tissue.

For simplicity and clinical convenience, in the subsequent sections of this chapter, we will revert to the approximation of mono-exponential disposition.

Half-life

What is half-life and how is it determined? Considering the events in Figs 21.3 and 21.8, half-life ($t_{1/2}$) describes the time required for the plasma concentration of a drug (reflecting the amount of drug in the body) to decline to half of its existing value. It is easier to determine half-life from data on semilogarithmic coordinates. For the data in Fig. 21.8, the plasma drug concentration extrapolated back to zero time (C(0)) is 6 mg/l and it took 6 h for the plasma concentration to decline to 3 mg/l. Thus, the half-life of this drug in this patient is 6 h. The same answer (6 h) would have been obtained for the data shown in Fig. 21.8 if we had determined the time for the plasma concentration to fall from 3 to 1.5 mg/l, from 4 to 2 mg/l, from 1 to 0.5 mg/l, from 0.08 to 0.04 mg/l, and so on.

Most commonly, we are interested in the half-life for the elimination of a drug from the body, sometimes referred to as the elimination half-life. It is the elimination half-life that we have calculated above for the data shown in Fig. 21.8. It should be appreciated, however, that other processes, such as the absorption of the drug from its site of administration, may also be described in terms of a half-life (absorption half-life); we will not consider this further in this chapter.

Returning to the plasma drug concentration versus time data shown in Fig. 21.8, it is evident that the decline in plasma concentration as a function of time is log-linear (a straight line on semilogarithmic coordinates). This behaviour is characteristic of a first-order kinetic process and may be described by a single- or mono-exponential equation of the form:

$$C(t) = C(0) \times e^{-k \times t} \quad (17)$$

where C(t) is the plasma concentration of a drug at a given time (t), C(0) is the initial plasma concentration at zero time and k is the first-order elimination rate constant. The fact that it is a first-order process simply means that the rate of elimination is proportional to the amount of drug in the body (or plasma drug concentration) at the same point in time; recall the earlier discussion of clearance.

What is the relationship between half-life $t_{1/2}$ and the first-order rate constant (k)? Given that $t_{1/2}$ is the time (t) that it takes for the plasma drug concentration to decline from C(0) to half of C(0), equation (17) may be rewritten as:

$$0.5 = e^{-k \times t_{1/2}} \qquad (18)$$

which may also be written as:

$$2 = e^{k \times t_{1/2}} \qquad (19)$$

and since the natural logarithm of 2 (ln 2) is 0.693, solving for $t_{1/2}$ yields the expression:

$$t_{1/2} = \frac{0.693}{k} \qquad (20)$$

Rearrangement of equation (20) gives:

$$k = \frac{0.693}{t_{1/2}} \qquad (21)$$

Thus, for the data shown in Fig. 21.8 where the half-life was determined to be 6 h, the first-order elimination rate constant must be 0.116 h^{-1} (i.e. 0.693 divided by 6 h). Note that the first-order rate constant has units of reciprocal time.

For the data shown in Fig. 21.8 (which may be described by equation 17), it is instructive to consider the relationship between the ratio of the time elapsed after drug administration to the half-life ($t/(t_{1/2})$)and the fraction of the initial amount in the body remaining at various times. As expected, after a time has elapsed equal to one half-life, 50% of the drug is eliminated from the body and 50% remains (Table 21.1). After a time corresponding to two half-life values, 75% is eliminated and 25% remains in the body, and so on. When a time equal to five half-life values for the drug has elapsed, only a little more that 3% of the drug amount originally in the body would remain. Hence, the pharmacokinetic 'rule of thumb' that it takes a time equal to about five half-lives for virtually all of the amount of drug present originally to be eliminated from the body.

What is the relationship between clearance, volume of distribution and half-life? Recall that *clearance* (CL) is the pharmacokinetic parameter that *best describes the efficiency of drug elimination* from the body, while *volume of distribution* (V) provides *a measure of the extent of distribution* of a drug within the body. Both CL and V are known as *primary pharmacokinetic parameters,* whereas elimination half-life $t_{1/2}$ is a *secondary pharmacokinetic parameter* whose magnitude is determined by the relative magnitudes of the primary parameters (CL and V), as shown in equation (22).

$$t_{1/2} = \frac{0.693 \times V}{CL} \qquad (22)$$

It is evident from equation (22) that a drug may have a long half-life either because the clearance of the drug is low or because the volume of distribution is large, or a combination of the two. It is relatively easy to accept that a drug having low clearance is likely to have a long half-life. Not so easily understood, however, is that a drug with a large volume of distribution is likely to have a long half-life. This can be more easily appreciated by recognising that for a drug with a large volume of distribution (a large fraction of drug in the body at any point in time is outside the vascular system), it will take a long time to deliver to the eliminating

Table 21.1 Fraction of drug remaining in the body as a function of time after drug administration. The fractions may be obtained by the use of a rearranged form of equation 17 ($\frac{C(t)}{C(0)} = e^{\frac{-0.693 \times t}{t_{1/2}}}$) where $\frac{0.693}{t_{1/2}}$ replaces k.

Time Elapsed After Drug Administration (multiples of $t_{1/2}$)	*Fraction of Amount Remaining in the Body*
0	1
1	0.5
2	0.25
3	0.125
4	0.0625
5	0.03125

organs (liver and kidneys) all of the drug in the body. Thus, even if the eliminating organs clear the drug efficiently, the drug may have a long half-life. It is also evident from equation (22) that an increase in half-life in an individual patient may arise from an increase in volume of distribution alone, while the efficiency of drug elimination (CL) may remain unchanged. These considerations indicate that *half-life should not be used to quantify the efficiency of drug elimination*.

Why is half-life important clinically? There are several reasons why half-life is important clinically. *First, half-life may be a determinant of the duration of action of a drug* after a single dose, as may be appreciated from a consideration of the profiles shown in Fig. 21.10. If, for example, the minimum effective plasma drug concentration to elicit the desired effect for this drug is 1 mg/l, the duration of action of the drug is likely to be longer in the patient having the longer half-life.

Secondly, half-life determines the time required to achieve steady-state plasma drug concentrations on chronic administration. This is most readily demonstrated by a consideration of a drug administered by constant-rate intravenous infusion, as shown in Fig. 21.5. The equation that describes the plasma drug concentration (C(t)) as a function of time during a constant-rate intravenous infusion (t) is:

$$C(t) = \frac{R_0}{CL}(1 - e^{-k \times t}) \qquad (23)$$

This equation may be re-written as:

$$C(t) = \frac{R_0}{CL}(1 - e^{\frac{-0.693 \times t}{t_{1/2}}}) \qquad (24)$$

Note that when the drug has been infused for a sufficiently long period such that $t >> t_{1/2}$, the exponential term approaches zero and the right-hand side of the equation collapses to (R_0/CL). Clearly, under these circumstances, the plasma concentration of the drug is constant with time, and we say that the plasma drug concentration is at steady state C^{ss}. That is:

$$C^{ss} = \frac{R_0}{CL} \qquad (25)$$

Note that equation (25) is exactly the same as equation (7) that was derived by recognising that at steady state, the rate of drug input into systemic circulation, R_0, is equal to the rate of elimination; and that the latter is equal to clearance (CL) multiplied by plasma drug concentration C^{ss}.

Substitution of equation (25) in equation (24) gives:

Figure 21.10 Plasma concentrations of a drug as a function of time in two hypothetical patients following the administration of an intravenous dose of 300 mg at zero time. In both cases, the volume of distribution is 50 l. For the patient whose data is depicted in the lower profile, the half-life is 6 h (same data as shown in Fig. 21.8) while for the other profile, the half-life is 12 h. The data is shown on semilogarithmic axes.

$$C(t) = C^{ss}\,(1 - e^{\frac{-0.693 \times t}{t_{1/2}}}) \qquad (26)$$

Re-arrangement of equation (26) allows determination of the time required to achieve various fractions of the steady state plasma concentration after commencing a constant-rate intravenous infusion (Table 21.2). Thus, it can be seen that after infusing for a time equivalent to one half-life, the plasma concentration will have reached 50% of the steady-state value; after a time equivalent to two half-lives, the concentration will have reached 75% of steady state, and so on. It can be seen that after infusing for a time equivalent to 3–5 half-life values, the plasma concentration will have reached about 88% and 97%, respectively, of the steady-state concentration (Table 21.2).

In a clinical setting, there is likely to be little difference between 88% and 97% of the steady-state concentration. Therefore, in this setting, it is acceptable to conclude that steady state is essentially achieved after a time of administration equivalent to about 3–5 half-lives. These principles are demonstrated graphically in Fig. 21.5; in that case, the drug had a half-life of 6 h and it can be seen that it took about 20–30 h for the drug to achieve the steady-state plasma concentration.

It should be noted that this pharmacokinetic 'rule of thumb' also applies when drugs are administered according to other regimens, including chronic oral dosing (as discussed in *Case Study 4*). For example, when a drug is administered to a patient as a fixed dose given at a set dose interval, it will take about

3–5 half-lives for the plasma concentration to reach steady state. This can be seen to be the case for the data shown in Fig. 21.6. In addition, if an existing dose regimen is altered, it will take a time equivalent to 3–5 half-lives for the new steady-state concentration to be achieved.

Thirdly, half-life needs to be considered when deciding on the dose interval in a multiple-dosing regimen. This is readily apparent from the plasma concentration time profiles shown in Fig. 21.11. The profiles have been generated for the same patient; in one case, 300 mg was administered orally every 6 h, while in the second, 600 mg was administered every 12 h. In accordance with equation (12), and because the daily dosing rate (1200 mg per day) and bioavailability and clearance were the same on both occasions, it is not surprising that the average steady-state plasma concentration (C^{ss}_{av}) was the same in both cases (4.3 mg/l). However, the 'peak to trough' fluctuations are substantially greater for the regimen with the longer dose interval; it may be expected that there would be greater swings in the intensity of the pharmacological/toxicological effect throughout a dose interval.

As a general 'rule of thumb', the ratio of 'peak to trough' concentrations will be less than two if a drug is administered by a conventional oral formulation at a dose interval no longer than a time equal to its half-life. If a suitable sustained-release formulation is used, it may be possible to limit the degree of fluctuations in the plasma concentration while extending the dose interval.

Table 21.2 Fraction of steady-state plasma drug concentration achieved at various times during a constant-rate intravenous infusion. The fractions may be obtained by use of a rearranged form of equation 26 $(\frac{C(t)}{C^{ss}}) = (1 - e^{\frac{-0.693 \times t}{t_{1/2}}})$.

Time Elapsed After Commencing a Constant-rate Infusion (multiples of $t_{1/2}$)	Fraction of steady state Plasma Drug Concentration Achieved
0	0
1	0.5
2	0.75
3	0.875
4	0.9375
5	0.9688

Fraction Excreted Unchanged in Urine

What is the fraction excreted unchanged in urine and how is it determined? As the name implies, the fraction excreted unchanged in urine (fe) is the fraction of the amount of the dose that reached the systemic circulation that is ultimately excreted in its unchanged (unmetabolised) form into urine. It is best determined after the intravenous injection of the drug because in this case the amount reaching the systemic circulation is known – it is the dose. Under these circumstances, collection of all urine voided over a period of about five half-lives after drug administration permits determination of the amount of unchanged drug excreted in urine to 'infinite' time (Ae(∞)); recall from our discussion of half-life that virtually all of the drug reaching the systemic circulation will be excreted after five half-lives have elapsed. Then, fe may be determined as:

$$fe = \frac{Ae(\infty)}{D} \qquad (27)$$

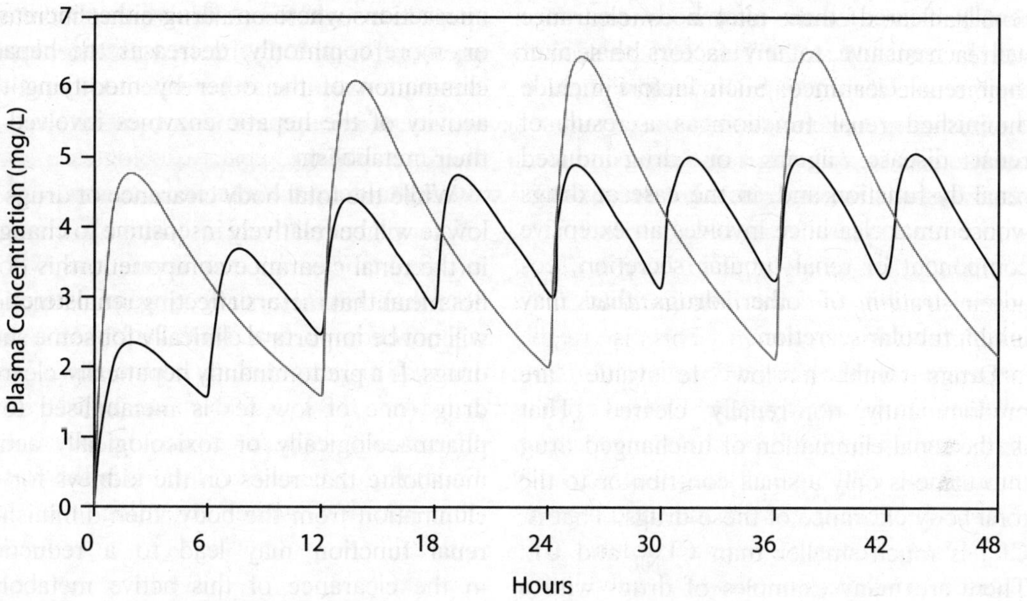

Figure 21.11 Plasma concentration–time profiles for a drug administered to a patient as a 300-mg oral dose given every 6 hours (same data as shown in Fig. 21.6) or as a 600-mg oral dose given every 12 hours. The total body clearance, half-life and bioavailability for this drug in this patient were 5.8 L/h, 6 h and 0.5, respectively.

where D is the intravenous dose administered. Since both the numerator and the denominator of equation (27) have units of amount, it is evident that fe is a dimensionless parameter. From an examination of equation (27), it is also obvious that the lower and upper limits for fe are zero and one.

Why is the fraction excreted unchanged in urine important clinically? The fraction excreted unchanged in urine (fe) is important because it points to the main organ involved in the clearance of the drug from the body (kidneys or liver, or a combination of the two). This, in turn, often provides a good insight into those factors that may modify the clearance of the drug in a patient.

While fe is determined using equation (27), from a consideration of Fig. 21.2 and equation (1), it is evident that fe is also equal to the ratio of the renal clearance of a drug to its total body clearance. That is:

$$\text{fe} = \frac{CL_R}{CL_R + CL_{NR}} \tag{28}$$

and, therefore:

$$\text{fe} = \frac{CL_R}{CL} \tag{29}$$

Thus, when fe is high, renal clearance of the unchanged drug in urine is the main contributor to total body clearance. Such a drug may be described as being predominantly renally cleared. Examples of drugs that belong to this category include aminoglycoside antibiotics, such as gentamicin (fe ≈ 1), and digoxin (fe ≈ 0.7). Because drugs of high fe are predominantly renally cleared, their total body clearance will be sensitive to any factors that alter their renal clearance. Such factors include diminished renal function as a result of renal disease, ageing or drug-induced renal dysfunction and, in the case of drugs whose renal clearance involves an extensive component of renal tubular secretion, co-administration of other drugs that may inhibit tubular secretion.

Drugs with a low fe value are predominantly non-renally cleared. That is, the renal elimination of unchanged drug into urine is only a small contributor to the total body clearance of these drugs. That is, CL_R is much smaller than CL_{NR} and CL. There are many examples of drugs with a low fe, including theophylline, phenytoin, carbamazepine, lignocaine and tricyclic anti-depressants. As indicated earlier, the main organ contributing to the non-renal clearance of drugs is the liver. Thus, in most cases, it is reasonable to assume that predominantly non-renally cleared drugs are predominantly hepatically cleared.

The total body clearance of these drugs will be sensitive to factors that modify the activity of drug metabolising enzymes in the liver and, in some cases, blood flow to the liver and the fraction of the drug unbound in plasma. Factors that may affect the activity of drug metabolising enzymes in the liver include genetic constitution that determines the level of expression of drug metabolising enzymes, liver diseases such as hepatic cirrhosis, environmental factors such as cigarette smoking that may induce drug metabolising enzymes and co-administration of other drugs that may either induce or inhibit the enzymes. Predominantly hepatically-cleared drugs are quite often involved in drug–drug interactions where one drug either increases or, more commonly, decreases the hepatic elimination of the other by modifying the activity of the hepatic enzymes involved in their metabolism.

While the total body clearance of drugs of low fe will be relatively insensitive to changes in the renal clearance component, this does not mean that factors affecting renal function will not be important clinically for some such drugs. If a predominantly hepatically-cleared drug (one of low fe) is metabolised to a pharmacologically or toxicologically active metabolite that relies on the kidneys for its elimination from the body, then diminished renal function may lead to a reduction in the clearance of this active metabolite (Fig. 21.2).

Pethidine is one such drug. This synthetic opioid analgesic is predominantly hepatically cleared (fe $\approx$ 0.1), with norpethidine being one of the metabolites formed. Norpethidine has little analgesic activity but it causes excitation of the central nervous system that may result in seizures. The renal route of elimination predominates for norpethidine and therefore its renal clearance and, as a consequence, its total body clearance, decreases in patients with impaired kidney function.

To avoid accumulation of this toxicologically active metabolite in renally impaired patients (and the risk of seizures), it would be necessary to decrease the dosing rate of pethidine. Unfortunately, this often leads to a decrease in analgesic effect because of the lower plasma concentration of pethidine achieved and the lack of analgesic activity of norpethidine. This explains why pethidine is a very poor choice of opioid analgesic in patients with impaired renal function.

Fraction Unbound in Plasma

What is the fraction unbound in plasma? Many drugs can bind reversibly to sites on plasma proteins. The proteins most commonly involved in plasma binding of drugs are albumin (especially for weak organic acid drugs) and α_1-acid glycoprotein (especially for weak organic base drugs). Rather than considering the fraction of drug in plasma that is bound to proteins, it is more useful in pharmacokinetics to consider the fraction of drug in plasma that is in the unbound form (fu). This may be expressed as:

$$fu = \frac{Cu}{C} \quad (30)$$

where Cu is the concentration of drug in the unbound form and C is the concentration of total drug in plasma at the same point in time. Major determinants of fu are the affinity of the protein for the drug and the concentration of the protein to which the drug binds.

Since both the numerator and the denominator of equation (30) have units of concentration, it is evident that fu is a dimensionless pharmacokinetic parameter. Furthermore, it is clear that fu will be one (the upper limit) when no binding occurs (Cu = C), while fu will be near zero when a drug is very extensively bound to plasma proteins (Cu <<< C).

Why is fraction unbound in plasma important clinically? At equilibrium after drug administration, the concentration of the unbound drug in plasma (Cu) is usually considered to be the same as (or at least reflective of) the concentration of the unbound drug in the biological fluids bathing the receptor site for the drug. Thus, the concentration of unbound drug in plasma often relates well to the intensity of the pharmacological and toxicological effects of a drug. *One of the most important things to recognise about fu* is that while it is related to Cu, it is not the same!

As is evident from equation (30), fu is simply a way of conveying information about the fraction of the total drug present in (a sample of) plasma that is in the unbound form. Thus, in a sample of plasma with a total concentration (C) of 5 mg/l and an fu of 0.2, the unbound concentration will be 1 mg/l.

Various factors may increase the fu of a drug. Such factors include a decrease in the concentration of the binding protein (as may occur for plasma albumin concentration in liver or renal disease) or the co-administration of another drug that binds extensively to the same binding site, leading to competition for binding between the two drugs. Obviously, the potential for an increase in fu will be greatest for those drugs that are most extensively bound (where fu is low).

Is an increase in fu likely to be important clinically? The answer to this question in most cases is no! The reason is that the main determinant of unbound concentration of drug (Cu) during therapy is usually the activity of the intrinsic clearance mechanisms for the drug. These mechanisms are the activity of drug metabolising enzymes in predominantly hepatically cleared drugs and, the glomerular filtration rate and possibly the activity of renal tubular secretory transport systems for predominantly renally cleared drugs. Thus, while an increase in fu may occur as a result of, for example, a plasma protein binding displacement drug interaction, the unbound *concentration* (Cu) of drug is not likely to change greatly (unless there is also a change in the efficiency of the intrinsic clearance mechanisms for the drug in question). It follows that, although the unbound concentration (Cu) may not change greatly when fu increases, the total concentration (C) will decrease (Fig. 21.12).

Phenytoin is an example of a drug where these concepts are important clinically. Care is needed when interpreting measured total plasma phenytoin concentrations during therapeutic drug monitoring in circumstances where fu may have changed.

Bioavailability

What is bioavailability and how is it determined? As mentioned previously, bioavailability (f) refers to the fraction of an administered dose that reaches the systemic circulation intact; it is a dimensionless parameter. In intravenous administration, the entire dose reaches the systemic circulation, and therefore, the drug is fully bioavailable (f = 1). With other routes of administration, however, absorption of the drug from the site of administration to the systemic circulation may be incomplete. Since oral administration of drugs is common, we shall briefly consider those factors that may lead to less than complete absorption into the systemic circulation with this route of administration.

The main factors that may lead to a decrease in bioavailability after oral administration are summarised in Table 21.3. Note that there are two categories of factors. Firstly, those that may decrease the fraction of the administered dose that reaches the hepatic portal vein as intact (unmetabolised) drug; we will refer to the fraction that is absorbed from the gut into portal circulation as f_G. There are several possible reasons for a low f_G value.

The second factor that may decrease oral bioavailability is hepatic first-pass metabolism. This will be most significant when the liver has very high efficiency for clearance of the drug such that there is a high fraction of drug that is delivered to the liver that is 'extracted' (metabolised) on each circulation through the liver, including the 'first pass' immediately following absorption into the portal circulation. We will refer to the fraction that escapes hepatic extraction as f_H.

The overall bioavailability (f) is the product of f_G and f_H. That is:

$$f = f_G \times f_H \tag{31}$$

Thus, if 50% of an orally administered dose is absorbed into portal circulation and 50% of these molecules escape hepatic extraction during 'first pass' through the liver, the bioavailability will be 0.25 (f = 0.5 x 0.5). For many drugs, low f_H is the main factor leading to low bioavailability after oral administration (for example, the bioavailability of morphine administered orally is only about 0.3 (30%), even though it is well absorbed from the gut).

Briefly, bioavailability (f) following extravascular (for example, oral) administration is most commonly determined from the area under the plasma concentration–time curve relative to that achieved with intravenous dosing on another occasion in the same subject, normalised for any differences in dose between the two routes of administration. That is:

$$f = \frac{AUC_{oral}}{AUC_{IV}} \times \frac{D_{IV}}{D_{oral}} \tag{32}$$

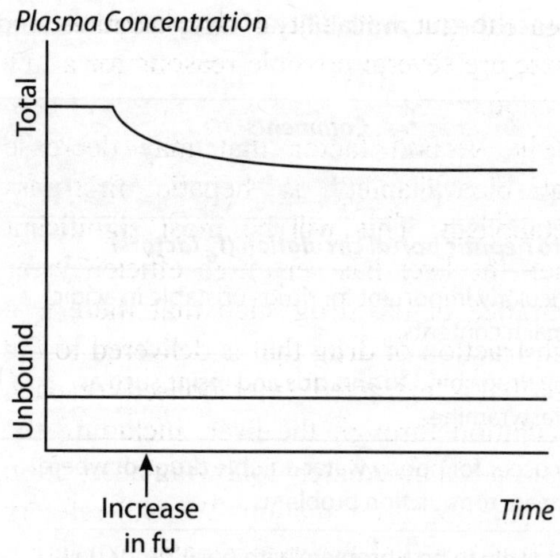

Figure 21.12 Diagrammatic representation of the impact of an increase in unbound fraction in plasma (fu) in a patient whose total and unbound concentrations in plasma were already at steady-state prior to the increase in fu. After the increase in fu occurs, the total concentration decreases to a new lower steady-state value. However, if there is no change in the activity of the intrinsic clearance mechanisms, there will not be a change in the steady-state concentration for the unbound drug in plasma. While the intensity of the pharmacological/toxicological effect is not likely to alter greatly (because the unbound concentration has not changed), there is much potential to misinterpret therapeutic drug monitoring data based on measurement of total plasma concentration.

where AUC_{oral} and AUC_{IV} are the areas under the plasma concentration–time curves after oral and intravenous administration, respectively, and D_{oral} and D_{IV} are the corresponding doses. Implicit in the use of equation (32) is that the total body clearance is the same on the two occasions on which the subject receives the drug; this requires careful control to avoid factors that could change the hepatic and/or renal clearance.

Why is bioavailability important clinically? As is evident from earlier discussions, bioavailability (f) is one of the pharmacokinetic determinants of plasma concentrations achieved after the administration of an extravascular dose; clearance is the other determinant (see equation (12)). It is also important to recognise that some of the factors that may contribute to low bioavailability through a low f_G (Table 21.3) are amenable to alteration in the clinic (for example, by using an enteric-coated formulation for acid-labile drugs, administering drugs at different times from antacids, etc.).

Conclusion

In the preceding sections, we have provided an overview of several pharmacokinetic parameters. In particular, we have demonstrated why these parameters are important clinically and provided the background theory as to how they may be used to individualise therapy in patients – in the *Case Studies*, you will have the opportunity of putting this theory into practice! As will be seen, sometimes it is possible to estimate some of these parameters for a specific patient in the clinic. However, many times this is not possible and it will be necessary to use 'population' estimates relevant to the type of patient you may be dealing with. 'Population' estimates of each of the parameters discussed above are available for many drugs and may be found in tabulations contained in the books in the section *Further Reading*.

Table 21.3 Summary of main factors that may decrease the bioavailability of drugs administered orally by alteration of f_G or f_H.

Factors That May Lead to Less Than 100% of an Orally Administered Dose Reaching Systemic Circulation	*Comments*
Less than complete absorption from intestinal lumen into hepatic portal circulation (f_G factors)	
• Degradation of drug in stomach or intestine	Particularly important for drugs unstable in acidic stomach contents.
• Complexation/binding to food or other drugs	Many drugs bind to antacids and resins such as cholestyramine.
• Insufficient time for dissolution before gastrointestinal transit is complete	May occur for poorly water-soluble drugs or where there are formulation problems
• Insufficient time for absorption across intestinal mucosa before gastrointestinal transit is complete	Most likely to be a problem with polar drugs (low solubility in intestinal epithelium cell membranes)
• Metabolism by bacteria in the gut or during absorption through the intestinal epithelial cells	Intestinal cells contain enzymes that may metabolise a drug during absorption
Removal of drug during transit from hepatic portal circulation to systemic circulation (f_H factor)	
• Hepatic 'first-pass' metabolism	Drug that has just been absorbed must pass through the liver for the first time to reach systemic circulation. Any drug that is metabolised during this first pass will decrease the amount reaching systemic circulation.

Table 21.4 Definitions for pharmacokinetic symbols

A	Amount of drug in the body
Ae(∞)	Amount of unchanged drug excreted in urine to infinite time
AUC	Area under the plasma drug concentration versus time curve
C	Plasma drug concentration of total drug (unbound plus bound drug)
Cu	Concentration of unbound drug in plasma
C(0)	Plasma drug concentration achieved just after administration of an intravenous injection
C(t)	Plasma drug concentration at a given time t
C^{SS}	Plasma drug concentration at steady state achieved with a constant-rate infusion
C_{av}^{ss}	Average plasma drug concentration at steady state achieved with a fixed dose given at a fixed dosage interval
CL	Total body clearance of drug
CL_R	Renal clearance of drug
CL_{NR}	Non-renal clearance of drug (clearance via pathways other than excretion into urine)
D	Size of drug dose
f	Fraction of administered drug dose that reaches systemic circulation intact
fe	Fraction of amount of the dose that reached systemic circulation that is excreted in unchanged form into urine
fu	Fraction of drug in plasma that is in unbound form
k	First-order rate constant for elimination of drug from the body
R_0	Rate of intravenous infusion of drug
t	Time elapsed after drug administration or after commencing drug administration
τ	Dosage interval
$t_{1/2}$	Half-life of drug
V	Volume of distribution of drug

CASE STUDY 1

RN, a 30-year-old male weighing 68 kg, has been admitted to the emergency room for the third time this year, complaining of severe dyspnoea and frequent coughing that has progressively worsened over the past two days. His medical history is significant for multiple admissions due to acute asthma. Following administration of salbutamol, RN's physical examination still revealed an anxious-appearing man in moderate to severe respiratory distress, with audible expiratory wheeze and frequent coughing. The attending physician has now requested you, as the clinical pharmacist, to estimate an intravenous loading dose of aminophylline that will produce a plasma theophylline concentration of 15 mg/l (usual therapeutic range: 10–20 mg/l). The volume of distribution for theophylline in normal adults is approximately 0.5 l/kg and the salt form factor for conversion of aminophylline to theophylline equivalents is 0.8.

Discussion

As discussed earlier, the principal application of volume of distribution is in determining the size of dose necessary to achieve the initial plasma concentration. This first dose, often termed the loading dose, is particularly important for dosing drugs such as theophylline, where the desired therapeutic response is required urgently and related to plasma concentration. The usual or 'population' volume of distribution for theophylline among adults like RN is approximately 0.5 l/kg; however, it may vary among other patient groups. You will recall that by using equation (16), a loading dose for theophylline may be calculated.

$$D = V \times C(0)$$

To achieve an initial plasma concentration (C(0)) of 15 mg/l for theophylline, that has an estimated volume of distribution of 34 l (0.5 l/kg multiplied by 68 kg), it will be necessary to administer an intravenous dose of theophylline of 510 mg (34 l multiplied by 15 mg/l). Theophylline is available for intravenous administration in a salt form, called aminophylline. Aminophylline contains 80% anhydrous theophylline and as intravenous aminophylline is to be used, the loading dose calculated must be divided by the salt form factor (S) of 0.8.

$$D = \frac{[V \times C(0)]}{S}$$

Therefore, in order to achieve an initial plasma concentration (C(0)) of 15 mg/l for theophylline, that has an estimated volume of distribution of 34 l, it will be necessary to administer an intravenous dose of aminophylline of 638 mg (510 mg divided by 0.8), or approximately 640 mg.

Another common scenario is how to calculate a loading dose of aminophylline in the setting where theophylline already exists in the body from an earlier administration. For example, imagine that RN had a plasma theophylline concentration of 2 mg/l determined in the emergency room. In this circumstance, rather than requiring a loading dose of aminophylline to increase theophylline concentrations from 0 mg/l to 15 mg/l (a 15 mg/l change), a dose is required to increase concentrations from 2 mg/l to 15 mg/l (a 13 mg/l change). In this case, the loading dose can be calculated as:

$$D = \frac{[V \times (C(0) - (C(1))]}{S}$$

where (C(0) – C(1)) is the difference between the desired plasma theophylline concentration (C(0), which is 15 mg/l) and the measured plasma theophylline concentration (C(1), which is 2 mg/l). In order to increase the plasma concentration of theophylline from 2 mg/l (C(1)) to 15 mg/l (C(0)) for theophylline, that has an estimated volume of distribution of 34 l, it will be necessary to administer an intravenous dose of aminophylline of 552 mg (34 l multiplied by (15 mg/l – 2 mg/l) divided by 0.8), or approximately 550 mg.

It is important to remember that by using these simple equations to calculate a loading dose, there is an assumption that the dose is administered as a bolus injection. In clinical practice, there are circumstances where it is not appropriate to administer a drug as a bolus injection. For example, aminophylline must not be administered as a bolus intravenous injection as toxicity involving the heart and central nervous system correlates with transiently high plasma concentrations of theophylline that occur with rapid administration. Therefore, loading doses of aminophylline should be administered slowly, over about 30 minutes.

CASE STUDY 2

RN received a loading dose of 640 mg of aminophylline to achieve a target plasma theophylline concentration of 15 mg/l. His signs and symptoms of acute asthma have started to improve. The attending physician would now like to know what continuous infusion rate of aminophylline should be used to maintain the theophylline concentration at 15 mg/l. During your patient interview, you established that RN smokes a packet of cigarettes most days.

Discussion

Whereas calculation of the loading dose requires volume of distribution, you will recall from the section ***Why is clearance important clinically?*** that steady-state plasma concentration (C^{SS}) is directly proportional to the rate of infusion (R_0) and inversely proportional to clearance (CL) (see equation (7)):

$$C^{ss} = \frac{R_0}{CL}$$

where C^{SS} is the desired concentration of 15 mg/L, the clearance (CL) is unknown, and the rate of infusion (R_0) is desired.

In the same fashion as in *Case Study 1*, where a usual or 'population' estimate of volume of distribution was used to calculate a loading dose, it would be convenient to also use a 'population' clearance value to calculate an initial maintenance infusion rate. However, it must be recognised that the clearance of theophylline and many drugs may be affected by other factors, including disease and drug interactions. This means that there will be a number of quoted 'population' clearances depending on the presence of disease, organ dysfunction or other conditions. For theophylline, the 'population' clearance value has been expressed in the following way:

$$CL_{theophylline} = 0.04 \text{ L/h/kg} \times \text{Body weight (kg)} \times \text{Factor}$$

where the 'factor' is dependent upon the presence of a disease, concomitant drug therapy or other condition that affects clearance, as listed in the table below.

Conditions affecting $CL_{theophylline}$ and the factor by which clearance is altered

Conditions Increasing or Decreasing Clearance	*Factor*
Conditions increasing $CL_{theophylline}$	
Smoking history	1.6
Cystic fibrosis	1.5
Paediatrics	1.6
Phenytoin	1.6
Phenobarbitone	1.3
Rifampin	1.3
Conditions decreasing $CL_{theophylline}$	
Congestive heart failure	0.4
Chronic obstructive pulmonary disease	0.8
Hepatic cirrhosis	0.4
Cimetidine	0.6
Ciprofloxacin	0.7

Adapted from Winter ME. 1998. *Basic Clinical Pharmacokinetics 3rd ed.* Applied Therapeutics Inc.: Washington.

Given that RN is a smoker, his estimated clearance would be 4.4 l/h ($CL_{theophylline}$ of 0.04 l/h/kg multiplied by 68 kg multiplied by 1.6 (from the table)). From equation (6):

$$R_0 = CL \times C^{ss}$$

an infusion rate (R_0) required to maintain a concentration of 15 mg/l C^{SS}), in a patient with an estimated clearance of 4.4 L/h (CL) would be 66 mg/h of theophylline, or 82.5 mg/h of aminophylline (R_0 divided by the salt form factor (0.8) for aminophylline). Approximately 24 hours after commencement of maintenance infusion, a plasma theophylline concentration of 15.6 mg/l was obtained. Assuming that the concentration at 24 hours approximated the 'steady-state' condition, the similarity between the observed (15.6 mg/l) and desired (15 mg/l) concentrations indicates that the 'population' estimate of clearance (4.4 l/h) must have been a good approximation of RN's individual clearance.

CASE STUDY 3

Three weeks later, RN is admitted to hospital yet again with an acute exacerbation of asthma. The attending physician initiates the same aminophylline loading dose and maintenance dose regimen that had been used last time (*Case Studies 1 and 2*). A few hours later, RN's respiratory function had significantly improved but he started to complain of headache and nausea. Twenty-eight hours after the maintenance infusion had been started, the plasma theophylline concentration was determined to be 25 mg/l. The physician has asked your advice on why RN is showing signs of theophylline toxicity, despite the same dosing regimen being used without incident, only a few weeks ago. Further, you are asked to design a maintenance infusion regimen for aminophylline to achieve a theophylline concentration of 15 mg/l. During a discussion with RN, you learn that he has abstained from smoking since his last admission.

Discussion

You will recall from equation (7) that the steady-state plasma concentration (C^{SS}) is directly proportional to the rate of infusion (R_0) and inversely proportional to clearance (CL):

$$C^{ss} = \frac{R_0}{CL}$$

Whereas in *Case Study 2*, a 'population' value of clearance was used to design the maintenance dose regimen, it is possible using the information presented above, and equation (8), to calculate RN's individual clearance ***relevant to the present hospital admission***.

$$CL = \frac{R_0}{C^{ss}}$$

In calculating the individual clearance, it will be necessary to assume that the plasma theophylline concentration determined 28 h after commencing the infusion represents the 'steady state'. RN's clearance can be calculated to be 2.6 l/h (82.5 mg/h (R_0 for aminophylline) multiplied by 0.8 (salt form factor for conversion of aminophylline to theophylline equivalents) divided by 25 mg/l (C^{SS})). This clearance estimate is 60% of the 'population' value (4.4 l/h) used to design the maintenance regimen in *Case Study 2*; also recall that during the earlier hospital admission, the same aminophylline maintenance infusion rate resulted in a 'steady-state' plasma theophylline concentration of 15.6 mg/l. Logically, it is not uncommon for individual patient clearances to differ from values determined from a population; however, the substantial difference observed in RN's clearance between admissions is likely due to his recent abstinence from cigarette smoking. Smoking induces the enzymes responsible for the metabolism of theophylline, leading to an increase in clearance (by a factor of about 1.6, as shown in the table above);

upon cessation of smoking, as occurred with RN between admissions, the enzyme activity and clearance of theophylline decreased. This should be discussed with the attending physician.

In your discussion with the physician, you suggest that it would be preferable to stop aminophylline infusion for a period of time sufficient for the plasma theophylline concentration to decline to 15 mg/l, and then to re-commence infusion at a suitable rate to maintain the desired plasma concentration. The time required for the plasma concentration to decline from 25 mg/l to 15 mg/l can be estimated using equation (17):

$$C(t) = C(0) \times e^{-k \times t}$$

While this equation was applied earlier to the mono-exponential disposition of a drug following intravenous injection, it may also be applied to the decline in plasma concentration following cessation of a constant-rate infusion. Since $k = \frac{0.693}{t_{1/2}}$ (equation (21)), the equation above may be re-written as:

$$C(t) = C(0) \times e^{\frac{-0.693 \times t}{t_{1/2}}}$$

which, upon re-arrangement, gives

$$\frac{C(t)}{C(0)} = e^{\frac{-0.693 \times t}{t_{1/2}}}$$

and

$$\frac{C(0)}{C(t)} = e^{\frac{0.693 \times t}{t_{1/2}}}$$

which may be expressed as:

$$\ln\left(\frac{C(0)}{C(t)}\right) = \frac{0.693 \times t}{t_{1/2}}$$

It can be seen that the time (t) necessary for the concentration to decrease from C(0) to C(t) is given by:

$$t = \frac{\ln (C(0) / C(t)) \times t_{1/2}}{0.693}$$

An estimate of $t_{1/2}$ may be obtained from equation (22):

$$t_{1/2} = \frac{0.693 \times V}{CL}$$

which gives a value of 9.1 h for theophylline half-life in RN during this admission (0.693 multiplied by 34 l (from *Case Study* 1) divided by 2.6 l/h; note that the volume of distribution is not affected by cigarette smoking). Thus, the time required for plasma theophylline concentration to decline from 25 mg/l to 15 mg/l is:

$$t = \frac{\ln(25/15) \times 9.1}{0.693}$$

which gives a time of 6.7 h. Thus, if the infusion is discontinued for approximately six and a half hours from the time of collection of the blood sample above, the plasma concentration would be expected to decline from 25 mg/l to about 15 mg/l. When performing any calculations like this, always convince yourself that the answer makes sense! In this case, it does – the estimated half-life in this case is 9.1 h, and so it will take a time less than one half-life for the concentration to decrease to 60% of its original value (15 mg/l divided by 25 mg/l = 0.6).

Now to the calculation of a new maintenance aminophylline infusion rate to maintain the plasma theophylline concentration at 15 mg/l. The infusion rate can be determined on the basis of RN's individual clearance using equation (6), as demonstrated in *Case Study 2*:

$$R_0 = CL \times C^{ss}$$

The new aminophylline infusion rate (R_0) required to maintain a theophylline concentration of 15 mg/l (C^{SS}) in a patient with a clearance of 2.6 l/h (CL) would be approximately 40 mg/hr of theophylline, or 50 mg/hr of aminophylline equivalents (R_0 for theophylline divided by the salt form factor for conversion of theophylline to aminophylline).

CASE STUDY 4

A medical intern has called you regarding JM, an 87-year-old woman of 54 kg, who is scheduled to be discharged home on digoxin for stage II congestive heart failure (CHF). The medical intern is seeking advice on an appropriate oral maintenance dose of digoxin that would maintain an average steady-state plasma digoxin concentration of 1.5 µg/l (usual therapeutic range: 0.5–2 µg/l). The intern has also asked when a plasma digoxin concentration should be measured to check the appropriateness of the regimen. JM's creatinine clearance (CLcr) was recently determined to be 30 ml/min.

Discussion

You will recall that the average steady-state plasma concentration (C^{ss}_{av}) achieved in a patient receiving a drug regularly by the oral route is determined by the dose regimen (the size of each dose (D) and how often it is given (τ)), and the pharmacokinetic parameters bioavailability (f) and clearance (CL) according to equation (12):

$$C^{ss}_{av} = \frac{f(D/\tau)}{CL}$$

The half-life of digoxin, a drug cleared mainly by the kidney, in patients with normal renal function is about 36 h; in patients like JM, who have diminished renal function, a longer half-life may be expected. Therefore, for maintenance dose regimens with digoxin, a dose interval of 24 h is appropriate to minimise 'peak-to-trough' fluctuations (see *Why is half-life important clinically?*). Using a dosing interval (τ) of one day, and an oral bioavailability (f) of 0.7, we are able to calculate the size of each daily dose (D) to achieve an average steady-state plasma concentration of 1.5 µg/l, provided we have information about clearance (CL).

As we saw with theophylline in *Case Studies 2* and *3*, the clearance of digoxin may vary considerably among patients due to a variety of reasons, including alteration of renal function and presence of CHF. In this case, the total clearance of digoxin may be estimated with the following 'population-based' equation:

$CL_{digoxin(CHF)}$ (mL/min) = (0.9) x (CLcr mL/min) + [(0.33 mL/min/kg) x Weight (kg)]

(This equation is taken from Winter ME. 1998). You will recall that the total clearance of a drug is the sum of both the renal and non-renal clearances (see equation (1)).

Using this equation, JM's estimated total digoxin clearance is 44.8 ml/min, which comprises the renal clearance (CL_R equal to 0.9 multiplied by CLcr of 30 ml/min) and the non-renal clearance (CL_{NR} equal to 0.33 ml/min/kg multiplied by 54 kg)].

By rearranging equation (12), it is possible to calculate the daily digoxin dose required to achieve an average steady-state plasma concentration of 1.5 µg/l:

$$D = \frac{C_{av}^{ss} \times CL \times \tau}{f}$$

where τ is 1 day, the desired C_{av}^{ss} is 1.5 µg/l, f is 0.7 and CL is 64.5 l/day (44.8 ml/min multiplied by 60 min/h multiplied by 24 h/day divided by 1000 ml/l). The change of dimensions for CL is necessary; it is always important to ensure that the dimensions used in the various parts of a pharmacokinetic equation are consistent! Thus, the required dose is 138 µg per day, or rounding down to the most convenient dose form of 125 µg per day (0.125 mg per day).

The intern still requires advice on when the first plasma digoxin concentration should be measured to check the appropriateness of the regimen. The answer to this question should include advice relating to when the drug concentrations are no longer increasing (or are relatively stable, or at steady state, as discussed under the section *Why is half-life important clinically?*) and advice describing the number of hours following a dose at steady state where a plasma digoxin concentration is most informative.

You will recall that after repeated dosing for approximately 3–5 half-lives, you can feel confident that drug concentrations are virtually at steady state. Equation (22), from the section *What is the relationship between clearance, volume of distribution and half life?* can be used to estimate the half-life of digoxin in this case.

$$t_{1/2} = \frac{0.693 \times V}{CL}$$

where CL is 64.5 l per day, and a 'population' estimate for digoxin volume of distribution for this case is 298 l (based on V (l) = 3.8 x Weight in kg + 3.1 x CLcr (ml/min), (from Winter ME 1998); thus, the estimated half-life for JM is 3.2 days. If a blood sample for determination of plasma digoxin concentration is collected in approximately 10–16 days from commencement of the dosage regimen, you can be reasonably confident that drug concentrations will be virtually at steady state. Of course, plasma concentrations can be determined earlier if there is concern about the possibility of a toxicological response; however, such concentrations are of little use for making adjustments to the maintenance regimen.

The second part of the intern's request requires consideration of when, in relation to a given dose at steady-state, a plasma sample should be collected for determination of digoxin concentration. As discussed in the section ***Is the rate of drug distribution important?***, digoxin is a drug that displays a prominent 'distribution' phase, and concentrations at the site of action (myocardial tissue) equilibrate slowly with those in plasma. It is necessary, therefore, to wait at least 12 hours after a dose before collecting a sample so that the plasma digoxin concentration can be interpreted correctly.

KEY MESSAGES

- Clinical pharmacokinetics is concerned with the process of using pharmacokinetic principles and pharmacodynamic criteria to assist in the selection of appropriate drug dose regimens for individual patients.
- Clearance is a primary pharmacokinetic parameter that describes the efficiency of drug elimination and is critically important for designing maintenance dose regimens that will achieve a desired steady-state concentration (continuous infusion regimens) or desired average steady-state concentration (intermittent regimens).
- Volume of distribution is a primary pharmacokinetic parameter that describes the extent of distribution and is important for calculating a loading dose to achieve a desired initial concentration.
- The secondary pharmacokinetic parameter, half-life, is directly related to the volume of distribution and indirectly proportional to clearance.
- Half-life is important because it may be a determinant of the duration of action of a drug; it determines the time required to achieve a steady-state plasma drug concentration on chronic administration and may be a determinant of the dosage interval in intermittent dosing regimens.
- Factors affecting pharmacokinetic parameters in individual patients include genetic constitution, impact of disease and co-administration of other drugs.
- When designing dose regimens, 'population' estimates of pharmacokinetic parameters are commonly used; however, pharmacokinetic parameters from individual patients are preferred if they can be calculated reliably.

Further Reading

Bauer LA. 2001. *Applied Clinical Pharmacokinetics.* McGraw-Hill Book Company: New York.

Evans WE, Schentag JJ and Jusko WJ. 1994. *Applied Pharmacokinetics. Principles of Therapeutic Drug Monitoring. 3rd ed.* Applied Therapeutics Inc.: Washington.

Hardman JG, Limbird LE and Gilman AG. 2001. *Goodman & Gilman's The Pharmacological Basis of Therapeutics, 10th ed.* McGraw-Hill: New York.

Shargel L and Yu ABC. 1999. *Applied Biopharmaceutics and Pharmacokinetics, 4th ed.* Appleton and Lange: New York.

Winter ME. 1998. *Basic Clinical Pharmacokinetics, 3rd ed.* Applied Therapeutics Inc.: Washington.

22 Therapeutic Drug Monitoring

Stefan Kowalski and Karin Nyfort-Hansen

Learning Objectives

Upon completion of this chapter, the reader should be able to:

- Explain the term therapeutic drug monitoring (TDM)
- List the drugs for which TDM is commonly used, and the target ranges for these drugs
- Explain the difference between the terms reference range, therapeutic range and target range
- Describe some common clinical situations where TDM may be useful
- List the factors that may affect serum drug concentrations and which should be considered when interpreting TDM results
- Describe the role of the pharmacist in the TDM team
- Discuss some limitations of TDM

A key component of clinical pharmacy practice is the establishment and monitoring of short- and long-term treatment outcomes for therapeutic agents. We aim to achieve the best health outcomes for a patient, but are always aware of the potential adverse effects of the drugs we use in clinical practice. How best to achieve the balance between obtaining optimal clinical effect and simultaneously minimising the chance of an adverse effect can be difficult to work out.

For most drugs, clinical effectiveness is usually assessed by directly observing changes in a patient's signs and symptoms, or by monitoring relevant laboratory data. For example, when we administer anti-hypertensive drugs, our primary short-term treatment goal is to reduce blood pressure. We assess effectiveness by checking blood pressure measurements. By contrast, the response to an oral hypoglycaemic agent is best monitored in the short term by measuring blood glucose concentrations, and in the longer term by measuring HbA1c.

Depending on the response, the dose of the hypoglycaemic agent can be adjusted to achieve the optimal balance between good control of blood glucose and risk of hypoglycaemia.

However, for some drugs, individualising the dose can be more challenging. The clinical consequences of prescribing an insufficient dose, and consequently not achieving the desired clinical effects, or by contrast, prescribing an excessive dose of a drug, may be catastrophic. For some of these drugs, therapeutic drug monitoring may be a useful addition to clinical observations and other investigations.

Therapeutic Drug Monitoring (TDM) refers to the measurement and interpretation of principally blood or plasma drug concentration measurements with the purpose of optimising a patient's drug therapy and clinical outcome while minimising the risk of drug-induced toxicity.

For TDM to be considered for routine clinical use, the following criteria should generally apply:

- The drug should have a narrow therapeutic index. For these agents, small changes in dose may result in loss of efficacy (if the dose is lowered) or toxicity (if the dose is increased). Examples of drugs with a narrow therapeutic index include digoxin, theophylline, lithium and phenytoin. The usefulness of TDM is reinforced if the drug has a narrow therapeutic index and also displays non-linear pharmacokinetics (for example, phenytoin), has potentially clinically important interactions, or is associated with large pharmacokinetic variations between individuals (for example, perhexiline).
- There should be a beneficial concentration–response relationship between the blood drug concentration and the pharmacological effects, preferably with respect to both clinical efficacy and toxicity. The therapeutic range represents drug concentrations that are effective for a particular indication in most patients, with a minimal risk of toxicity.
- There should be no other easily measurable physiological parameter. As mentioned previously for drugs such as anti-hypertensives and hypoglycaemic agents, it is much more convenient, cheaper and clinically appropriate to use measures such as blood pressure and glucose level rather than plasma drug concentrations.

The drugs for which TDM is most commonly performed are shown in Table 22.1. Other drugs where TDM may be used less commonly include other immunosupressants, analgesics (paracetamol, methadone), anti-depressants, anti-psychotics, anti-retrovirals, anti-fungal agents and anti-neoplastic agents.

How Effective is TDM?

In many countries, TDM has become a routine investigation over the last 40 years. However, there is only limited data to indicate that TDM improves a patient's response to therapy and health-related quality of life. For example, a 2009 Cochrane Review of the TDM of anti-epileptic drugs for epilepsy found only one relevant randomised controlled trial. In this study, 180 patients with newly-diagnosed untreated epilepsy were randomised to anti-convulsant therapy either with or without TDM as an aid to dose adjustment. Twelve-month remission from seizures was achieved in 60% of patients in the TDM group and in 61% in the control group.

Evidence suggests that the greatest benefits from TDM are in defined patient populations, for example, in children or elderly patients, or in patients with severe renal impairment. For example, there is evidence of improved patient outcome for aminoglycoside TDM, with reduced adverse effects such as nephrotoxicity. Pharmacoeconomic studies have examined the cost justification for TDM, but the results are inconclusive. TDM has become a standard of care in certain high-risk clinical situations, and cost is generally not a consideration in countries with well-resourced healthcare systems.

When Should TDM be Requested?

Drug assays are expensive, so your reason for performing TDM should always be clear. Routine monitoring of many drugs is not required in a clinically stable patient. TDM is most commonly used to assist the optimisation of drug therapy.

The decision if, and when, to perform TDM typically depends on a variety of considerations. Appropriate indications for TDM include:

- A patient with an inadequate clinical response. For some drugs, a minimum serum concentration is needed to ensure efficacy. TDM can be used to assess whether the dosing regimen is achieving this minimum concentration. For example, TDM may be useful in a transplant patient to ensure cyclosporine concentrations are adequate.
- A patient with signs or symptoms which may indicate drug toxicity. For example, a patient who complains of persistent nausea while on theophylline.
- To minimise the risk of drug toxicity. Ensuring that the concentration of a drug remains within a targetted range can help minimise the risk of toxicity. The most common example here is the use of TDM to minimise the risk of nephrotoxicity and ototoxicity associated with aminoglycoside therapy.
- To individualise dosing for some drugs with an unpredictable dose–response curve. For example, phenytoin has non-linear kinetics, and an increase in dose may lead to a disproportionate increase in serum drug concentration.
- To help predict a patient's dose requirements. TDM combined with an understanding of a drug's pharmacokinetic profile can allow individualised rapid dose titration to be undertaken while minimising the risk of toxicity.
- To assess medication compliance. For example, TDM for anti-convulsants in patients with poor seizure control.
- To identify poisons and to assess the severity of poisoning in a poisoning emergency (for example, paracetamol poisoning). The effectiveness of antidotes and the excretion of poisons can be monitored by measuring the concentration of the poison in body fluids.

Table 22.1 Relevant data for drugs for which TDM is used commonly (Adapted with kind permission of Pharmacy Department, Repatriation General Hospital, Adelaide)

Drug	*Therapeutic or target range*	*Adult half-life (t1/2)*	*Average time to reach steady state*	*Sample collection time*	*Drug interactions*	*Principal route of elimination and Comments*
Amiodarone	Ventricular tachyarrhythmias 1–2.5 mg/L 1.6–4 micromol/L Atrial tachyarr-hythmias: 0.5–1.5 mg/L 0.8–2.4 micromol/L	27–105 days	3–6 months (if not loaded)	Anytime once steady state is reached		Hepatic metabolism Loading regimen usually indicated because of long half ife. Consider reloading patients over a 1–2-week period if increasing dose.
Carbamazepine	4–12 mg/L 17–50 micromol/L	20–30 hours	3–5 days	Pre-dose trough	Plasma concentrations may be **elevated** by: cimetidine, diltiazem, clarithromycin, erythromycin, fluoxetine, nefazodone, fluvoxamine, danazol, isoniazid, ritonavir and verapamil.	Hepatic metabolism Carbamazepine induces its own metabolism and the half-life may decrease over the first three weeks of therapy. In the management of bipolar disorder and neuralgia, monitoring of plasma concentration serves as a guide to toxicity rather than to establish therapeutic concentrations.
Cyclosporin	100–300 mcg/L (see comments)	19 hours	3–4 days	Pre-dose trough	Plasma concentrations may be **decreased** by rifampicin, carbamazepine, phenytoin and phenobarbitone, **increased** by azole anti-fungals, diltiazem, macrolide antibiotics, nefazodone and fluoxetine.	Hepatic metabolism Defined therapeutic range depends on indication for use. Diurnal variation in clearance occurs, so samples taken for therapeutic drug monitoring should be taken at a specific time of the day.
Digoxin	Heart failure: 0.6–1.0 nmol/L 0.5–0.8 mcg/L AF: 0.6––2.6.nmol/L 0.5–2 mcg/L	30–50 hours	7–12 days	Pre-dose trough (preferred or at least 6 hours post-dose)	Plasma concentrations may be **elevated** by amiodarone, quinidine, verapamil and diltiazem.	50–75% renal Therapeutic range depends on indication. Low serum potassium may potentiate toxicity despite a serum digoxin concentration within the therapeutic range.

Drug	Therapeutic or target range	Adult half-life (t1/2)	Average time to reach steady state	Sample collection time	Drug interactions	Principal route of elimination and Comments
Gentamicin	Trough <0.5 mg/L (once daily dosing)	2–5 hours	<24 hours	Pre-dose trough		Renal Consider alternate daily dosing in patients with renal impairment.
Lithium	Acute mania: 0.5–1.2 mmol/L Prophylaxis: 0.4–1 mmol/L	14–30 hours	5–8 days	Pre-dose trough	Plasma concentrations may be **elevated** by diuretics, NSAIDs and ACE inhibitors.	Renal Serum lithium concentrations below the therapeutic range may be satisfactory for antidepressant augmentation.
Phenytoin	10-20 mg/L 40–80 micromol/L	Dose dependent (10–30 hours)	Dose dependent (8–21 days)	Anytime once steady state is reached	Plasma concentrations may be **elevated** by amiodarone, azole anti-fungals, cimetidine, diltiazem, fluoxetine, fluvoxamine and isoniazid. Plasma concentrations may be **decreased** by rifampicin.	Hepatic metabolism Dose dependent elimination; small increases in dose can give rise to disproportionate increases in plasma concentration. Consider measuring free phenytoin concentrations in patients with hypoalbuminaemia and severe renal failure (therapeutic range: 1–2 mg/L or 4–8 micromol/L)
Theophylline	10–20 mg/L 55–110 micromol/L	Non-smoker: 7–11 hours Smoker: 3–5 hours	24–36 hours OR 3-4 days (with slow release preparations)	Pre-dose trough	Plasma concentrations may be elevated by cimetidine, diltiazem, fluvoxamine, mexiletine, oral contraceptives, erythromycin and ciprofloxacin. Plasma concentrations may be **decreased** by rifampicin, phenobarbitone carbamazepine, smoking.	Hepatic metabolism Increased plasma concentrations may be seen in hepatic insufficiency, CCF and hypoxia. Concentrations in the range of 10–20 mg/L may be required for bronchodilatory effect, but lower concentrations may be effective in COPD.
Valproate	40–100 mg/L 280–700 micromol/L	6–20 hours	3–5 days	Pre-dose trough	Plasma concentrations may be **decreased** by carbamazepine, phenytoin, phenobarbitone and primidone.	Hepatic metabolism Therapeutic range for bipolar disorder is not well defined however 50–100 mg/L serves as a guide.
Vancomycin	Trough 10–20 mg/L	3–8 hours	24–48 hours	Pre-dose trough		Renal

Target Drug Ranges for TDM

When we quote a 'normal' reference range for routine electrolytes such as sodium and potassium, we are quoting a value that has been determined by testing a large number of healthy individuals. We use a range based on the mean value obtained, plus or minus 2 standard deviations from this mean. Any electrolyte value that is outside this normal reference range can have severe health implications for a patient, for example, severe hypo or hyperkalaemia.

If we take a group of healthy volunteers and perform TDM using the same criteria then the normal reference range for a drug is zero! Remember we administer drugs to patients! Therefore, when we quote a target drug reference range, we are using a concentration range that has been obtained by observing the effects of the drug for a particular indication in a group of patients who did not develop dose-related toxicity. Therapeutic or target ranges are often based on observations in small groups of patients only. Ranges are only a guide. Rigid adherence to a target range in individual patients is often not appropriate.

Timing of the Blood Sample

If we return to the example of plasma sodium or potassium concentration in a healthy individual, we would not expect significant variation during a 24-hour period. Therefore, the exact time when the plasma sample is collected will not be critical to the interpretation of the electrolyte result. Contrast this with the variability in plasma concentration obtained following the administration of an oral digoxin tablet (Fig. 22.1). The measured concentration will differ significantly throughout the day depending on when the sample was taken. In addition, in the days preceding the achievement of steady state, the maximum and minimum concentration attained each day will also vary.

In general, blood samples for TDM should be trough samples, that is, collected at the end of the dose interval and immediately before the next dose (a trough concentration). This is particularly important for drugs with a short half-life, such as theophylline or vancomycin where there is large variation in drug concentrations over the dose interval.

For drugs with long half-lives (more than 24 hours) such as digoxin, phenytoin, phenobarbitone and amiodarone, samples can be collected at any time once the distribution phase is complete. For example, a blood sample for a digoxin assay can be obtained 6–24 hours after dose administration. Although this practice is acceptable, it should be stressed that a trough concentration is still nearly always preferred.

Steady state: Unless toxicity is suspected, TDM should be performed after sufficient time has elapsed to allow for a steady-state plasma concentration to be reached (the situation when drug intake equals drug clearance). Without a loading dose, this means waiting for a period of time approximating four to five elimination half-lives of the drug after commencement of therapy or a change in dose. In some emergency situations, TDM may be performed before steady state has been reached; for example, in poisoning cases, or where an additional loading dose may be useful because of poor therapeutic response to an initial dose. An example of the latter would be a patient who continues

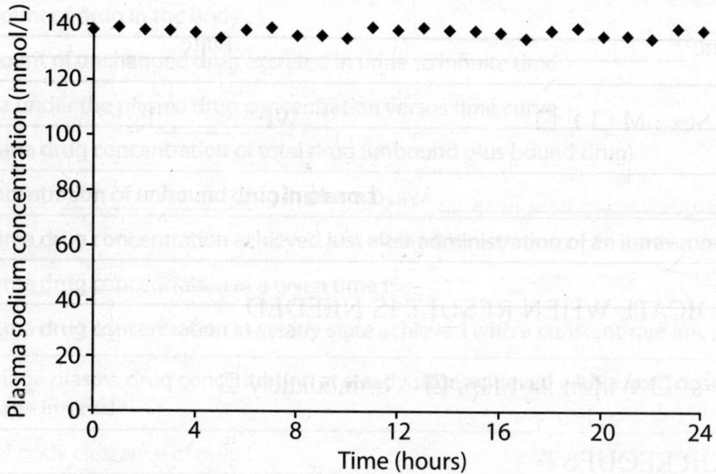

(a) The plasma sodium concentration does not vary greatly in a 24-hour period in a healthy individual

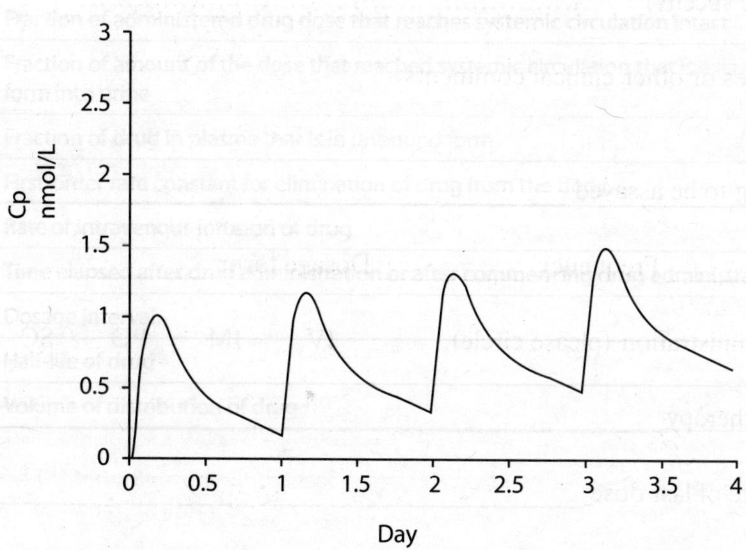

(b) The plasma digoxin concentration varies throughout a dosage interval and during the days preceding achievement of steady state. The maximum and minimum concentrations attained each day also vary.

Figure 22.1 Comparison of the effect of sampling time on plasma sodium measurement vs plasma digoxin concentration following oral dosing

Therapeutic Drug Monitoring Request

Patient's name ____________________ Date ______

Age: ______ Sex : M ☐ F ☐ Wt: ______ kg

Hospital : ____________ Ward or clinic: ____________

PLEASE INDICATE WHEN RESULT IS NEEDED

Within 24 Hrs ☐ Within 2–4 Hrs ☐ Immediately ☐

REASON FOR REQUEST

Suspected toxicity ☐ Possible drug interaction ☐

Therapeutic confirmation ☐ Lack of therapeutic response ☐

Other (please specify) ....

Co-morbidities or other clinical comments

Name of drug to be assayed ____________________

Dose ________ Frequency ________ Dosage form ________

Route of administration (please circle): IV IM PO SC

Duration of therapy____

Time and date of last dose ______________________________________

Time and date when sample was drawn ____________________________

Doctor's signature ______________________________ Date ________

Contact details for urgent results ____________________

Figure 22.2 Example of a TDM request form

to experience seizures after an initial loading dose of intravenous phenytoin.

Aminoglycoside monitoring: For a once-daily dose of aminoglycoside, the timing of the blood sample depends on the monitoring method. A common approach is to take a trough sample to ensure that the concentration is less than a range which may be associated with drug accumulation and toxicity. If a nomogram method is used then the sample may be taken 6–14 hours post-dose. Some hospitals monitor therapy by using computer programmes which calculate the area under the concentration–time curve, in which case, two blood samples over the dosing interval are required.

Usually plasma or serum from samples of venous blood is used for drug assays. Whole blood is used for cyclosporine assays due to the movement of drug between red cells and plasma depending on storage conditions. If a drug is being administered by intravenous infusion at the same time as a blood sample is drawn, the sample should be taken from a distant site, such as the other arm.

Some blood collecting tubes may be unsuitable for some drugs. For example, tubes containing lithium heparin as an anti-coagulant are not suitable for lithium samples.

Interpreting TDM Results

Many factors need to be considered when interpreting TDM results. The minimum information needed is the indication for therapy, dosing regimen, duration of therapy, time of the last dose, time of the sample and the reason why TDM has been requested. This information is routinely requested on TDM order forms (Fig. 22.2). However, drug concentrations should always be interpreted taking into account the clinical circumstances of the individual patient.

Rigid adherence to a target range may not be appropriate. For example, if a patient has well-controlled bipolar disorder, but has a lithium concentration just below the recommended therapeutic range, an increase in dose would not usually be indicated. Conversely, high concentrations of a drug in some patients may still be associated with a lack of response. For these patients, prescription of an alternative drug from another chemical/pharmacological category would be the best clinical decision.

An algorithm for the interpretation of TDM results for drugs used as prophylactic therapy is presented in Fig. 22.3.

Factors which need to be considered when interpreting TDM results include:

- **Patient data**: Age, sex and lean body weight are particularly important for renally cleared drugs, as this will allow calculation of the estimated creatinine clearance.
- **Dosage regimen (dose, dosing frequency and route of administration) and duration of therapy**: For a drug which has recently been started, sufficient time should elapse to allow steady state to be achieved before TDM is performed.
- **Sampling time**: The serum or plasma concentration of a drug depends on the time when the blood drawn for a TDM assay was sampled in relation to the last dose. The time and date of the last dose and the time and date of blood sampling need to be known. Many TDM assays are wasted due to omission of these details. For drugs with short elimination half-lives, samples should

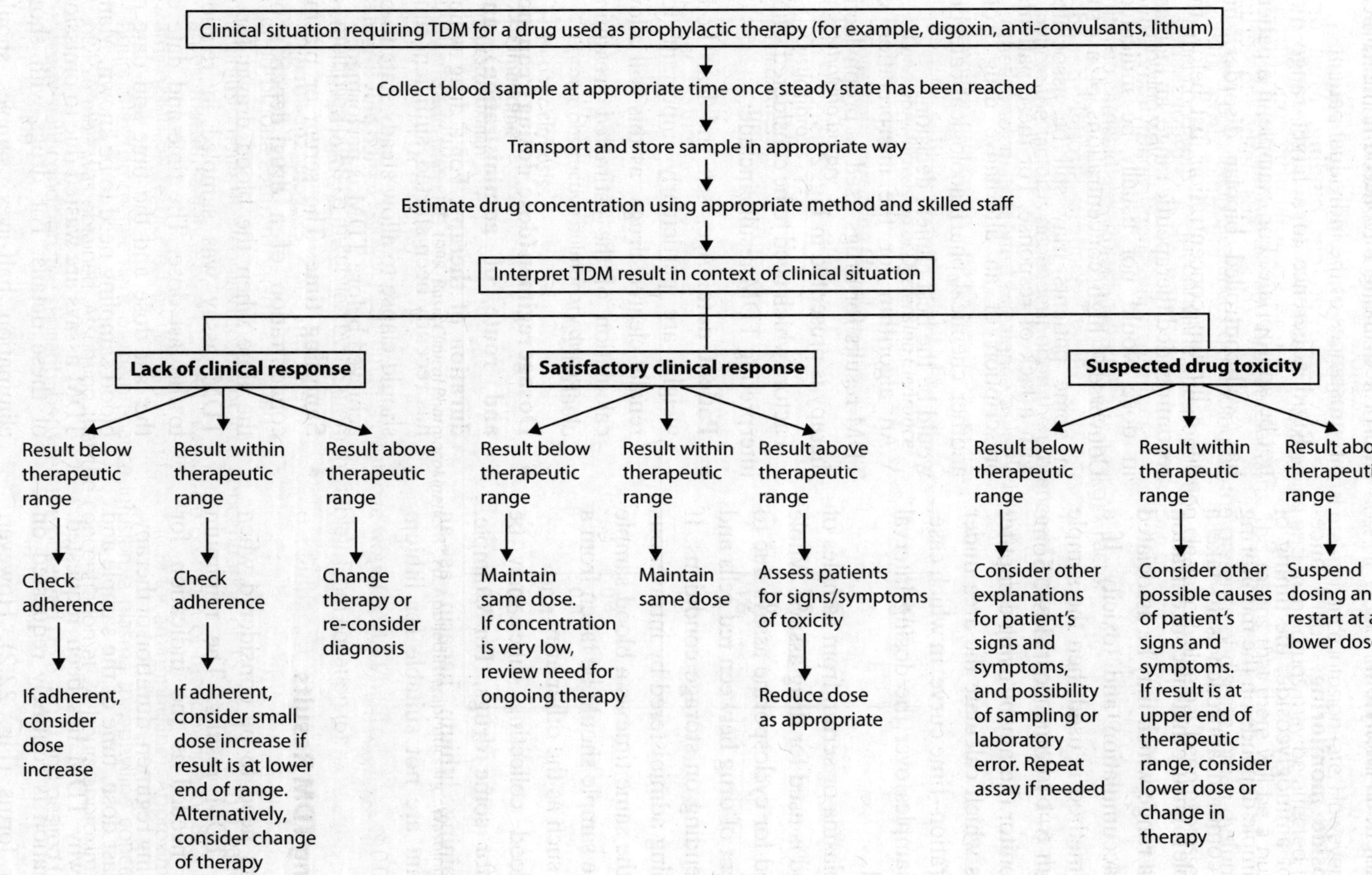

Figure 22.3 Algorithm for interpretation of TDM results for drugs used as prophylactic therapy (adapted with kind permission of Pharmacy Department, Repatriation General Hospital, Adelaide)

be drawn immediately before the next dose (a trough level). For drugs with long elimination half-lives, samples may be drawn at any time during the post-distribution phase, once steady state has been achieved. However, since the time to reach peak concentrations can vary, peak levels are usually not monitored routinely in clinical practice.

- **Indication for therapy**: Digoxin is an example of a drug prescribed for two different clinical indications (rate control of atrial fibrillation and for an inotropic effect in heart failure). Although the reference range is usually quoted as 0.5–2 micrograms/L, if a patient is in sinus rhythm and is being treated for heart failure, we usually aim for a lower reference range (0.5–0.8 micrograms/L). Amiodarone also has two target ranges depending on the clinical indication, one for ventricular tachyarrythmias (1.0–2.5 mg/L) and one for atrial fibrillation (0.5–1.5 mg/L). For vancomycin, a higher trough therapeutic range of 15–20 mg/L may be recommended for serious MRSA infections compared to the usual range of 10–20 mg/L.
- **Patient adherence**: If the concentration of the drug is lower than expected, the possibility of non-adherence should be investigated before a dose increase is recommended. This is more likely to be a problem in patients who are unable to afford the cost of medication. Asking the patient in a non-judgemental way about their recent medication compliance is the simplest way to check for non-adherence. However, in some situations, for example, an elderly patient with dementia, this may not be a reliable method.
- **Reduced protein binding**: Most drug assays measure total drug concentration (protein-bound plus unbound drug), but only the unbound drug interacts with its receptor. Conditions such as malnutrition or nephropathy may reduce the concentration of plasma proteins. For drugs which are strongly bound to plasma proteins, such as phenytoin, a reduced albumin level may result in a higher concentration of unbound (free) drug. The measurement of both total and free drug concentrations can be useful in these situations.
- **Drug interactions**: TDM results should be interpreted in light of the patient's other drug therapy. For example, patients on digoxin may have unexpectedly high digoxin serum concentrations and develop digoxin toxicity if drugs such as amiodarone or verapamil are started without a reduction in the digoxin dose. The serum concentrations of some hepatically cleared drugs may be affected by the commencement or cessation of drugs which either induce or inhibit hepatic cytochrome P450 isoenzymes.
- **Pathological factors which may affect the patient's capacity to absorb, distribute, metabolise or excrete the drug**: The patient's co-morbidities should be taken into consideration when interpreting TDM results. Conditions such as vomiting, diarrhoea and inflammatory bowel disease can alter the absorption of drugs, which in turn can alter serum drug concentrations. Gastric or small-bowel surgery and infections such as *Giardia lamblia* may cause malabsorption. In

patients with hepatic cirrhosis and tuberculosis, administration of normal doses of rifampicin and isoniazid can lead to elevated concentrations of drugs along with increased hepatotoxicity.

- **Tobacco use**: Cigarette smoking increases the hepatic clearance of clozapine and theophylline, and patients who have recently stopped smoking may have unexpectedly high concentrations of these drugs. For example, theophylline clearance falls by 35% within 7 days of smoking cessation.
- **Alcohol use**: Chronic alcohol consumption may cause non-specific hepatic microsomal enzyme induction, resulting in increased clearance and decreased serum concentrations of hepatically cleared drugs.
- **Medication or sampling errors**: For inpatient situations where the TDM result is inconsistent with drug administration records, the possibility of a medication or sampling error should be considered. For example, a wrong dose of gentamicin may have been given, or blood may have been mistakenly drawn from another patient with the same name.
- **Laboratory errors**: If all other causes of an unexpected result have been ruled out, a laboratory error may be the explanation. The laboratory should be contacted and asked to repeat the assay, or a new blood sample can be taken and sent to a different laboratory.

Drug Analysis

Most common drug assays are now performed using automated immunoassay methods. Manual assays using high performance liquid chromatography (HPLC) and gas liquid chromatography (GLC) may also be used for some drugs. Drug assay methods should have adequate specificity and sensitivity for the drug or metabolites to be measured, and suitable accuracy and precision.

In India, TDM is available either through biochemistry departments in large teaching hospitals or through private medical laboratories, using automated equipment and ready-to-use kits. Many laboratories do not provide clinical interpretation of results, and in effect are providing a therapeutic drug 'measuring' service rather than therapeutic drug 'monitoring'.

Communication of TDM Results

TDM results should be communicated to the clinical staff caring for the patient as quickly as possible. Ideally, the result should be returned before the next dose is due so that appropriate clinical interventions (dose adjustment or change in therapy) can occur without delay.

Common methods of communicating with the clinical team include:

- **By telephone**: If a drug concentration is significantly above the therapeutic range, the result should be conveyed over the telephone to the doctor to allow rapid intervention in patients at risk of toxicity. Factors which may need to be considered when interpreting the result should be explained at this time.
- **By hard copy reports**: As the full clinical context is usually not known to laboratory staff, written comments from the TDM laboratory are usually 'generic' comments using the limited information supplied on the request form. A more useful example of a hard copy TDM

THERAPEUTIC DRUG MONITORING
CLINICAL PHARMACY INTERPRETATION

PATIENT NAME: ....*MR B. PATEL*............................... MRN:...xxxxxx...............

Drug: ......*Digoxin*..................................... Indication: .....*AF*...................

Dose: *125 mcg daily*................................. Duration of therapy on this dose: *Uncertain.*

Indication for TDM:

Dose adjustment	☐	Inadequate response	☐
Suspected toxicity/poisoning	☐	Potential drug interaction	☐
Recent loading dose	☐	Routine monitoring	☐ √

Date and time of last dose: 21/...12...../...10...... at ...0800..............

Date and time of TDM sample: 22....../...12..../...10........ at ...0520..............

Drug concentration: ...2.4 mcg/L........... Target range: ...0.5–2.0 mcg/L.......

Comments and suggested clinical action:

Trough concentration above therapeutic range for AF on background of acute on chronic renal failure and concurrent amiodarone. No reported signs or symptoms of digoxin toxicity. Consider ceasing digoxin if rate/rhythm control are satisfactory on amiodarone alone. If continuing therapy suggest hold dosing for 2–3 days, then recommence at 62.5 mcg daily.

Suggested timing of next drug assay if applicable:

If continuing therapy, reassay 7–10 days after dose change (earlier if renal function remains impaired).

Pharmacist's Signature: Ms P. Veena Pager:xxxxx Date: 22/9/11

Figure 22.4 Example of a completed hard copy TDM report (sticker) designed to be completed by clinical pharmacists and attached to patient case notes (adapted with kind permission of Pharmacy Department, Repatriation General Hospital, Daw Park, South Australia)

report designed for clinical pharmacists to communicate TDM results is shown in Fig. 22.4. Written reports should include the dosing and sampling details supplied on the assay request form. Assay results may be reported in mass or molar units, although mass units are preferable. Different analysers may vary in their validated target concentration ranges, and the target range should always be included with results. In addition, the same drug may have more than one therapeutic range depending on the indication. For example, amiodarone has two ranges, one for ventricular tachyarrythmias (1.0–2.5 mg/L) and one for atrial fibrillation (0.5–1.5 mg/L).

- **By online pathology reporting systems**: Sometimes, computer-generated default comments are provided which often have limited value as they do not take into account the clinical situation of the patient.

Clinical pharmacists are ideally placed to interpret TDM results as they have knowledge of the patient's clinical condition and can gather missing information which may not have been provided on the request form.

Role of the Pharmacist

A reliable and responsive TDM service depends on team work between nurses, doctors, pharmacists, scientists and technical staff. The clinical pharmacist should provide advice to medical staff on the appropriate use and timing of TDM and assist with the interpretation of results. In addition, the pharmacist may be involved in:

- Initial selection of drug regimen. This may involve decisions about drug choice, dose, dosing interval, route of administration and dosage form of the drug, taking into account factors such as sex, age, body weight, race, metabolism status, renal function, plasma albumin concentration, use of other drugs and laboratory results.
- Adjustment of the dosage regimen based on TDM results and the patient's clinical response.
- Assessment of possible causes for unexpected results, such as non-compliance, bioavailability problems, medication errors, drug interactions or pharmacogenetic variability.
- Dose adjustment for patients on haemodialysis or peritoneal dialysis.
- Provision of poisons information.

Limitations of TDM

TDM is available only for a limited number of drugs, and for each drug there are inherent limitations associated with their use. These include the analytical accuracy of the drug assay method and the validity of recommended target ranges. The standard therapeutic ranges are derived from studies in small groups of Caucasian patients. Inter-ethnic differences in the pharmacokinetics of some drugs are well-established, particularly in Chinese and Afro-Caribbean patients. Research is needed to define therapeutic ranges in various Indian sub-populations.

In many countries, government regulatory authorities give accreditation to laboratories which meet the required standards. In India, the increasing number of private medical laboratories has raised concerns about quality control of pathology testing, including TDM assays. Accurate measurement of drug concentrations depends on the use of appropriate techniques by skilled and trained personnel. Individual laboratories should develop their own quality assurance programme. This should assess staff competency at regular intervals, and measure and document the accuracy, precision, sensitivity and specificity of each assay. In addition, assay performance should be evaluated using an external quality assurance programme such as that provided by the American College of Pathologists. Each analytical run should be performed with the appropriate number of calibration standards and quality controls. Laboratory IT systems can also be employed to reduce the need for data transcription and to improve the timeliness and reliability of result dissemination.

The widespread use of over-the-counter and non-allopathic medicines reinforces the need to obtain a full medication history for all patients whenever TDM is ordered. Medicines prescribed by Ayurveda, Unani and Siddha practitioners and some herbal and tribal medicines may have pharmacodynamic and pharmacokinetic interactions with allopathic drugs. This may make it more difficult to assess the clinical outcomes of drug therapy and apply the results of TDM assays. Interference with some TDM assay methods may occur. On occasion, some so-called 'Ayurvedic' medicines have been found to contain allopathic drugs such as phenytoin.

Nutritional deficiencies are common among Indian patients and may affect drug pharmacokinetics. For example, low serum albumin concentrations may lower the protein binding of drugs such as phenytoin, resulting in higher concentrations of the unbound 'free' drug. In these patients, measuring free phenytoin concentrations should be considered if they are clinically indicated. Pharmacists also need to consider the possibility of formulation variations between different brands of the same drug; these may account for variable or unexpected TDM results. In addition, counterfeit or substandard drugs may not contain the specified amount of drug or may contain contaminants which may interfere with the assay.

Conclusion

Used appropriately, TDM can help optimise drug therapy and contribute to improved health and quality of life. Clinical pharmacists have an important role to play in advising on the appropriate use of TDM and in the interpretation of assay results. The cost–benefit of assays should be carefully considered especially in cases of economic hardship. A sound knowledge of clinical pharmacokinetics, pharmaceutical analysis and applied therapeutics is required by pharmacists wishing to become a member of the 'TDM team'.

CASE STUDY

A 74-year-old obese female patient with a history of asthma and heart failure was admitted to hospital complaining of increased shortness of breath. Her medical history also included type 2 diabetes, osteoporosis, hypertension and osteoarthritis. On admission, she was diagnosed with an exacerbation of asthma and heart failure, and was started on hydrocortisone IV 50 mg qid, salbutamol via nebuliser 2.5 mg 4 hourly and her frusemide dose was changed from 40 mg oral daily to 80 mg IV daily. About 12 days after admission, she was observed to be confused and her temperature spiked to 38.4 °C. Urine culture identified *Pseudomonas aeruginosa*, and gentamicin 320 mg IV once daily was prescribed. TDM was requested on the third day of therapy and her gentamicin concentration was 3.0 mg/L.

Discussion

Is TDM indicated in this patient? Explain your answer.

Yes, TDM is appropriate in this patient. Aminoglycosides such as gentamicin have a narrow therapeutic index and are associated with nephrotoxicity and ototoxicity. This patient has a urinary tract infection caused by *Pseudomonas aeruginosa* on a background of significant heart and lung disease and type 2 diabetes mellitus. It can therefore be anticipated that the patient will require multiple doses of gentamicin, which may lead to drug accumulation and toxicity if an inappropriately high dose is used. Factors which may increase the risk of toxicity in this patient include age-related renal impairment and the use of frusemide.

If so, when should the first TDM measurement be made?

TDM is generally recommended for patients who have received two doses of gentamicin in order to assist further dose adjustment and to minimise toxicity. Alternatively, if further doses are planned after the first dose, TDM may be performed before the second dose. In both situations, a blood sample should be taken just before the next dose is due, that is, a trough sample.

What information should be supplied on the TDM request form?

Apart from the patient's name, age, gender, medical record number and indication for therapy, the following information should be supplied:

- Dose of gentamicin and duration of therapy
- Date and time of last dose
- Date and time of blood sample

What clinical factors need to be considered when interpreting the TDM result?

Clinical pharmacists are ideally placed to collect and assess clinical data which should be considered whenever TDM results are interpreted. Gentamicin dosing is based on body weight, but in this case, dosing should be based on ideal body weight because of the patient's obesity. Calculation of ideal body weight requires the patient's actual weight and height. Gentamicin is renally cleared, so serum creatinine and urea should be measured daily to identify changes in renal function. Creatinine clearance should be estimated using the Cockcroft–Gault equation and the patient's ideal body weight. The patient's response to therapy should be assessed by observing changes in laboratory markers of infection (WCC and CRP), temperature, urinary symptoms, mental status and abdominal pain/nausea/vomiting, if present initially. Changes in the doses of other nephrotoxic drugs such as frusemide also need to be considered.

The TDM blood sample was drawn 18 hours after the second dose of gentamicin. What recommendations would you make to the medical team?

The recommended trough concentration for gentamicin is <0.5 mg/L. If the trough concentration is <0.5 mg/L, it indicates that the kidneys are clearing the drug adequately and accumulation and toxicity are unlikely. However, in this case, the TDM blood sample was not a trough sample, but was instead drawn 18 hours after the second dose. This makes interpretation more difficult as you now need to use your clinical experience and knowledge of gentamicin pharmacokinetics to predict whether the gentamicin concentration after another 6 hours will be <0.5 mg/L. The usual half-life of gentamicin is 2–3 hours, but this will be longer in patients with renal impairment. You estimate the patient has a creatinine clearance of 45 ml/minute and therefore judge that the gentamicin concentration will be above 0.5 mg/L in six hours' time when the next dose is due. You advise the medical team accordingly and recommend that the dosing interval be every 36 hours. This will allow clearance of gentamicin before the third dose is given. As the dosing interval is changing, you advise repeating TDM before the fourth dose if therapy continues, together with daily monitoring of serum creatinine and urea.

KEY MESSAGES

- Pharmacists can help ensure the appropriate use, timing and interpretation of TDM.
- Routine monitoring of many drugs is not required in a clinically stable patient.
- Many factors influence serum drug concentration, including renal function, medication compliance, sampling time, genetic variability, protein binding, other drug therapy and co-morbidities.
- TDM results must always be interpreted taking the above factors into account and in the context of the patient's clinical situation.

Further Reading

Ghiculescu RA. 2008. Therapeutic drug monitoring: Which drugs, why, when and how to do it. *Australian Prescriber* 31(2):42–44.

Gogtay NJ, Kshirsagar NA and Dalvi SS. 2001. Therapeutic drug monitoring in a developing country: An overview. *Br J Clin Pharmacol* 52(Suppl 1):103–109S.

Gross AS. 1998. Best practice in therapeutic drug monitoring. *Br J Clin Pharmacol* 46(2):95–99.

Soldin SJ and Steele BW. 2000. Mini-review Therapeutic Drug Monitoring in Pediatrics. *Clinical Biochem* 33:333–5.

Website of Interest

International Association of Therapeutic Drug Monitoring and Clinical Toxicology (check here for regional meetings held in India)

http://www.iatdmct.org

23 Continuing Professional Development

David Cosh

Learning Objectives

Upon completion of this chapter, the reader should be able to:

- Understand the importance of continuing professional development (CPD) in maintaining the competency to practice as a clinical pharmacist
- Identify a range of activities which may contribute to a CPD programme
- Understand that a pharmacist's personal CPD programme should be tailored to meet specific goals for knowledge and skill development
- Access reputable online CPD activities of relevance to clinical pharmacists

Key competencies for effective clinical pharmacy practice are attained and maintained by experiential training in therapeutics during both undergraduate and postgraduate education, and from a commitment to continuing education for the duration of professional life. For many diseases, the rate at which treatment recommendations change and new drugs are introduced into practice can be bewilderingly rapid. Prescribers and pharmacists are faced with the constant challenge of how best to stay abreast of new developments in disease state management and how to evaluate evidence that underpins new treatment strategies. This chapter summarises some of the common routes pharmacists can use to meet these challenges.

Continuing Education versus Continuing Professional Development

The term continuing professional development (CPD) is increasingly used when continuing education (CE) is discussed. Is this just another way of saying the same thing or is there a meaningful difference between the two terms?

Continuing professional development suggests an individual rather than a collective approach to ongoing education. The concept of tailoring education to the individual's particular needs is recognised as an important factor in generating a commitment to ongoing learning. People quickly lose interest when asked to assimilate information that has little or no perceived relevance to their immediate needs. A pharmacist working in a large teaching hospital will have different ongoing educational needs to a colleague working in a rural clinic with no on-site medical staff and a restricted range of health services on offer.

Properly structured, CPD has the flexibility to allow all practitioners to access the information they need in their own practice. A series of formal lectures that addresses disease state management and which is provided by a professional society is an example of a CE programme. Individual members of that society who are planning their own CPD programme may choose to attend all, several or none of these lectures depending on their assessment as to how relevant the topics are to their own practice. They may include other activities such as journal readings, specialist seminars and online training to create a CPD programme that suits their own specific needs.

The International Pharmaceutical Federation, (FIP) recognising the importance of CPD, has issued a statement that is offered as a framework for pharmacists to consider their own ongoing educational needs (available at www.fip.org).

Professional Responsibility and Competency

Sociologists have defined the core elements of a profession as the 'possession of a specialised body of knowledge and commitment to service'. This definition acknowledges the demands of a better-informed community seeking transparency and sound professional standards. In many countries, the bodies responsible for the registration of pharmacists have been considering ways in which the ongoing competency of pharmacists can be established as a condition of re-registration. CPD is now a mandatory professional requirement for registration as a pharmacist in many countries. In the United Kingdom and Australia, pharmacists must maintain a personal record of their CPD activities, and these records are subject to regular auditing.

The willingness of regulatory bodies to increase their demands on those wishing to maintain their professional status is based on the belief that it is unethical for a pharmacist to falsely proclaim to be a provider of accurate and current therapeutic knowledge. This is a situation analogous to a surgeon who continues to operate knowing that he is no longer capable of doing so in a safe and effective manner. By advocating compulsory CPD, the regulators of the pharmacy profession are meeting their responsibility to the consumers of pharmacy services. Pharmacists who seek to avoid their responsibilities to remain competent to practice demonstrate their unsuitability to remain active in the profession.

Professional Organisations

There are many professional associations that provide useful support to pharmacists in their practice. The Royal Pharmaceutical Society of Great Britain, the American Society of Health System Pharmacists, the Pharmaceutical Society of Australia, The Society of Hospital Pharmacists of Australia and many others see the provision of continuing education and continuing professional development as a core role. They provide services such as conferences, seminars, workshops, journals and an increasing number of online courses.

It is difficult for clinical pharmacists to operate effectively in isolation but no matter how geographically isolated a pharmacist may be, belonging to a relevant professional association provides contacts and links with peers through newsletters, journals and meetings. Many pharmacists with specialist interests join relevant medical and scientific associations and attend conferences on their specialty. However, there are excellent free websites which provide relevant information across an almost unlimited range of health topics.

Conferences are excellent forums for networking with colleagues. While the ease with which information can be accessed online has increased, face-to-face discussions with colleagues remains an invaluable way to gain information, generate enthusiasm and break down barriers imposed by isolation. Some pharmacists join overseas organisations to broaden their exposure to the professional activities of colleagues in other countries. But for all pharmacists, the first priority should be to join and support local professional organisations, which provide educational services that support local practice. The Indian Pharmaceutical Congress provides an annual forum for all pharmacists and includes sessions devoted to clinical pharmacy practice.

Keeping Up-to-date with the 'Literature'

We are all told that we must stay abreast of the 'literature', meaning the wealth of material available in journals. Many of these are now also accessible online. To be successful in using the literature as a practice support, pharmacists needs to accept that no one can ever truly keep up with all the information on offer, and that knowing how to quickly access information by using effective search strategies is an essential skill. Many online databases are relevant to disease state management, and searching these databases is becoming increasingly user friendly.

Clinical pharmacy practice has spawned a number of journals, and these may contain useful articles on practice research and how others go about instituting clinical services. The Annals of Pharmacotherapy and the American Journal of Health-System Pharmacy are publications emanating from the USA; the Royal Pharmaceutical Society of Great Britain publishes both The Pharmaceutical Journal and Clinical Pharmacist. The Journal of Pharmacy Practice and Research (formerly the Australian Journal of Hospital Pharmacy) is published by the Society of Hospital Pharmacists of Australia. The Australian National Prescribing Service provides a number of publications, all of which are available free to users online (www.nps.org.au).

While pharmacists need to keep abreast of their own profession's body of literature, they also need to read what prescribers are reading if they are to understand and influence prescribing decisions. Medical decision-making is influenced by a number of factors including peers, specialists, the pharmaceutical industry and the medical literature. The pharmacy literature is not likely to be a factor in medical prescribing decision-making. However, many pharmacy journals provide abstracts from the medical literature and this makes them useful sources of clinical information for pharmacists. There is, however, no substitute to sourcing original references, and the availability of many major medical journals online is making this a feasible option for many practitioners, no matter where their practice may be based.

Indian pharmacists should always look to the Indian medical and pharmacy literature to keep abreast of practice in their own country. For example, an Indian pharmacist with an interest in infectious diseases needs to read Indian journals that deal with infectious disease and antibiotic use in India, where disease presentation, drug availability and resistance patterns may be very different to those seen elsewhere.

Nevertheless, it is important for all clinical pharmacists, irrespective of where they practice, to access mainstream medical and scientific journals where the results of large multicentre trials that have such an influence on drug use are published. While the findings of these landmark studies are often abstracted by other journals, the primary articles, editorials and letters to the editor found in the mainstream journals are all very useful in allowing pharmacists to formulate their own opinions on how research findings may be applied in practice.

The professional maturity to recognise when you do not know the answer to a question is an essential developmental step in becoming an effective practitioner. It is unrealistic to expect that saying 'I don't know' can become a remote possibility. Those three words have been described by Richard Smith, former Editor of the British Medical Journal, as the three most important words in medical education. Very few questioners will be critical if a clinical pharmacist admits to not having the necessary information at hand but offers to find out. This again emphasises the need to be able to effectively search the literature for answers.

Communication Skills

Effective communication skills, a key competency previously mentioned and discussed in *Chapter 5*, are generic skills required by all clinical pharmacists. Communication skills, once mastered, have a much longer currency than therapeutics where, as has previously been stated, treatment recommendations can change rapidly. If communication skills are lacking, then recognition of the need to improve and doing something to achieve this are important elements of CPD. Personal study of communication texts may be of benefit, but there is no substitute for training that involves communication with others in a supportive structure that can include role plays and objective assessment of progress.

Information Technology

Today's clinical pharmacist must work within a very rapidly changing and evolving information technology (IT) environment. Some computer literacy, including the ability to retrieve information from the worldwide web and communicate electronically, is essential in many settings. There are many reputable online CPD activities on offer and some organizations provide these free of charge (Table 23.1; websites at the end of the chapter). However, in some practice settings, pharmacists may be expected to provide clinical services without sophisticated IT

Table 23.1 Some reputable sources of free online CPD

Medscape for pharmacists	www.medscape.com/pharmacists
National Prescribing Service	www.nps.org.au/health_professionals
Cancer Learning	www.cancerlearning.gov.au
Veterans Mates Modules	www.veteransmates.net.au

and library support. In this context, clinical pharmacy is no different from the practice of medicine and surgery in the developing world. The addition of ingenuity to a good working knowledge of therapeutics relevant to local medical problems and simple pharmaceutical formulation skills can allow for a meaningful contribution to local healthcare.

Practice Guidelines

An increasing number of educational resources fall somewhere between a standard textbook and a journal, and these are best referred to as practice guidelines. The most useful ones to pharmacists are those produced by organisations independent of the pharmaceutical industry, and written by expert groups that often include pharmacists and other allied healthcare professionals. The best guidelines are revised frequently and, because of their portability (they usually fit into a white apron pocket) and currency of information, are very popular with practitioners and students alike. They will reflect current best practices in the setting in which they are written so that they are perhaps of most use to practitioners working in the country of guideline origin. However, providing local factors are taken into consideration, well-written guidelines from other countries can be very useful reference sources. Increasingly, such guidelines are available in the electronic format and online (for example, see www.nice.org.uk).

Abstracting and E-mail Services

Structured abstracts conforming to a standard format are demanded of prospective authors submitting papers by many medical, pharmaceutical and scientific journals. Many online medical information providers will make these abstracts available and some actually provide full-text articles. Some journals devote themselves to publishing only concise summaries of research and clinical papers.

Major journals recognise the need for rapid publication of important findings to assist practitioners to stay abreast of medical advances, and provide a service whereby pharmacists can receive automatic email notification of the contents of each new edition. Where the public interest is at stake, many journals will issue press releases on important issues prior to the publication of the relevant article in the journal, and these may be available free online. Publishing policy and access rules do change from time to time but an online search of the relevant subject or journal will allow the searcher to easily find out the necessary information.

Evidence-based Medicine

Evidence-based medicine (EBM) refers to a practice that is directed by evidence rather than an ad hoc approach to treatment. Its primary objective has been described as an attempt to bolster clinical decision-making by providing better scientific evidence as a complement to clinical skills. This is a useful description because it recognises the primacy of clinical skills and in doing so also accepts that medicine remains both an art as well as a science.

Therapeutics that depends on treatment algorithms to guide practice in a quasi-mathematical fashion, hoping that such an approach will make up for a lack of experience and knowledge, will fail. To take advantage of the evidence, one must have the clinical acumen to be able to apply that evidence to an individual patient's treatment, recognising when a course of treatment that may have the imprimatur of evidence may in fact be unsuitable for the patient in question. Experience-driven clinical acumen is as important to the clinical pharmacist as it is to the prescriber, and this again reinforces the need for bedside teaching and life-long learning.

The Cochrane Library (www.cochrane.org) is a source of evidence-based information online. It contains databases that include systematic reviews of medical treatment, a controlled trials register and other evidence-based information on the treatment of a wide range of diseases. It is updated on a quarterly basis and is a valuable source of evidence for the pharmacist.

Journal Clubs

A journal club refers to a gathering of a group of professionals who meet regularly to discuss recently published articles in their field of interest, which for clinical pharmacists would be the medical and pharmacy literature. The usual way that a club operates is for the chairperson or organiser to develop a roster where each participant is allocated a meeting date when they are responsible for selecting an article to be discussed. Other participants are either informed ahead of time about which article is to be discussed, or copies of the article may be distributed to all members of the club. The articles chosen are usually recently published papers dealing with important developments in the club's area of interest, and for clinical pharmacists these would be the papers that are likely to influence prescribing practice, those that describe experience with new drugs and papers that describe new indications for established drugs. Papers that generate editorials and letters to the editor are often very valuable, especially where the subject has generated controversy and debate.

The key to success is to create a non-threatening environment where both presenter and those present are encouraged to offer opinions and exchange ideas without fear of ridicule. Having members with a range of experience makes for a very good learning opportunity, especially for younger and less-experienced members of the club. A journal club can be a way of combining a useful educational experience with a social occasion by locating the club at participants' homes on a rotational basis and ensuring that some refreshments are provided. There are obviously many formats that can be used, but the fundamental objective is to learn through a critical evaluation of the literature.

Courses to Assist Specialisation

While community pharmacists spend relatively little time in conversation with medical practitioners and most of their time talking with their customers, clinical pharmacists devote more time discussing therapeutic issues with colleagues, prescribers, nurses and patients. In this setting, a pharmacist whose knowledge of current therapeutics is inadequate will not be able to conceal such a shortcoming for long.

Some pharmacists may specialise in certain areas of clinical practice and develop expertise in areas such as cardiology, respiratory medicine, psychiatry, oncology or geriatrics. Online access to many courses offered by tertiary institutions and professional organisations makes distance learning a feasible proposition. The American Pharmaceutical Association's Board of Pharmaceutical Specialties (BPS) provides a range of specialty certification qualifications by examination accessible to qualified pharmacists from other countries. Five specialties are currently offered, including general pharmacotherapy, nuclear pharmacy, nutrition support pharmacy, oncology pharmacy and psychiatric pharmacy. If there are sufficient candidates wishing to take a BPS examination at the same time, they can be conducted in the candidates' home country. The American College of Clinical Pharmacy (AACP) provides a range of educational resources that assist candidates in preparing for the BPS certification.

The US Commission for Certification in Geriatric Pharmacy also offers pharmacists from other countries the opportunity to undertake studies and examination in geriatric pharmacotherapy. This is a generalist programme to recognise pharmacists who have the knowledge and skills to provide pharmaceutical care to the elderly.

KEY MESSAGES

- Education gained at an undergraduate level is only a foundation upon which life-long learning can take place.
- Effective clinical pharmacy practice is not possible without a commitment to ongoing professional development.
- Technological advances mean that very few practitioners need be truly professionally isolated.
- As well as remaining up-to-date with disease state management and drug treatment, pharmacists must develop and maintain the skills necessary to retrieve and store information.

Websites of Interest

Board of Pharmaceutical Specialties
www.bpsweb.org

Commission for Certification in Geriatric Pharmacy
www.ccgp.org

American Society of Consultant Pharmacists
www.cgpreview.com

The Cochrane Library
www.cochrane.org

National Prescribing Service
www.nps.org.au

Australian Adverse Drug Reactions Bulletin
www.tga.gov.au/adr/aadrb.htm

mdBriefcase
www.mdbriefcase.com.au

Rural Health Education Foundation
www.rhef.com.au

24

Ethical Issues in Clinical Research

Urmila Thatte

Learning Objectives

Upon completion of this chapter, the reader should be able to:

- Discuss the importance of autonomy, beneficence and justice in clinical research
- List the elements of an informed consent document and the criteria which need to be fulfilled when obtaining informed consent
- Identify some common barriers which may increase the difficulty of obtaining informed consent
- Define the term 'therapeutic misconception' as it relates to clinical research
- Summarise the roles and responsibilities of an Ethics Committee before, during and after research takes place

Ethics is not definable, is not implementable, because it is not conscious; it involves not only our thinking, but also our feeling.

–Valdemar W Setzer

The word 'ethics' derives from the Greek, *ethos*, which means custom or character and is the study of principles relating to right and wrong conduct and also defines the standards that govern the conduct of a person (especially in a profession). Ethics comes from within in contrast to law and regulations, which are essentially external controls and mandatory.

Clinical research is defined as a systematic investigation in humans designed to discover or contribute to a body of generalisable knowledge. As clinical research involves human participants, researchers and their teams are legally and ethically obligated to protect them. In clinical practice, a physician would be expected to use interventions that have a reasonable expectation of success and are designed solely to enhance the well-being of an individual. As against this, clinical research is designed to test a hypothesis, permit conclusions to be drawn and thereby develop or contribute to generalisable knowledge – here, the participant may not get the best known treatment and therefore the obligations on the researcher are greater.

This chapter reviews some ethical aspects that arise while designing and conducting clinical research. After discussing some historical milestones, the key issues elaborated in some of the codes, declarations and other documents that govern the ethical conduct of clinical research will be covered, followed by the basic principles of ethical research, critical elements of informed consent and the roles and responsibilities of Ethics Committees. Finally some special challenges in India are discussed.

Historical Perspective

In the eighteenth century, clinical investigations were exemplified by self-experimentation. The work of Edward Jenner (1749–1823) is illustrative as he tested his ideas about the smallpox vaccine on his own son and other neighbourhood children! Later, US Army doctors from Walter Reed's research team in Cuba, including James Carroll, Aristides Agramonte and Jesse Lazear, infected themselves with yellow fever. Incidentally, Jesse Lazear died from yellow fever complications in 1900. These efforts ultimately resulted in proof of the mosquito-borne nature of yellow fever transmission and saved countless lives. Accounts describe that only 'the healthiest specimens' were 'experimented upon' and in the words of Agramonte, 'A written consent was obtained from each one, so that our moral responsibility was to a certain extent lessened'.

In the absence of codes, guidelines, rules or laws, there was much scope for what we would recognise today as exploitation. Due to implicit faith in the treating physicians, and no recognition of the vulnerable sections of society, it required major mishaps to push the medical fraternity into developing ethical guidelines and codes for research.

The twentieth century witnessed the experiments conducted by Nazi physicians during the Second World War; these were unprecedented in their scope and the degree of suffering and harm they caused. Horrific experiments were performed on 'worthless' individuals – testing their limits of toleration of altitude and temperature.

Essentially, four types of medical experiments were performed: *racial-anthropologic research* (for example, Mengele's experiments in Auschwitz to show racial factors in immune response to infections); *brain research and neurology,* where research on the brains of Austrians and Germans was performed; *military medical research* in which wounds were studied and vaccines developed; and *medical and genetic experiments*.

Joseph Mengele's scientific research was informal and appeared to be a hobby. He found 1,500 sets of imprisoned twins and conducted genetic experiments on them including injection of chemicals into their eyes to see whether they would change colour, and literally sewing twins together in attempts to create conjoined twins. Less than 200 individuals survived.

At the end of the Second World War, in December 1946, 23 physicians and administrators were brought to trial before the War Crimes Tribunal at Nuremberg for their willing participation in such experiments. Sixteen of them were found guilty and imprisoned, while seven were hanged in 1948. Disturbingly, several of the accused had argued that their 'experiments' differed little from pre-war ones and more importantly that there was no law that differentiated between legal and illegal experiments.

As appalling as the Nazification of medicine was, the Asian Holocaust was not any less horrifying. The Imperial Japanese experiments conducted in China around the same time included human experimentation that defied imagination, especially those conducted in Unit 731 under Shirō Ishii. For example, prisoners were taken out in freezing weather and left with exposed arms, periodically drenched with water until frozen solid. The arm was later amputated. The doctor would repeat the process on the victim's upper arm, up to the shoulder. After both arms were gone, the doctors moved on to the legs until only the head and torso remained. The victim was then used for plague and pathogen experiments.

Under an 'immunity arrangement' with US officials, many researchers were never brought to trial – in return, the US got access to the results of biological warfare experiments that had been performed on prisoners. On the other side of the globe, in the August 1947 verdict of Nuremberg, the judges included a section called 'Permissible Medical Experiments'; this section became known as the *Nuremberg Code*. This was the first clear guidance document describing ten points that governed ethical human experimentation.

The history of human experimentation does not end with the Nazi war crimes or even the declaration of the Nuremberg Code. The studies on hepatitis performed in children at the Willowbrook State School illustrate the continued need for overseeing clinical research. This was an institution for mentally challenged children in New York and Krugman began his experiments in hepatitis here in 1954. In fact, Krugman even published his intentions in the *New England Journal of Medicine,* stating that the purpose of his studies was threefold: to study the natural circumstances in which the disease occurred, the effects of γ globulin on the disease and whether passive-active immunity could be induced by feeding the virus to treated individuals.

In today's context, several ethical principles were compromised; for example, children who were mentally challenged were chosen as subjects: the children were deliberately infected and parents consented under coercion without adequate knowledge of risks. Researchers defended the deliberate infection of these children by stating that most of them anyway acquired the infection while at Willowbrook, a fact which in itself is unacceptable.

At the other end of life's spectrum, in the summer of 1963, Southam and Custodio together injected live, cultured cancer cells into 22 chronically ill and debilitated patients. This was the Jewish Chronic Disease Hospital Study, where patients had been told that they were receiving a skin test. No consent was documented.

The most notorious example of prolonged and knowing violation of the rights of a vulnerable group of research participants was the long-term study of black males conducted at Tuskegee by the United States Public Health Service. Leading to the Belmont Report and the declaration of the basic principles of ethical research in humans, the Tuskegee study was initiated in the 1930s to examine the natural history of untreated syphilis. Continued till 1972, the study recruited more than 400 black men suffering from syphilis. Several ethical violations punctuated this 40-year-long study, the most dramatic being that these participants were not given access to penicillin which would have cured them. The study resulted in 28 deaths, 100 cases of disability and 19 cases of congenital syphilis.

The ethics debate continues even today as society becomes empowered and newer ethical issues occupy us. HIV research is perhaps one of the most challenging, ethically speaking, that is relevant today. A vulnerable population, this set of individuals raises new ethical dilemmas – the most important being that of access (or lack thereof) to therapy. Research on molecules to treat cancer also offers newer challenges, including the fact that terminally ill individuals are perhaps at their most vulnerable.

Ethical aspects of gene transfer (and especially clinical research in this area) are illustrated by the recent Gelsinger case that highlights several issues in the ongoing clinical research debate. The death of Jesse Gelsinger (18) in 1999 at the University of Pennsylvania School of Medicine raised profound questions about patient protection, protocol adherence, reporting of adverse events, informed consent and financial conflicts.

History is a good teacher and from these tragedies emerged many of the codes and guidelines that now govern ethical research in India as in the world.

Codes, Declarations and Guidelines

The Nuremberg Code (available at http://ohsr.od.nih.gov/guidelines/nuremberg.html) was the first international standard laid down for the conduct of research, and contains ten clear principles to be followed by researchers while conducting human experiments. The need to obtain 'voluntary consent of the human subject' before recruitment in a study, was clearly mandated for the first time formally in this Code. The Code emphasises safety of research participants with a need for animal experimentation to precede human experimentation, and specifies that risk should never exceed the expected benefit to either the participant or to society. The right to withdraw from experiments is also clearly mandated.

The Declaration of Helsinki (available at http://www.wma.net/en/30publications/10policies/b3/index.html), first accepted by the 18th World Medical Assembly (WMA) in 1964, has been revised six times and the latest version with 35 points was published in 2008 at the 59th WMA, Seoul, South Korea. This new version addresses important aspects like emphasising the need to provide access to research to otherwise under-represented populations, registration of clinical trials, post-study access and compensating subjects with research-related injuries, which have great implications for all stakeholders in clinical research today. It was the Declaration of Helsinki that first required that 'all protocols must be submitted to an Ethics Committee for review, which must be independent of the investigator, the sponsor or any other kind of undue influence'. The informed consent process is reiterated as a central requirement for ethical research and

Table 24.1 Guidelines for Ethical Conduct of Research in Human Subjects

1.	Nuremberg Code 1947 (http://ohsr.od.nih.gov/guidelines/nuremberg.html)
2.	Declaration of Helsinki, 1964 (http://www.wma.net/en/30publications/10policies/b3/index.html)
3.	The Belmont Report, 1979 (http://ohsr.od.nih.gov/guidelines/belmont.htm)
4.	International Ethical Guidelines for Biomedical Research Involving Human Subjects, 1982, 1993, 2002 (http://www.cioms.ch/frame_guidelines_nov_2002.htm)
5.	The Ethics of Research related to Healthcare in Developing Countries, Nuffield Council, 2002 (http://www.nuffieldbioethics.org/go/screen/ourwork/developingcountries/publication_309.html)

emphasis laid on the need to protect the vulnerable, while at the same time elaborating on the need to perform research in these very populations, lest they (as a population) not obtain any benefit from the research.

The US Congress established the National Commission for the Protection of Human Subjects of Biomedical and Behavioral Research in 1974 to identify ethical principles and develop guidelines to govern the conduct of clinical research. After 43 meetings, on April 18, 1979, the *'Ethical Principles and Guidelines for the Protection of Human Subjects'* (available at http://ohsr.od.nih.gov/guidelines/belmont.html) was published. This report is known as the **Belmont Report** after the place where the foundation for this 'analytical framework' for ethical research was laid (at the Smithsonian Institution's Belmont Conference Centre, Elkridge).

The Belmont Report specified the fundamental Principles of Ethical Research, namely, *autonomy* (respect for persons), *beneficence* and *justice.* The principle of autonomy is applied through the informed consent process, while that of beneficence is addressed in the risk–benefit assessment and justice in the selection of participants.

The Council for International Organizations of Medical Sciences (CIOMS) was formally constituted by the World Health Organization (WHO) and the United Nations Education, Scientific and Cultural Organization (UNESCO) in 1949. In 1982, CIOMS first published its Proposed International Guidelines which were meant to describe how to effectively apply the principles set out in the 1975 version of the Declaration of Helsinki. A decade later, in 1993, the *International Ethical Guidelines for Biomedical Research Involving Human Subjects* was published.

In keeping with advances in medicine as well as new social, ethical and public health challenges, the 2002 (http://www.cioms.ch/frame_guidelines_nov_2002.htm) revision was published. The CIOMS guidelines were designed to be particularly relevant for research planned in developing countries, especially for defining national policies on the ethics of clinical research, applying ethical standards in local circumstances, and establishing or improving ethical review mechanisms. The conditions and needs of low-resource countries and the implications for multinational or transnational research in which they may be partners are also addressed.

The CIOMS recently published the updated International Ethical Guidelines for Epidemiological Studies with 24 guidelines with commentaries as its core. An Appendix lists the items to be included in a research protocol to be submitted for epidemiological research involving human subjects.

The Indian Council for Medical Research (ICMR) Policy Statement on Ethical Considerations involved in Research on Human Subjects was promulgated in 1980 where several ethical issues were addressed, including the role of the Ethics Committees, informed consent, research on traditional medicine and publications-related issues. By the mid-90s, a need was felt for revision of this statement as critical issues in the area of biogenetic research were emerging and it was becoming mandatory for clinical trials to be conducted for new drugs. Hence, the Central Ethics Committee for Human Research (CECHR) comprising 27 members was set up under the chairmanship of Justice Hon'ble MN Venkatachaliah in August 1996. Five sub-committees of experts were set up for drawing up the guidelines in respective areas, namely, clinical evaluation of drug/devices/diagnostics/vaccines/herbal remedies, epidemiological research, human genetic research, transplantation research including fetal tissue transplantation and assisted reproduction technologies. A draft consultative document was prepared in December 1997 which was given nation-wide circulation in January 1998. Regional public debates were held between 1998 and 1999 and meetings of the sub-committees for special issues were held in 1999 and the document (ICMR Ethical Guidelines for Biomedical Research on Human Subjects) was published in 2000 (Table 24.2). This version has been replaced by the 2006 version (http://www.icmr.nic.in/ethical_guidelines.pdf) and covers several ethical issues including the informed consent process, compensation for participation and compensation for research-related injury, conflict of interest, vulnerable or special groups as research participants, post-trial access, international collaboration and research on drugs, devices, diagnostics, vaccines and herbal remedies. Principles for epidemiological studies are covered as well

Table 24.2 Indian Guidelines for Ethical Conduct of Research in Human Subjects

1.	Ethical Guidelines for Biomedical Research on Human Participents (IMCR), 2006 (http://www.icmr.nic.in/ethical_guidelines.pdf)
2.	Ethical Guidelines for Social Science Research in Health in 2000 by CEHAT (http://www.cehat.org/publications/ethical.html)
3.	Ethical Guidelines for Stem Cell Research, DBT+ICMR: (http://www.icmr.nic.in/stem_cell/stem_cell_guidelines.pdf)
4.	Guidelines for Ethical Practices in Studies Involving Animals, ICMR (http://icmr.nic.in/bioethics/Guidelines_medicalcollege.pdf) INSA, (http://icmr.nic.in/bioethics/INSA_Guidelines.pdf)
5.	Guidelines for Vaccine Trials, DBT (http://dbtindia.nic.in/publication/publicmain.html)
6.	Guidelines for Genetics and Genomics by DBT (http://dbtindia.nic.in/publication/publicmain.html)
7.	Guidelines for Good Clinical Laboratory Practices (http://www.icmr.nic.in/guidelines/GCLP.pdf)

as those for human genetics and genomics research, and transplantation research.

Currently, it is expected that all institutions in India which carry out any form of biomedical research involving human beings will follow these guidelines in letter and spirit to protect the safety and well-being of all individuals. The guidelines have been submitted for legislation.

The Indian Good Clinical Practice (GCP) guidelines were published in late 2001 (www.cdsco.nic.in) and the current Schedule Y, dated 20th January 2005, gives timely legal support to these GCP guidelines. It is the investigator's responsibility to ensure GCP compliance of the approving Ethics Committee.

BASIC PRINCIPLES OF CLINICAL RESEARCH

Clinical research (the word 'clinical' derives from the Greek word *klinikos,* meaning 'pertaining to a bed') is research involving humans designed to advance the goals of medicine, including the development of new prophylactic, diagnostic and therapeutic interventions.

Autonomy (derived from the Greek *auto* or 'self', and *nomos,* meaning 'law'; 'one who gives oneself their own law') is a concept found in moral, political and bioethical philosophy. It refers to the capacity of a rational individual to make an informed, un-coerced decision and is the first principle of ethical research described in the Belmont Report. When we respect autonomy, we give weightage to a person's considered opinions and choices while refraining from obstructing their actions unless they are clearly harmful to others. The principle of autonomy implies two separate moral requirements: firstly, to acknowledge an individual's autonomy (independence) and secondly, the requirement to protect those with diminished autonomy.

Autonomy may be diminished due to medical or legal reasons. For example, a person with a psychiatric illness may have lost insight and is incapable of reasoned logic, or a child (legally below 18 years in India) is not considered legally capable of consenting. Protecting such people becomes an important task and is actually closely linked to the assessment of risk and benefit.

Protection may mean excluding them from the study altogether (although this must be balanced with the need to give them access to research and to generate research data on them) or designing the research in such a way that adequate protections are in place commensurate with the risk of harm and the likelihood of benefit. Although respect for the autonomy of patients is an important goal, it can conflict with a competing ethical principle, namely, beneficence.

While respecting a person's choice to participate in research and making efforts to minimise harm, the researcher must also ensure their well-being. This is the principle of beneficence, which, as per the Belmont Report, is an obligation. This principle is linked to two complementary statements. While minimising harm, it is important to maximise possible benefits. The benefits have to be looked at from the point of view of the individual as well as society. The application of this principle is the overriding responsibility of the investigator and applies to many different kinds of harms, namely, physical, psychological, social, economic, legal or harm to communities/society/ well-being of the research participant.

This principle is applied by using the best possible research design to minimise harm and maximise benefits, making sure the researchers are able to perform procedures and handle the risks and prohibit research without a favourable risk–benefit ratio, all ensured by appropriate ethical review of the proposal.

The third basic principle of ethics relates to who should bear the burden of research and who ought to or does receive its benefits. This is the principle of justice. If a person is entitled to a benefit and is denied it without reason, or some participant bears risk without benefit either to him or to the society he comes from, then injustice is done. How should people be treated equally? The Belmont Report says according to individual need, individual effort, according to societal contribution and merit.

We have seen historically that the burden of serving as research subjects fell largely upon poor or underprivileged patients, while the benefits of improved medical care went to moneyed patients. Patients should not be selected because of their 'easy availability' (exemplified in research among students or employees) or their social or financial vulnerability (where poor patients who cannot afford a routine standard of care take part in research). This principle is applied practically by ensuring that selection of subjects is done equitably (distribute risks and benefits), taking special care to avoid exploitation of vulnerable populations.

The two important pillars that support the application of these basic principles of clinical research are review by ethics committees and the informed consent process. One of the common questions raised is 'Which studies require the use of these patient protection methods?'. To answer this, it is necessary to define 'Who is a research participant?'.

The human participant is a living individual about whom a researcher obtains data through intervention or interaction or from identifiable private information. Thus, protection of participants covers a wide range of research, including that which involves tissue specimens, medical records, genetic material, behavioural and/or biomedical assessments, and treatments. Further, research involving residual diagnostic specimens, including specimens obtained for routine patient care that would have been discarded if not used for research, private information, such as medical data that can be readily identified with individuals, even if the information was not specifically collected for the study in question also requires safeguards. Research on cell lines or DNA samples that can be associated with individuals falls in this category.

Informed Consent

To honour the principle of autonomy or respect for persons, it is necessary that potential research participants (to the extent that they are capable) be given the opportunity to choose whether or not to take part in the research. This is ensured though the informed consent process. When a competent (medically or legally) individual agrees to participate in research when he or she has received the necessary information, has understood this information and having understood it (perhaps after discussion with family members or the family doctor) has arrived at a decision about participation without having been under any coercion, undue influence, inducement or intimidation, it is called informed consent. By all standards, it is necessary to document this consent as a written, informed consent. It must be obtained from every subject before any study-related procedure and documented on a form approved by the Ethics Committee.

It is always preferable that the research participant give consent. If the subject is unable to give consent (for example, in the case of a child, a patient with dementia or an unconscious patient), the subject's legally acceptable representative (LAR) is expected to consent. However, the subject should be informed to the extent compatible with his/her understanding and assent to participate should be sought and documented.

It is at all times the investigator's responsibility to obtain consent. Either the Principal Investigator or his delegate (who must be qualified to administer consent) should discuss all pertinent aspects of the study, including the informed consent form, answer any queries/doubts, request consent and if given, document it on the Ethics Committee approved form. The consent should be signed and dated by the subject or the subject's LAR, the person conducting the informed consent discussion and if the subject or subject's LAR is illiterate, an impartial witness. It is important to ensure that no coercion/undue influence is used and the subject is given ample time for decision, and adequate opportunity to discuss issues.

If a subject does not understand English, a vernacular consent form (approved by the Ethics Committee) must be administered in the language he understands. In the case of an illiterate individual, consent is administered in the presence of an impartial witness. The subject can give a thumb impression in place of the signature. It is important to document the method of obtaining consent in all these cases. A signed and dated copy of the consent form must be provided to the subject or his LAR.

In older children, Schedule Y now mandates obtaining assent as well as the consent of the parents.

There are three basic elements in any consent form: *information, voluntariness* and *competence,* and the contents of a consent form have to be approved by the Ethics Committee. Of relevance to our country is the need to provide information in the language the person is best able to understand. This information should be scientifically accurate as well as sensitive to the local social and cultural context. Schedule Y (Appendix XI) specifies the content of the informed consent document and these are the minimum elements that must be part of this, including the fact that the trial involves research and that his participation is strictly voluntary.

The purpose of the study including the interventions and procedures, risks, benefits and alternative treatments must be mentioned. Compensation or treatment for injury is an important part of the consent form. The subject's responsibilities must be delineated and, if any payment is to be made, this should be clarified. How the confidentiality of patient data will be protected must be specified, as well as whom to contact for study-related information including the Ethics Committee details.

If important new information is obtained during the study, the informed consent form must be revised, Ethics Committee approval obtained before use and the subject or subject's LAR informed in a timely manner and consent obtained to continue in the study.

Informed consent may be waived if it is justified that the research involves not more than minimal risk, when the participant and the researcher do not come into contact or when it is necessitated in emergency situations. Such studies should have protection in place for both privacy and confidentiality and must not violate the rights of the participants. The ICMR guidelines state that Ethics Committees may waive the requirement for informed consent:

- when the confidentiality of personally identifiable information has to be maintained throughout research (for example, a study on the disease burden of HIV/AIDS)
- when research is to be conducted on publicly available information, documents, records, works, performances, reviews, quality assurance studies, archival material or third-party interviews, service programmes for the benefit of the public having a bearing on public health programmes, and consumer acceptance studies
- when research is planned on anonymised biological samples from deceased individuals, left-over samples after clinical investigation, cell lines or cell-free derivatives like viral isolates, DNA or RNA from recognised institutions or qualified investigators, samples or data from repositories or registries etc., in emergency situations when no surrogate consent can be taken.

Interestingly, a lot of research is being carried out about the process of informed consent. Most of these studies indicate that the level of understanding of participants about the purpose of the study varies widely, but is generally rather poor. Similarly, many studies have documented that strikingly few participants understand that they did not have to participate or that they had a right to withdraw (sometimes less than half understood these issues). Studies show that participants feel obligated to continue in the trial. Thus, the freedom and voluntariness participants should experience and exercise, the very epitome of ethical research, may not be adequately understood.

A criticism that is often levelled at informed consent documents pertains to their complexity. The number of pages and technicalities included in them sometimes make it difficult for the community representative in the Ethics Committee, leave alone the patient, to understand the document. Studies have shown that fewer than half the participants understand the concepts of placebo control and randomisation (in one study conducted in children, only 7% of the parents understood that treatment assignment would be random, for example). Whether this is because of therapeutic misconception or due to the complexity of the concept is not well known.

Participant comprehension of the risks and benefits of the trial is central to the process of consent. Many studies have shown a definite trend towards excessive optimism about benefits – one study showed that 43% of patients had no doubts at all about the benefits they were likely to get from the treatment, when the consent form actually said that no benefit could be assured. In a Phase I oncology trial, only 22% of the participants actually understood that there may be no benefit to them by participating.

Similarly, a patients' ability to evaluate the risks of participation are sometimes suspect. Many studies have shown that patients are unable to recollect even three of the side effects listed in a consent form.

Poverty is often mistakenly believed to be associated with reduced understanding; however, studies have proven that this is not so. Similarly, the sex, age and disease type do not seem to affect understanding. However, the extent of education does significantly influence the level of understanding of the consent form.

Several interventions have been tested to enhance understanding of the consent process, including audio-visual and multimedia interventions, enhanced consent forms, extended discussions and tests/feedback. However, results have not been conclusive with any intervention, although the use of multimedia has been shown to be effective, especially in patients with a mental health disorder.

An important concept that must be appreciated by the physician-investigator is that of therapeutic misconception. When a patient agrees to participate in a trial, he may harbour a mistaken belief (therapeutic misconception) that the physician treating him will, by default, take decisions about his treatment based solely on his condition and clinical needs, and not according to what the protocol requires. This is believed to be an important obstacle to ethically valid consent as the patient fails to appreciate that his physician is now wearing the 'investigator's hat'. It may sometimes be useful to have counsellors or the study nurse conduct the consent process, to minimise therapeutic misconception. The responsibility of reducing this misconception rests squarely on the investigator.

What emerges from this discussion is that the consent process is difficult and may be a multi-step procedure involving more people that just the investigator and the participant. An informed consent is not a piece of paper or a signature. It is a process by which we ensure that our subject's right to be informed and right to consent to research is protected, and by which we document our efforts to protect the subject's rights to the satisfaction of independent observers.

Roles and Responsibilities of Institutional Review Boards

The Declaration of Helsinki and the ICMR Guidelines have mandated that all proposals on biomedical research involving human subjects undergo ethical review. This activity is generally performed by an Ethics Committee which is required to protect the study subjects' well-being, rights and confidentiality, to meet the mandate of the Declaration of Helsinki and to make clinical research socially respectable and acceptable to regulatory authorities and journal editors.

Ethics Committees could be institutional or independent. The Ethics Committee (EC) is made up of a reasonable number of members, who collectively have the qualifications and experience to review and evaluate the science, medical aspects and ethics of the proposed trial. Generally, members should be aware of local, social and cultural norms, and this is why approval of local ECs is required even if central or international ECs have already approved the proposal.

The ICH-GCP guidelines (available at http://www.ich.org) recommend that an EC may contain an odd number of members (at least five members familiar with GCP), including at least one member whose primary area of interest is not science, and one member independent of the institution. The ICMR Guidelines suggest, and Schedule Y mandates, that the Chairperson should be from outside the institution and not the head of the same institution to maintain the independence of the Committee. The Member Secretary, however, belongs to the same institution to facilitate administration of the EC.

Schedule Y (2005 amendment) specifies in Appendix VIII that the EC should have at least seven members, being a mix of medical/non-medical, scientific and non-scientific persons, including a lay person. The quorum for an EC meeting has been specified as at least five members consisting of a basic medical scientist (preferably one pharmacologist), a clinician, a legal expert, a social scientist/representative of a non-governmental voluntary agency/philosopher/ethicist/theologian or a similar person and a lay person from the community.

An investigator can be an EC member although he/she cannot opine or vote on a proposal in which he or she is the investigator. The EC can invite *ad hoc* subject experts for a meeting if they feel a lack of expertise within themselves. However, these experts can only offer expert advice or opinion on a scientific, legal or any such issue and they cannot vote on a proposal. They must be named, their participation justified in writing, and their opinion or advice recorded.

It is necessary for an EC to function according to written standard operating procedures (SOP) which define the composition of the EC and the authority under which it is established, the scheduling, notification and conduct of meetings, as well as the process of conducting initial and continuing review of trials. A list of members and their signed and dated CVs must always be available for audit or inspection.

The investigator, not the sponsor, always communicates with the EC although the sponsor can help the investigator to respond to the issues raised by the EC, supply additional information required and amend the study plan if necessary as well as comply with the EC's other requirements.

The EC's responsibilities extend from before the start of research, including review and approval of the proposal (Table 24.3 lists the documents the Ethics Committee is expected to review as per the ICMR Guidelines and Schedule Y before taking a decision on a proposal), while research is in progress to monitor the study and review serious adverse events, to after completion of research including publication and archiving.

A clinical study cannot be initiated before approval is obtained from an Ethics Committee and it is important that ECs provide independent, competent and timely review of the science, ethics and medical aspects of the proposed studies according to an established review procedure. The elements of review have been well described in the WHO's Operational Guidelines for Ethics Committees That Review Biomedical Research (available at http://www.who.int/tdr/publications/publications/pdf/ethics.pdf).

The scientific design and conduct of the study has to be reviewed at the outset as poor science is poor ethics. The appropriateness of the study design in relation to the objectives of the study, the statistical methodology (including sample size calculation), and the potential for reaching sound conclusions with the smallest number of research

Table 24.3 Documents an Ethics Committee must review

- Trial protocol(s)/amendment(s), with date and version
- Written informed consent form(s) and consent form updates that the investigator proposes for use in the trial
- Subject recruitment procedures (advertisements)
- Written information to be provided to the subjects (Patient Information Sheet and Informed Consent Form, including updates if any) in English and/or the vernacular language
- Investigator's Brochure (IB), available safety information
- Information about payments and compensation available to subjects
- Investigator's current curriculum vitae and/or other documentation evidencing qualifications
- Any other document that the EC may require to fulfill its responsibilities
- May request more information be given to subjects when, in the judgment of the EC, the additional information would be meaningful to the protection of the rights, safety and/or well-being of the subjects
- Insurance Policy/Compensation for participation and for serious adverse events occurring during study participation
- Investigator's Agreement with the sponsor
- Investigator's Undertaking (Appendix VII of Schedule Y)

participants has to be assessed. There must be a justification for the predictable risks and inconveniences weighed against the anticipated benefits for the research participants and the concerned communities. The justification for the use of control arms, criteria for prematurely withdrawing of research participants and for suspending or terminating the research as a whole may be assessed. The EC should also review the policies for monitoring and auditing conduct of research, including the constitution of a data safety monitoring board (DSMB). The adequacy of the site, including the qualifications of the Principal Investigator and supporting staff, available facilities and emergency procedures, are also assessed by the EC before approving a study.

The recruitment of research participants is a central aspect to be reviewed by the EC. The characteristics of the population from which the research participants will be drawn, the means by which recruitment is to be conducted, and how full information will be given to the potential research participants must be reviewed.

Any plans in the protocol to withdraw or withhold standard therapies for the purpose of the research, and the justification for such action, needs careful review. What medical care will be provided to research participants during and after the course of the research is another important facet to be assessed, including adequacy of medical supervision and psycho-social support for the research participants. Plans for post-trial access to the study product must be evaluated. It is crucial to assess the description of any financial costs to research participants, rewards and compensations for research participants (including money, services and/or gifts) as well as provisions made for compensation/

treatment in case of injury/disability/death of a research participant attributable to participation in the research (including insurance and indemnity arrangements)

Maintaining confidentiality of patient information is important in the study, and the EC must review the plans to protect this.

The informed consent process has to be studied in detail, including the identification of those responsible for obtaining consent. The adequacy, completeness and understandability (including vernacular forms) of information to be given to the research participants must be reviewed. The EC must be satisfied regarding the justification to use a vulnerable population and special attention paid to the process of informed consent and assent should be clarified.

The EC may evaluate the impact and relevance of the research on the local community, and study, where relevant, proposed community consultation during the course of the research. The manner in which the results of the research will be made available to the research participants and the concerned communities may also be addressed.

When reviewing proposals, the EC must assess whether the anticipated benefit of the research (new knowledge or improved health for the research participant) justifies undertaking the risks. The EC should not approve research in which the risks are believed to be unreasonable in relation to the anticipated benefits. Risks can be physical, psychological, social, legal and economic and can be graded as less or greater than minimal risk. The EC must ensure that risks to participants are minimised. ECs should assess the degree of therapeutic misconception that may occur in a protocol.

The EC must review proposals within a reasonable time, document its views in writing, clearly identifying the trial, documents reviewed and the dates for approval/favourable opinion, modifications required prior to its approval/favourable opinion, disapproval/negative opinion or termination/suspension of any prior approval/favourable opinion.

An expedited review may be conducted if the research proposal involves less than minimal risk to the study subjects, or involves a minor amendment to a study already approved by the EC. A written approval containing the date of the meeting, documents reviewed (versions and dates), list of members present indicating that quorum was complete should be given. It is mandated that no clinical study can be started without EC permission and no deviations or changes initiated without prior written EC approval except when necessary to eliminate immediate hazards to the subjects.

During a trial, the Principal Investigator must submit updated documentation, written summaries of the trial status annually or more frequently if requested, serious adverse events within seven working days (and provide additional information as requested), a summary of the trial's outcome upon completion as well as amendments to the protocol or informed consent document.

Some Issues with Ethics Review

The most common problem the EC faces is that of scientific and ethical review. Investigators do not appreciate scientific review and EC members often lack training in ethics review. Often, investigators submit incomplete protocols, the level of evidence generated using the proposed design is low and many of the planned studies are of a 'me-too' variety. Efficacy and failure end points are also often not specified. In practical terms, it is useful to have a checklist for members related to major scientific and ethical aspects while reviewing a proposal so that such issues are covered.

As new members are recruited into any EC, it becomes necessary for training in the review process as well as to inculcate an understanding of their roles and responsibilities so that the EC becomes compliant with relevant guidelines in letter and spirit. Further, as guidelines and laws change, it becomes necessary to have continued training of members. ECs are also often overburdened. Increasing number of projects per meeting and the 'size' of each proposal leads to superficial reviews. The time available for discussions is also limited, leading to inadequate review.

An aspect that is never addressed and for which there are no guidelines is how EC members should be compensated for their expertise and time.

ECs usually perform a preliminary review of the proposal, and then no further monitoring is performed. Investigators submit serious adverse events or SAEs (often not in prescribed formats, and with incomplete data) and the ECs often only acknowledge that these SAEs have been received. Further follow-up action is rare. Naturally, again the question of time, expertise and funds is crucial.

The EC must have an independent office with open communication lines. The role of the Chairperson cannot be emphasised enough – this individual has to knit together a number of (very busy and often senior) individuals from diverse backgrounds and ensure compliance with GCP guidelines. The Secretary and Secretariat also have a very important role. The Secretary acts as a liaison between the investigator and the committee and therefore needs to ensure appropriate communication between them.

It is necessary to increase communication between ECs to prevent the phenomenon of 'EC shopping', where sponsors may change investigators because of rejection by the EC of a proposal at one site. There is also a strong need for national audits of ECs and a functioning accreditation system. It would also be useful to create awareness and provide training to researchers and EC members, sponsors, administrators and policy makers in this area.

Special Challenges

Research in India carries some special ethical challenges which need to be addressed:

- *The consent process:* With its reams of material and technical terms, the informed consent document can be daunting. Vernacular translations pose a special challenge as many technical terms like ECG or placebo are difficult to translate. Some translations lose the meaning in the process and every effort needs to be made to have translations that mean the same thing as the original. Documentation of consent is also fraught with challenges; in the case of illiterate participants, it is necessary to provide the consent form in a language that the participant understands and the witness can read. Issues relating to confidentiality (for example, in HIV studies), individual versus community consent and cultural influences are other challenges.

- *Standard of care:* What should be the control arm is an issue that worries many ECs. Should it be the best current treatment currently available anywhere in the world or treatment based on an alternative standard (the best care available locally) or placebo? Although the appropriate answer to this question would be that patients be offered a universal standard of care, this is sometimes impractical and could also act as an undue inducement for participation. In any case, the final approval rests with local ECs which should be aware of the local scenario.
- *Post-trial access:* Should post-trial access to the study drug or treatment always be provided or would it be undue inducement? Will the drug be registered in India and should research be permitted if not? Who is responsible for providing post-trial access? Such questions need to be addressed.

Conclusions

Conducting ethical clinical research is challenging, particularly so because it is a multi-disciplinary activity. Just as it is the responsibility of the physician to honour the three principles of ethical research, *autonomy, beneficence* and *justice*, it is also important for other healthcare workers like pharmacists who are invariably associated with clinical research to internalise these concepts. In addition, attention to guidelines and appropriate regulatory supervision can greatly enhance participant protection.

KEY MESSAGES

- Clinical research is a systematic investigation in human beings designed to discover or contribute to a body of generalisable knowledge.
- One of the primary legal and ethical obligations of researchers and their teams is to protect the human participants who take part in the research.
- Most ethical guidelines have evolved after tremendous human tragedies, but today these form the foundation for clinical research.
- The three fundamental principles of ethical research are autonomy (respect for persons), beneficence and justice.
- The two pillars that protect human participants in clinical research are voluntary, informed consent and independent ethics review of the protocol.
- A wide range of research is considered as 'clinical research', including that which involves tissue specimens, medical records, genetic material, behavioural and/or biomedical assessments, and treatments.
- Informed consent is given when a competent (medically or legally) individual agrees to participate in research when he or she has received the necessary information, has understood this information and having understood it (perhaps after discussion with family members or family doctor) has arrived at a decision about participation without having been under any coercion, undue influence or inducement or intimidation.

- If the subject is unable to give consent (for example, a child, or a patient with dementia, an unconscious patient), the subject's legally acceptable representative (LAR) is expected to consent.
- The three basic elements in any consent form are information, voluntariness and competence, and the contents of a consent form have to be approved by the Ethics Committee.
- It is necessary for an EC to function according to written standard operating procedures (SOP).
- The EC's responsibilities extend from before start of research, including review and approval of the proposal, while research is in progress to monitor the study and review serious adverse events, and after completion of research including publication and archiving.

Further Reading

The Oxford Textbook of Clinical Research Ethics. 2008. Emanuel EJ, Grady C, Crouch RA, Lie RK, Miller FG and Wendler D. Oxford University Press.

25
Research in Clinical Pharmacy

Milap C Nahata

Learning Objectives

Upon completion of this chapter, the reader should be able to:

- Understand the role of pharmacists in conducting research
- Describe the types of clinical research
- Indicate the knowledge and skills needed to perform clinical research
- Discuss the guidelines for conducting various types of clinical research

The main purpose of clinical research is to generate new knowledge for improving the health of individuals and populations. The results of clinical research should provide information about the prevention and treatment of diseases that can be used to improve health outcomes and the quality of life of humans. Clinical research involves human subjects and can include a broad spectrum of research; for example, pharmacokinetics, clinical trials to evaluate drug efficacy and safety, epidemiological studies, and health services and outcomes research.

Clinical research is essential to determine the efficacy, adverse effects, interactions and cost-effectiveness of drug therapy in various patient populations. It is important to conduct clinical trials with various pharmacotherapeutic modalities to determine which one should be preferred in a specific patient. Optimal dosage regimens (dose, frequency and route of administration, and duration of therapy) have not been established for many drugs for a variety of diseases.

Pharmacists have a unique educational background in medicinal chemistry (drug discovery), pharmacognosy, pharmaceutics (drug delivery, pharmacokinetics), basic and clinical pharmacology (mechanism of drug action, pharmacodynamics, efficacy and adverse effects), social, behavioural and administrative pharmacy, and clinical pharmacy or pharmacy practice (pathophysiology and pharmacotherapy). They may also have substantial clinical experience through educational training and employment. Thus, pharmacists with an appropriate background should be able to conceive research ideas, design and conduct studies, analyse data and disseminate the findings through presentations and publications.

Types of Clinical Research

As described in Table 25.1, pharmacists can contribute to various types of clinical research. Pharmacists should not only participate in research projects but must also lead some as principal investigators, with adequate support of co-investigators from other disciplines, for example, physicians, nurses and other scientists or practitioners.

The *pharmacokinetics* of a drug describes what the body does to the drug. Pharmacokinetic studies are performed to characterise the process of absorption (rate and extent of absorption, bioavailability), distribution, metabolism and elimination of drugs in humans. The results of these studies are useful in estimating doses and frequency of administration.

Pharmacodynamics is what a drug does to the body. Such responses may include biochemical, physiological, pharmacological and therapeutic effects. Pharmacodynamic evaluations are performed to correlate plasma or serum concentration and pharmacokinetics with the parameters of efficacy or safety (for example, changes in blood pressure or kidney function). Such evaluation may be performed initially in healthy individuals and later in patients with specific illnesses. The effect of disease on the pharmacokinetics and pharmacodynamics of drugs in patients must also be studied. These studies assist in refining the dose requirements in efficacy and safety studies.

Efficacy or effectiveness studies are done to determine therapeutic or clinical response to drug therapy in patients. Efficacy may be evaluated using objective or subjective end points and may be measured at cellular, tissue, organ and whole body level. *Adverse effects* and safety studies are also performed in patients to assess the potential risks of drug therapy. Drug–drug, drug–disease and drug–food interactions may take place in healthy persons (volunteers or subjects) or in patients. *Pharmacogenetic*/genomic studies are conducted to understand the influence of genetics on drug response (for example, efficacy, safety).

Pharmacoeconomics, health outcomes, quality of life and health service studies are carried out in patients, generally to evaluate an individual drug treatment or compare

Table 25.1 Types of clinical pharmacy research

• Pharmacokinetics	• Pharmacoeconomics
• Pharmacodynamics	• Health outcomes/quality of life
• Efficacy	• Drug use studies
• Adverse effects or safety	• Stability or compatibility
• Interactions	• Pharmacoepidemiology
• Pharmacogenetics/genomics	

different drug therapies. Drug use studies research the patterns and determinants of drug use in institutions or communities. Examples include studies of drug-related benefits, drug-related risks and problems, adverse drug reactions, adverse drug events, drug-related hospitalisations, patient adherence and the quality of drug use in health services. The WHO indicators used in the latter type of study are presented in *Chapter 8, Essential Medicines and Rational Drug Use.*

A drug use evaluation or review is conducted to assure the quality of drug use through the use of predetermined standards (such as guidelines or protocols), with the goal of improving drug use, consistent with the standards. The effectiveness of corrective actions is measured periodically to assure continued optimal use of drugs.

Stability studies are done to assure that at least 90% of the drug remains in a modified dosage form (for example, a suspension prepared from a commercially available tablet form). Finally, compatibility studies are performed to make sure that two or more drugs are chemically and physically stable during co-administration from the same delivery system (such as intravenous tubing) to patients.

Skills for Conducting Clinical Research

There is a logical progression of steps involved in the successful completion of clinical research (Table 25.2). Clinical research should be done to address specific clinical questions.

Many clinical questions need to be answered for providing optimal patient care. For example, what should be the dose and frequency of administration for a new drug in patients with asthma; which of three

Table 25.2 Steps in clinical research

1. Identify a clinical problem
2. Confirm the need to conduct research
3. Formulate a research question
4. Develop hypotheses and specific objectives
5. Assess feasibility (availability of patients, collaborators and funding)
6. Design the study with appropriate methods to address objectives and test hypotheses
7. Submit the proposal to Human Subjects Research (Ethics) Committee and for funding
8. Assign specific responsibilities for conducting the study to collaborators and support personnel
9. Perform the study
10. Analyse the results to determine the statistical and clinical significance of the findings
11. Discuss the results, possible interpretations and potential conclusions with collaborators
12. Prepare an abstract for presentation at a national meeting
13. Prepare a manuscript for publication in a refereed journal

preferred drugs on the formulary should be used in patients with hypertension; or, what is the association between the use of protease inhibitors and CD4 count, viral load and clinical outcomes in patients with HIV/AIDS.

A study should not be undertaken simply because it has not been done previously – clinical observation should determine the need to conduct clinical research. Once a problem has been identified, the need for study should be confirmed by discussions with colleagues and through evaluation of the existing literature. A research question, specific objectives and hypotheses should then be formulated by the principal investigator with input from collaborators or co-investigators.

The feasibility of conducting studies should be carefully assessed or reassessed before investing additional time and effort. This assessment should include the availability of an adequate patient population, sufficient financial resources, and the qualification and support of collaborators (physicians, nurses or other researchers). The study should be designed with the use of validated methodology to address specific objectives and test hypotheses. A biostatistician may be consulted.

The study proposal is then submitted to the Institutional Review Board (IRB) or Human Subjects Research (Ethics) Committee to assure that the potential benefits outweigh potential risks to humans and that all appropriate rights of patients are protected. This process must be followed for all studies (retrospective, concurrent and prospective) involving humans. The approved proposal may also be submitted to funding agencies to acquire grant funds to perform the study.

The principal investigator must convene all individuals (collaborators and supportive personnel) to clearly identify the role of each participant. This is an important step to minimise confusion and ensure that all procedures are followed correctly. Examples of activities include recruitment of patients into the study, obtaining signed informed consent from patients or guardian(s), administering drugs, collecting blood samples from patients, measuring the drug concentration, assessing clinical, humanistic and economic outcomes, analysing data, presenting research papers at meetings, and publishing research articles in peer-reviewed journals.

The study should be performed while adhering to the protocol approved by the Ethics Committee. Any unexpected finding and/or harmful effects from drug therapy should be communicated to the patient and the family, Ethics Committee, collaborators, drug manufacturer, funding source and the governmental regulatory agency (such as the Food and Drug Administration in the US). In some cases, it may be necessary to modify or terminate the protocol before completion of the study. For example, it would be unethical to continue a study of a drug versus a placebo when the drug is clearly more effective than the placebo in the initial group of patients.

After study completion, the data should be analysed to determine clinical and statistical significance. A biostatistician may be consulted, if necessary, to assure the use of appropriate statistical tests. In some cases, data may show clinically important differences in the absence of statistically significant differences; the reverse may also be true in certain situations.

When the data has been fully analysed, the principal investigator should discuss the results with all collaborators to seek their input about the study findings. The results may have to be re-analysed to answer new questions. It is important to decide what should be emphasised in the study report and what conclusions are fully supported by the data.

It is critical to disseminate study results through abstracts to be presented at national meetings and through manuscripts to be submitted for publication in refereed (peer-reviewed) journals. The journal should be on indexing services (such as MEDLINE or EMBASE) and should preferably have a high impact factor (number of citations divided by number of articles published over a two-year period) and ranking within the field. The authorship should be offered only to those who have made substantial contributions to the project.

Guidelines for Conducting Studies

Pharmacokinetic studies: Demographic information for all patients should be collected. The entire dose of the drug should be fully administered to patients and the time of administration should be recorded. Multiple blood samples should be collected to adequately characterise absorption (for drugs not given by the IV route), distribution, metabolism and elimination. If a drug or active metabolite is excreted by the kidneys, total urine volume at timed intervals should also be collected during the dosage interval to calculate the percentage of drug excreted and renal clearance. For drugs used in treating meningitis, samples of cerebrospinal fluid are also collected to determine the drug concentration, with the goal of assuring adequate drug concentration at the disease site to achieve a favourable outcome.

The analytical method used to measure drug concentration in biological fluids or tissue samples should be validated demonstrating sensitivity, specificity and reproducibility. The data should be analysed to determine the correlation between the demographic data (such as age, gender) and the pharmacokinetics of the drug. Similarly, an attempt should be made to correlate the pharmacokinetics of a drug to clinical response (such as blood pressure, blood glucose). Maximum plasma drug concentrations (Cmax), time to achieve maximum concentration (Tmax), area under the plasma concentration-time curve (AUC), clearance (total, renal, oral), apparent distribution volume and elimination half-life of the drug are the most commonly determined parameters.

Efficacy/Safety Studies: Clinical trials should be conducted with appropriate controls; for example, by using a randomised, double-blind or single-blind study design. A new drug may be compared to a previously accepted drug of choice or to a placebo if there is no established therapy and if the drug may be no better than the placebo.

During drug development (pre-marketing), clinical studies are done in three phases (Phase I–III) by the industry. A phase I trial is done to determine the pharmacokinetics and safety of a drug in humans. It usually includes 20–100 individuals on the drug: normal, healthy volunteers. A phase II trial is performed in a small number of patients with a disease for which the drug is intended. Data from in vitro and animal studies and the phase I trial are used to identify the groups of patients most likely to benefit from the new drug. A phase II trial generally has 100–300 patients.

Phase III trials are usually conducted in 300–3000 patients at multiple medical centres and/or clinics to establish the efficacy and safety of a drug. The data from these studies forms the basis for preparing a new drug application (NDA) for submission to governmental regulatory agencies such as the US Food and Drug Administration to seek approval for marketing. Phase IV studies are performed after the drug has been on the market as part of a post-marketing surveillance programme, to learn more about the efficacy and safety of the marketed drug.

All demographic and disease data, drug administration, clinical and laboratory parameters of efficacy and safety should be documented in the detailed case report form for each patient. These studies are most expensive to perform but are crucial to receive drug approval from the regulatory agencies for specific indications. A common problem with these studies is that the number of patients enrolled may be too small to detect a true difference between treatments (type II error).

Further, the new treatment may appear safe under strict guidelines of the protocol (such as no concurrent drugs allowed) but in fact may be associated with serious toxicity when used under normal clinical conditions in a large group of patients taking multiple drugs. Many drugs like cerivastatin, cisapride, grepafloxacin, terfenadine and trovafloxacin had to be withdrawn from the US market following reports of serious adverse effects associated with them, either directly or due to interactions with other drugs.

Drug use evaluation (DUE): These studies are commonly performed in hospitals as well as in ambulatory (outpatient) clinics. The goal is to assess the patterns of drug use under routine clinical situations, to maximise efficacy and minimise adverse effects and cost of therapy. For example, one may perform a drug use evaluation of vancomycin to prevent its use without indication to assure efficacy, prevent the development of microbial resistance and to reduce costs.

Such studies may be done retrospectively or prospectively by collecting demographic and disease data, dosage regimens of all drugs, efficacy and safety parameters (clinical and laboratory) and clinical outcomes. The results are compared with established therapeutic guidelines. Deviations from the guidelines are identified and communicated to the medical department and appropriate institutional committees. Evaluations may also be done for expensive drugs to ascertain that these are being used appropriately. Further information about the conduct of DUEs is presented in *Chapter 26, Drug Utilisation Evaluation*.

Stability/Compatibility studies: Many drugs have to be used outside of labelled indications or approved guidelines. For example, two intravenous (IV) drugs may have to be administered through the same IV tubing due to limited access to IV sites, or the contents of a tablet or capsule may have to be reformulated in an oral suspension due to the inability of a young child or an elderly patient to swallow it. In such cases, the chemical and physical stability and compatibility must be documented to avoid undesirable therapeutic or toxic effects.

Chemical stability studies require the use of a specific, accurate, reproducible and stability-indicating analytical method (such as high performance liquid chromatography).

The studies are conducted while simulating clinical use for appropriate drug concentration, storage containers and temperature. While validating the assay method, the reformulated or extemporaneously prepared dosage form is intentionally degraded under extreme temperature or pH conditions to make sure the degraded products would not interfere with the measurement of the active drug during actual study.

Physical stability or compatibility is determined by visual inspection. A reformulated drug in a prescription bottle or two drugs to be combined in IV tubing are placed against white and black backgrounds to detect any changes in physical appearance. Presence of flocculation, turbidity or precipitation for an IV drug, and separation or caking in a suspension would indicate that the drug is physically unstable. Changes in colour and odour may also imply (but not confirm) lack of physical stability.

Transition from Research Project to Research Programme

The administration (Director or Chief Pharmacist) of the department should clearly communicate the importance of clinical research by pharmacists. It should be an essential part of the mission of the department. No health profession can survive, let alone thrive, without its ability to create new knowledge for achieving improved health outcomes. A culture for multidisciplinary research should also be created and enhanced.

Pharmacists should start with a single research project which has high clinical impact and probability of successful completion. It should be taken all the way from conception of an idea to publication of an article. It is equally important to sustain the research effort by identifying additional clinical problems. Support from physician collaborators and the Department of Pharmacy, however, is essential for success. This will also increase the chances of successful funding applications for financial support. Important funding agencies in India include the All-India Council for Technical Education, University Grants Commission, Indian Council for Medical Research, Department of Science and Technology and the Council for Scientific and Industrial Research. The International Pharmaceutical Federation also supports research in the area of pharmacy practice.

Preparing Clinical Researchers

Most first-generation clinical pharmacists had to learn clinical research on the job, since there were few education and training programmes during the 1960s and '70s. During the '80s in the USA, two-year postdoctoral fellowship programmes were developed for Pharm D graduates with or without residency experience. In 2001, there were about 60 fellowship programmes available in the USA in various areas of clinical pharmacy (such as cardiology, infectious diseases, paediatrics). This is still a small number, considering the need for clinical researchers.

Many pharmacy schools in the US are unable to find well-trained researchers to take faculty positions today. Some graduate (MS or PhD) programmes have also been developed but the number of pharmacy graduates focusing on clinical research is small. Fellows or graduate students should obtain experience in all steps of clinical research to develop confidence.

Attracting students from bachelor's degree programmes to seek careers in clinical research through additional education and training should be a high priority, if we are to succeed as a profession in having a nucleus of qualified clinical researchers to generate new knowledge. This may involve providing financial assistance or offering an option for graduation with Honours or Distinction.

In India, skills in clinical and pharmacy practice research are taught as part of the Masters programmes in pharmacy practice, where students undertake a significant research project in the second year. Some students may go on to PhD studies in clinical pharmacy or pharmacy practice, and further develop their research skills. Skilled clinical research pharmacists are urgently needed as relatively little is known about many epidemiological and clinical aspects of drug use in the Indian population. To achieve this, pharmacists should take up opportunities for training in research methodology, biostatistics, epidemiology, public health, pharmacoeconomics and grant writing.

Conclusion

The ultimate goal of clinical research is to make an impact on patient care. Our efforts should clearly contribute towards achieving improved quality of life through prevention and treatment of diseases in the most cost-effective manner. This can best take place when research findings are widely shared through presentations at national or international meetings and publications in peer-reviewed journals indexed on databases including MEDLINE/PubMed and EMBASE.

CASE STUDY 1

Title of study: Pharmacokinetics and safety of tobramycin after once-daily administration in patients with cystic fibrosis

Type of study: Pharmacokinetics and safety

Clinical problem or rationale for conducting study: An aminoglycoside antibiotic (gentamicin or tobramycin) is commonly used in patients with respiratory tract infections caused by Gram-negative pathogens. It is normally given three times daily by intravenous infusion. The peak and trough serum concentrations are monitored to maximise efficacy and minimise toxicity. Animal studies indicated that administration of the total daily dose as a single dose was at least as effective as multiple daily doses and was associated with less toxicity compared with the multiple dose regimens. A single daily dose would also be less expensive to administer and monitor compared to multiple daily doses.

Objective of study: To determine the pharmacokinetics and safety of once-daily dosing of tobramycin in patients with a genetically inherited disease, cystic fibrosis.

Methods: The initial single dose was the same as the combined multiple daily doses for each patient used during the last hospital admission. For the first admission, the once-daily dose was 10 mg/kg. Subsequent doses were adjusted based on pharmacokinetic monitoring. At steady state, blood samples were collected just before starting an infusion with the next dose, at the end of infusion, and at 1, 2, 4 and 8 hours thereafter, to characterise the pharmacokinetics of tobramycin. Renal function (BUN and serum creatinine) tests were done to assess nephrotoxicity. Audiometric (masked bone conduction and pure tone air conduction) studies were performed at various frequencies to evaluate potential ototoxicity associated with tobramycin. Microbiological studies were evaluated to assess antimicrobial response. Clinical evaluation was done to assure efficacy and document safety.

Results: The peak serum concentrations were substantially higher, as expected, after once-daily dosing. Total body clearance, apparent volume of distribution and elimination half-life were similar to those after multiple doses. The time above the minimum inhibitory concentration (MIC) was five times longer with once daily dosing. No nephrotoxicity, ototoxicity or other adverse effects occurred in any patient. Once-daily dosing led to a saving in cost compared with multiple daily doses.

Conclusion: Tobramycin may be used safely in once-daily doses to treat exacerbations of respiratory tract infections in patients with cystic fibrosis. Additional randomised studies in a large population are needed to determine its efficacy and safety.

CASE STUDY 2

Title of study: Efficacy of amlodipine in paediatric patients with hypertension

Type of study: Efficacy and safety

Clinical problem and rationale: Amlodipine is a commonly used calcium antagonist in adults with hypertension. It offers a convenient once-daily dosing and is relatively well tolerated. An increasing number of children were diagnosed with hypertension and were uncontrolled on existing ACE inhibitors. There were no studies available for any calcium antagonist in children with hypertension.

Objective: To determine the efficacy and safety of amlodipine in children with hypertension.

Methods: Twenty-one children were enrolled in an open label study after confirming that they had hypertension by a 24-hour ambulatory blood pressure monitor (ABPM), with blood pressure (BP) measured every 20 minutes. Oral amlodipine therapy was initiated at 0.05 mg/kg/day. The subsequent dose was titrated based on BP measurements at home monitored by ABPM. The dose was reduced or discontinued if significant adverse effects occurred during therapy. Patients or caregivers were given BP measuring equipment and requested to record BP twice daily on the right arm in the sitting position and maintain a diary. An investigator contacted the caregiver or patient twice weekly to monitor therapy and adjust the dose. All adverse effects were recorded. At the beginning and end of the study, patients and caregivers completed a quality of life questionnaire consisting of 52 global and specific questions about psychological well-being, health perception and physical ability. Compliance was measured by pill count, pharmacy records and telephone interviews.

Results: The starting mean dose was 0.07 mg/kg/day (equivalent to 5 mg/day in an adult weighing 70 kg). The mean titrated dose to control BP was 0.29 mg/kg/day in patients below the age of 13 years and 0.16 mg/kg/day in those at or above 13 years of age. BP control was achieved and quality of life improved in most patients. Adverse effects occurred in a number of patients but the drug was well tolerated by most patients.

Conclusion: Amlodipine is an effective anti-hypertensive agent with an acceptable safety profile. Younger patients may often require higher doses, as has been observed for other drugs.

CASE STUDY 3

Title of study: Development of two stable oral suspensions of levodopa-carbidopa for children with amblyopia

Type of study: Stability of extemporaneously prepared drugs

Clinical problem and rationale: The levodopa-carbidopa combination has been shown to improve visual function in children with amblyopia. The drug combination is commercially available in tablets. Since younger patients cannot swallow tablets and their dose is based on mg/kg of body weight, a liquid dose form would be most suitable for administration. However, no stability studies were available to document the physical and chemical stability of levodopa/carbidopa under clinically simulated conditions.

Objective: To determine the physical and chemical stability of levodopa/carbidopa in two oral suspensions stored in plastic prescription bottles over a three-month period at 4 °C under (refrigeration) and at 25 °C (room temperature).

Methods: Levododopa and carbidopa tablets were used to prepare two suspensions containing syrup and carboxymethylcellulose – one without an antioxidant and another with ascorbic acid as an antioxidant. Each suspension was stored in 10 bottles – five at 4 °C and five at 25 °C. Samples were drawn at 0, 7, 14, 28, 42, 56, 70 and 91 days after preparation and analysed by a validated and stability-indicating HPLC method.

Patients or caregivers completed a questionnaire over a four-week study to determine the safety of the two drugs in the two suspensions. The questionnaire was completed just before starting the study and at 2 and 4 weeks during the study.

Results: The mean concentrations of levodopa and carbidopa exceeded 90% of the initial concentrations for 42 days at 4 °C and 28 days at 25 °C. The drugs were less stable in the suspension containing ascorbic acid. The adverse effects were similar in children receiving suspension to those in older patients receiving tablets of the same drugs.

Conclusion: Levodopa/carbidopa can be administered safely in extemporaneously prepared suspensions to children with amblyopia.

KEY MESSAGES

- Pharmacists, as professionals, must contribute new knowledge to the literature through research.
- Pharmacists can perform various types of clinical research, for example, pharmacokinetics/ pharmacodynamics, efficacy, safety, stability and usage evaluations of drugs, in collaboration with other healthcare professionals.
- Successful completion of research requires knowledge and skills in designing studies, writing proposals, performing studies, analysing data, and presenting and publishing papers.
- Pharmacists must be knowledgeable about the guidelines applicable to various types of clinical research.

Further Reading

Hulley SB, Cummings SR, Browner WS, Grady D, Hearst N and Newman TB. 2001. *Designing clinical research*, 2nd ed. Lippincott, Williams & Wilkins: Philadelphia, USA; 1–336.

Browner WS. 1999. *Publishing and presenting clinical research*. Lippincott, Williams & Wilkins: Philadelphia, USA; 1–206.

Rosen B. 2000. *Fundamentals of biostatistics*, 5th ed. Duxbury: Pacific Grove, CA, USA; 1–792.

Bates RD, Nahata MC, Jones JW, McCoy K, Young G, Cox S and Barson WJ. 1997. Pharmacokinetics and safety of tobramycin after one-daily administration in patients with cystic fibrosis. *Chest* 112:1208–13.

Nahata MC, Morosco RS and Leguire LE. 2000. Development of two stable oral suspensions of levodopa-carbidopa for children with amblyopia. *J Pediatr Opthalmol Strabismus* 37:333–337.

Tallian KB, Nahata MC, Turman MA, Mahan JD, Hayes JR and Mentser MI. 1999. Efficacy of amlodipine in pediatric patients with hypertension. *Pediatr Nephrol* 13:304–310

Website of Interest

The ethics of research related to healthcare in developing countries, report published by the Nuffield Council on Bioethics, 2002

www.nuffieldbioethics.org/developingcountries

26 Drug Utilisation Evaluation

BS Sathvik

Learning Objectives

Upon completion of this chapter, the reader should be able to:

- Define the term drug use evaluation (DUE)
- List the objectives of DUE
- Describe the steps in the DUE cycle
- Classify different types of DUE
- Describe ways in which drug use problems can be identified
- Provide examples of strategies which may be used to improve drug use
- Identify the resources and tools required for a DUE study
- Summarise the pharmacist's role in DUE

Drug use is a complex process. Uncertainties in diagnosis, treatment and medication adherence contribute to wide variations in the way drugs are used for any given condition. In any country, a large number of sociocultural factors also contribute to the way drugs are used. In India, these include national drug policy, illiteracy, poverty, use of multiple healthcare systems, drug advertising and promotion, sale of prescription drugs without prescription, competition in the medical and pharmaceutical marketplace and limited availability of independent, unbiased drug information. The complexity of drug use means that optimal benefits of drug therapy in patient care may not be achieved because of underuse, overuse or misuse of drugs. Inappropriate drug use may also lead to increased cost of medical care, anti-microbial resistance, adverse effects and patient mortality. One method to evaluate and improve drug use is conducting drug use evaluation studies.

What is Drug Use Evaluation?

Drug use evaluation (DUE) is an ongoing, authorised and systematic quality improvement process, which is designed to:

- review drug use and/or prescribing patterns
- provide feedback of results to clinicians and other relevant groups
- develop criteria and standards which describe optimal drug use
- promote appropriate drug use through education and other interventions

Drug use/usage/utilisation evaluation (DUE) was originally known as drug utilisation review (DUR) in the 1970s and early '80s. The terms drug utilisation review (DUR) and drug use evaluation (DUE) are interchangeable. Medication use evaluation (MUE) is another term that has been used in place of DUE by some authors since 1994. According to the World Health Organization (WHO), MUE is similar to DUE in all respects, except that it is patient outcome–oriented and places emphasis on assessing clinical outcomes. MUE mainly aims at assessing and improving patient outcomes and thereby improving the individual patient's health-related quality of life (HRQOL). Regardless of the terminology, the main aim of DUE studies is to promote rational drug use (Table 26.1).

DUE is a discipline that aims to understand how and why drugs are used as they are, so that drug use and health outcomes can be improved. DUE can play a key role in helping the healthcare system understand, interpret and improve the prescribing, administration and use of medications. DUE information may assist healthcare systems and hospitals to design educational programmes that may improve prescribing and drug use. Some DUE programmes may provide physicians with feedback on their performance and prescribing patterns compared to predetermined criteria or treatment protocols. DUE information may also allow physicians to compare their approach to treating certain diseases with their peers. The 'peer pressure' generated by these comparisons may be useful in motivating physicians to change their prescribing habits in an effort to improve care.

Types of DUE

DUE studies are often drug-focused, where the use of a single drug (such as amikacin) or class of drugs (such as third-generation cephalosporins) is examined. Less commonly, DUE studies are indication-focused, where the use of a drug or drugs (for example, intravenous omeprazole for bleeding peptic ulcers) for a specific indication is examined.

Table 26.1 Aims of DUE

The main aim of any DUE study is to promote rational drug use by:
• reducing drug- and health-related treatment costs
• improving health-related quality of life
• improving quality of medical treatment
• improving coordinated healthcare
• decreasing the number of medication-related problems and medication errors
• decreasing the number of hospital admissions
• improving prescriber awareness and practice towards appropriate prescribing

DUE studies have also been described as quantitative or qualitative. Quantitative studies involve the collection, organisation and display of estimates or measurements of drug use. This type of data is often used for making purchasing decisions or other financial activities such as preparing drug budgets. However, data from quantitative drug use reviews should generally be considered suggestive, but not conclusive, with respect to the quality of drug use. Quantitative DUE studies may or may not be an ongoing activity and are almost always a unilateral pharmacy function.

Qualitative DUE studies, on the other hand, are multidisciplinary operations, which collect, organise, analyse and report information on actual drug use. They are usually one-off examinations of narrowly defined areas of drug use, usually specific drugs or specific conditions. The main difference between qualitative and quantitative DUE studies is that qualitative DUE includes the concept of criteria. Criteria are the predetermined elements against which aspects of the quality, medical necessity and appropriateness of medical care may be compared. Drug use criteria may be based on such items as indications for use, dose, dosing frequency and duration of therapy.

It is possible to combine both quantitative and qualitative DUE studies into a single study, which yields information about the patterns and amount as well as the quality of drug use.

Establishment of a DUE Programme

Although individuals may conduct DUEs in both hospital and community settings, the more common approach in hospitals is to develop a co-coordinated DUE programme. The body responsible for planning and implementing DUE programmes in hospitals is the DUE Committee.

DUE Committee

The DUE Committee should be composed of physicians, pharmacists and other relevant healthcare professionals. The Committee must include professionals with an interest in improving drug therapy in the hospital, and have ready access to experts in medicine, surgery and major hospital specialties. This body may be the hospital's drug and therapeutics committee or a specific DUE Committee, depending on local resources, inter-professional relationships and administrative structures. Pharmacists generally play a major role in the delivery of DUE and it is usual for the Committee to include Pharmacy department representation. The members of the DUE Committee should take sufficient time to read published articles, which provide information regarding the aims of DUE, staffing requirements and accepted standards of practice.

The administration of a DUE programme should be multi-disciplinary to avoid the common problems that can occur if the DUE Committee is administered by the Pharmacy department. These problems are listed below:

- Medical staff may be more likely to perceive the DUE programme as a pharmacy budget measure rather than a tool for improving clinical care.
- The involvement of medical and nursing staff may be more restricted, which may reduce the effectiveness of the DUE programme.

Table 26.2 Phases and steps involved in conducting a DUE

Phase I: Planning	
STEP 1	Identify drugs or areas of practice for possible study
STEP 2	Design the study
STEP 3	Define criteria and standards
STEP 4	Design the data collection form
Phase II: Data collection	
STEP 5	Collect data
Phase III: Evaluation	
STEP 6	Collate data and evaluate results
Phase IV: Feedback of results	
STEP 7	Feed results back to clinicians and other hospital staff
Phase V: Interventions	
STEP 8	Develop and implement interventions
Phase VI: Re-evaluation	
STEP 9	Re-evaluate to determine if drug use has improved
STEP 10	Re-assess and revise DUE programme as needed
Phase VII: Feedback of results	
STEP 11	Feed results back to clinicians and other hospital staff

- DUE may be given a lower priority than other Pharmacy department activities and DUE staff may be forced to relinquish their DUE activities when the department is short-staffed.

Functions of the DUE Committee: The DUE Committee has several functions to perform before, during and after completion of a DUE study. The Committee should draft and approve the policies and procedures that will govern its work, and establish and maintain adequate means of communication with the hospital's administration and other relevant hospital committees. Medical and other hospital staff should understand that the DUE programme is a continuous quality improvement activity designed to ensure safe and effective drug use. The Committee should prepare a schedule, including a yearly planning meeting, and meetings for selecting and approving criteria, evaluating data, designing interventions and reviewing the programme.

One of the key functions of the DUE Committee is to develop or review the standards and criteria of DUE studies based on their knowledge, experience and literature findings. Reviewing the data generated from the study is also the responsibility of the Committee. Initially, monthly meetings may be necessary to discuss start-up problems and make corrections in the programme. Later, quarterly meetings may be sufficient. If the hospital is starting a DUE programme for the first time, the DUE Committee may decide to complete one drug evaluation. Using that experience, the Committee can then establish an ongoing DUE schedule. Obviously, as interventions and re-evaluations begin, the workload of the Committee will increase. It is also important that the DUE Committee ensure compliance with good clinical research guidelines, such as maintaining the confidentiality of all patient data.

The DUE Cycle

It is important to keep in mind that DUE operates in a repeating cycle (Fig. 26.1). The DUE process is a continuous one and will be most valuable if the cycle is completed rather than performing different steps in isolation. The DUE cycle should include the following seven major activities or phases (Table 26.1):

I. Planning
II. Data collection
III. Evaluation

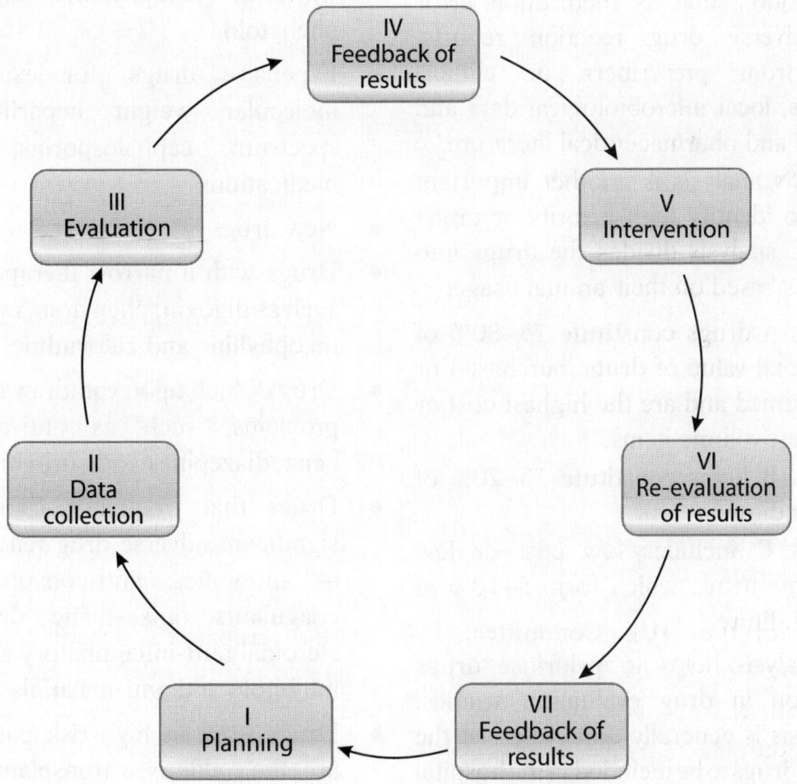

Figure 26.1 DUE cycle

IV. Feedback of results
V. Interventions
VI. Re-evaluation
VII. Feedback of results

Steps Involved in Conducting a DUE

Step 1: Identify drugs or therapeutic areas of practice for possible inclusion in the programme

It is not possible and also unnecessary to examine and evaluate every drug used in a hospital. Hence, the DUE Committee must identify priority drugs or areas of practice where improvement in use will result in the greatest clinical impact. These areas can be identified through various sources of information, such as medication error reports, adverse drug reaction reports, feedback from prescribers or clinical pharmacists, local microbiological data and the medical and pharmaceutical literature.

ABC/VEN analysis is another important tool used to identify high priority or target drugs. ABC analysis divides the drugs into three classes based on their annual usage:

- Class A drugs constitute 75–80% of the total value of drugs purchased or consumed and are the highest cost or highest volume items.
- Class B items constitute 15–20% of expenditure.
- Class C includes low cost or low volume items, which form 5–10% of expenditure.

ABC analysis helps to prioritise drugs for inclusion in drug evaluation studies. VEN analysis is generally done to assist the selection of drugs to be included in the hospital formulary. In VEN analysis, the drugs are generally classified as vital (V), essential (E) and non-essential (N). Based on the VEN analysis, one can identify the drugs that are of priority and require possible inclusion in the programme. DUEs have largely focused on drugs with a high volume of use (such as antibiotics), high cost (such as proton pump inhibitors) or high frequency of adverse drug events (for example, anti-coagulants). DUEs may also focus on areas where drugs are underused, such as with aspirin in patients with diabetes.

Common targets for DUE include:

- Commonly prescribed drugs, such as antibiotics and proton pump inhibitors
- Drugs associated with potentially significant drug interactions, such as warfarin, theophylline, digoxin and phenytoin
- Expensive drugs, for example, low molecular weight heparins, broad-spectrum cephalosporins, anti-HIV medications
- New drugs
- Drugs with a narrow therapeutic index, such as digoxin, phenytoin, cyclosporine, theophylline and zidovudine
- Drugs which upon withdrawal may cause problems, such as anti-depressants, benzodiazepines and anti-convulsants
- Drugs that frequently cause serious/significant adverse drug reactions, such as antibiotics, anti-convulsants, anti-coagulants, anaesthetic drugs, non-steroidal anti-inflammatory agents, ACE inhibitors and anti-malarials
- Drugs used in high-risk patients, such as the elderly, transplant patients, cancer chemotherapy and intensive care patients, neonates or children

- Drugs used in the management of common conditions, such as chronic pain, respiratory tract infections or urinary tract infections
- Drugs used in areas of practice which are not well performed, such as the prescribing of antibiotics for surgical prophylaxis
- Drugs which have been recently added or which are under consideration for addition to the hospital formulary
- Complex areas of prescribing, such as anti-thrombotic and post-transplantation therapy

More drugs or practice areas will usually be identified in Step 1 than can be included in a typical one-year DUE cycle. The final choice will ultimately be determined by evidence of a medication use problem within the institution, the severity of harmful effects resulting from inappropriate drug use, the resources available for criteria development, data collection and evaluation, and the likelihood of interventions being successful in improving drug use.

Step 2: Design of study

A variety of research methods have been used in DUE studies. Observational research methods are more commonly used than experimental methods such as randomised controlled trials. Cross-sectional studies, where drug use is examined at a single point in time, are useful for problem identification. The pre–post design where drug use is examined before and after interventions to improve prescribing is another commonly used observational method. Based on the design of the study, DUE studies may also be categorised as prospective, concurrent or retrospective, depending on the timing of data collection.

Prospective review involves evaluating a patient's planned drug therapy before a medication is administered. Depending on the study design, interventions may be provided if necessary before the patients receive the prescribed drug. Identification of drug–drug interactions is one issue commonly addressed by a prospective DUE. For example, a patient who is on warfarin for atrial fibrillation may be prescribed an NSAID by another physician. This increases the risk of gastrointestinal bleeding in the patient. Thus, a DUE of concurrent use of warfarin and NSAIDs should be designed in a way that allows the pharmacist to advise the treating doctor of the risks with this drug combination.

Concurrent review is performed during the course of treatment and involves the ongoing monitoring of drug therapy. This may involve consideration of laboratory test results and other monitoring data when appropriate, and usually does not offer immediate benefit to the patient. It differs from prospective review in that data collection does not have to occur prior to the administration of a first dose.

This method of data collection is convenient when pharmacists perform a daily review of medication charts as part of routine clinical care. For example, in the setting of a DUE evaluating aminoglycoside dosing, a patient with reduced renal function may be prescribed a high dose of gentamicin, which may be inappropriate for the patient based on the patient's estimated creatinine clearance. The clinical pharmacist identifies the dose as inappropriate during their regular treatment chart review and alerts the prescriber about the problem.

During a *retrospective DUE,* drug therapy is reviewed after the patient has completed a course of therapy. The patient's medication sheets (including discharge prescriptions), daily progress notes, nursing observations, pathology/biochemistry results and therapeutic monitoring results are screened to determine whether drug therapy met pre-determined criteria. The main advantage of this method is that prescribers and others are unaware of data collection and results may therefore be less biased. Another advantage is ease of data collection, as records are accessed at the data collector's convenience. A disadvantage is that some information may be unclear or missing and that reviewed patients do not gain immediate benefit, as interventions are delayed until the intervention phase.

Step 3: Define criteria and standards

After the DUE target has been selected, it is important to conduct a comprehensive literature review. The extent of work involved in this step depends on what has been done previously, or what is already available; for example, local, reliable and authoritative guidelines, or previous DUE criteria. The steps involved in literature review are:

- Perform an exhaustive literature search for the chosen drug or therapeutic area, using multiple search mechanisms such as medical (Medline, Micromedex, Drugdex, Cochrane Library, Embase) and pharmacy-based systems (IOWA Drug Information Service, International Pharmaceutical Abstracts).
- Assemble full copies (not just the abstracts) of all the relevant original research papers.
- Critically evaluate the studies directly relevant to the chosen drug or therapeutic area. This includes identifying strengths and weaknesses in the study design and deciding whether appropriate conclusions have been made from the data presented.
- Briefly summarise the literature review, identifying the 'key' papers in the chosen area and the drug use criteria that can be derived from evidence-based literature.

Criteria are predetermined statements describing optimal drug use, against which the quality of actual drug use is compared. Standards are professionally developed expressions of the range of acceptable variation from a criterion. The concept of standards was introduced to take into account the subjective nature of some aspects of medical practice and unusual clinical circumstances. Standards should also be based on published literature and should describe exceptions when deviation from criteria is acceptable.

Criteria should be scientifically based and be supported by clinical or research literature. They must be valid, unambiguous, realistic, easily measured and outcome oriented. The Committee itself may develop criteria with input from hospital specialists and clinical staff, or use established criteria from unbiased drug reference literature. The involvement of medical staff is recommended to ensure local agreement and acceptance of DUE results and interventions.

It is often needless and impossible to evaluate all the aspects of drug use in a hospital. Hence, it is the primary responsibility of the DUE Committee to select, decide or review criteria for DUE. For example, the DUE Committee of a tertiary care hospital may identify that inappropriate use of intravenous proton pump inhibitors (such as pantoprazole) takes place in the hospital. The DUE Committee may then adopt the following prescribing criteria for a DUE study based on extensive literature review using medical- or pharmacy-based systems and with the consensus of the hospital's gastroenterologists:

- Patients who are unable to take any oral proton pump inhibitors and must be nil per oral (NPO)
- Patients with a history of active upper GI tract bleeding
- Patients with pathological hypersecretion associated with Zollinger–Ellison syndrome or other neoplastic conditions
- Patients with bleeding or erosive gastritis
- Stress-ulcer prophylaxis of critical care patients
- Contraindication to using histamine-2 receptor antagonists

After identifying these criteria, the DUE Committee identifies the process indicators and evaluates the percentage of adherence or non-adherence to these criteria by performing a retrospective, prospective or concurrent review. Later, the percentage of adherence or non-adherence to these criteria is determined.

Step 4: Design the data collection form

Just as it is impossible to monitor and evaluate all the drugs used in a hospital, it is also impossible to address all aspects of use for each drug. Time and staffing constraints mean that it is important to limit data collection to only the most important and relevant aspects of drug use and to factors which may influence these. These will vary greatly depending on the type and objectives of the DUE. Some aspects of drug use, which are commonly surveyed during DUEs, are presented in Table 26.3 and data sources commonly available within hospitals are summarised in Table 26.4.

For example, third-generation cephalosporins are expensive, broad-spectrum antibiotics and have been the subject of many DUEs. In some hospitals, they are known to be frequently prescribed for minor infections or infections where a narrower spectrum antibiotic is more appropriate. Culture and sensitivity tests may not be ordered and they may be frequently prescribed concurrently with other antibiotics, providing unnecessary dual cover. Widespread usage has significant cost implications and may also lead to bacterial resistance.

In the treatment of community-acquired pneumonia, many guidelines now recommend restricting the use of third-generation cephalosporins to patients with severe pneumonia who are allergic to penicillin, or who have renal impairment where aminoglycosides should be avoided. For these reasons, a DUE of third-generation cephalosporins commonly involves the collection of data relating to patient demographics, prescriber identification, indications for use, disease severity, dosing data, concurrent use of other antibiotics, allergy history and laboratory results such as microbiology data and serum creatinine.

The success of any audit is only as good as the data collected. Hence, the more specific the information, the more useful it will be. To ensure that data reflects the end points to be evaluated and is consistent between audits, careful attention must be given to the design of the data collection form. This form should have a user-friendly format to encourage completion by data collectors. The appropriateness of the collection form can

Table 26.3 Common aspects of drug use studied in DUEs

- Patient demographics
- Prescriber details
- Disease severity
- Co-morbidities
- Indications for drug use
- Drug-disease contraindications
- Side/adverse effects
- Dosing information
- Duration of drug treatment
- Drug or drug class duplication
- Therapeutic duplication
- Preparation and administration
- Drug–drug and drug-food interactions
- Monitoring of drug therapy
- Patient education/instructions
- Cost of therapy
- Over/under utilisation of drugs

Table 26.4 Sources of data for DUEs in hospitals

I. Clinical data

- Patient treatment charts
- Patient admission (re-admission) records
- Departmental audits (surgical or discharge audits)
- Pathology records
- Microbiological data
- Medication charts
- Medical notes
- Observation charts
- Patient interview
- Nursing progress notes

II. Demographic data

- Breakdown of patient population by age, disease, average length of stay, etc.

III. Administrative data

- Drug purchasing and trends data
- Drug utilisation and trends data
- Cost per adjusted hospital bed stay (if available)

Figure 26.2 Data collection form for a DUE assessing the appropriateness of ciprofloxacin use

Hospital Name

Drug Use Evaluation assessing the appropriateness of ciprofloxacin use

Patient Data Collection Form

Patient Name : Age : Gender : ☐Male ☐Female

In Patient No : Weight (Kg): BMI:

Department : Name of the consultant :

Date of admission : ..../..../2011 Date of discharge : ..../..../2011

Renal function details :

Previous history of impaired renal function : ☐Yes ☐No

Serum creatinine and date : Estimated CrCl (mg/dl):

Details of ciprofloxacin therapy :

Indication : ☐UTI ☐Hospital Acquired Pneumonia ☐Community Acquired Pneumonia
☐Abdominal infection ☐Sepsis ☐Meningitis ☐skin and soft tissue Infection ☐Diarrhoea ☐Typhoid
☐fever ☐Surgical site infection ☐Acute Exacerbation of Bronchitis ☐Other (Specify)..........
Indeterminate: (Inadequate information in patient case note)........................

Dose (mg) : ☐Route : ☐oral IV

Frequency: ☐OD ☐BD ☐TDS ☐QID ☐Other (specify)..................

Date started : ..../..../2011 Date ceased : ..../..../2011

Reason for Ceasing: ☐Infection resolved ☐Side effects ☐Other (specify) ....

Renal function monitoring	Date	Remarks
Serum Creatinine	..../..../2011	
	..../..../2011	
	..../..../2011	

Other antibiotics given concurrently with ciprofloxacin :

Details on culture and sensitivity : Specimen collected Specimen not collected

Type of Specimen Collected	Date	Remarks
	..../..../2011	
	..../..../2011	

Data collectors name and Signature :

be easily tested by performing a pilot audit on a small number of patients, similar to a sample of the patients who will be studied in the DUE. A DUE patient data collection form for the DUE described in Example 1 is shown in Fig. 26.2.

Step 5: Data collection

Data collectors should be chosen carefully, and should be familiar with how information is arranged in the patient's case notes. Knowledge of drug names, strengths and the way orders are written is also important. Depending on their availability, physicians, pharmacists and nurses make ideal data collectors.

Another concern is the timing of data collection. This should be done in a period that is likely to be representative of the usual patterns of drug use. For example, a DUE examining the use of prophylactic antibiotics prior to surgery should be done when the usual surgeons are in attendance, taking care to avoid a period when key surgeons are on leave.

Step 6: Evaluate results

Data evaluation is one of the most critical steps in a DUE. The data obtained should be collated using available resources such as spreadsheeting, databasing and word processing. The next step is to summarise the main categories of results and to identify where exactly the data shows deviation from the guidelines and usage criteria that are previously identified. Then the reasons for this deviation should be evaluated. If there is a true reason for deviation, it may be necessary to redefine the criteria. The reasons may not be evident from the DUE data and may require further investigations, surveys or interviews. Reasons for deviation may include:

- Drug being used for new indication
- Outdated procedures
- Inadequate resources
- Gaps in knowledge or misinformation/misunderstanding

Step 7: Provide feedback of results

The success of any DUE strategy depends on feedback of the results to prescribers, other hospital staff involved in the study and to administrative heads. The presentation of any report is also very important. The report should be a well-presented and well-reasoned document, with no grammatical or typographical errors. It is important to prepare a scientific interpretation of the results rather than a value judgment. The results can also be circulated to hospital staff through newsletters, DUE meetings or the hospital's academic meetings.

Step 8: Develop and implement interventions

If a drug use problem was identified, the next step is to consider how the problem can be addressed. Interventions to improve drug use can be educational or operational, and can target groups or only those prescribers who did not meet drug use criteria.

Educational interventions consist of educational meetings, academic detailing circulation of protocols, feedback of study results, letters to individual physicians, newsletters and other informational materials such as posters and guidelines. Operational interventions include the development/ modification of drug order forms, manual or computerised reminders, prescribing restrictions, formulary additions/deletions, automatic stop orders or re-allocation of staff. Some interventions may be both educational and operational in nature, such as improving the availability of information and resources to support clinical decision-making. An example of the latter would be the addition in case notes of a protocol outlining how to reverse over-anticoagulation as an intervention to improve performance in this area.

The choice and development of interventions requires careful planning. The primary causes of the drug use problem need to be identified, together with key influencing factors. No one type of intervention is inherently effective, and more than one intervention is often needed. Interventions should be chosen based on their likely success, ease of application, cost, resources required and sustainability. Interventions, which have been found to be effective in improving drug use, include academic detailing, routine reminders, prescribing restrictions, structured prescription forms/ treatment charts and interactive educational meetings.

In academic detailing and interactive educational meetings, it is important to use skilled staff to deliver the intervention, select and repeat a limited number of key messages, provide positive prescribing alternatives and encourage interaction. Distribution of educational materials alone has been shown to have little or no impact on prescribing practices.

Step 9: Re-evaluate to determine if drug use has improved

Drug use and prescribing patterns need to be monitored to determine the success of interventions. Typically, the re-evaluation is done 3–12 months after the introduction of the intervention, and should involve collecting the same data as in the original DUE evaluation. If a complete evaluation with several criteria uncovered only a few problems, the focus may be narrowed to problematic criteria.

Step 10: Re-assess and revise the DUE programme

At the conclusion of a DUE evaluation cycle, an evaluation of the DUE programme is necessary. The questions addressed should include the following:

- Did the programme address important aspects of care?
- Were the criteria developed appropriate?
- Were drug use problems identified?
- Were the interventions made appropriate?
- Did the interventions have any unexpected or adverse effects?
- Were drug use problems solved?
- Did the DUE have an impact on the incidence of adverse drug reactions, drug–drug interactions, or medication errors?
- Did the DUE programme have a financial impact on the hospital?

The DUE process involves cooperation and coordination between various hospital staff. It is understandable that sometimes things may not happen as planned. Hence, lessons learnt from the first DUE cycle should be used to improve the quality, efficiency and effectiveness of future DUEs.

Step 11: Feedback results

It is important to circulate the results of the DUE to clinicians and other involved hospital staff. This is also a suitable time to obtain their opinions about the success or otherwise of the interventions, and how these can be improved.

Resources and Tools Required for DUE

The success of any drug evaluation study also depends on the type and quality of the resources and tools used to design and evaluate the study. The most important DUE resources are the 'human resources', as discussed earlier in this chapter. Some of the other essential resources and tools required for designing and managing DUEs include:

a) Key resources for the development of DUE criteria:

- Professional literature and up-to-date reference texts
- Guidelines: Locally developed or national and international treatment guidelines
- Published consensus statements, protocols and criteria

b) Tools for the measurement of quality use of medicines:

- Indicators, such as those published by the Joint Commission on the Accreditation of Healthcare Organizations (JCAHO)

c) Resources for documentation, management, evaluation and reporting of data:

- Computer databases
- Specially designed DUE software programs

The Pharmacist's Role in DUE

Pharmacists play a key role in the overall process of a DUE programme because of their experience in the area of pharmaceutical care. DUE affords pharmacists the opportunity to identify trends in prescribing within groups of patients such as those with asthma, diabetes or high blood pressure. Pharmacists can then, in collaboration with physicians and other members of the healthcare team, initiate action to improve drug therapy for both individual patients and patient populations. In addition to assisting in the performance of individual reviews, the suggested roles and responsibilities of pharmacists in a DUE programme are shown in Table 26.5.

Table 26.5 Possible roles for pharmacists in DUE

- Planning, organising and implementing a DUE programme
- Programme development, supervision and coordination
- Education of hospital staff about DUE in conceptual and practical terms
- Promotion of the goals and objectives of DUE
- Development/review of audit criteria, guidelines, study protocols and educational material
- Development of data collection instruments
- Pilot testing, data collection, analysis and report writing
- Documentation of programme outcome, effectiveness and cost benefits
- Participation on hospital committees concerned with quality assurance in general and drug usage
- Presentation of DUE results at meetings and conferences
- Publication of results in peer-reviewed journals

PRACTICE SCENARIO 1: SUMMARY OF A DUE TO ASSESS THE APPROPRIATENESS OF CIPROFLOXACIN USE

Step 1: Identify target drug or therapeutic area of practice

The Drug Utilisation Evaluation (DUE) Committee of a 1200-bed tertiary care teaching hospital decided to evaluate the appropriateness of ciprofloxacin use. The DUE Committee has noticed that there is widespread and inappropriate use of ciprofloxacin. In addition, the hospital Microbiology department has reported a significant increase in the number of Gram-negative organisms showing resistance to ciprofloxacin.

Step 2: Design of study

A concurrent observational prospective study design was selected. Clinical pharmacists were assigned to collect data during their routine clinical practice over a 12-week period. It was decided to carry out the study in the Internal Medicine, Paediatrics, Surgery and Respiratory departments where the use of ciprofloxacin is highest.

Step 3: Defining criteria and standards

The criteria and standards for appropriate use of ciprofloxacin were developed after extensive literature review and referring to local and international antibiotic guidelines. After consensus with senior medical consultants, the criteria adopted for appropriate use of ciprofloxacin were:

- *Appropriate Indication:* Suspected or proven infection caused by aerobic Gram-negative bacilli.
- *Appropriate Dose:* 500–750 mg PO twice daily or 400 mg IV (intravenous) twice daily in patients with normal or mild renal impairment. In patients with creatinine clearance, 30–50 ml/minute: oral: 250–500 mg every 12 hours. In patients with creatinine clearance 5–29 ml/minute: oral: 250–500 mg every 18 hours or 200–400 mg every 18–24 hours intravenously.
- *Appropriate Duration:* Duration of therapy is 1–2 weeks, except for infections such as prostatitis, osteomyelitis and endocarditis.
- *Appropriate Regimen:* Additional antibiotics are given only in mixed infections and to cover other microorganisms apart from Gram-negative bacilli.
- Monitoring of renal function during treatment with ciprofloxacin for two weeks if the baseline serum creatinine levels are normal.
- Appropriate cultures and sensitivities are obtained within 48 hours before the initial ciprofloxacin dose.

Step 4: Design data collection form

A study data collection form was designed to be user-friendly and to assist data analysis (see Fig. 26.2). The data collection form was piloted in 10 patients prior to finalisation.

Step 5: Data collection

Data collection was scheduled to run over a 12-week period when all clinical pharmacists in the hospital were available.

Step 6: Evaluation

A total of 200 patients received ciprofloxacin therapy during the audit period. Concordance with individual DUE criteria was as follows:

Criteria	Concordance n (%)	Non-concordance n (%)
Appropriate Indication	140 (70%)	60 (30%)
Appropriate Dose	160 (80%)	40 (20%)
Appropriate Duration	148 (74%)	52 (26%)
Appropriate Regimen	135 (67.5%)	65 (22.5%)
Renal Function Monitoring	67 (33.5%)	174 (65.5%)
Appropriate Cultures and Sensitivity Test	86 (43%)	11 (57%)

Most of the criteria showed moderate–high rates of appropriateness (67.5% to 80%) with the exception of monitoring of renal function and culture sensitivity tests prior to the initial ciprofloxacin dose.

Step 7: Feedback results

The results of the initial DUE were analysed and summarised in a form or report (Fig. 26.3) and circulated to relevant medical staff, the Drug and Therapeutics Committee and the Medical Director of the hospital.

Step 8: Develop and implement interventions

The DUE Committee met to review the results and to consider remedial action. Clinical pharmacists were asked to identify possible factors contributing to the non-checking of renal function during ciprofloxacin therapy. Reasons identified were the patient's inability to pay for additional tests, lack of awareness amongst prescribers about the necessity of monitoring renal function tests and dosage adjustment, or planned short duration of treatment. The reasons for inappropriate culture and sensitivity testing could be not ordering the test due to the patient's inability to pay or anticipated short-term therapy.

Hence, it was decided that these two factors should be targetted for intervention. As patients were admitted under different medical units, it was decided to use an academic detailing approach with doctors in these units. During detailing, a copy of fluroquinolone guidelines were given to all the treating physicians of the medicine ward. In addition, it was decided to

Figure 26.3 Hospital summary data for a DUE assessing the appropriateness of ciprofloxacin use

Hospital Name
Drug Use Evaluation assessing the appropriateness of ciprofloxacin use
Summary Data Documentation Form

Number of patient case notes reviewed:

Period of review: From .../.../2011 To .../.../2011

Patient characteristics:

Mean age of the patients: No. of females (%) ☐ No. of males (%) ☐

No. (%) on specified department: Medicine : Surgery ☐ Paediatrics ☐ Respiratory ☐

Details of Ciprofloxacin Treatment: Criteria 1:

No.(%) of patients with suspected or proven infection with aerobic Gram-negative bacilli:

Indication for ciprofloxacin (specify the number of patients (%) with each diagnosis):

UTI ☐ Hospital Acquired Pneumonia ☐ Community Acquired Pneumonia ☐
Abdominal infection ☐ Sepsis ☐ Meningitis ☐ Skin and soft tissue infection ☐
Surgical site infection ☐ Diarrhoea ☐ Acute exacerbation of bronchitis ☐ Typhoid fever ☐
Other (Specify)..........

Criteria 2:

No.(%) of patients receiving an appropriate dose based on renal function:

Criteria 3:

Mean days of treatment:
Number of patients treated <1 week: Number of patients treated <1 week:

Number of patients treated 1-2 weeks: Number of patients treated > 2weeks:

No. (%) of patients receiving appropriate duration of therapy:

Criteria 4:

No. of patients(%) receiving different concomitant antibiotics:
No. of patients receiving other antibiotics in concordance with criteria:

Criteria 5: Assessment of Renal Function during Treatment

No (%) in whom renal function (Scr) was measured:
Week 1............ (%)
Week 2............ (%)
Week 3............ (%)

Criteria 6: Details on Culture and Sensitivity

No. (%) of patients in whom culture and sensitivity testing was ordered prior to the initiation of ciprofloxacin dose:
Other details:

Name and Signature of Data Evaluator:

develop a reminder sticker about testing for culture and sensitivity and renal function to be placed on treatment charts by clinical pharmacists whenever ciprofloxacin was ordered.

Step 9: Re-evaluate after intervention

Three months after the introduction of reminder stickers and delivery of the academic detailing programme, a repeat DUE audit was performed using the same data collection form as in the pre-intervention audit. During the second audit period, a total of 212 patients received ciprofloxacin therapy. Analysis of the data indicated improved monitoring of renal function (33.5–56.5%) and appropriateness of culture and sensitivity testing (43–55%).

Step 10: Re-assess and revise the DUE programme

Improvement was most marked for renal function monitoring. Separate meetings and academic detailing was given to all the doctors in departments with the highest rate of inappropriate ciprofloxacin use.

Step 11: Feedback results

The results of the DUE were summarised in a report and distributed to clinicians, the Medical Director and the Drug and Therapeutics Committee.

KEY MESSAGES

- Drug use problems are common and have significant clinical and economic implications.
- A variety of research methods can be used in DUE studies.
- The support and involvement of medical staff is essential for the success of a DUE programme.
- Criteria are predetermined statements describing optimal drug use against which the quality of drug use is compared.
- A range of effective strategies can be used to improve drug use.
- Pharmacists play a key role in the overall operation of a DUE programme.

Further Reading

Chan A, Lim LLC and Tao M. 2009. Utilisation review of epoetin alfa in cancer patients at a cancer centre in Singapore. *Singapore Med J* 50(4):365.

Chatterjee S, Mandal A, Lyle N, Mukherjee S and Singh AK. 2007. Drug utilization study in a neonatology unit of a tertiary care hospital in eastern India. *Pharmacoepidemiol Drug Saf* 16(10):1141–5.

Fulda TR, Lyles A, Pugh MC and Christensen DB. 2004. Current status of prospective drug utilization review. *J Manag Care Pharm* 10(5):433–41.

Ghiculescu RA, Kubler PA and Gleeson P. 2007. Drug utilization evaluation of i.v. paracetamol at a large teaching hospital. *Intern Med J* 37(9) 620–23.

Gregoire JP, Moisan J, Potvin L, Chabot I, Verreault R and Milot A. 2006. Effect of drug utilization reviews on the quality of in-hospital prescribing: a quasi-experimental study. *BMC Health Services Research* 6:33.

Hing WC, Bek SJ, Lin RT and Li SC. 2004. A retrospective drug utilization evaluation of vancomycin usage in paediatric patients. *J Clin Pharm Ther* 29(4):359–65.

Hoover JG, Schumaker AL and Franklin KJ. 2009. Use of intravenous proton-pump inhibitors in a teaching hospital practice. *Dig Dis Sci* 54(9):1947–52.

McFarland MS, Cross LB, Gross B, Gentry C, Tunney J and Patel UP. 2009. Drug use evaluation of sitagliptin dosing by pharmacist versus nonpharmacist clinicians in an internal medicine department of a private physician-owned multispecialty clinic. *J Manag Care Pharm* 15(7):563–7.

Peng CC, Glassman PA, Marks IR, Fowler C and Castiglione B. 2003. Retrospective Drug Utilization Review: Incidence of Clinically Relevant Potential Drug-Drug Interactions in a Large Ambulatory Population. *J Managed Care Pharm* 9(6):513–22.

Raveh D, Muallem-Zilcha E, Greenberg A, Wiener-Well Y, Schlesinger Y and Yinnon AM. 2006. Prospective drug utilization evaluation of three broad-spectrum antimicrobials: cefepime, piperacillin-tazobactam and meropenem. *QJM* 99(6):397–406.

Sakhaiyan E, Hadjibabaie M, Gholami Kh, Fahimi F, Shamshiri AR, Alimoghaddam K et al. 2009. Drug Utilization Evaluation of Imipenem in Patients Undergoing Bone Marrow Transplantation. *International Journal of Hematology-Oncology and Stem cell Research* 3(2):10–13.

Starner CI, Norman SA, Reynolds RG and Gleason PP. 2009. Effect of a retrospective drug utilization review on potentially inappropriate prescribing in the elderly. *Am J Geriatr Pharmacother* 7(1): 11–9.

Zulkarnain BS. 2004. The adherence to prescribing guidelines: A drug utilization evaluation of tramadol (A study at the Royal Brisbane Hospital-Australia). *Folia Medica Indonesiana* 40(1):28–34.

Websites of Interest

World Health Organization (which provides information on drug utilisation evaluation)
http://apps.who.int/medicinedocs/en/d/Js4876e/4.6.html

The Society of Hospital Pharmacists of Australia (describes standards of practice for drug utilisation evaluation in Australian hospitals
http://www.shpa.org.au/lib/pdf/practice_standards/drug_use_ro.pdf

University of Wyoming (a useful site that consists of newsletters on drug utilisation review)
http://uwacadweb.uwyo.edu/DUR/Newsletters.asp

The European Drug Utilisation Research Group (information about Eurodrug, national groups, a bulletin and links to useful addresses and websites)
http://www.eurodurg.com

Division of Medical Assistance and Health Services Home, State of New Jersey
http://www.state.nj.us/humanservices/dmahs/boards/durb/newsletters/

27

PHARMACOEPIDEMIOLOGY

Jayashri Sankaranarayanan and Thomas R Einarson

Learning Objectives

Upon completion of this chapter, the reader should be able to:

- Define pharmacoepidemiology and describe its place in drug development and healthcare
- List the advantages and disadvantages of pharmacoepidemiological study designs over randomised controlled trials
- Identify the two major pharmacoepidemiological study designs used to test the relationship between drug exposure and patient outcomes
- Identify two common statistical measures used to describe the relationship between drug exposure and outcome
- Interpret a confidence interval for an odds ratio

Introduction to Pharmacoepidemiology

With about 1.21 billion inhabitants in 2011, India has the world's second largest population. The most recent reported annual spending by India on healthcare is said to be about 1% of its gross national product (GNP), or 6% of its gross domestic product (GDP). For the population below the poverty line, the cost of government insurance was about Rs 400 per person per year. For all persons other than those below the poverty line in India, the cost of private insurance was about Rs 1,200 per person per year. Out of India's spending of 6% of its GDP, 1.3% comes from the public (government) sector and 4.7% from the private sector. Further, the out-of-pocket spending for healthcare is about 80% in India. In contrast to a life expectancy of about 80 years in Western countries, India has a life expectancy of 63.2 years for men and 66.4 years for women, according to the United Nations.

In 2011, the value of the global pharmaceutical market was expected to grow by 5–7%, exceeding \$80 billion (Source: IMS Health). The Indian pharmaceutical market was estimated to reach \$ 9.77 billion in 2007–08. The Indian pharmaceutical industry grew at 13% during 2003–2007, driven by rising consumption levels in the country and strong demands from export markets. In 2007, 71% of oncology product sales came from the US and Europe's top five markets – France, Germany, Italy, the UK and Spain.

In 2008, the seven 'pharmerging' markets of China, Brazil, Mexico, South Korea, India, Turkey and Russia were expected to grow by 12–13% to $85–90 billion. Generics producing companies Barr, Ranbaxy, Mylan, Teva, Actavis and Dr Reddy's Labs have become dominant as they continue launching an increasing number of generics. According to a joint report published by the Federation of Indian Chambers of Commerce and Industry (FICCI) and Ernst & Young, India's growing pharmaceutical industry is expected to touch $20 billion by 2015 and feature among the global top 10.

India has the fourth largest pharmaceutical market by volume (8% of the global total) and the thirteenth largest by value (less than 1% of the global total). Between 1996 and 2006, sales of pharmaceuticals rose 9% annually. Of the $13 billion Indian pharmaceutical industry (valued in 2006–07), the domestic formulation segment accounted for almost 48%, the formulation export market for about 25%, and bulk drug exports represented 27% (Source: Crisil Research).

For pharmaceuticals, demand in India is growing faster than the global market because of the country's rising population, increasing number of senior citizens and growing personal income. India has emerged as a key destination for global pharmaceutical companies because of its high growth prospects led by an ageing population, changing disease profile, improved patent regulations and socioeconomic conditions as well as the availability of highly skilled personnel. With the amendment of the Indian Patent Act in January 2005, India started to comply with the World Trade Organization's Trade Related Aspects of Intellectual Property Rights (WTO-TRIPS) agreement and recognised product patents. Indian companies are capitalising on other initiatives across the world to promote generic drugs to reduce healthcare costs.

In 2008, India supplied 2% of all global pharmaceuticals from more than 20,000 companies. The domestic Indian companies supply about 70% of the pharmaceutical market in India. Table 27.1 lists the top 10 companies in India based on recent estimates. The leading players in the Indian pharmaceutical market comprise both India-based and multinational companies (MNCs). The top 10 companies in the highly competitive and fragmented Indian pharmaceutical market accounted for 41.2% of the total retail, institutional and doctors' sales audit in 2011. Among these 10 companies, seven are Indian-based, and account for 26.5% of the domestic market.

Table 27.2 shows the top 10 classes of drugs in India by sales volume from combined retail (distributors/stockists), institutional (hospitals and pharmacies in their vicinity) and doctors' sales audit. It shows that the anti-diabetic drug class is growing at a rate greater than 20%.

Rationale for Pharmacoepidemiolgy

There are concerns about the hazardous and irrational use of drugs and drug combinations. In addition, there is evidence of misuse of prescription drugs, often sold

Table 27.1 Top 10 pharmaceutical companies in India according to sales volume in 2011

Rank	***Total market***	***Company Type***	***% Share for 12-month period (May 2010–April 2011)***
			100.00
1	Abbott	Multinational	6.8
2	Cipla	India-based	5.2
3	Ranbaxy	India-based	4.6
4	Glaxo SmithKline	Multinational	4.4
5	Sun	India-based	3.8
6	Zydus Cadila	India-based	3.8
7	Alkem	India-based	3.3
8	Pfizer	Multinational	3.3
9	Mankind	India-based	3.2
10	Lupin Limited	India-based	2.8
	Total (Top 10)		41.2%
	Others		58.8%

**Source:* IMS Health Total Sales Audit (TSA) April 2011 based on Moving Annual Total (MAT) size of Rs 57,466 crore (Rs 574.66 billion ~ US $12.8 billion at average 2011 dollar to rupee conversion of 45) for a 12-month period from May 2010 to April 2011 from combined retail (distributors/stockists), institutional (hospitals and pharmacies in their vicinity) and doctors' sales audit

Table 27.2 Top 10 classes of drugs in India by sales volume in 2011

No.	***Drug class***	***% growth rate****	***% Share****
1	Systemic Anti-bacterials /Antibiotics	14.4	17.8
2	Anti-diabetic therapy	23.6	5.8
3	Antacids and Anti-flatulents	18.2	5.6
4	Hypotensives	17.6	4.3
5	Vitamins	14.2	4.3
6	Anti-inflammatory and Anti-rheumatics	8.6	4.1
7	Cough and Cold preparations	6.0	3.9
8	Cardiac therapy	12.8	3.1
9	Sex hormones and Stimulants	12.5	3.9
10	Anti-anaemic preparations	14.9	2.6

*Source: IMS Health Total Sales Audit (TSA) April 2011 based on Moving Annual Total (MAT) size of Rs 57,466 crore (Rs 574.66 billion ~ US $12.8 billion at average 2011 dollar to rupee conversion of 45) for a 12-month period from May 2010 and ending April 2011 from combined retail (distributors/stockists), institutional (hospitals and pharmacies in their vicinity), and doctors' sales audit

inappropriately without prescription and without enough information.

Thus, India is a major player on the world stage with many suppliers and great product diversification when it comes to pharmaceuticals. As healthcare professionals involved in assuring appropriate drug use, pharmacists must become involved in the study of drugs and their effects at the population level to ensure better therapy at the patient level. Pharmacoepidemiology, therefore, is an integral part of the pharmacists' role in society.

Definitions

Hartzema et al. have defined pharmacoepidemiology as 'the application of epidemiologic reasoning, methods, and knowledge to the study of the uses and effects (beneficial and adverse) of drugs in human populations'. Populations are large groups of people, which may include thousands or even millions of people.

The methods used in the study of drug use in populations are borrowed from the field of epidemiology, which is the research discipline concerned with the distribution and determinants of disease in populations. Thus, the field of pharmacoepidemiology is the application of the methods of epidemiology to the study of the uses and effects of drugs.

Waning and Montague state that the basics of pharmacoepidemiology are to measure the source, diffusion, use and effects of drugs in large populations and to determine the frequency and distribution of drug use outcomes in those populations. Pharmacoepidemiological research in practice includes:

- evaluation of specific drug use in certain conditions,
- patterns of drug use, that is, how it is being used – how much, where, when and by whom and
- drug-taking behaviours in society.

The World Health Organization (WHO) targets its pharmacoepidemiological efforts to ensure the quality, safety and efficacy of drugs and their use in specific patient populations about:

- describing patterns of drug use,
- changes in use over time,
- measuring effects of information, education, promotional activities and price on drug use,
- identifying inappropriate drug use and related problems,
- predicting drug needs in disease outbreaks and
- planning the selection, supply and distribution of drugs.

Place of Pharmacoepidemiolgy in Drug Development

The results of drug use may be either positive or negative. Positive outcomes refer to the efficacy or effectiveness of the drugs. Efficacy refers to the clinical effect of the drug when used under ideal conditions. These ideal conditions include complete compliance or adherence to advice from medical and pharmacy professionals, ideal patient monitoring and complete control of interfering factors. Those conditions occur only in randomised controlled trials (RCTs). On the other hand, effectiveness refers to the use of drugs under normal conditions of everyday life, where adherence to prescribed regimens (compliance) is often less than 100% and patients have co-morbid conditions and take several drugs at the same time. In addition, some patients may have compromised kidney, liver or lung function. The only way to study drug effectiveness is through pharmacoepidemiology studies.

Negative outcomes are referred to as adverse drug events (ADEs). They involve a relationship between drug ingestion and a subsequent negative outcome that has been observed, but for which causation cannot be established for certain. When there is a causal association with the drug, it is referred to as an adverse drug reaction (ADR). For further details, see *Chapter 9, Adverse Drug Reactions and Pharmacovigilance.*

Pharmacoepidemiology operates on three distinct levels, referred to as the macro, meso and micro levels. The standard level is the macro level, which refers to that of the population. The *macro level* deals with such phenomena as patterns of drug use in populations, the overall net benefit of drug use in society, expenditure on drugs at the national or international level and drug policy. The *meso level* is that of groups of people who are clustered together by a common factor such as age (for example, geriatric people >65), geography (such as the people in India), drug use (for example, patients who take penicillin within the country), disease (for example, diabetics), service (for example, hospitalised patients) or insurance coverage (for example, people belonging to a specific drug plan). The *micro level* reflects the measurement of drug use at the level of the individual patient, prescriber or pharmacist.

Thus, all studies of drugs and their effects may be classified as pharmacoepidemiological studies. The field is concerned with identifying patterns of drug use, the consequences of that use, and factors that may help explain these phenomena.

Origins and Evolution

One of the first pharmacoepidemiological studies occurred in 1902. It involved an investigation into two outbreaks of tetanus in 1901 in the USA because of contaminated vaccines. In St Louis, the outbreak was due to contaminated diphtheria antitoxin, and in New Jersey, because of contaminated smallpox vaccine. That investigation prompted the 1902 Biologics Control Act in the USA. A similar event in 1937 led to the requirement for manufacturers to test drugs for toxicity and provide clinical safety data before drugs could be marketed. Thus, pharmacoepidemiology prompted protective legislation.

Reports of serious adverse drug effects, such as aplastic anaemia and grey baby syndrome from chloramphenicol use, began to appear in the early 1950s. Soon after, the first textbook on ADRs was published. These events, among others, gave rise to pharmacovigilance, the study of the adverse effects of drugs. The 1960s were formative years for pharmacoepidemiology. In 1966, one of the largest and perhaps the most famous pharmacoepidemiological study, the Boston Collaborative Program, began. Perhaps the most dramatic adverse consequence of drug use was reported in 1961 by McBride who identified phocomelia in infants born to mothers who had taken thalidomide. That report is credited with giving rise to the field of teratology, which is the study of birth defects.

In the intervening time, great strides have been made. In 1986, a series of articles in the Annals of Pharmacotherapy precipitated the first textbook on pharmacoepidemiology. In the same year, the International Society of Pharmacoepidemiology (ISPE) was formed.

The field continues to develop with new research methods and new studies creating new knowledge.

Evidence-based Medicine (EBM) and the Need for Pharmacoepidemiology

The role of the pharmacist is to assure the optimal use, in terms of safety and effectiveness, of drugs in society. The pharmacist has the primary responsibility for the supply of medications, which involves procurement and storage of drugs, preparation and dispensing of prescriptions, and sometimes drug administration. The role also involves the provision of adequate information and instruction to the patient or agent (for example, the spouse, parent or family member) so that the patient or caregiver has the requisite knowledge, information, skills and attitudes to successfully participate in the drug use process. In addition, communication and feedback to physicians about prescribing problems encountered is essential. The outcome, if done properly, is appropriate drug utilisation.

Currently, educators in the health professions, including pharmacy, have been emphasising the importance of *evidence-based medicine* (EBM) as one of the cornerstones of appropriate drug use. Sackett and colleagues defined evidence-based medicine as 'the integration of best research evidence with clinical expertise and patient values'. Therefore, to determine the state of the art in pharmacotherapy, the pharmacist must be able to access and evaluate the primary literature on drugs.

It is essential that the best available evidence be used in patient care. Table 27.3 lists the types of study design in a hierarchy. Evidence includes information from randomised controlled trials (RCTs) and other studies, virtually all of which fall within the field of pharmacoepidemiology. Thus, the pharmacist must be familiar with various pharmacoepidemiological study designs and be able to critique their strengths and weaknesses.

RCTs, especially double-blind assessments, are considered to provide the highest level of evidence for use in patient care. It is the only design that can truly assess causation, since all factors and influences are controlled. Randomising patients to groups assures (at least in the long run) equivalence between those groups and, therefore, differences found between treatments (usually active drug and placebo) can be attributed to the drug and not to other factors.

However, there are many limitations to consider. RCTs are not performed for every drug in every indication in all populations; therefore, Level 1 data may not be available. Often, it is unethical (for example, in pregnant women) or impractical (for example, in life and death emergencies) to perform RCTs. Sometimes, it may be difficult or impossible to perform comparative trials because of the nature of the product (for example, homeopathy).

Market factors often play a major role in the decision-making process. One reason why RCTs are not conducted is that the market may be too small to generate adequate return (for example, in rare diseases). Another very important consideration is patent protection and the amount of time before its expiry. If a new indication is discovered late in the product cycle, there may not be adequate time for the manufacturer to perform the requisite testing and prepare for marketing before the drug patent expires. If adequate opportunity is not available to recover those

Table 27.3 Levels of evidence for clinical decision-making

Level	*Study Design Properties*	*Examples*
I*	Randomised + Comparative trial	Randomised controlled trial (RCT)
	Ia: double-blind Ib: single-blind Ic: open-label	
II*	Comparative trial	Non-randomised comparative trial
		Cohort study
		Case control study
		Comparative database study/chart review
III	Non-comparative study	Non-comparative clinical trial
		Observational cohort
		Database analysis
		Chart review
		Case series
		Case report, N-of-1 trial
IV	Expert opinion	

*Within levels, meta-analysis of studies is considered to have the greatest credibility, confirmed trials are next, then single trials. Larger trials are given more weight than smaller ones.

costs, the sponsor may have no interest in doing the research. Therefore, data from RCTs may not be available. In such cases, other forms of evidence are required to inform a clinical decision.

Further, RCTs have their own problems. Researchers are highly selective when recruiting patients for RCTs, excluding those who have co-morbidities or are taking other drugs. Sometimes, they treat only people who are experiencing their first episode of illness; those with prior episodes or who have had prior treatment are not considered. Specific patient groups are usually not entered into primary research studies, including geriatric patients (especially the very old), children (especially the very young), premature infants, the malnourished and women (in general, but especially, of child-bearing age). Consequently, little is known about excluded groups.

RCTs which are usually conducted in the pre-marketing phase of drug development have many inadequacies. The total number of patients examined in these trials is approximately 6,000, which is too small to identify adverse reactions that occur less often than about 1/2000. The duration of these trials is often short; data from RCTs for one year or more are rare. Long-term effects require more time, often with many persons exposed over many years (often referred to as person-years of exposure) before they become apparent.

Within the clinical trials, conditions are quite different from those normally encountered in daily life. All patients are constantly monitored, with nurses checking that all medications have been taken and laboratory tests administered, at their proper time. Therefore, results are only valid for comparable patients under comparable conditions and are not generalisable to the real-world use of these medications. Many trials use only surrogate outcomes, such as blood cholesterol levels or blood pressure, rather than actual patient outcomes such as stroke, myocardial infarction or death. One is forced to look elsewhere for effectiveness data.

Finally, RCTs are not designed for the detection of new indications. Therefore, we must rely on data from observational studies to signal 'new indications' for drug use.

Aims and Applications of Pharmacoepidemiology

Generalising evidence from short-term RCTs that have been designed primarily to test efficacy outcomes, to routine practice settings is controversial. However, Bridge and Axelson have stated that 'Pharmacoepidemiological studies complement RCTs by using observational methods to examine safety and effectiveness of medications in the general population'. The aims of pharmacoepidemiology fall into three main domains:

- The first is to identify new ADRs and new indications for drugs. This is done through signal generation, often arising from case reports, which result from a single observation. Others may emerge during the course of a patient follow-up study specifically designed to detect signals.
- The second aim is to qualify the nature of ADRs or clinical effects, identifying and describing factors associated with the drug's risk/benefit.
- The final aim is to quantify outcomes. By using larges samples of patients, it is possible to achieve a high degree of precision in estimating rates of risk or the beneficial effects of drugs. Also, by testing hypotheses, we are able to quantify the degree of association between an exposure and an outcome.

Sources of Data on Drug Use

The many sources of drug data include:

- Institutionalised medical records and databases like hospital and pharmacy claims databases
- System-wide databases from health insurance claims or pharmaceutical organisations or commercial data mining vendors
- National databases like pharmacoepidemiological surveillance systems, government-sponsored studies like Medical Expenditure Panel Survey (www.meps.ahrq.gov/mepsweb/), National Ambulatory Medical Care Survey or National Hospital Ambulatory Medical Care Survey (www.cdc.gov/nchs/ahcd.htm) from the United States
- Field data like records from dispensers, sellers or distributors or from small groups
- Experimental clinical trial data

Measurement of Outcome

Classifying drugs: To study drugs, it is essential that we have a system for classifying them. One reason is that drugs with similar chemical structures usually have similar therapeutic and toxic effects, often referred to as *class effects*. For example, all benzodiazepines have tranquillising effects and all produce withdrawal syndromes. However, individual drugs within this group have different propensities for producing these effects, so they are not all identical or necessarily interchangeable for all patients.

Presently, the most useful drug classification scheme is that developed by the WHO. It is known as the ATC system, the letters standing for Anatomic, Therapeutic and Chemical, which represent the three axes along which drugs are classified.

The first axis, Anatomic, is categorised according to the body system that is affected, as presented in Table 27.4. Within this classification, drugs are next categorised by their main therapeutic use. The final sub-classification is by the chemical class of the drug. Each drug is assigned a unique identifying number, in order of appearance on the market. For example, omeprazole is classified as A02BC01, where A stands for Alimentary, 02 is the therapeutic class 'Drugs for treatment of peptic ulcer', and BC refers to the chemical class 'proton pump inhibitors'. Since omeprazole was the first in that class, it was assigned the number 01. Pantoprazole and lansoprazole, arriving later, were assigned the numbers 02 and 03, respectively.

Measuring drug use – units of use: Drug use is usually expressed as a proportion. The

Table 27.4 The Anatomic Therapeutic Chemical (ATC) classification system

Code	*Definition (System of Interest)*
A	Alimentary tract and metabolism
B	Blood and blood-forming organs
C	Cardiovascular system
D	Dermatologicals
G	Genito-urinary system and sex hormones
H	Systemic hormonal preparations, excluding sex hormones
J	General anti-infectives for systemic use
L	Anti-neoplastic and immunomodulating agents
M	Musculoskeletal system
N	Nervous system
P	Anti-parasitic products
R	Respiratory system
S	Sensory organs
V	Various

The first level of the code indicates the anatomical main group and consists of one letter. There are 14 main groups.

Source: Anonymous Anatomic Therapeutic Chemical (ATC) classification index with Defined Daily Doses (DDDs). WHO Collaborating Centre for Drug Statistics Methodology. Oslo, Norway January 2002. Available at: www.whocc.no/atcdddaccessed 15 October, 2009

numerator is expressed in utilisation units and a variety of units are employed as the denominator. Perhaps the simplest unit of measure is monetary, that is, dollars, pounds or rupees. Money has the advantage of being a universally acknowledged medium for comparison. Everything can be translated into monetary terms (for example, drugs, services, labour and benefits) and it, in turn, may be translated into other units (for example, euros). It is very flexible and can be discounted over time, and is commonly used throughout the world.

On the other hand, there are many problems with monetary measures of drug use. First, they do not measure actual drug use. One cannot determine how many people are taking how much of a drug. Drugs have different strengths, and sell at different prices with price fluctuations over time and geography. It is impossible to know exactly what the money value of drug sales means in terms of the quantity of drugs consumed. Nonetheless, it is widely accepted.

The prescription is another unit of measure that is widely used. It is straightforward and easily understood. The disadvantage is that the quantity of drugs dispensed varies, as does the strength of the drug, the intended duration of treatment and a host of other factors. The assumption is that, with chronic therapy, the amount of drug dispensed should average out over the long run, making comparisons valid.

Another measure is the number of units of drug (that is, tablets, capsules, etc.) dispensed. The problems with this are similar to those found with prescriptions, in that quantities may vary with patient characteristics such as weight, age and disease severity. Also, many different forms of the drug may exist.

To overcome the various problems with traditional units of measurement, the WHO developed the concept of defined daily doses (DDDs). This is a technical unit of measurement that is based on the average daily dose of the drug when used in adults for its major indication. Utilisation is most often reported in countries as DDD/1000 inhabitants, while in hospitals, it is DDD/100 bed-days. The DDD/1000 patients and DDD/100 bed-days approaches were used by Kotwani and colleagues to asscss antibiotic utilisation in patients at pharmacies and by Uppal and colleagues in a hospital in India, respectively.

The advantage of DDD is that it is a uniform concept that can be applied to a large number of drugs. It provides a unit of measurement that can be used to compare utilisation between regions or countries and over time. The disadvantages are that DDDs are not available for all drugs or for paediatric use. Also, there may be more than one indication for a drug.

Outcome measures of drug use: The three classic measures of drug use are prevalence, cumulative incidence and incidence rate.

Prevalence: Prevalence is the proportion of people affected by or exposed to a drug at a given time. It is a cross-sectional statistic that is usually determined by a survey. Prevalence can vary between 0 and 1 and is usually expressed as cases per 1000 exposures or per 1000 inhabitants. The prevalence at any given time is the point prevalence, and for a year is the annual prevalence. For example, if 2,000 persons in a city of 1 million inhabitants suffered from peptic ulcer disease (PUD), the prevalence would be 2,000/1,000,000 = 0.2%, or 2/1000 inhabitants.

Cumulative incidence: The cumulative incidence is often referred to simply as 'incidence'. It is the number of new cases of disease/outcome that occur in a population in a defined time period divided by the number of people in that population. It is a longitudinal measure that is time dependent and is normally measured with an inception cohort study. That is, a large group of people is observed over time, and the number of cases of disease/outcome is noted. The cumulative incidence is expressed either as a percentage or proportion per unit time (cases per 1000 population per year). In the example above, suppose 200 new people developed PUD. The incidence for that year would be 200/1,000,000 or 2 per 10,000.

There is a mathematical relationship between prevalence and incidence:

Prevalence ≈ Incidence × Average duration of disease

the prevalence ≈ 2/10,000 × 10 = 2/1000.

$\sum$ (Persons * Time exposed)$_i$.

Incidence rate: A variant of the cumulative incidence is the incidence rate (IR), also known as the incidence density. It is the number of new cases that appear over the amount of person-time at risk, and is most commonly expressed as cases/person-year exposure. For the denominator, the time each person was at risk (that is, taking the drug) is summed: $\sum$ (Persons*Time exposed)$_i$.

For example, suppose 5,000 people had taken NSAIDs for 7 years, 10,000 for 4 years, and 5,000 for 1 year and that 1,000 of them developed bleeding. The total exposure would be: 5,000*7 + 10,000*4 + 5,000*1 = 80,000 person-years. Since 1000 developed bleeding, the IR would be 1000/80,000 = 0.0125, or 12.5 bleeds per 1000 person-years of exposure to NSAIDs.

Risk: When studying drugs, it is important to understand the idea of risk. It is the probability of developing an outcome when exposed to a drug. It is independent of seriousness, severity or harm. Each outcome has its own risk, which is a probability that is dependent on a number of factors, such as patient age, physical condition, co-morbidities, concomitant drug use, drug absorption patterns, pharmacogenetic makeup, and several that are unknown. For example, nicotine gum carries a risk of producing hiccups, but the result would generally not be considered as harmful to the patient.

Harm is hurt or damage that is suffered by the patient due to an adverse effect of the drug. Its impact is a composite of the frequency, severity and duration of symptoms produced. Readers can refer to *Chapter 9, Adverse Drug Reactions* for further details.

Attributable risk: When assessing drug effects, it is essential that they be considered within a context. For example, if the incidence of gastrointestinal bleeding in people taking NSAIDs is 0.5%, we cannot attribute all of it to the drugs since some of the patients may have had spontaneous bleeding unrelated to the drug. One way to assess the relationship is to subtract the baseline risk from the rate observed in the sample. We call this measure the attributable risk; it is also referred to as the risk difference or rate difference. Mathematically, it is expressed as follows:

$$AR = R_{\text{exposed}} - R_{\text{non-exposed}}$$

where R is the rate of the outcome of interest.

Suppose the rate of spontaneous bleeding was 0.1% in the same population. Thus, the attributable risk would be 0.5% – 0.1% =

0.4%, or 4/1,000 exposures. In other words, if 1,000 people took NSAIDs and 1,000 did not, we would expect there to be 5 cases of bleeding in the former group and 1 in the latter. Thus, we would attribute 4 bleeding cases to drug exposure that were in excess of the 1 case expected in a non-exposed population.

The attributable risk is a statistic that is simple to calculate and to understand. When used to describe clinical outcomes, it is referred to as the rate difference. It simply quantifies how much higher one rate is than that of its comparator. For example, if one drug is 80% successful and another is 65% successful, the rate difference is 80% – 65% = 15%, or 0.15 when expressed as a decimal fraction.

Outcomes from epidemiologic studies

2x2 tables for outcomes: Research studies most often include a study group and a comparison group of some sort. To facilitate understanding of results, they may be cast into a 2 x 2 table (Fig. 27.1). The four cells are labelled A, B, C and D. The marginals (e_1, e_0, c_1 and c_0) represent the total number of persons exposed to the drug, the number not exposed, the number who had the outcome of interest, and the number who did not have the outcome, respectively, and N is the total number in the study.

Relative risk: One of the most important coefficients in pharmacoepidemiology is the relative risk (RR), also known as the risk ratio. The term originated in the field of pharmacovigilance, hence the use of negative terminology (such as, risk of adverse events). When used to compare success rates, it is sometimes referred to as the rate ratio. It is the ratio of the rate of outcome (for example, risk or success) from exposure to a drug to the rate of outcome in a non-exposed comparison group, or $Rate_{Exposed} / Rate_{Non\text{-}exposed}$.

Using the terminology in Fig. 27.1:

$$RR = \frac{A/(A+B)}{C/(C+D)}$$

Since RR is a ratio of rates, it will equal unity (1) when the rate in the exposed group is equal to the rate in the comparison group. Thus, an RR of 2 means that the rate in the exposed group is two times that in the non-exposed group. Conversely, an RR of 0.5 means that the rate in exposed individuals is half that in non-exposed individuals.

The RR is used only in large cohort studies, which is the only way to measure incidence accurately. It requires large samples so that the comparison group can provide an accurate estimate of the baseline risk in the population of interest. The RR compares what we observe in a typical sample of

	Outcome	No Outcome	Total
Exposed	A	B	e_1
Not exposed	C	D	e_0
Total	c_1	c_0	N

Fig. 27.1 Presentation of results from pharmacoepidemiological studies

exposed persons with what we expect in the unexposed population.

For example, if 40 out of 1,000 people receiving a drug develop a rash, as compared to 20 out of 1,000 who did not take the drug, the RR would be: 40/1000 ÷ 20/1000 = 2.0. That means people who take the drug develop a rash twice as often as do people who do not take the drug. The assumptions are that the comparison group rate accurately reflects the baseline risk rate in the general population and that all other factors are similar between groups.

Odds ratio: This is another commonly used estimator of risk. It provides a rough estimate of the RR and is interpreted similarly. The OR is used in case control studies, but may be used with other types of studies including RCTs and cohort studies, and is often the statistic chosen when studies are combined in meta analysis. The formula is as follows: OR = AD/BC

Confidence intervals for risk estimators: When risk estimators such as RR or OR are calculated, they are usually presented along with a confidence interval (CI). Most commonly, a 95% CI (sometimes written as $CI_{95\%}$) is calculated. The $CI_{95\%}$ is interpreted as meaning that we are 95% certain that the true value lies between these limits. Alternately, if we did 100 studies, 95 of the results would fall within those limits.

For the risk ratio, a confidence interval may be calculated as follows: CI = RR*exp (± Z* SE), where Z is the standard normal deviate (1.96 for a 95% CI) and SE is the standard error. For the risk ratio, the SE is calculated as follows:

$$SE = \sqrt{B/A^*(A+B) + D/C^*(C+D)}.$$

The odds ratio has a parallel formula:

$$CI = OR^*\exp(\pm Z^*\ SE),$$

where

$$\sqrt{SE = [1/A + 1/B + 1/C + 1/D]}.$$

Occasionally, a problem arises in calculating the standard error for an odds ratio because one or more of the cells has a zero entry. In that case, Sheehe has recommended adding 0.5 to each cell in the 2 × 2 table. For example, if we have cells A = 0, B = 100, C = 2 and D = 100, the cells would be adjusted by adding 0.5 to each of them.

Thus, the standard error would be

$$\sqrt{1/0.5+1/100.5+1/2.5+1/100.5}=1.56.$$

Depicting and interpreting CIs graphically: The ideal presentation of the above statistics (risk estimators and their $CI_{95\%}$) is on a semilog scale. Figure 27.2 depicts the presentation of the OR or RR and their 95% confidence intervals. Since RR and OR are ratios, they are distributed exponentially. Therefore, it is best to use their natural log or to plot them on a semilog scale, which produces symmetrical CIs.

Figure 27.2 depicts three possible scenarios. In the first, Drug A is associated with a significantly greater outcome than Drug B. Note that the 95% confidence interval does not cross the line of unity; that may be interpreted as a (statistically) significant difference between the two groups. If the outcome is positive (a cure), then Drug A cures more patients than does Drug B; if negative, then Drug A is associated with more ADRs than is Drug B.

In the second scenario, the confidence interval overlaps with the line of unity, therefore, there is no difference between them. In the third case, Drug A produces

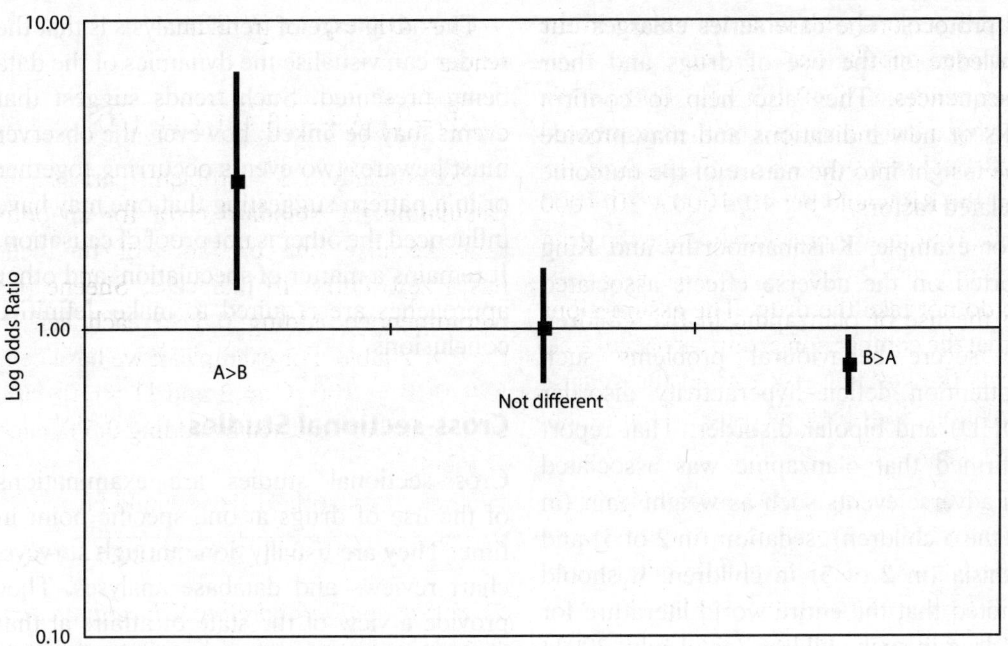

Figure 27.2 Depiction of odds ratios (or risk ratios)

statistically less outcome than Drug B. If the outcome is positive, drug A is not as beneficial as B; if the outcome is adverse, then Drug A is protective against that outcome.

Pharmacoepidemiological Study Designs

Case Report

The case report is the simplest form of observational study. During their daily routine, practitioners notice the emergence of an outcome and relate it to a drug exposure. The reporting of that event through an official reporting system or medical/pharmacy journal generates a signal that alerts others to the possibility of causal association.

One of the most influential case reports was that by McBride, which generated a signal, later confirmed, that drugs could produce foetal abnormalities. That report is responsible for the creation of teratology as a field of study.

New indications for drugs have also been identified through case reports. For example, Zappacosta presented a case report of a patient treated with minoxidil that was discovered to stimulate hair growth. Subsequently, a topical formulation of minoxidil was developed to take advantage of that effect. It is now a successful product on the market.

Case Series

A case series is a set of sequential case reports identified either by exposure or by outcome, such as the first 100 patients treated with a drug or the first 100 cases of an outcome seen by a practitioner. It resembles an open trial of a drug, except that it lacks a formal trial protocol. The case series enlarges our knowledge of the use of drugs and their consequences. They also help to confirm ADRs or new indications and may provide some insight into the nature of the outcome or related factors.

For example, Krishnamoorthy and King reported on the adverse effects associated with the use of olanzapine in five children with severe behavioural problems such as attention deficit hyperactivity disorder (ADHD) and bipolar disorder. That report confirmed that olanzapine was associated with adverse events such as weight gain (in 3 of the 5 children), sedation (in 2 of 5) and akathisia (in 2 of 5) in children. It should be noted that the entire world literature for that drug in such children (as of July, 2001) consisted of case reports and case series involving only 30 children in total.

Trend Analysis

Trend analysis involves the plotting of data over time. By inspecting the plot, patterns may emerge that can help explain events that have occurred. For example, if a new pharmacy law is passed or a drug policy is implemented, we can plot drug usage over time and note what happens before and after the change. Any shift in the trend line suggests that the change in law or policy may have an impact on drug utilisation.

When two separate sets of data are displayed together and show a consistent pattern, we refer to it as an ecological correlation. For example, if we plot the use of antibiotics over time and numbers of resistant strains of bacteria developing over the same time frame, the relationship would be an ecological correlation.

The advantage of trend analysis is that the reader can visualise the dynamics of the data being presented. Such trends suggest that events may be linked; however, the observer must beware: two events occurring together or in a pattern suggesting that one may have influenced the other is not proof of causation. It remains a matter of speculation, and other approaches are required to make definitive conclusions.

Cross-sectional Studies

Cross-sectional studies are examinations of the use of drugs at one specific point in time. They are usually done though surveys, chart reviews and database analyses. They provide a view of the state of affairs at that time, and an estimate of the prevalence of utilisation and (possibly) of outcomes. Such information can be used for formulary management and policy development.

These types of studies have been used to compare drug use between countries or regions within a country (such as, states). Very large differences suggest that reasons for those differences should be investigated and policies examined to determine whether outcomes and costs also differ and whether changes should be made.

An example of a cross-sectional study was published by Dua and colleagues, who examined antibiotic use in pharmacies in Nagpur. Among other things, they found evidence of inappropriate prescribing by physicians and inappropriate sales of antibiotics by pharmacists, often without having received a prescription, contrary to the Indian Pharmaceutics and Cosmetics Act. Such studies can identify problem areas and suggest where remedial action should be directed.

Database Studies

An ideal database would have all the requisite data for conducting pharmacoepidemiological research, including information on the patient, diagnosis, drug and outcomes. With the appropriate linkages, databases are versatile, and the advantages are many. Researchers can conduct any type of observational study, especially longitudinal cohort studies. Databases can contain data from literally millions of patients. These large numbers allow for reasonably accurate estimates of ADR incidence, rates of drug effectiveness and comparative patient outcomes such as death or cost of care.

On the other hand, there are limitations and disadvantages. Few databases are linked and those with links tend to be fairly small or do not have data for long time periods. Other limitations include missing or miscoded data. However, that is a problem for any database, whether it is paper-based, like a patient chart, or electronic.

Also, databases often lack important information because they were developed for purposes other than pharmacoepidemiological research. For example, drug insurance databases have a great deal of information, but seldom have the diagnosis or patient characteristics. Thus, it is not possible to do much more than the most elementary study. A further problem is that databases record only prescriptions filled; they do not measure how much was actually ingested by the patient.

Drug Utilisation Studies

Drug utilisation studies are considered to be a form of pharmacoepidemiological study (see *Chapter 26, Drug Utilisation Evaluation*).

Epidemiological Studies

The two main types of epidemiologic study are the cohort study and the case control study. Both utilise a comparison group. The principle behind these studies is that we take a sample of patients for whom we determine both their exposure status and their outcome status. We then compare the results with those from a group that represents the non-exposed population.

The comparison provides an estimate of the relative merits of the drug(s) in question. Thus, we are able to test hypotheses about proposed relationships between drug exposure and patient outcome. Cohort and case control studies differ in their approach to assembling a comparison group.

Cohort study: A cohort study is one into which patients are entered according to their exposure status. That is, we assemble a group of patients who are exposed to a drug and a non-exposed comparison group similar to them in all other important aspects. The two groups are then followed through time, and outcomes are observed and recorded. When the trial is completed, rates are compared between the two groups, and hypotheses may then be tested.

A variant is the historic cohort study, which is the same in all respects, except that the data is collected retrospectively from patient charts or databases. Because patients are identified and grouped according to exposure status, it is a cohort study. However, since data is collected after the fact, it is termed historic, rather than prospective. Thus, the cohort study has considerable flexibility in that data may be collected from a variety of sources including directly from patients, patient charts or computerised databases.

The cohort study is used in situations where the outcome is not rare. If exposure to the drug is rare, then the sample size must be increased, but the model is still valid. Cohort studies have the advantage of being able to actually measure outcome incidence. In addition, effectiveness data can be collected. With one study, many different outcomes to a single exposure may be examined. For example, the Nurses' Health Study followed more than 160,000 American nurses over time, starting in 1976. The exposure of interest was oral contraceptive use. The researchers on that project were able to prospectively examine different outcomes such as cancer (breast, colon, skin), deaths, thromboembolism and skeletal problems. They also determined patient status with respect to many other factors such as diabetes, smoking and nutrition and were therefore able to prospectively monitor the effects of several risk factors simultaneously on several important outcomes.

Although cohort studies can produce a lot of useful information, their disadvantages are many. Large sample sizes may be required, often numbering in the tens of thousands or more (as in the Nurses' Health Study). These numbers require large investments of money and in highly skilled management teams. Studies often take years to complete, by which time the results may be meaningless as the study drugs may have become obsolete. Also, dropouts are many and follow-up is difficult. Even with large numbers, there may still not be sufficient patients to assess rare events. As with all observational studies, we cannot truly establish causation, and we cannot guarantee that all of the confounders have been ruled out.

Case control study: The case control study may be seen as the mirror image of the cohort study. That is, we start by assembling a group of patients having the outcome of interest. We then match them on important variables (age, sex or disease severity) with a similar group of individuals who did not have that outcome. Matching is important because we are not able to randomise patients into groups as in an RCT. Then, we determine whether the patients had been exposed to the drug in question, and compare the groups.

Case control studies are used when outcomes are rare, but only if exposure to the drug is not too uncommon. For a rare outcome and rare exposure, there may be no effective model for examining the issue. Such may be the case with orphan (rarely used) drugs causing unusual events. The best approach would be to study case reports and apply clinical judgment.

An advantage of case control study designs is that we can assess rare outcomes and multiple exposures on a single outcome. Hypotheses can also be tested. Compared to cohort study designs, it is quite inexpensive and usually involves far fewer participants. If results can be obtained from a database, then a study may be undertaken very quickly.

An example of a case control study is that of Chan and co-workers, who examined cases of admissions to hospital due to GI haemorrhage and matched them with admissions for other reasons. They compared rates of NSAID exposures to those in non-exposed controls, and also in people who had taken ulcer healing drugs, and paracetamol. Odds ratios were 14.0 for non-exposed controls, 12.5 for other ulcer drugs and 2.5 for paracetamol, all of which were statistically significant.

Conclusion

Pharmacoepidemiology is a field of study whose importance is constantly growing. It is useful especially in post-marketing effectiveness and safety surveillance of pharmaceutical drugs. Many significant contributions have been made to pharmacotherapy using observational data. When used wisely, results can serve to inform public policy and assist in treating groups of people.

Limitations should always be kept in mind. More efforts are required to develop new and useful methods to help in patient care. Students are encouraged to become familiar with this field and its tools and use them appropriately.

Pharmacoepidemiology is a major part of drug therapy, and all pharmacists should be aware of this field and its potential.

KEY MESSAGES

- Pharmacoepidemiology is the study of the use of drugs in large groups of people.
- It involves the study of both adverse and beneficial effects of drugs.
- Pharmacoepidemiological studies provide evidence that can answer clinical questions not addressed in randomised controlled trials.
- Pharmacoepidemiological studies are observational studies that provide valuable information about the use of drugs and their effects in real life that can be applied in practice.
- A major weakness with observational studies is that, usually, causation cannot be determined with certainty.

Further Reading

Anonymous Anatomic Therapeutic Chemical (ATC) classification index with Defined Daily Doses (DDDs). 2002. *WHO Collaborating Centre for Drug Statistics Methodology,* Oslo, Norway (available at www.whocc.no/atcddd/)

Anonymous. Guidelines for DDD. *WHO Collaborating Centre for Drug Statistics and Methodology,* Oslo, Uppsala 2009. (available at http://www.whocc.nmd.no/)

Bhattacharjya AS and Sapra PK. 2008. Health insurance in China and India: Segmented Roles for Public and Private Financing. *Health Affairs* 27:1005–1015.

Bridge JA and Axelson DA. 2008. The contribution of pharmacoepidemiology to the antidepressant-suicidality debate in children and adolescents. *Int Rev Psychiatry* 20:209–14.

Census India Posts (available at http://censusindia.gov.in) accessed 15 August 2011

Chan TY, Critchley JA, Lau JT, Sung JJ, Chung SS and Anderson DC. 1966. The relationship between upper gastrointestinal hemorrhage and drug use: a case control study. *Int J Clin Pharmacol Ther* 34:304–08.

Cluff LE, Thornton GF and Seidl LG. 1964. Studies on the epidemiology of adverse drug reactions. I. Methods of surveillance. *JAMA* 188:976–83.

Colditz GA, Manson JE and Hankinson SE. 1997. The Nurses' Health Study: 20-year contribution to the understanding of health among women. *J Women's Health* 6:49–62.

Dua V, Kunin CM and vanArsdale Wright L. 1994. The use of antimicrobial agents in Nagpur, India. A window on medical care in a developing country. *Soc Sci Med* 38:717–724.

Einarson TR and Einarson A. 1997. Hiccups following nicotine gum use. *Ann Pharmacother* 31:1263–4.

Gatyas G. Press Room. IMS Forecasts Global Pharmaceutical Market Growth of 5–7% in 2011; *Reaching 880 Billion* (available at http://www.imshealth.com)

Gupta H. 2007. The role of insurance in health care management in India. *Int J Health Care Qual Assur* 20:379–391.

Hepler CD and Strand LM. 1990. Opportunities and responsibilities in pharmaceutical care. *Am J Hosp Pharm* 47:533–543.

Hartzema AG, Tilson HH and Chan KA (eds). 2009. *Pharmacoepidemiology and Therapeutic Risk Management*. Harvey Whitney Books: Cincinnati, USA.

IMS releases first Total Sales Audit (TSA) report. Express Pharma, 16 june 2011 (available at http://www.expresspharmaonline.com/20110630/market04.shtml) accessed 15 August 2011.

India Healthcare Indicators (available at http://www.trade.gov/td/health/india_indicators05.pdf)

India Source: World Statistics Pocketbook | United Nations Statistics Division. 2009. (available at http://data.un.org/CountryProfile.aspx?crName=India)

India's Pharmaceutical Industry on Course for Globalization. 2008 (available at http://www.dbresearch.com/PROD/DBR_INTERNET_EN-PROD/PROD0000000000224095.pdf)

Indian Pharmaceutical Industry. 2009. (available at http://www.researchandmarkets.com/reports/660350)

Kotwani A, Holloway K and Chaudhury RR. 2009. Methodology for surveillance of antimicrobials use among out-patients in Delhi. *Indian J Med Res* 129:555–60.

Krishnamoorthy J and King BH. 1998. Open-label olanzapine treatment in five preadolescent children. *J Child Adoles Psychopharmacol* 8:107–113.

Mangla B. 1993. India to modify drug policy. *Lancet* 342:608.

McBride WG. 1961. Thalidomide and congenital abnormalities. *Lancet* ii:1358.

Morris JA and Gardner MJ. 1988. Calculating confidence intervals for relative risks (odds ratios) and standardised ratios and rates. *Stat Med* 296:1313–16.

Myler L. 1952. *Side effects of drugs*. Elsevier: Amsterdam.

Penna RP. 1990. Pharmaceutical care: pharmacy's mission for the 1990s. *Am J Hosp Pharm* 47:543–549.

Pillai AM. 1995. Impact of GATT agreement on drug prices. *J Indian Med Assoc* 93:113–120.

Poddar A. 2009. Indian pharma industry a lucrative destination for MNCs, to feature among global top 10 by 2015 (available at http://www.ibtimes.co.in/articles/20090921/indian-pharma-industry-lucrative-destination-mncs-feature-among-global-top-ten-2015-report.htm)

Sackett DL, Straus SE, Richardson WS, Rosenberg W and Haynes RB. 2002. *Evidence-based medicine: how to practice and teach EBM*. Churchill Livingstone: Toronto.

Sankaranarayanan J and Puumala SE. 2007. Anti-psychotic use at adult ambulatory care visits by patients with mental health disorders in the United States, 1996–2003: national estimates and associated factors. *Clin Ther* 29: 723–41.

Sheehe PR. 1966. Combination of log relative risk in retrospective studies of disease. *American Journal of Public Health* 56:1745–50.

SOHM India Highlights Population, Geographical Information and Market Potential for India's Generic Pharmaceutical Market. 2009 (available at http://www.pharmacychoice.com/News/article.cfm?Article_ID=463412)

Strom BL (ed). 2005. *Pharmacoepidemiology*, 4th ed. John Wiley: Sussex, UK

Sundaram VM. 2008. Pharma Industry in India. *Drug News Perspect* 21:59.

The Top 10 Pharmaceutical Companies in India: Growth Strategies, Performance and SWOT Analyses. 2009. (available at http://www.reportlinker.com/p0137687/The-Top-10-Pharmaceutical-Companies-in-India-Growth-strategies-performance-and-SWOT-analyses.html)

Uppal R, Khanna S, Sharma SK and Sharma PL. 1991. Antimicrobial drug use in urology. *Int J Clin Pharmacol Ther Toxicol* 29:366–8.

Wallerstein RO, Condit PK and Kasper CK. 1969. Statewide study of chloramphenicol therapy and fatal aplastic anemia. *JAMA* 208:2045–2050.

Waning B and Montagne M. 2001. *Pharmacoepidemiology: Principles and Practice*, 1st ed. McGraw-Hill.

Zappacosta AR. 1980. Reversal of baldness in patient receiving minoxidil for hypertension. *New Eng J Med* 303:1480–81.

Websites of Interest

International Society for Pharmacoepidemiology
www.pharmacoepi.org

International Society for Pharmacoeconomics and Outcomes Research
www.ispor.org

See also Appendix I: Bibliography of Pharmacoepidemiologic Studies Done in India

28 Medication Errors and Adverse Drug Events

Philip J Schneider

Learning Objectives

Upon completion of this chapter, the reader should be able to:

- State what percentage of adverse medical events are caused by medications
- List the five steps in the medication use process
- List and define the twelve types of medication errors
- Distinguish between medication errors, adverse drug events and potential adverse drug events
- List the most common systems failures that cause adverse drug events

Improving medication safety has been an important part of the history and professional attention of pharmacists for several decades, even though this has been a topic of public interest only recently. Research by pharmacists as long as forty years ago documented the incidence of drug administration errors in hospitals in the United States as being 10% or higher. This provided the evidence and impetus to develop drug distribution systems that were safer, including unit dose drug distribution systems and intravenous admixture programmes. These systems were demonstrated to be at least twice as safe as the floor stock system that they replaced. Systems where the responsibility for preparing, distributing and administering medications was transferred to pharmacy personnel further improved medication safety. These integrated systems were shown to reduce medication error rates to less than 1%. This is the lowest medication error rate ever documented in a hospital.

Despite the long history of work in Pharmacy, research related to patient safety and medical errors began to be published in the medical literature only recently. One of the most important of these was the Harvard Medical Practice Study. In this study, it was shown that 3.7% of patients admitted to hospitals in the state of New York experienced injury resulting from medical care. It was also shown that 19% of these injuries were caused by the use of medicines. Medication-related injuries were more common than infections, which caused 14% of the events. Many injuries (42%) were judged preventable. While the publicity of medical research in this area has been a source of some frustration to pharmacists, given their earlier work in this area, there are some important differences between studies published in the pharmacy literature and those published in the medical literature.

Research reported in the medical literature has focused on the adverse clinical outcomes of medications. These adverse medical events are much less common than medication errors but generate more interest among prescribers, nurses, administrators and risk managers, because injury occurs. Medication errors often do not result in injury, and are often associated with blame and punishment. Thus, medication errors are often ignored or not treated as important. Research published in the medical literature has more impact than that published in the pharmacy literature. Based on both bodies of literature, medication safety is an important issue to the public and an important opportunity for pharmacists.

Medication Use Systems

A system is a combination of related steps intended to achieve a common goal. The use of medicines in healthcare is an example of a system. It consists of as many as forty to fifty small steps but is often described as having five major steps, each of which involves different healthcare professionals. These major steps include:

- Selecting and procuring – establishing a formulary of accepted medicines
- Prescribing – assessing the patient, determining the need for drug therapy, electing and ordering the medicine
- Preparing and dispensing – purchasing and storing medicines, reviewing and confirming the order, preparing the medicine, and distributing it to the patient location
- Administering – reviewing the dispensed medicine and order, assessing the patient and administering the medicine
- Monitoring – assessing the patient's response to the medicine and reporting reactions and errors

Different healthcare professionals perform each of these steps in the medication use system. For example, clinicians and administrators typically perform the selecting and procuring step. Physicians usually prescribe the medicine. Pharmacists most often prepare and dispense medicines. Nurses and patients most frequently administer them. All healthcare professionals, patients and their families monitor the patient's response to medicines.

While these traditional professional roles continue to evolve and blur, the medication use system involves many different people, with many 'hand-offs', including the transfer of information and medicines. This creates the potential for errors.

Medication Errors

A medication error is an episode associated with the use of a medicine that should be preventable through effective control systems. Pharmacists have had a long-standing interest in improving medication safety and have studied ways to reduce medication errors. The definition used in medication error studies conducted by pharmacists was a more restricted one of error. In these studies, a medication error was defined as any deviation from the prescriber's order. This definition does not consider the clinical outcome of the error.

The American Society of Health-System Pharmacists' (ASHP) definition of medication errors includes prescribing, dispensing, medication administration and patient compliance errors. They define the following categories of medication errors:

- Prescribing errors
- Omission errors
- Wrong time errors
- Unauthorised drug errors
- Improper dose errors (administration of a dose that is greater or less than the amount prescribed)
- Wrong dosage form errors (administration of a drug product in a different dosage form from that prescribed)
- Wrong drug preparation errors (drug product incorrectly formulated or manipulated before administration)
- Wrong administration or technique errors (inappropriate procedure or improper technique in the administration of the drug)
- Deteriorated drug errors (administration of a drug that has expired or whose physical or chemical dosage form integrity has been compromised)
- Monitoring errors (failure to review a prescribed regimen for appropriateness or failure to assess response to prescribed therapy)
- Compliance errors (failure of the patient to adhere to the prescribed medication regimen)
- Other medication errors (any error that does not fall into one of the above categories)

The National Coordinating Committee on Medication Error Reporting and Prevention (NCCMERP) in the United States is an interdisciplinary healthcare group consisting of representatives of fourteen healthcare organizations. Their purpose is to promote the reporting, understanding and prevention of medication errors and focus on ways to protect patient safety through the coordinated efforts of associations and agencies. NCCMERP defines medication errors as any preventable event that may cause or lead to inappropriate medication use or patient harm while the medicine is in the control of the healthcare professional, patient or consumer. Such events may be related to professional practice, healthcare products, procedures and systems, including prescribing; order communication; product labelling, packaging and nomenclature; compounding; dispensing; distribution; administration; education; monitoring; and use.

It has been shown that only a small percentage of medication errors actually result in harm to the patient. The current definition of medication error focuses on breaks in performing any step in the medication use system, not just the drug administration step. As previously noted, the incidence of medication errors in most hospitals is approximately 10%.

Adverse Drug Events

The term adverse drug event (ADE) is a newer term that emerged as studies of the epidemiology of adverse medical events were published. The Harvard Medical Practice Study identified medications as the most common cause of injury resulting from medical care. This represented a shift in focus to the preventable adverse outcomes associated with drug therapy, and errors as one cause of these adverse outcomes.

Bates et al. defined an ADE as an injury resulting from medical interventions related to a medicine. They noted that most ADEs are dose-dependant and potentially predictable and constitute the greatest percentage of errors that result in clinical harm. They also noted that a smaller number of ADEs are unpredictable, idiosyncratic or allergic reactions to medicines (note that this resembles a category of events that could be defined as adverse drug reactions). These authors introduced another term, *'potential ADE'*, which is defined as a medication error with the potential for injury, but in which no injury occurs (note the relationship between medication errors and ADEs). ADEs may therefore result from medication errors or from adverse drug reactions in which there was no error.

The relationship between medication errors, adverse drug events and potential adverse drug events is shown in Fig. 28.1.

The terms adverse drug event and adverse drug reaction (ADR) may be confused. An *adverse drug reaction* is a 'response to a drug which is noxious and unintended and which occurs at doses normally used in humans for prophylaxis, diagnosis or therapy of disease or for the modification of physiologic function'. In other words, an ADR is harm directly caused by the drug at normal doses, during normal use.

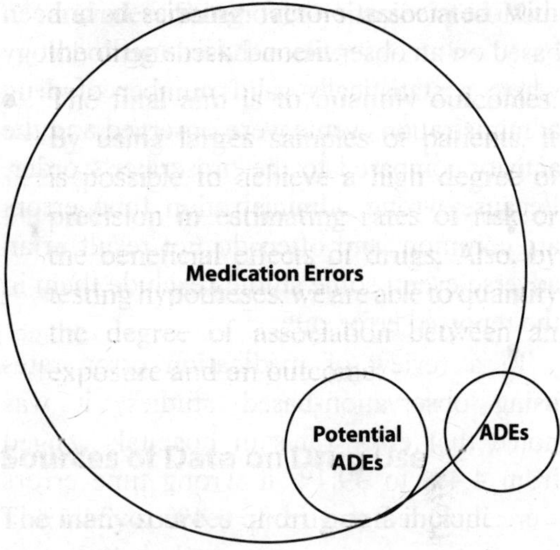

Figure 28.1 The relationship between medication errors, adverse drug events and potential adverse drug events

An example of an ADR is nausea resulting from chemotherapy. A death associated with a prescribed overdose of chemotherapy that was not detected and corrected before a fatal dose was administered to a patient is an ADE.

Epidemiology of Medication-related Problems

Almost every patient receiving healthcare receives medicines as part of their care. Literally, millions of doses per year are administered to patients in the average hospital, and billions of doses are self-administered in the outpatient setting. How often do medication-related problems actually occur? What is the cause of such problems? How much unnecessary cost results from adverse drug events, particularly those that are preventable?

Most medication error studies have been based on an observation-based methodology where a statistically valid number of drug administration events were observed and the activity compared to the prescriber's order. Because wrong administration time errors are common, and often do not result in an adverse event, some studies exclude them in the reported error rate.

In a review of medication error rates using observation-based studies, it was noted that error rates in hospitals ranged from 4.4% to 59.1% if wrong time errors were included and from 0.4% to 24.7% if wrong time errors were excluded. It was further noted that lower error rates were consistently noted (typically 50% lower) in hospitals using unit dose drug distribution systems compared to those using floor stock systems. The lowest medication error rate ever reported (0.6%) was in hospitals with pharmacy-coordinated unit dose and drug administration programmes.

Despite safety considerations, the unit dose drug distribution system makes it difficult for nurses to respond to rapidly changing drug therapy orders. As a result, automated dispensing cabinets (ADCs) that enable secure storage of medications in the patient care area have been developed. In fact, hospitals in the US are increasingly changing from centralised unit dose drug distribution systems to decentralised systems using ADCs. A large majority of US hospitals (83%) now use ADCs as part of their medication distribution systems. Studies have confirmed that if access to medications is possible before the pharmacist reviews the medication order, ADCs are error-prone.

Barker and Allen compared error rates in a system where medications were available for administration from a unit-based ADC that was not integrated with a computerised medication profile to a traditional unit dose system. The error rate in the unit-based, ADC was 16.3% compared to 5.4% with the unit dose system. Borel and Rascati compared medication error rates before and after implementing a medication profile-linked version of an ADC. The error rate with the unit dose system used before the ADC system was implemented was 16.9%. The error rate for the profile-linked, unit-based system was 10.4%. Therefore, an important safe medication use practice is to require a pharmacist review of orders for medicines before they can be obtained from any supply and the dose is administered to a patient.

It would appear therefore that medication errors are relatively common, and error rates are influenced by the drug distribution system. Unit dose systems are still considered safer than floor stock systems. ADCs that place medicines in the patient care area can be less safe if not properly configured with links to computerised medication profiles that include a pharmacist review. The safest system is an integrated unit dose, drug administration programme with a high level of procedural standardisation and double checks, such as reviewing transcription accuracy, rescheduling missed doses, and regular review of the medication administration record to verify that medications have been administered as scheduled.

Causes of Medication Errors

In an analysis of the systems failures associated with ADEs and potential ADEs, errors were classified according to proximal cause by a multidisciplinary team of physicians, nurses and pharmacists. In the review, 334 errors were detected as the cause of 264 preventable ADEs and potential ADEs. Sixteen major systems failures were identified as the underlying cause of the errors. The most common systems failure (29%) was in the dissemination of drug knowledge, particularly to prescribers. The next most common system failure was inadequate availability of patient information (18%) such as laboratory tests. Seven systems failures accounted for 78% of all errors, all of which the authors state could be improved by better information systems.

The stage of the medication use process associated with these ADEs was also determined. Problems at the prescribing stage were most common (39%), followed by drug administration (38%) and dispensing (11%).

The most common error type was wrong dose (28%) followed by wrong drug (9%), known allergy (8%), missed dose (7%) and wrong time (7%).

Lesar et al. have studied medication prescribing errors in a teaching hospital. From a total of 289,411 medication orders written during a one-year period, 905 prescribing errors were detected and averted by pharmacists. The overall detected error rate was 3.13 errors for every 1000 orders written and a rate of 1.81 significant errors per 1000 orders. The most common medication classes involving errors were antimicrobials (28.5%), cardiovascular (10.7%), gastrointestinal (8.8%) and benzodiazepines (7.7%). The types of medication errors detected included:

- Overdose – 28.7%
- Missing information – 22.3%
- Underdosing – 17.8%
- Wrong dose form ordered – 7.3%
- Allergy to ordered drug – 6.7%
- Duplicate therapies – 5.5%
- Wrong drug ordered – 5.5%
- Wrong route ordered – 3.4%
- Wrong patient – 1.1%

A subsequent study by Lesar found the prescribing error rate to be 3.99 errors per 1000 orders. The most common specific factors associated with errors included: decline in renal or hepatic function requiring alteration of drug therapy (13.9%), patient history of allergy to the same medication class (12.1%), using the wrong drug name, dosage form or abbreviation (11.4%), incorrect dose calculations (11.1%), and atypical or unusual and critical dosage frequency considerations (10.8%). The most common groups of factors associated with errors were those related to the knowledge and application of knowledge regarding drug therapy (30%) or patient factors that affect drug therapy (29.2%), use of calculations, decimal points or unit and rate expression factors (17.5%), and nomenclature factors (13.4%). These data highlight the importance and need for a review of drug orders by pharmacists to detect and prevent errors before a dose is obtained and administered to the patient.

Cost of these Problems

Schneider et al. studied the cost of medication-related problems at a university hospital. The charts of patients who had experienced an ADE were reviewed and the cost of treating the events was tabulated. Mean cost incurred for the management of ADEs included: additional laboratory tests ($95), non-invasive procedures ($184), additional medication treatment ($227), invasive monitoring or procedures ($2,505), increases in length of stay ($2,596), and transfer to an intensive care unit ($2,640). It was estimated that the annualised total cost of ADEs was $1.5 million.

- Classen et al. used a matched, case control model to compare the length of stay, added costs and attributable mortality associated with ADEs. They found that mortality in cases where there was an ADE was 3.5% compared to 1.05% in matched control cases that did not. Mean length of hospital stay was 7.69 days compared to 4.46 days in control patients. The mean cost of hospitalisation was $10,010 in patients who experienced an ADE compared to $5,355 in case controls who did not. The extra length of stay attributable to an ADE was 1.74 days, resulting in added costs of $2,013. They noted that based on the number of ADEs detected in one year, the direct hospital costs were $1,099,413.
- Bates et al. assessed the additional resource utilisation associated with ADEs. They also used a case control method and compared the cost of care for patients who experienced an ADE to matched control cases with the same diagnosis who were on the same service, but did not experience an ADE. They too found an increase in length of stay, with patients who experienced an ADE being in the hospital for 2.2 additional days. The increase in cost associated with an ADE was found to be $3,244. For preventable ADEs, the increase in length of stay was longer (4.6 days), and increase in costs was higher ($5,857). They estimate the cost of ADEs and preventable ADEs in their 700-bed teaching hospital to be $5.6 million and $2.8 million, respectively.

Tools to Measure the Performance of the Medication Use Process

How do we detect medication errors so that safety improvement goals can be established and the changes made to improve medication safety be evaluated? Errors occur at all steps in the medication use process, and measurement systems should be designed to evaluate each step. Voluntary medication error reports often focus only on the drug administration step, making the assumption that there are no errors at the prescribing step. Nurses can be very sensitive that medication error reporting programmes focus only on what they do when they administer a medicine, and ignore errors at other steps. In reality, errors can occur at all steps in the medication use system.

Voluntary, self-reporting systems also often miss medication errors. Investigators have evaluated other ways to detect medication errors and ADEs, including chart reviews, computer screening and combinations of methods that can improve detection. Even the best combinations of reporting systems miss many errors and events. As long as problems with the use of medicines are discovered and opportunities to improve the medication use system can be identified, it is a method that has value.

In spite of the limitation of under-reporting, a voluntary reporting system can still be a very good method to monitor performance because it is not time consuming and it engages the staff. When healthcare professionals report errors or adverse events, there is recognition that a mistake has happened and a willingness to improve the process. Observation-based studies are often perceived as 'catching people doing things wrong'. It can be difficult to motivate the staff to admit that they have made an error because of the fear of punishment.

In contrast to voluntary reporting programmes, observation-based studies are much more quantitative – they detect all errors that occur during an observation period. They do not, however, detect rare events. If really serious events only happen five or six times a year, these errors are not likely to be detected from a small statistical sample when activities are observed. On the other hand, if the impact of a change made to reduce medication errors is being studied, a more quantitative measurement method than voluntary reporting is needed.

A way to do this is a 'before and after' evaluation of the impact of the change to see if there are fewer medication errors. An example of a medication safety goal might be to reduce the number of intravenous antibiotics administered at the wrong time ('late doses'). A voluntary reporting system would be much less likely to be able to show that improvement resulted from change(s) compared to an observation-based study of the administration of intravenous antibiotics.

Criteria-based audits, also known as medication use evaluation studies, are a third way to find opportunities for improvement. When a problem is suspected, a study using chart review to collect data can provide a quantitative assessment of the problem. An example is a warfarin medication use evaluation study. It might be found for example through chart review that many physicians use the wrong laboratory test to monitor warfarin therapy (for example, partial thromboplastin time or PTT instead of prothrombin time (PT) or International Normalised Ratio (INR)) or that patients with high INR values are treated too often with fresh frozen plasma instead of safer and less expensive vitamin K. These types of findings would provide excellent examples of medication safety problems that need to be solved.

Computerised detection programmes have emerged as an effective way to detect medication errors and ADEs. Classen et al. have described a computer ADE monitor that integrates clinical and drug information in a way that allows physicians and pharmacists to detect errors more quickly. Alerts are built into their rules base that identifies medication errors. Examples include orders for naloxone, vitamin K, fresh frozen plasma and potassium exchange resins. These orders are very likely to be associated with medication errors. This method is sometimes called the '*trigger tool*' because certain laboratory tests or drug orders 'trigger' an alert that an ADE might have occurred. It is also important to note that computer ADE monitoring systems only detect events that result in abnormal laboratory values or the use of antidotes. Not all ADEs result in this and are therefore not detected by computer detection systems. These are all good ways to identify errors without waiting for an incident report, but build on a voluntary reporting system.

Jha et al. compared the rate and type of ADEs identified using a computer-based monitor to those discovered by chart review and by asking physicians, pharmacists and nurses for voluntary reports of ADEs. The computer-based monitoring programme identified alerts, which were situations suggesting that an ADE might be present – for example, an order for an antidote such as naloxone. A trained reviewer examined the chart to determine whether an ADE had actually occurred. The number and types of ADEs discovered with this system was compared to those discovered by chart review alone and by voluntary reports by nurses and pharmacists. The computer monitoring programme identified 2,620 alerts in eight months for patients on nine medical and surgical wards in a tertiary care hospital. Chart review alone found 398 ADEs and there were 23 voluntarily reported.

Of the 617 ADEs detected by at least one method, only 76 were detected by both computer and chart review methods. The types of events detected by chart review were different from those detected by computer monitoring. Chart review was more effective in detecting symptomatic events, such as a change in mental status, nausea and vomiting, and hypotension. The computer monitor was more reliable in identifying events associated with changes in laboratory monitoring or events that required treatment with medications. Using a combination of these techniques, the incidence of ADEs was found to be 17.8 per 1000 patient days.

What Can Pharmacists Do to Improve Medication Use Safety?

Traditional methods

Unit dose drug distribution systems: The first study to demonstrate that medication errors were a relatively common occurrence was published in 1962. The error rate in this study was found to be 16.2%. Subsequently, these investigators and others studied the impact of providing medicines that were packaged, labelled and distributed to the point of care for administration within 24 hours or less (the unit dose drug distribution system). It was shown that significant improvement could be achieved by a unit dose system, if fully implemented. Studies cited in this review have shown that error rates can be paradoxically *higher* when compromises such as dispensing multidose containers, increasing cart exchange rates and increasing floor stock were made. With the increased interest in ADCs, the unit dose drug distribution system has been challenged as the standard of practice in hospitals. Improperly configured, these dispensing cabinets can be less safe than unit dose drug distribution systems (see below). Until the safety of properly configured systems can be demonstrated, unit dose drug distribution systems remain a fundamentally safer system than floor stocked medications.

Intravenous admixture systems: Concerns about the safety of medicines administered by the intravenous route also began to be expressed in the 1960s. Patterson and Nordstrom reported that 60% of IV solutions being infused to hospitalised patients contained more than one medicine – some as many as five drugs. More than half the medicines were prepared more than an hour before administration. A pharmacy-based, intravenous admixture programme was proposed. Thur et al. reported an error rate of 21% in a system where nurses prepared and administered IV medicines. An error rate of 7.24% in a pharmacy-based IV admixture service has been described. It has also been shown that physicians and nurses make more errors in dosage calculations compared to pharmacists. The uniformity of mixing when IV solutions are prepared at the bedside is lower than that when they are prepared in the pharmacy. Schneider has reviewed the safety of intravenous drug delivery using the following systems:

- IV push (nurses prepare and administer the dose directly using a syringe)

- Volume control chambers (a container between an IV solution and the IV tubing into which medicines can be added for infusion)
- Pharmacy prepared minibags/glass bottles (medicines are added to a small volume of IV fluid under sterile conditions in the pharmacy)
- Spring-loaded syringe-based system (a device that uses a spring to put pressure on the plunger of a syringe to facilitate delivery of a dose)
- Point-of-care activated system (ADD-Vantage[R], Minibag Plus[R]) (a plastic bag containing IV fluid and a special port for directly attaching a vial of medicine for mixing at the bedside)
- Outsourced piggyback systems (a central pharmacy prepares IV containers containing medicines and delivers these to the hospital for use)
- Manufacturer's container (a glass vial that allows for reconstitution of the dose and direct administration to the patient from the vial using an IV set)
- Premixed and frozen minibags (pre-made IV solutions containing the medicines, some of which are frozen because of limited stability)

Using a decision analysis model derived from the consensus development method used by the US National Institutes of Health, these systems were compared by an independent, interdisciplinary panel of experts. Their recommendations were based on comparing these systems using four criteria: safety, cost, simplicity and training. Three systems were ranked as being safer – manufacturer prepared (premixed and frozen minibags), point-of-care activated and pharmacy-based IV admixture systems. Systems ranked less safe included IV push, syringe pumps and volume control chambers. It was noted that clinical circumstances may require a less safe system (for example, during a medical emergency). In those cases, increased vigilance is needed to assure safety.

The results of a summit on preventing patient harm and death from IV medication errors was recently published. It lists priority IV medication safety practices along with barriers to implementation and actions to overcome these barriers. Some examples of priority practices according to steps in the medication use system include:

- Formulary management and medication use policy
  - Implement standardised infusion concentrations based on local and national practices that are appropriate for most practice settings
  - Establish comprehensive IV medication administration policies with standardised administration times, upper and lower dosage limits, and administration rates
- Prescribing and ordering
  - Use standardised orders (paper or electronic) for IV medicines
  - Prescribe standardised infusion diluents, concentrations and units (preferably commercially available products)
- Storage
  - Differentiate look-alike medicines, including separate storage locations
  - Prohibit or impose tight security precautions on stocking concentrated injectable products and more than one concentration of an IV medicine on patient care units

- Preparation and dispensing
  - Dispense IV medicines in a ready-to-administer form that does not require manipulation before administration to the patient
  - Standardise the process for compounding sterile preparations, with procedures to minimise unnecessary interruptions and distractions, trace and verify the accuracy of compounding, and provide for pharmacist checking of accuracy
- Administering
  - Require independent double-checks and documentation of administration of selected high-alert medicines, including IV pump settings
  - Standardise IV medication administration with provisions to minimise unnecessary interruptions, focus on one patient at a time, refer to an accurate medication administration record, engage the patient or family member in the medication administration process, and use two patient identifiers before administering the medicine
- Monitoring medication use
  - Have antidotes, supportive medicines, dosing and administration information and resuscitation equipment immediately available in patient care areas
  - Establish standard operating procedures for communication at the time of patient transition from one care setting to another to provide for continuity of care and medication reconciliation

Clinical Pharmacy Programmes

The positive impact of pharmacist participation on medical rounds in an intensive care unit on the rate of preventable ADEs caused by ordering errors has been reported. In this study, a pharmacist made rounds with the ICU team and remained in the ICU for consultation in the morning and on call throughout the day. The rate of prescribing errors decreased by 66% from 10.4 per 1000 patient days before the intervention to 3.5 per 1000 patient days after the intervention. In a control unit, the incidence of ADEs did not change. In eight months, 366 recommendations were made by the pharmacist, of which 362 (99%) were accepted by the prescribers.

There is also evidence of improved patient safety by clinical pharmacists practicing in the outpatient setting. Lee and Schommer documented a five-fold decrease in bleeding complications and re-admission to the hospital associated with anti-coagulation management, comparing a pharmacist-run anti-coagulation management service to regular medical care. Pharmacists have also been able to reduce the number of errors of omission (improve adherence to medication treatment regimens) to improve the outcomes of patients taking medications to lower cholesterol and treat diabetes in the outpatient setting.

Application of Technology

The emergence of new technology offers great potential to improve both the efficiency and the accuracy of care, resulting in improved patient safety. Technology and automation also have the potential to worsen patient safety or simply change the type of patient safety problems if not properly used.

Computer prescription order entry (CPOE) system: This is a computer application that accepts the prescriber's orders for diagnostic and treatment services electronically rather than recording them in writing on an order sheet or prescription pad. This includes orders for medications. The computer can compare the orders against standards for dosing, check for allergies or interactions with other medications and warn the prescriber about potential problems. Thus, CPOE systems address two of the most common systems failures causing errors: lack of information about the medicine and lack of information about the patient.

CPOE has been widely recommended as a way to improve patient safety. A medication safety expert panel assembled by ASHP recommended this as the top-priority action to prevent ADEs in hospitals. There are several advantages of CPOE that have the potential to improve medication use safety. Handwriting problems are solved, resulting in fewer transcription errors. The prescription can be quickly transferred to providers, reducing delays in dispensing and initiating therapy. Decision support logic and integration with other relevant clinical information can be built into a computer order entry system to assist physicians in avoiding errors.

The impact of a computer order entry system on antibiotic therapy has been documented by Evans et al. They studied the prescribing of antibiotics in an intensive care unit where orders were entered into a computer program that was linked to clinical information and provided the prescriber with recommendations and warnings about drug therapy. Significant reduction was observed in antibiotic susceptibility mismatches before and after the computer program was implemented (12 vs. 206). Fewer antibiotics were prescribed for patients with known allergies to those drugs (35 vs. 146). The incidence of overdoses and mean number of days of excess treatment were lower (87 vs. 405 and 2.7 vs. 5.9), as was the incidence of ADEs (4 vs. 28). Most importantly, a safer system reduced the total hospital cost to the patient ($26,315 vs. $44,846).

Bates et al. reported the effect of computer order entry and team intervention on the prevention of serious medication errors. They found that providing a computerised order entry system along with a team-based intervention programme that increased the availability and role of the pharmacist reduced serious medication errors by 55%, from 10.7% per 1000 patient days to 4.86 events per 1000 patient days.

If improperly configured or implemented, CPOE systems may facilitate the risk of medication errors. Koppel et al. reported about 22 types of medication error risks resulting from a CPOE system, including:

- Fragmented CPOE displays that prevent a coherent display of patients' medications
- Pharmacy inventory displays mistaken for dosage guidelines
- Ignored antibiotic renewal notices placed on paper charts rather than in the CPOE system
- Separate functions that facilitate double-dosing and incompatible orders
- Inflexible ordering formats generating wrong orders

CPOE, like all technologies, is a tool, not a solution to medication errors, and must be designed and implemented carefully to realize benefits.

The use of CPOE systems in US hospitals has grown slowly but steadily. In 2007, 17.8% of US hospitals had a CPOE system. The rate of adoption of CPOE differed significantly by type and size of facility. Clinical decision support systems (CDSSs) are important components of CPOE, directing prescribers toward evidence-based drug therapy. Of those hospitals with CPOE, 67.2% had CDSSs in use to improve prescribing. Nearly one-third of hospitals with CPOE systems did not have a CDSS. In these facilities, clinicians entered orders into electronic systems that did not have rules that integrated order information, patient information and clinical practice guidelines into computer system logic to provide feedback to prescribers. Therefore, it was estimated that 12% of US hospitals at the end of 2007 had CPOE with a CDSS.

The use of computer order entry systems in the outpatient setting has been limited by the lack of a network of providers and an electronic infrastructure connecting them. Workflow does not favour having prescribers enter prescriptions in the office setting. The increase in networking providers and the rapid growth of wireless communication will very likely fuel the development of computer order entry in the outpatient setting.

Despite the seeming consensus that this is an important change concept, rapid implementation has been, and will continue to be, limited by expense, design of decision support systems and the difficulty in changing the habits of prescribers.

Bar code, bedside care systems: The second recommendation from the medication safety expert panel assembled by ASHP to recommend top-priority actions for preventing ADEs in hospitals was evaluating the use of machine readable coding (for example, bar coding) in their medication use processes. In 2008, 24% of hospitals used some form of machine readable coding to verify doses before dispensing, and 21.5% of US hospitals had barcode medication administration systems (BCMA) at the bedside in place.

Bar code systems are particularly suited for efficient and accurate checking functions. It has been suggested that the checking and documentation functions that occur when medications are dispensed and administered could be done more efficiently and accurately if aided by bar code scanning. This application would include having bar codes on the package of each medication dispensed and administered, on a patient identifier (such as a wristband), and on the person dispensing and administering the dose (such as a name badge). A BCMA can be linked to clinical information and the medication profile, so that when the dose is dispensed and administered to a patient, an automatic check could be made to ensure that the drug was prescribed for the correct patient, the dose, time and route of administration is correct, and that the patient does not have an allergy to the medication being dispensed and administered. The nurse could even be reminded to administer a dose with such a system.

In addition to improving safety through these series of automatic double-checks, the documentation of the dose dispensed and administered would be improved. Furthermore, performance measurement systems such as late doses and doses omitted could automatically be tracked, reducing the dependence on voluntary reporting or observation-based studies.

Poon et al. reported that a bar code-assisted dispensing system decreased dispensing errors by 86% and potential ADEs by 97%. Paoletti et al. reported a 54% reduction in medication administration errors after implementing a new medication administration system that included BCMA.

Barriers to implementation of the bar code bedside care system include cost, the need to use cumbersome equipment, lack of universally bar-coded medication packages, lack of standardisation of bar code languages, and problems linking bar code systems to other hospital computer databases and programs.

Integrated clinical information systems: Information systems within healthcare are often configured as standalone systems that meet the needs of individual departments, but can be difficult to integrate. The healthcare industry has under-capitalised information systems in comparison to other industries. The result is fragmented information and difficulty obtaining the complete clinical information needed to care for patients. Physicians often do not have access to medication profiles. Pharmacists often do not have access to diagnosis, weight, organ system function or allergy history. As a result, medication-related problems occur.

Advances in technology and increased consolidation and integration among healthcare providers are resulting in rapid integration of clinical information systems. Two examples of advances in technology are the Internet and smart cards. Each of these technologies is enabling the storage and transfer of large quantities of clinical information efficiently among caregivers. Concerns about confidentiality of information have been raised as efforts to transmit clinical information have increased.

It is imperative that clinical information among caregivers who do not practice in contiguous sites and see patients at different times be integrated. Only with access to complete information about why the patient is being treated, previous experiences with medications, and conditions, medications and foods that may affect the choice or responses to pharmacotherapy, can medication safety be improved.

Implications for Pharmacists in India

India is a rapidly developing country but may still not have the resources that exist in countries that have created and evaluated safe medication use systems. It is unrealistic to expect the rapid adoption of expensive technologies that can improve patient safety, such as CPOE and bar code systems. It is also a country with more variation in how healthcare is provided, including the use of homeopathic and ayurvedic medicines in addition to the allopathic medications used more commonly in the West. This variation might result in even more problems with medication errors resulting from interactions among these different medications. While there are more pharmacists in India than most other countries, most do not practice in settings where they can work closely with prescribers or nurses to discuss medication-related problems and develop safer medication use systems.

Where should pharmacists in India begin? Perhaps some lessons can be learned from the experience of other countries. Some suggestions include:

- *Acknowledge that medication errors and ADEs occur and are a problem in India.* Part of this realisation might include studying the problem of medication use safety and developing methods to detect errors and ADEs in hospitals and clinics.

- *Declare that improving medication use safety is a serious and dedicated aim for pharmacists in India*. This might be accomplished by adding this topic to coursework in pharmacy colleges and as a focus for discussion at meetings of the pharmacy associations in India.
- *Use your experience to identify medication errors that frequently cause patient harm and focus attention on finding ways to improve the system so that those errors are less likely to happen again*. Attention should be directed to errors that are most common, most likely to cause harm and least likely to be detected before harm occurs. An example of such an error is having toxic medications (like concentrated solutions of potassium chloride) available as floor stock in a hospital. An example of a medication that can result in harm if errors occur in outpatients is the anti-coagulant warfarin.
- *Critically examine each step of the medication use process in your hospital or pharmacy and identify areas where the risk of medication errors can be minimised*. For example, transcription of drug orders is common in many Indian hospitals and is a well-recognised cause of medication errors. Some other potential causes of medication errors in India are listed in Table 28.1.
- *Begin by making the improvement of medication use safety an individual pharmacist's duty, day by day and patient by patient*.

Conclusion

Concerns about the safety of the healthcare system are now a matter of public concern. Studies show that the most common type of medical error is medication errors. Pharmacists have a long history of developing systems that have improved medication safety. Pharmacists need to build on this record of contribution to improve medication safety even more, by working more closely with prescribers, nurses and patients, using new technologies to help build a safer health system.

Table 28.1 Potential system-based causes of medication errors in India

• Dispensing of drugs without labels to indicate the patient's name or directions for use
• Returning original prescriptions to patients once medications have been dispensed
• Transcription of hospital treatment chart orders onto prescription forms before dispensing
• Recording of drug administration in hospitals on separate stationery from treatment chart orders
• Use of treatment charts which do not include a space for documentation of drug allergies or adverse reactions
• Use of treatment charts which do not include a separate space for route of administration
• Separate medical records for inpatient and outpatient visits
• Lack of drug information references and guidelines for parenteral administration on wards

Taking a leadership role in this multidisciplinary process will require careful definition of improvement goals, creating measurement systems to document improvement and testing innovative change concepts. It will also require creating the environment for improvement – no easy task.

As traditional roles in drug preparation, packaging and distribution fall away from the traditional practice of pharmacy, there will not only be ample opportunity to tackle these roles, but it might be considered part of a more contemporary definition of the practice of pharmacy – the profession that is responsible for the effectiveness, safety and appropriate use of pharmacotherapy.

CASE STUDY

A 32-year-old mother of three, in her fourth pregnancy, was admitted to hospital for delivery of her baby. She had received prenatal care through an obstetrician/gynaecologist and had a history of syphilis dating back 10 years. There was no documentation of whether she had received treatment. The laboratory tests for syphilis (RPR and FTA) were positive during her pregnancy. She was not treated during the prenatal period.

A baby boy was delivered. The mother indicated that she had been treated for syphilis before the prenatal period, but this could not be confirmed. A neonatologist was consulted, and he discussed the case with a paediatric infectious diseases specialist. They recommended that evaluation and treatment of possible congenital syphilis was indicated because of the undocumented treatment of the mother.

All tests were negative for congenital syphilis.

A prescription was written for a single dose of benzathine penicillin G, 50,000 units/kg. by intramuscular injection. It read: 'Benzathine Pen G. 150,000 u IM, X 1.' The order was hand-delivered to the pharmacy by a nurse. The pharmacist received the order, looked up the dose to confirm that it was correct, and called the nursery to confirm the baby's weight of 3 kg. Another pharmacist verified that the physician's order was correct. What the pharmacist thought she had done was to dispense penicillin that was available in the pharmacy – two syringes of 120,000 units of benzathine penicillin – and have them delivered to the nursery in a small plastic bag with a warning label for the nurse to note the strength of the medicine dispensed from the pharmacy. What the pharmacist really did was to misread 'u' as '0' and thus, prepare and send 1,200,000 units (1.2 million units) in each syringe to the unit. The penicillin was stocked in the pharmacy in syringes of 600,000 units/cc and 1.2 million units/2 cc and the pharmacist thought to dispense what was available.

The nurse saw the medication on the counter after it was delivered from the pharmacy and thought it was a lot of medication (high dose), but did not give the dose at that time, or look at the package or syringes. When another nurse came to administer the dose, it was determined that five intramuscular injections would be required to give the medication on the counter, since the label indicated the total dose required was 2.5 cc. of penicillin. The standard practice is to administer 0.25 to 0.5 cc per intramuscular injection to newborns.

The nurses conferred about how to give this large volume of medication and it was suggested that it be given by the intravenous (IV) route. None of the nurses had given this type of penicillin before. They looked for information about penicillin in reference books kept in the patient care area and found that penicillin could be given by slow IV push. The nurses did not know that there were two different types of penicillin: aqueous for IV administration and suspension for IM administration. This was not clear in the reference book that was consulted.

In the interest of the comfort of the infant, the nurses decided to administer the benzathine penicillin by IV injection. After administering 1.8 cc, or 1,050,000 units, the baby became limp and dusky and experienced cardiovascular arrest. Resuscitation was started, and after 50 minutes, the baby had a heart rate of 120 beats/min, but was severely acidotic. The baby suffered a second cardiac arrest and expired. The baby died of massive pulmonary emboli, oedema and congestion.

Questions

1. Is this an example of an ADE, an ADR or a medication error? Explain your answer.

This is an ADE because it resulted in injury to the patient. The event was caused by several medication errors – at the prescribing, dispensing and drug administration steps in the medication use process.

2. What type of medication errors contributed in this case?

There were several prescribing errors – writing an order for a medicine that was not needed, and using an unacceptable abbreviation ('U' instead of writing out the word 'unit'). There was a dispensing error in that a ten-fold dose was dispensed for the patient. There were several drug administration errors – changing the route of administration from IM to IV without talking to the prescriber, and administering a ten-fold overdose.

3. At what steps of the medication use process did these errors occur?

There were errors in three steps in the medication use process: prescribing, dispensing and administration.

4. What suggestions can you make to improve the medication use process in this hospital so that similar outcomes are avoided in the future?

Some suggestions include: a policy prohibiting the use of dangerous abbreviations, having medicines double-checked before dispensing, dispensing medicines as unit doses, and a policy prohibiting changing orders without calling the prescriber.

KEY MESSAGES

- There are significant opportunities to improve medication use safety by reducing medication errors.
- Much is known about how to reduce the frequency of medication errors by improving pharmacy systems and increasing the role of clinical pharmacists.
- The role of clinical pharmacists to improve medication safety includes a role in reducing errors in prescribing and drug administration, not just dispensing.

Further Reading

Allen EA and Barker KN. 1990. Fundamentals of medication error research. *Am J Hosp Pharm* 47:555–71.

American Society of Hospital Pharmacists. 1993. ASHP guidelines on preventing medication errors in hospital. *Am J Hosp Pharm* 50:305–14.

Barker KN and Allen EL. 1995. Research on drug-use system error. *Am J Health-Syst. Pharm* 52:400–3.

Barker KN, Heller WM, Brennan JJ et al. 1962. The problems of detecting medication errors in hospitals. *Am J Hosp Pharm* 19:360–9.

Bates DW, Boyle DL, Vander Vliet MB et al. 1995. Relationship between medication errors and adverse drug events. *J Gen Intern Med* 10:100–205.

Bates DW, Cousins DD, Flynn E et al. 2000. Consensus development conference statement on the safety of intravenous drug delivery systems: balancing safety and cost. *Hosp Pharm* 35:150–5.

Bates DW, Leape LL, Cullen DJ et al. 1998. Effect of computerized physician order entry and a team intervention on prevention of serious medication errors. *JAMA* 280:1311–16.

Bates DW, Spell N, Cullen DJ et al. 1997. The cost of adverse drug events in hospitalized patients. *JAMA* 277:307–11.

Bluml BM, McKenney JM, Cziraky MJ and Elswick RK, Jr. 1998. Interim report from Project ImPACT: Hyperlipidemia. *J Amer Pharm Assoc* 38:529–534.

Borel JM and Rascati KL. 1995. Effects of an automated, nursing unit-based drug-dispensing device on medication errors. *Am J Health-Syst Pharm* 52:1875–9.

Brennan TA, Leape LL, Laird NM et al. 1995. Incidence of adverse events and negligence in hospitalized patients – results of the Harvard Medical Practice Study I. *N Engl J Med* 324:370–6.

Classen DC, Pestotnik SL, Evans RS et al. 1991.Computerized surveillance of adverse drug events in hospital patients. *JAMA* 266:2847–51.

Classen DC, Pestotnik SL, Evans RS et al. 1997. Adverse drug events in hospitalized patients – excess length of stay, extra costs, and attributable mortality. *JAMA* 277:301–6.

Cohen MR. 2007. *Medication Errors, 2nd edition*. American Pharmacists Association: Washington, DC.

Cranor CW, Bunting BA and Christensen DB. 2003 The Ashville Project: Long-term clinical and economic outcomes of a community pharmacy diabetes care program. *J Am Pharm Assoc* 43:173–84.

Evans RS, Pestotnik SL, Classen DC et al. 1998. A computer-assisted program for antibiotics and other antiinfective agents. *N Eng J Med* 338:232–8.

High-Alert Medications. 2008. Joint Commission Resources: Oakbrook Terrace, IL.

Jha AK, Kuperman GJ, Teich JM et al. 1998. Identifying adverse drug events: developing a computer-based monitor and comparison with chart review and stimulated voluntary report. *J Am Med Inform Assn* 5:305–14.

Koppel R, Metlay, Cohen A et al. 2005. Role of computerized physician order entry systems in facilitating medication errors. *JAMA* 293:1197–1203.

Leape LL, Bates DW, Cullen KJ et al. 1995. Systems analysis of adverse drug events. *JAMA* 274:35–43.

Leape LL, Cullen DJ, Clapp MD et al. 1999. Pharmacist participation on physician rounds and adverse drug events in the intensive care unit. *JAMA* 82:267–70.

Leape LL, TA Brennan, NM Laird et al. 1995. The nature of adverse events in hospitalized patients – results of the Harvard Medical Practice Study II. *N Engl J Med* 324:377–84.

Lee YP and Schommer JC. 1996. Effect of pharmacist-managed anticoagulation clinic on warfarin-related hospital admissions. *Am J Health-Syst Pharm* 53:1580–3.

Lesar TS, Briceland L and Stein DS. 1997. Factors related to errors in medication prescribing. *JAMA* 277:312–17.

Lesar TS, Briceland LL, Delcoure K, et al 1990. Medication prescribing errors in a teaching hospital. *JAMA*. 263:2329-34.

Manasse HR and Thompson KK. 2005. *Medication Safety: A Guide for Healthcare Facilities*, American Society of Health-System Pharmacy: Bethesda, MD.

Medication Reconciliation Handbook. 2006. Joint Commission Resources: Oakbrook Terrace, IL.

Medication use: A system approach to reducing error, 2nd ed. 2008. Joint Commission Resources: Oakbrook Terrace, IL.

Must-have information for pharmacists about quality and patient safety. 2007. Joint Commission Resources: Oakbrook Terrace, IL

Nazdam DM. 1998. A System Approach to Medication Use, in: DD Cousins, (Ed) *Medication use – A Systems Approach to Reducing Errors*. Joint Commission on Accreditation of Healthcare Organizations, Oakbrook Terrace.

NCCMRP taxonomy of medication errors. Rockville, MD. USA: The National Coordinating Council for Medication Error Reporting and Prevention. http://nccmrp.org.

Paoletti RD, Suess TM, Lesko MG et al. 2007. Using bar-code technology and medication observation methodology for safer medication administration. *Am J Health-Sys . Pharm* 64:536–43.

Patterson TR and Nordstrom KA. 1968. An analysis of IV additive procedures on nursing units. *Am J Hosp Pharm* 25:134–7.

Pedersen CA and Gumper KF. 2008. ASHP national survey on informatics: Assessment of the adoption and use of pharmacy informatics in U.S. hospitals – 2007. *Am J Health-Syst Pharm* 65:2244–64.

Pedersen CA, Schneider PJ and Scheckelhoff DJ. 2009. ASHP National Survey of Pharmacy Practice in Hospital Settings: Dispensing and Administration – 2008. *Am J Health-Syst Pharm* 66:926–46.

Perlstein PH, Callison C, White M et al. 1979. Errors in drug computations during newborn intensive care. *Am J Dis Child* 133:376–9.

Poon EG, Cina JL, Churchill W et al. 2006. Medication dispensing errors and potential adverse drug events before and after implementing bar code technology in the pharmacy. *Ann Int Med* 145: 426–34.

Proceedings of a summit on preventing patient harm and death from i.v. medication errors. 2008. *Am J Health-Syst Pharm* 65:2367–79.

Sanders LH, Mabadeje SA and Avis KE. 1978. Evaluation of compounding accuracy and aseptic technique for intravenous admixtures. *Am J Hosp Pharm* 35:531–6.

Schneider PJ, Gift MG, Lee YP et al. 1995. Cost of medication-related problems at a university hospital. *Am J Health-Syst Pharm* 52:2415–8.

Schneider PJ. 1999. A review of the safety of intravenous drug delivery systems. *Hosp Pharm* 34: 1044–56.

Shultz S, White SJ and Latiolais CJ. 1973. Medication errors reduced by unit dose. *Hospitals - JAHA* 47(6):106–12.

Thompson WL and Feer TD. 1980. Incomplete mixing of drugs in intravenous solutions. *Crit. Care Med* 8:603–7.

Thur MP, Miller WA and Latiolais CJ. 1972. Medication errors in a nurse-controlled parenteral admixture program. *Am J Hosp Pharm* 29:298–304.

Top-priority actions for preventing adverse drug events in hospitals. 1996. *Am J Health-Syst Pharm* 53:747–51.

United States Department of Veterans Affaris (http://www.pbm.va.gov/vamedsafe/Adverse%20Drug%20Reaction.pdf) (accessed August 10, 2009).

Websites of Interest

Institute of Safe Medication Practices
http://www.ismp.org/

American Society of Health-System Pharmacists
http://www.ashp.org/

National Patient Safety Foundation
http://www.npsf.org/

Institute for Healthcare Improvement
http://www.ihi.org/ihi

American Pharmaceutical Association
http://www.pharmacist.com/

Hospital Pharmacy
www.factsandcomparisons.com/hospitalpharm/

Agency for Healthcare Research and Quality
www.ahrq.gov

US Food and Drug Administration
http://www.fda.gov/CDER/drug/MedErrors/default.htm

American Society of Medication Safety Officers
http://www.asmso.org/

The Joint Commission
http://www.jointcommission.org/

29

Pharmacoeconomics: Theory, Research and Practice

Duska Franic, Anandi V Law and Dev S Pathak

Learning Objectives

Upon completion of this chapter, the reader should be able to:

- Explain the need for pharmacoeconomics in the current environment of pharmacy practice
- Define the term pharmacoeconomics
- Distinguish between the five types of pharmacoeconomic evaluations
- Attain familiarity with pharmacoeconomic terminology
- Conduct a basic pharmacoeconomic evaluation of two or more drugs, therapies or programmes
- Evaluate published studies in the area of pharmacoeconomics

Scenario: You are the clinical pharmacist member of the Pharmacy and Therapeutics Committee at a mid-sized hospital, and have been given the responsibility of evaluating a new beta-blocker product Ezehart® for inclusion in the hospital drug formulary. Currently, your hospital already has a drug from the same class listed on the formulary – Bpblock®. Both beta-blockers are regarded as breakthrough products with new, but similar, mechanisms of action to reduce blood pressure in hypertensive patients. In addition to preventing myocardial infarction, your literature search reveals nominal clinical advantages with the newer agent. However, unlike other beta-blockers, there are substantial benefits in terms of quality of life.

Patients receiving Ezehart® versus Bpblock® for a three-month trial period reported less sleepiness, faintness and fatigue. In addition, sexual function, work well-being, and mental and emotional health were improved for patients on the newer agent. What type of pharmacoeconomic analysis would you conduct to determine whether

Ezehart®should be added to the formulary? Alternately, if you were the manufacturer of Ezehart®, what would be your plan of action to ensure that your product is chosen by physicians over the competitor, given the similarities?

Introduction

The scenario presented above is very familiar to individuals in Western countries, and is equally applicable to Indian clinical pharmacy and the pharmaceutical industry. In clinical settings, consideration must be given to:

- The therapeutic effectiveness of the agent for the patient sub-population
- The impact of therapeutic agent cost or impact on the hospital pharmacy budget, in addition to nursing care costs and lab costs
- Quality of life

In the industry, while there is stiff competition for market share, drug price control is also seen. There are numerous scenarios where decision making of this type, whether in clinical pharmacy or the pharmaceutical industry, requires understanding and balancing of clinical and economic knowledge and tools. Pharmacoeconomics is one such tool that aids in decision making using the combination of cost (economic) and consequences (clinical or humanistic endpoints).

Definition of Terms

Economics is the study of the allocation of **limited (scarce)** resources or **inputs** among **alternative uses** to satisfy unlimited wants for **outputs**. Thus, the three major elements of any economic analysis for the purpose of rational decision-making by individuals and societies are identification and choice among alternatives, assessment of costs and consequences, and decision-making within limited (or fixed) budgets.

The International Society for Pharmacoeconomics and Outcomes Research (ISPOR) defines the terms health economics and pharmacoeconomics as follows:

Health economics: 'The field of study that evaluates the behavior of individuals, firms, and markets in health care, and that usually focuses on the cost (inputs) and consequences (outcomes) of health care interventions, such as the use of drugs, devices, procedures, services and programs.'

Pharmacoeconomics: 'The field of study that evaluates the behavior of individuals, firms and markets relevant to the use of pharmaceutical products, services and programs, and which frequently focuses on the costs (inputs) and consequences (outcomes) of that use.'

Thus, pharmacoeconomics (PE) is a subfield of health economics. Operationally, the field of pharmacoeconomics consists of comparing outcomes (clinical, economic or humanistic) and costs (resource consumption) of pharmaceutical products, programmes and/or services to the next best alternatives from selected perspectives. The aim of this approach is to identify, measure, value and establish a link between both resource consumption and outcomes so that relative worth of selected pharmaceutical products, programmes and/or services can be established. The combination of cost and outcomes analysis may take many forms including cost minimisation analysis (CMA), cost–benefit analysis (CBA), cost effectiveness analysis (CEA), cost utility analysis (CUA) and/or cost–consequences analysis (CCA). The discipline of pharmacoeconomics draws upon various areas such as economics, epidemiology, medicine, pharmacy and the social sciences.

Four Es of Health Programme Evaluation

Most health programme evaluations have one or more of the following four objectives:

- Efficacy: Can it work? Does it do more good than harm under ideal conditions?
- Effectiveness: Does it work? What can be achieved under realistic conditions?
- Equity: Is it reaching those who need it (access)? Who gains and who loses (distribution)?
- Efficiency: Is it worth doing?

The economic evaluation of any healthcare or pharmaceutical normally limits itself to evaluating the efficiency of the programme relative to other programmes. However, economic evaluations are most useful to decision makers when they are preceded by studies investigating the other three objectives. It should be also noted that efficiency evaluation should not be superimposed on any programme or treatment that is not efficacious or effective. Readers interested in learning more about the principles and methods to conduct the other three types of evaluation studies are directed to Sackett's work.

History

Although the economic underpinnings of economic evaluation can be traced back to the works of Dupuit (1844), Wilfred Pareto (1906), Kaldor (1939) and Hicks (1939, 1941), the roots of pharmacoeconomics developed in the 1970s, following the evolution of pharmacy as a clinical discipline and the incorporation of the pharmaceutical sciences into the pharmacy curriculum. The concepts of cost–benefit and cost effectiveness analyses were first introduced in the pharmacy literature in 1978 by McGhan, Rowland and Bootman. Bootman et al. also published an early research article in 1979 in which cost–benefit analysis was used.

In 1983, Pathak offered a graduate-level course to provide 'an overview of the application of cost-benefit and cost-effectiveness analysis in health care with special emphasis on the application of these techniques to the delivery of pharmaceutical care' at the Ohio State University (OSU) College of Pharmacy. In 1984, the Merrell Dow Professorship, the first of its kind, was established at the OSU College of Pharmacy 'to initiate and direct a program of research and development addressing major issues confronting the delivery of pharmaceutical care. Some of these major issues are: cost effectiveness of pharmaceuticals for the health care delivery system; cost-benefit analysis of provision of high quality of information and counseling by pharmacists for the 'wellness' of the American public; and socio-economic impact analysis of major public policy decisions from a retrospective basis.'

Finally, the term pharmacoeconomics itself first appeared in 1986 in print when a presentation by Townsend was published, describing the need to develop research activities in this emerging discipline. The popularity of pharmacoeconomics resulted in a journal of the same name in 1992. The discipline (and the term) has now been adopted by the pharmaceutical industry, academia and practitioners worldwide as a part of health science.

Misperceptions about Pharmacoeconomics (PE) and Other Selected Terms

Misperception 1: PE = Cost containment. While PE analysis may result in cost containment, it is not its only goal. Full PE analysis considers clinical, economic and humanistic outcomes and not just cost containment.

Misperception 2: PE = Cost effectiveness. While many PE studies use cost effectiveness analysis, CEA is but only one tool of PE analysis.

Misperception 3: PE = Medication Utilisation Evaluation (MUE). MUE (formerly known as drug utilisation evaluation or review, DUE or DUR) focuses on assessing the appropriateness of drug use and it may use quantitative and/or qualitative approaches. Sometimes, MUE studies have considered resources utilised and other economic variables. But this is not always the case.

Misperception 4: PE = Outcomes research. These two terms are sometimes used interchangeably within the field of pharmacy. However, outcomes research is a broad discipline that involves evaluating the impact of healthcare interventions. Depending on the perspective, the outcomes could be clinical, economic or humanistic. Pharmacoeconomics is one of the tools used in evaluating the impact of a drug or healthcare intervention on health outcomes and in guiding decision-making.

Misperception 5: Cost savings = Cost–benefit analysis. These two terms are often used interchangeably; however, they are fundamentally different. Cost–benefit analysis incorporates all benefits by including individual preferences using the contingent valuation or willingness to pay method. Dollars saved, although an important consideration in instituting a programme, does not incorporate individual preferences as a benefit measure. Studies measuring only cost savings, thus, are in effect cost analyses since they do not incorporate all benefits based on individual preferences.

Need for Pharmacoeconomics in Indian Pharmacy Practice

The need for this tool is not so different in the context of Indian pharmacy practice from its need elsewhere, since it offers assistance under resource constraints, tight budgets and competing programmes. However, some of the applications may be specific to the Indian environment for various reasons such as priorities of the populace, drug price controls, lack of specific product patents and the relatively limited spread of the concept of health insurance. However, the following reasons are important in increasing the relevance of pharmaceoeconomics in the Indian context:

- As Indian pharmaceutical research and manufacturing firms expand into world markets and globalisation increases, evidence from pharmacoeconomic studies in drug launches and in a competitive drug market may become imperative.
- The advent of the clinical PharmD curricula in Indian colleges of pharmacy signals a changing era

where drug selection by a pharmacist into a formulary and therapeutic recommendations for patients will use evidence-based pharmacotherapy – evaluation of cost and consequence will then become essential.

- Even with drug price controls, in a populace that has reduced access to costly medications, the ability to provide lifesaving medications at a low cost is important from a public health/policy angle, especially for diseases with fast spread and high morbidity and mortality. In such cases, pharmacoeconomic projections help governments, public health institutions and commercial firms that are called upon to provide medications.

Thus a solid conceptual understanding and application of this field is of increasing importance.

Pharmacoeconomics can aid in decision making in evaluating the affordability of and access to the right medication to the right patient at the right time, comparing two drugs in the same therapeutic class or drugs with similar mechanisms of action (as with the beta-blocker example presented at the beginning of the chapter) and in establishing accountability that the claims by a manufacturer regarding a drug are justified.

Some specific scenarios may involve deciding a) whether a drug should be included in a hospital formulary, b) which drug would provide net positive benefits to a particular group of patients, c) which would be the best drug for a pharmaceutical manufacturer to develop and the right price to market it, and d) what is the expected quality-of-life improvement with a certain drug when trading-off its side effects. Some of these scenarios will be presented in case format at the end of the text.

In addition, many of the statements contained in the Vision 2010 statement prepared by the sub-group of the Prime Minister's Task Force on Pharmaceutical and Knowledge Based Industries and published in the IDMA Bulletin (Indian Drug Manufacturers Association Bulletin), June 2001, clearly indicate that PE tools will be needed in evaluating some of the objectives included in these statements. Following are a few selected statements:

For the People of India: To build a 'Healthy India' by 2010 with: Wide-spread availability of therapeutic drugs and medical services of acceptable quality at affordable rate to all citizens.

For the Indian Pharma(ceutical) Industry: Create a brand image for India as a cost-economic supplier of quality pharmaceuticals; to synergize the scientific principles of traditional systems of medicine, with those of modern systems of medicine and to thereby launch innovative and inexpensive products for public healthcare. Create an enabling Environment for Research and Innovation – promote and fund research on special tropical diseases of interest to India and other developing countries through innovative public/private partnerships.

De-control of Prices: Gradually decrease the span of price control over the Pharmaceutical Industry by encouraging indigenous manufacturers and competition.

Pharmacoeconomic principles and tools can assist in measuring and evaluating each of the above statements. It is obvious that pharmacoeconomic training will be needed to evaluate many of these objectives in the future. This is evidenced by recently developed postgraduate courses on pharmacoeconomics in India by the Pharmaceutical and Allied Manufacturers and Distributors Association (PAMDEL) jointly with the Bombay College of Pharmacy. This was shortly followed by the formation of the India Chapter of International Society of Pharmacoeconomics and Outcomes Research (ISPOR-INDIA) in 2006 (for more information about the chapter, go to www.ispor.org)

Pharmacoeconomic Evaluations

All pharmacoeconomic evaluations are based on answers to two basic questions: 1) Are there two or more alternatives? 2) Do the interventions examine costs and health effects?

Based on the answer to each of these questions, a classification of pharmacoeconomic evaluation studies is developed and presented (Fig. 29.1). If only one treatment or drug or programme is examined then it is simply a descriptive analysis of that treatment, drug or programme and hence, can be classified as a partial economic evaluation. If the pharmaceutical programme evaluation consists of two or more alternatives but limits itself to a discussion of costs or effects only, then this type of study is also considered a partial economic evaluation. However, if a PE evaluation comprises a comparison of two or more alternatives and attempts to link both

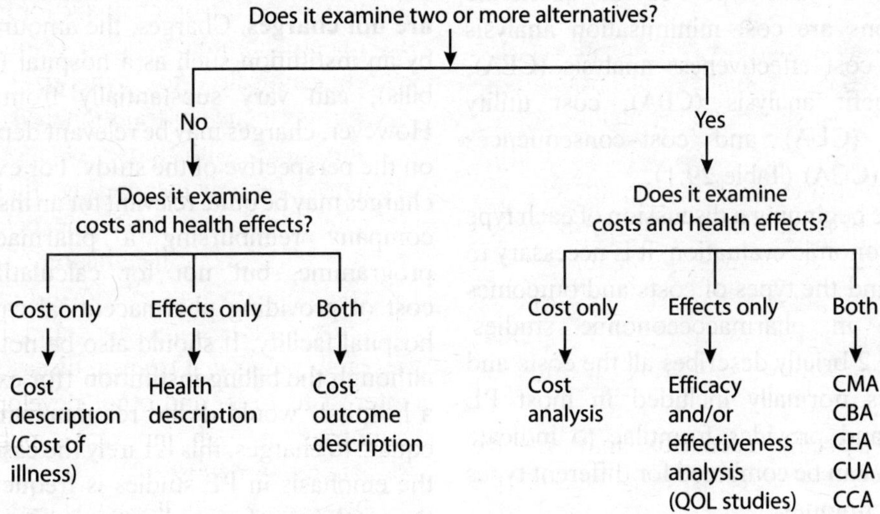

Figure 29.1 Classification of pharmacoeconomic evaluation studies

Source: Adapted from Drummond et al. 2005

CMA: Cost minimisation analysis
CBA: Cost–benefit analysis
CEA: Cost effectiveness analysis
CUA: Cost utility analysis
CCA: Cost–consequences analysi

Table 29.1 Types of pharmacoeconomic evaluation techniques

Method	Cost measurement	Outcome measurement	Decision rule
Cost Minimization Analysis (CMA)	Monetary	Outcomes of alternatives assumed identical	Lowest monetary cost
Cost–Benefit Analysis (CBA)	Monetary	All outcomes translated into monetary units	Net monetary gain
Cost Effectiveness Analysis (CEA)	Monetary	Non-monetary physical units of effectiveness	CE ratios using incremental or marginal analysis
Cost Utility Analysis (CUA)	Monetary	Utility values and Quality Adjusted Life Years (QALY)	Cost per QALY and League Tables
Cost Outcomes Analysis (COA) or Cost–Consequence Analysis (CCA)	Monetary	Combination of quality of life and natural units	Choice left to the decision maker

Source: Adapted from unpublished notes of DS Pathak.

costs and effects, then these evaluations are considered full economic evaluations.

The five main types of full economic evaluations are cost minimisation analysis (CMA), cost effectiveness analysis (CEA), cost–benefit analysis (CBA), cost utility analysis (CUA) and cost–consequences analysis (CCA) (Table 29.1).

Before beginning a discussion of each type of full economic evaluation, it is necessary to understand the types of costs and outcomes included in pharmacoeconomic studies. Table 29.2 briefly describes all the costs and outcomes normally included in most PE studies and provides formulae to indicate how they can be combined for different types of PE techniques.

There are four main types of costs: those incurred by the health sector; those incurred by the patient and the family, external costs and productivity losses (Table 29.2). This classification follows recommendations by Drummond et al., instead of using the typical economic classification of direct, indirect, intangible and external costs (see *Glossary*).

Furthermore, it should be noted that **costs are not charges**. Charges, the amount billed by an institution such as a hospital (patient bills), can vary substantially from costs. However, charges may be relevant depending on the perspective of the study. For example, charges may be quite relevant for an insurance company reimbursing a pharmaceutical programme, but not for calculating the cost of providing pharmaceutical care in a hospital facility. It should also be noted that although the billing institution (for example, a hospital) would desire reimbursements to equate to charges, this is rarely the case. Also, the emphasis in PE studies is frequently on the total cost of providing a pharmaceutical programme since many studies take a societal perspective in evaluating programmes.

Finally, the real (or 'economic') cost of any programme is not only monetary, it also includes the health outcomes forgone in another project by taking the current project,

Table 29.2 Types, costs and outcomes used in pharmacoeconomic studies

Inputs: Costs (Resource Utilization)	*Outputs (ECHO)*
Healthcare Sector (C1): Cost of providing care by the programme (that is, organising and operating costs within the health sector) as well as the cost of continuing care such as treatment of infections or other side effects. It may include 'direct' costs such as overhead, capital and variable costs such as drug costs, laboratory tests and physician visits.	Economic (Monetary) Outcomes: Reduction in resource use or savings is included in this category. This may accrue to the healthcare sector (S1), patients and family (S2), non-health sector (S3) and productivity gains (S4). This may include savings due to treatment (direct monetary benefits) as well as production gains to return to work (indirect monetary benefit).
Patient and Family (C2): This includes 'direct' costs such as out-of-pocket costs, co-payment, travel cost to hospital, costs to accommodate the patient. and time consumed by patient (and family) receiving treatment.	Clinical Outcomes/ Physical effects E = Changes in physical effects in natural units, for example, lab values, # of lives saved, # of deaths averted, # of disability days reduced etc. H: Humanistic outcomes
External costs (C3): This category includes all resources consumed in other (non-health) sectors. Items such as resources consumed by the volunteer sector, church kitchens, homemaker services, etc. are included here. Productivity Losses (C4) Inclusion of 'indirect' costs or 'productivity costs' due to loss of leisure or work time due to sickness is appropriate only in some circumstances.	V: Changes in other values not necessarily related to health, such as the process of care, information received and reassurance. U: Changes in QALY (quality adjusted life years) based on valuation of health state preferences W: Willingness to pay or contingent valuation W': Global willingness to pay (includes all outputs listed above)

CMA: (C1 – S1) or (C1 + C2 + C3 + C4) – (S1 + S2 + S3 + S4)
CEA: (C1 – S1) / E; [(C1 + C2 + C3+ C4) – (S1 + S2 + S3+ S4)] / E
CUA: (C1 – S1) / U; [(C1 + C2 + C3+ C4)] /U
CBA: (W') – (C1 + C2 + C3+ C4); [(W + V + S1 + S2 + S3+ S4) – (C1 + C2 + C3+ C4)]
CCA: List all relevant parameters in an array format.
Source: Adapted from Drummond et al 2005

that is, the opportunity costs. Economic costs are not easy to measure and in many analyses are ignored in favour of accounting costs. Interested readers are referred to the ISPOR Drug Standards Task Force which is currently developing standards on assessing drug costs in pharmacoeconomic studies at the ISPOR website (see *Websites of Interest*).

'Outcomes research is the scientific discipline that evaluates the effect of health care interventions on patient-related, if not patient-specific, clinical, humanistic and economic outcomes' (Table 29.3). The formula provided to link costs and outcomes for the purpose of using various PE techniques (Table 29.2) are not described

Table 29.3 Types of outcomes

Clinical outcomes	*Economic outcomes*	*Humanistic outcomes*
Final *Mortality* (examples) ♦ Number of deaths/lives saved ♦ Life-years gained ♦ Cure rate *Morbidity* (examples) Strokes, myocardial infarctions, days of hospitalisation, days of disability **Intermediate** *Mortality* (examples) ♦ Cases identified ♦ Response rate *Morbidity* (examples) BP, serum cholesterol, drugs correctly prescribed	*Utilisation of health resources* (examples) ♦ Hospital days ♦ Physician visits ♦ Medications ♦ Services such as nursing or food delivery *Non-monetary* ♦ Absenteeism ♦ Job changes ♦ Time for returning to work ♦ Productivity	♦ Intangibles ♦ Quality of life ♦ Utility including QALY

in detail, but it should be recognised that the perspective adopted in conducting such analysis plays a major role in what is included in the costs or outcomes side of the equation. Perspective is an important consideration in PE because costs and consequences and thereby, the results of the PE evaluation, can differ based on whose point of view is taken. There are no rules for which is the correct perspective to select, although the societal perspective is preferred because of its broad implications. It is possible to select more than one perspective but that is not usually done because it increases complexity and confounds decision making. This may become more apparent in the discussion of each type of pharmacoeconomic evaluation. For more details, please consult Drummond, O'Brien, Stoddard and Torrance.

Types of PE Evaluations

PE evaluations are divided into four types, based on differences in measuring the outcome (Table 29.2).

Cost minimisation analysis (CMA): When two or more drugs or alternative programmes or interventions have demonstrated equivalent impact in terms of the consequences of an intervention, only the costs of the alternatives need to be compared. Such a cost analysis is referred to as a CMA. In effect, such an analysis identifies the least costly alternative in terms of monetary value (rupees or other currency) and hence, can be considered as a special case of CEA.

Since the primary assumption for the CMA is that the outcomes of the alternatives are not different, it is imperative that the equivalency of outcomes be established based on valid information such as concurrent trials, published studies in peer-reviewed articles or information available from clinical trials. It is important to consider what happens when two drugs have demonstrated similar efficacy/effectiveness but have different adverse effect profiles.

Tighe and Goodman, for example, reported their experiences with carboplatin as compared to cisplatin in treating stage II/IV ovarian cancer. They found that while carboplatin was more expensive per dose than cisplatin, it was cheaper when the total cost was taken into account because of lower toxicity encountered with its use. Further, treatment with cisplatin required hospital admission because of the need for intensive hydration before and after the procedure. Since the effects of these two drugs were considered equivalent, this is an example of CMA (Table 29.4).

Cost–benefit analysis (CBA): This compares the total cost of each alternative to resultant consequences or benefits of the intervention, measured in monetary units. Benefits are measured using the human capital approach or contingent valuation, also commonly referred to as the willingness to pay method (WTP). The human capital approach equates benefits with productivity gain or earnings. It is measured using a wage rate and the time missed due to illness or intervention. Although ideally it can measure the value of employed and unemployed individuals, it tends to discriminate against homemakers and the unemployed since they are not 'productive' in wage-earning terms. It also discriminates against low wage earners since their human capital is assumed to be lower than that of a high wage earner.

Example: Assume 240 working days; # days (365) – #weekend days (104) – vacation days (14) – #sick leave days (7).

WTP measures an individual's desirability or 'utility' for a programme by determining how much money (rupees) he or she is willing to lose to purchase access to improved health. In healthcare, CBA is the least popular method of pharmacoeconomic analysis.

It can be used to compare the value of alternatives whose outcomes are in different

Table 29.4 Comparative cost (£) for the treatment of Stage II/IV ovarian cancer with carboplatin and cisplatin: An example of CMA

Drugs	*Carboplatin £*	*Cisplatin £*
Carboplatin (450 mg) or Cisplatin (100 mg)	205.71	17.90
Dexamethasone	2.34	—
Metoclopramide (150 mg IV)	—	3.60
Domperidone tablets	3.47	—
0.9% IV Saline	0.55	3.30
Total drugs (+ 15% value added tax)	243.88	28.50
Hospital bed	8.00	324.00
Senior registrar's time (1 hr)	8.70	—
Total	260.58	352.60

Source: Tighe M and Goodman S 1998. Carboplatin versus cisplatin. *Lancet* 1372–1373

units. The monetary value of the consequences and costs are converted to their net present value (by a process called discounting) and then compared as net benefit (benefit minus costs) or as a ratio (benefits/costs). The alternative with the largest net benefit (or benefit to cost ratio) is evaluated as the best economic alternative. For example, the benefit of a programme can be measured by asking a patient the maximum amount of money he or she would be willing to give up in order to have access to an intervention (that is, willingness to pay or WTP). Thus, the WTP for a benefit can and often does exceed the actual cost of therapy. If the benefits exceed the cost, the intervention is regarded worthwhile; however, if the cost exceeds the benefits, the programme should not be accepted since it results in an overall loss of dollars or rupees.

In the 1980s and early '90s, the surge of PE articles published resulted in some

Table 29.5 Cost analysis of preconception care versus prenatal care for women with established diabetes mellitus

Cost	Preconception care	Prenatal care
Programme costs	$11,294,100 (3)	$9,296,900 (1)
Adverse outcomes		
maternal	1,989,749	3,191,425
neonatal	7,665,300	10,181,367
subtotal	9,655,079 (4)	13,372,792 (2)
Total Cost	20,949,179	22,669,692

Net cost savings= 22,669,692 – 20,949,179 = $1.72 million

Source: Adapted from Elixhauser A, Weschler JM and Kitzmiller JL et al. 1993. Cost-benefit analysis of preconception care for women with established diabetes mellitus. *Diabetes Care* 16(8):1146–1157.

confusion between the terms cost savings and cost–benefit analysis (see *Misconception* 5 for more details). As a result, readers cannot assume that an article entitled CBA truly is a CBA. For example, Elixhauser et al. published an article labelled CBA. Economists would argue since individual preferences were not measured using contingent valuation, this paper is in fact a cost analysis. The cost analysis study was performed to 'determine whether the additional costs of preconception care are balanced by the savings from averted complications'. The study compared two alternatives of obstetric care for diabetic mothers: preconception care (women seek obstetric care prior to pregnancy) and prenatal care (current standard of care). The results, as reported in Table 29.5, indicate that the prenatal care programme for high-risk populations could result in significant monetary savings to the third party (insurance companies). However, these results should be viewed as summarising cost savings, not a CBA.

From Table 29.5, authors estimated a cost/benefit ratio where 'benefits' = (2–4) and 'costs' = (3–1), therefore B/C = (2–4)/(3–1) = 1.86. The terms cost–benefit and benefit–cost analysis are both used in healthcare literature, depending on how the ratio is calculated. Both terms are acceptable. Thus, a B/C ≥1 or a C/B < 1 are considered beneficial programmes. In other words, authors listed the cost savings of the programme as a benefit. Although cost savings is obviously financially beneficial, this measure is not consistent with the economic use of all benefits or incorporation of patient preferences. This will be explicated in the next example.

An example of benefits measured using willingness to pay was presented by O'Brien et al. Authors estimated the value of a new anti-depressant, moclobemide, in comparison to tricyclic anti-depressants (TCAs) which have equivalent efficacy but a higher incidence of adverse events. In the study, respondents/patients with a history of mild to moderate depression were asked to rank, from most to least bothersome, a list of seven common side effects associated with the use of TCAs. Next, they were asked to assume they had two choices: they could continue taking their TCA with specified probability of side effects or they could take a new drug with a lower incidence of these side effects. However, the new drug was more expensive and not covered by their health insurance. Respondents were asked what was the maximum they were willing to pay for the extra benefits of the new drug per month? Respondents were also informed that access to the newer agent would require them to pay out of pocket. Table 29.6 presents the monthly cost of moclobemide versus four TCAs, the net cost of switching from TCA to moclobemide (a negative cost is a cost savings), WTP for reduction in incidence of adverse events (the monetary value of the benefits, and the resultant cost–benefit ratio. In this example, instead of calculating B/C ratios, the authors presented the net benefit of the programme (B–C); thus, for a programme to be beneficial, B–C ≥ 0.

Ideally, all costs and benefits of the programme should be identified and valued for a CBA. However, more often than not, it is difficult to measure and assign a monetary value to various benefits such as patient satisfaction, or impact of the programme on caregivers. In such cases, these variables are defined as 'intangible benefits' and are used as additional inputs for decisions, or the analysis is changed to a cost effectiveness

Table 29.6 Costs, benefits and net benefit switch from tricyclic anti-depressant (TCA) to moclobemide (Adapted from Table VI, O'Brien et al. 1995)

Drug	*Drug cost per month*	*Net cost for switch* [a]	*WTP Range*		*Net benefit**
			WTP_U [b]	*WTP_L* [c]	*(a–b and a–c)*
moclobemide	61.5				
TCAs					
amitryptyline	9.9	51.6	117.6	36.2	indeterminant
imipramine	10.8	50.7	117.6	36.2	indeterminant
desipramine	75.6	–14.1	117.6	36.2	>0
clomipramine	76.8	–15.3	117.6	36.2	>0

[a] Calculated by subtracting average patient monthly cost of moclobemide from average patient monthly cost of TCA.

[b] Upper bound of WTP.

[c] Lower bound of WTP.

*Net benefit less than zero does not support changing over from TCA to moclobemide. Net benefit greater than zero supports the conversion of TCA to moclobemide.

Indeterminant means that depending on whether the upper or lower bound of WTP range was used the net benefit will be greater than or less than zero, therefore, data is too broad to support a decision regarding conversion.

analysis or cost–consequences analysis. The type of costs and benefits considered in the analysis depends on the perspective or objective of the study.

Cost effectiveness analysis (CEA): Cost effectiveness analysis is a technique used to aid in decision making between alternatives; when the costs are measured in monetary terms but the consequences are measured in natural unit changes in health (life-years increased or number of side effects decreased).

The definition of cost effectiveness used in this chapter is 'having an additional benefit worth the additional cost'. In a comparison of two drugs, X and Y, the decision is straightforward if X is less costly and more effective (X becomes the drug of choice) or more costly and less effective than Y (X will be dropped from the selection). In other scenarios, careful analyses and decision rules are necessary.

Table 29.7 presents nine possible scenarios for a cost effectiveness analysis. Here, the alternative with the lower cost to effectiveness ratio is thought preferable. A caveat to be considered at this time is that these analyses only present quantitative ratios to the decision maker. A low cost effectiveness ratio (CER) may not be considered to be equally favourable by two decision makers, because of differing perspectives and affordability.

In general, in cost effectiveness analyses, the effectiveness metric of the two comparators should be the same; that is, they should have a common measurable unit. Demonstrations of effectiveness must be comparative: they should measure the outcomes of the control and experimental groups. The evidence should result in a quantitative estimate of the relative effectiveness of the experimental group that is both reliable (reproducible) and valid (a true, unbiased measure of effectiveness).

Table 29.7 Scenarios in cost-effectiveness analysis

Change in effectiveness	*Change in cost*		
	Positive	***Zero***	***Negative***
Positive	C. More effective and more costly	B. More effective but same cost	Adopt
Zero	Avoid*	Not C/E: Neutral on both*	A. Less costly and as effective
Negative	Avoid*	Avoid*	D. Less effective and less costly

A strategy is viewed to be more cost-effective if it is:

A: At least as effective at less cost

B: More effective at the same cost

C: More effective and more costly but additional effectiveness more than offsets the increase in cost

D: Less effective and less costly but additional cost reductions more than offset the reduction in effectiveness. This is not particularly useful if the reduction in effectiveness is great and the difference clinically relevant. However, if it less toxic, that may be a significant offset.

Note: * = If in these instances, effectiveness is defined only clinically, intangible or humanistic measures may be investigated before a final decision.

Table 29.8 Guidelines for evaluating evidence of effectiveness

Level of evidence	*Type of evidence*	*Recommendation grade*
I	Large randomised trials with clear-cut results and low risk of error (includes meta-analysis)	A
II	Small randomised trials with uncertain results (and moderate to high risk of error)	B
III	Non-randomised concurrent cohort studies	C
IV	Non-randomised historical cohort studies	C
V	Case series without controls	C

Source: Cook DJ, Guyatt GH, Laupacis A and Sackett DL . 1992. Rules of evidence and clinical recommendations on the use of antithrombotic agents. *Chest* 102(4): 305S–311S.

Sometimes, prospective studies are either expensive or premature. In such cases, the evidence can be demonstrated by using retrospective data from published studies. Evidence of effectiveness in a CEA can be evaluated using guidelines, as provided in Table 29.8. Although CEA are criticised more so for their effectiveness data, guidelines for levels of evidence for economic analysis are also available and can be categorised from 1 (multi-level sensitivity analysis) to 5 (expert opinion).

Most studies using CEA report average cost effectiveness ratios (CER) as well as incremental CER (ICER). Average CER is the total cost divided by the total effectiveness for each group. ICER is the added cost per additional effect gained for one alternative as compared to another. If a new therapy costs less and is more effective than the original therapy, it is called the dominant therapy and hence, no incremental CER is considered necessary.

An example of how CEA can be used in deciding cost effectiveness in a pharmacy

Table 29.9 Cost effectiveness analysis for cholesterol reduction

Alternatives	*C*	*ΔCost*	*E*	*ΔE*	*ICER=ΔC/ΔE*
Diet alone	13.44	—	(1.73)	—	—
Drug A	289.32	275.88	12.65	14.38	19.18
Drug C	723.73	434.41	13.71	1.06	409.82
Drug E-2	1,315.21	566.09	19.57	5.86	471.74
Drug E-3	4,916.61	3615.21	26.81	7.24	499.34

Key: C=cost, Δ=Change, E=effect (Reduction in total cholesterol level mg/dl), ICER=incremental cost effectiveness analysis ratio.

Source: Based on, Hakim Z, Pierson JF and Pathak DS. 1996. A proposed model for conducting institutional-specific cost-effectiveness analysis: a case study of lipid-lowering agents. *Pharmacy Practice Management Quarterly* 16(1):79–97.

setting is provided in Table 29.9. The results reported are slightly modified from the original study by Hakim, Pierson and Pathak. The original study was conducted at a Veterans Affairs Outpatient Clinic (VAOC) in a large Midwestern city, from the perspective of the pharmacy department of VAOC, to evaluate the cost effectiveness of four lipid-lowering agents. These four drugs were consuming a large percentage of the pharmacy budget but had varying costs and degrees of effectiveness. The alternatives considered were: No drug treatment, or 'diet' recommendation alone and four lipid lowering agents – drugs A, C and two different doses of drug E.

The study was conducted using four measures of effectiveness: changes in total cholesterol level, high density lipids (HDL), low density lipids (LDL) and triglycerides. Table 29.9 reports results based on the measures of total cholesterol level only and treatment alternatives are listed from lowest to highest cost (second column). The results indicate that all four combination treatments (drug and diet) were more effective than diet alone, having varying cost effectiveness ratios. Diet alone actually resulted in higher total cholesterol levels, leading to a negative or undesirable effect. Which drug therapy to use, thus, become the decision of affordability and the clinically relevant target of effectiveness.

Decision analysis and CEA: If we assume that total cholesterol was the most important clinical outcome, a decision could be made based on drug costs and total cholesterol levels with the use of a 'decision tree'. This is designed to help the decision-maker make decisions by incorporating all the possible choices, probabilities and resultant outcomes. Since diet alone resulted in higher cholesterol levels, we will examine the remaining four drug therapies (combination treatments) in Table 29.9.

Decision trees are read from left to right and can be used to estimate CEA ratios. In this example, as shown in *Appendix A*, costs are measured in dollars and effects in total cholesterol levels. The tree provides summary data by informing the decision-maker which alternative is most cost effective (which alternative has the lowest CEA ratio). The tree was developed using a software program called Treeage® (see *Websites of Interest*).

As can be seen in Fig. 29.2a, we first start with a decision. In this case, the decision to treat high cholesterol levels is presented by the square node or box. At this point, the decision-maker can choose one of four therapies. Each of these four therapies is followed by a circle or 'chance' node, which represents probabilities beyond the control of the decision-maker – either a side effect occurs or it doesn't. The probabilities were obtained from the literature. Note that the sum of the probabilities at each circle is 1 and the probabilities are mutually exclusive and exhaustive.

Next, the tree branch is followed by a triangle or 'terminal node'. This is the end of the outcome measurement of interest and is presented by two numbers separated by a '/'. The first number is the cost associated with that branch: note how all costs associated with side effects are higher than the comparator without side effects since side effects require further treatment. The second number after the separator is the 'effect'. Note that for each treatment alternative the effect number is the same – this means that whether a side effect occurs or not, the impact on total cholesterol levels will be the same. In this

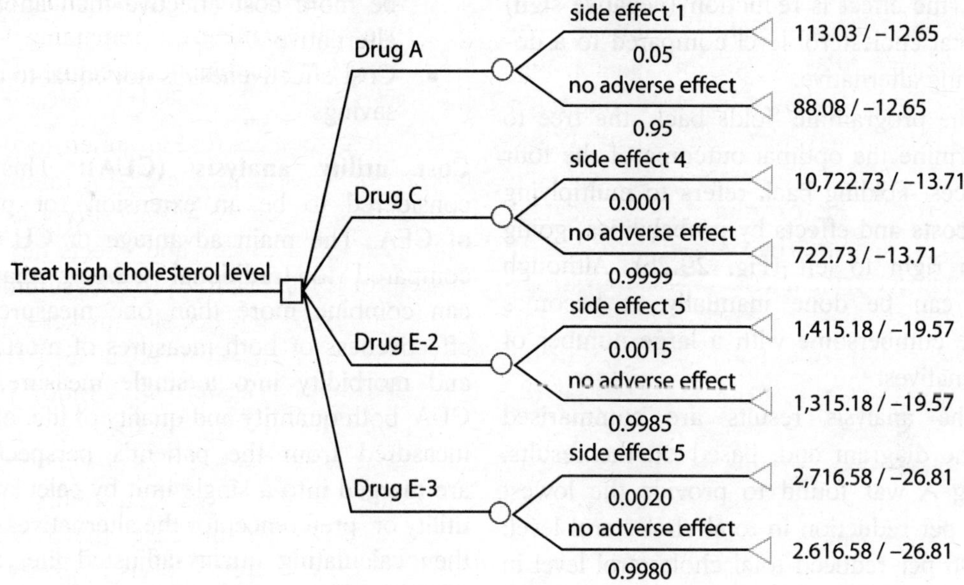

Figure 29.2a Decision tree comparing four drug treatments for high cholesterol level treatment. All costs are measured in US dollars and all effects are cholesterol level reduction (hence negative sign) measured in mg/dl: Presentation of raw data (*Adapted from Hakim, Pierson and Pathak 1996*)

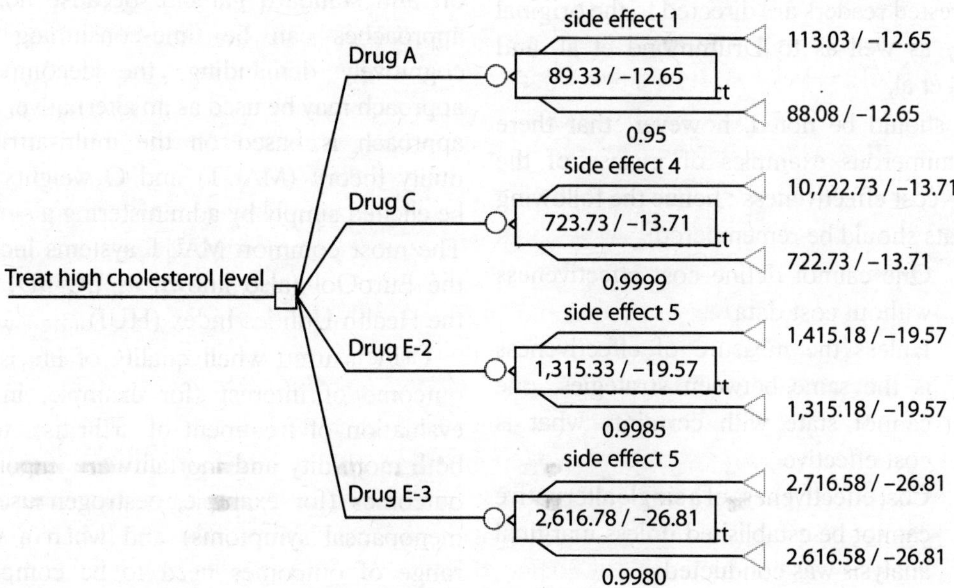

Figure 29.2b 'Rolled back' decision tree. (*Adapted from Hakim, Pierson and Pathak 1996*)

case, the effect is reduction (negative sign) in total cholesterol level compared to a do-nothing alternative.

The programme 'folds back' the tree to determine the optimal outcome of the four choices. Folding back refers to multiplying the costs and effects by probabilities, going from right to left (Fig. 29.2b). Although this can be done manually, it becomes quite cumbersome with a large number of alternatives.

The analysis results are summarised in the diagram and, based on the results, Drug A was found to provide the lowest cost per reduction in total cholesterol level: $7.06 per reduced total cholesterol level in mg/dl (89.33/–12.65 = –7.06). Drug C rates second at $52.79 per mg/dl of total cholesterol reduction (723.73–13.71); however, based on this analysis, Drug A is preferred. The other implications of CEA ratios are beyond the scope of this chapter. Interested readers are directed to the original study as well as to Drummond et al. and Gold et al.

It should be noted, however, that there are numerous examples of misuse of the term 'cost effectiveness'; hence the following caveats should be remembered:

- One cannot define cost effectiveness without cost data
- Unless the measure of effectiveness is the same between strategies, one cannot state with certainty what is cost effective
- Cost effectiveness of a single alternative cannot be established unless marginal analysis was conducted
- One cannot state that an alternative is the 'most cost effective', it can only be more cost effective than another alternative
- Cost effectiveness is not equal to cost savings

Cost utility analysis (CUA): This is considered to be an extension (or part) of CEA. The main advantage of CUA as compared to traditional CEA is that it can combine more than one measure of effectiveness or both measures of mortality and morbidity into a single measure. In CUA, both quantity and quality of life, often measured from the patient's perspective, are merged into a single unit by calculating utility or 'preference' for the alternatives and then calculating quality-adjusted life-years (QALY). These preferences or Q weights can be measured using the 'holistic' or 'decomposed' approaches.

Holistic approaches include the rating scale (also known as the visual analogue scale and thermometer scale), time trade-off and standard gamble. Because holistic approaches can be time-consuming and cognitively demanding, the decomposed approach may be used as an alternative. This approach is based on the multi-attribute utility theory (MAUT) and Q weights can be elicited simply by administering a survey. The most common MAUT systems include the EuroQol (also known as EQ-5D) and the Health Utilities Index (HUI).

CUA is used when quality of life is the outcome of interest (for example, in the evaluation of treatment of arthritis), when both morbidity and mortality are important outcomes (for example, oestrogen use for menopausal symptoms) and when a wide range of outcomes need to be compared across programmes. CUA should not be used if single intermediate outcomes will

Table 29.10 CUA of maintenance treatments of recurrent depression

Therapy	*Direct costs (Lifetime) US$*	*QALY*	*ΔCost*	*ΔQALY*	*ICER*
Placebo	21,204	9.56			—
Imipramine	19,573	14.98	(1631)	5.42	Lower cost and higher QALY values. Incremental analysis not necessary
IPT-M[1]	34,316	15.18	$14,743	0.20	$73,715/ QALY[2] $2,333/QALY[3]
IPT-M and Imipramine	48,390	15.61	$14,074	0.43	$32,730/QALY[4] $45,741/QALY[5]

Δ=change, QALY=quality adjusted life years, CER=cost effectiveness ratio – comparison of therapies to placebo, ICER=incremental cost effectiveness ratio (here the 'effect' is measured in QALYs)= ΔCost/ΔQALY

Source: Kamlet MS, Paul N, Greenhouse J and Kupfer D et al. 1995. Cost-utility analysis of maintenance treatment for recurrent depression. *Controlled Clinical Trials* 16:17–40.

[1] IPT-M = Interpersonal Therapy – Maintenance

[2] Incremental ratio as compared to Imipramine

[3] Incremental ratio as compared to Placebo. Interpretation: the expected increase in cost of IPT-M over placebo is $2,333 per additional QALY

[4] Incremental ratio as compared to IPT-M

[5] Incremental ratio as compared to Imipramine

be enough to measure the effectiveness of a therapy, or when natural units can do as good a job (for example, restricted days due to disability), or if the cost of the analysis is projected to be too high simply because conducting a CUA is more complex than conducting a CEA.

Table 29.10 summarises the results of a CUA study comparing placebo therapy and three maintenance therapies for recurrent depression. The three maintenance therapies were imipramine maintenance (drug), interpersonal therapy maintenance (IPT-M), and a combination of the two. Results indicated that the drug therapy was dominant over placebo therapy since it had lower cost of treatment (by $1,631) and higher effectiveness in terms of QALYs (by 5.42 quality-adjusted life-years). Because of this result, IPT-M was compared against drug therapy. The results of the comparison indicate that the IPT-M cost was an additional $73,715 for a gain of one extra QALY. When the combination of IPT-M and drug therapy was compared to IPT-M alone, it was found that it had the incremental cost per QALY ratio of $32,730/QALY. The lower incremental ratio, as compared to the ICER of IPT-M versus drug therapy alone, can be interpreted as 'extended dominance' of the combination therapy over IPT-M therapy alone. Hence, the combination therapy should be compared to drug therapy alone. The results of that analysis indicate that the incremental cost to QALY ratio was $45,741. In other words, the use of combination therapy as compared to the use of drug therapy will result in an additional cost of $45,741 for a gain of one additional QALY.

Cost–consequences analysis (CCA): Cost–consequences analysis simply calculates costs and varying outcomes (such as the number of disability days, changes in functioning, total cholesterol level, QALYs, etc.) and reports them in a table comparing each alternative therapy without calculating ratios (as in CEA or CUA) or net benefits (as in CBA). It is the responsibility of the decision-maker to review all possible costs and consequences of each therapy and then use his/her own decision rules to combine the values of varying costs and effectiveness and make the decision.

The decisions made using this approach may be less than optimum because they are based on the heuristic used by the decision-maker which may vary from person to person. However, it does make the calculation of costs and effectiveness explicit. If the decision process is verbalised and recorded in writing or electronically, it does provide insight into how decision-makers combine multiple factors to arrive at decisions. Although many CCA studies have been published, there are no CCA studies in pharmacoeconomic evaluations that address the issues of how decision-makers arrive at their decision once they are presented with the costs and consequences.

Patient Reported Outcomes

A more recent term in the outcome nomenclature is 'patient reported outcomes' (PROs). PROs encompass all outcome data reported by the patient; hence, the patient is the data source. Therefore, PROs include health-related quality of life, satisfaction, adherence to treatment, symptoms and reported adverse effects to treatment. However, the same challenges exist as for (CCA): treatment may improve one PRO but reduce another; a decision must therefore be made as to which is more important.

There is a significant body of literature on this subject in consumer behaviour and in cognitive psychology that can be adopted to advance the application of CCA in pharmacoeconomic literature. The reader is referred to the citation and readings on PROs through the ISPOR website and the US Food and Drug Administration.

Guidelines for Conducting or Evaluating a Pharmacoeconomic Evaluation

The prerequisite for conducting or evaluating a pharmacoeconomic evaluation is advanced knowledge of research methods and biostatistics, both of which are essential to design a protocol or evaluate the validity of a published study. In addition, a basic understanding of economics and finance is required to conduct the cost analysis. Economics is also useful in understanding utility-based outcomes such as QALYs. Finally, a grounding in psychometric analysis is essential for measuring outcomes pertaining to health-related quality of life.

The basic steps in any pharmacoeconomic analysis are outlined below and are described in the form of questions that need to be answered when undertaking an analysis:

- **Definition of the study question**: What is the purpose of undertaking the study? What perspective does the study use? The perspective is crucial in a pharmacoeconomic analysis because it dictates the type of data to be collected and how the variables are to be analysed. There are generally four types of perspectives used: the patient or consumer, the provider or institution, the payer or insurance company and society (in which case, all costs need to be considered).

- **Other questions to be asked**: Are alternatives identified and realistic? Are clinical management pathways specified in a logical manner?
- **Identification, measurement and valuation of costs and consequences**: What types of costs are considered? How are they enumerated? Measured? Valued? What sources were used in this process? What types of consequences are considered? How are they enumerated? Measured? Valued? And using what sources?
- **Selection of study protocol and design**: What type of economic evaluation will be used? Is this the most appropriate technique? What is the study design? Is this internally valid?
- **Methods of data collection and adjustment**: Are future costs and consequences discounted? What was the rationale for the discounting factor chosen? Is the sensitivity analysis conducted for the appropriate variables? Sensitivity analysis is used to test the robustness of assumptions to uncertainties in the measurement of costs and consequences. Is marginal or incremental analysis conducted (if necessary)?
- **Selection of decision rules**: How are the alternatives compared?
- **Presentation and interpretation of findings (for evaluation)**: Are the results clearly presented? Does the presentation address the research questions? Based on the information provided, can you replicate the study? Are conclusions or generalisations based on the results? Are comparisons with previous studies, implications and/or recommendations presented? Is the report unbiased and unaffected by the sources of funding for the study?

From Theory to Practice

There are several approaches by which pharmacoeconomic strategies can be translated into practice. These include: 1) evaluating, interpreting and using results of published studies, 2) using economic modelling and/or simulation studies and 3) conducting pharmacoeconomic studies specific to the institution and scenario using retrospective or prospective data.

Each of these strategies has its own advantages and disadvantages. For example, the first alternative appears to be the simplest to conduct. It is also inexpensive, easy and quick to access, and the results have already been evaluated previously by peer review. The disadvantages are that the data may be specific to the situation and hence not generalisable or comparative and there may be variations in the quality of published data from different sources (including authors or journals).

Using an economic modelling technique can also be relatively inexpensive and quick. In addition, these models can be devised to be specific to the situation and institution; and present effectiveness rather than efficacy data. The chief disadvantage of this technique is that the model is dependent on assumptions made by the researcher, and hence subject to bias. These assumptions should be tested using sensitivity analysis.

Conducting a pharmacoeconomic study specific to the situation and institution is advantageous for various reasons (comparative, reflects reality, data quality can be monitored), but this method can be costly in terms of time and resources.

Population-based Pharmacoeconomics

All of the pharmacoeconomic evaluations discussed in this chapter are based on the impact of treatment at the patient level. This type of patient level analysis is described as incidence-based evaluation because it focuses on 'the impact of a new treatment on a health condition from onset until cure or death'.

Incidence-based pharmacoeconomic evaluation is very useful for establishing the value of a new drug therapy or any new medical technology; however, it may be at odds with a decision-maker who is faced with the dilemma of cost containment in the short run or the impact of including a 'cost effectiveness' treatment on the one-year budget. Leidle argues that the 'cost-effectiveness of a medical intervention at the population level may deviate from that reported for evaluations at the patient level. (Thus,) it is important for decision makers and researchers to know the relevance of externalities, phasing-in effects, treatment effectiveness in the community, capacity issues, and different time perspectives in the evaluation of an intervention'.

This is the reason why it is now suggested that when the decision-maker is faced with considering the adoption of a new, expensive, but cost-effective technology based on the patient level analysis (or incidence-based evaluation), the manufacturer (or seller) of the technology could work with the decision-maker in generating additional data on prevalence-based evaluation. This type of evaluation focuses on the impact of the new technology on the health condition of specific populations of interest and on healthcare expenditure during one year (or specified) period.

CASE STUDIES

For each case, briefly answer the following questions. Justify your answer to each question based on the information provided in the case.

1. Whose perspective should be adopted?
2. What are the relevant alternatives?
3. What should be considered (costs, outcomes or both)?
4. Which healthcare evaluation technique should be used (CMA, CEA, CBA, CUA, CCA)?

Case 1

You are an AstraZeneca Pharmaceuticals representative and you are giving a presentation to the Pharmacy and Therapeutics Committee of a large hospital in India. Many of the committee members are attending physicians. Currently, Prevacid® is on the formulary for the treatment of acid reflux. Your presentation today should convince the committee members that the hospital adopt Prilosec®, a less expensive drug to save money. The side effect profile and efficacy is similar for both drugs.

Solution:

1. Hospital perspective (Note: The broader perspective of the hospital and not the pharmacy department is of interest because cost savings to the hospital are the primary objective).
2. Prevacid® and Prilosec®
3. Only costs, as the efficacy and safety profiles are similar
4. CMA

Case 2

You are the director of a large hospital, located in Mumbai. Currently, there are a couple of anti-psychotic medications available on your hospital formulary for the treatment of schizophrenia: haloperidol and the atypical anti-psychotic risperidone. A new atypical anti-psychotic, sertindole, has been approved by the Food and Drug Administration of India. You are questioning whether to add the drug to your formulary. Clinical trials for sertindole comparing the product to haloperidol and risperidone are available and it is found that the new drug is more effective but has additional side effects. The new drug is significantly more expensive.

Solution:

1. Hospital
2. Haloperidol, risperidone and sertindole
3. Cost and outcomes
4. CEA or CUA

Case 3

The city planning department of Bhavnagar, Gujarat, was recently informed by the city budget office that money is available to fund a new programme for the city of Bhavnagar. In light of the recent downturn in the economy, the planning department is constrained to choose one of the three proposals presented. The first proposal is for 'commit to be fit programme' to enhance awareness about health and fitness. The second is for new highway overpasses to reduce traffic problems on the highways. The third proposal is for a mobile immunisation programme for poor children and the elderly in the city. The planning department wants to select a proposal that would result in the greatest net financial benefit to the city of Bhavnagar.

Solution:

1. City
2. Health and fitness programme, highway overpasses, and mobile immunisation programme

3. Cost and outcomes (citizens' willingness to pay for the new programme)
4. CBA (cost and consequences of proposals analysed in rupees) because the planning department is interested in the largest 'net financial benefit' to the city. Also a CBA will enable comparison of different outcomes in monetary units.

Case 4

You are the chair of the Pharmacy and Therapeutics Committee at a 300-bed hospital. It has been brought to your attention that many physicians at your hospital are using ampicillin-sulbactam for intra-abdominal infections. The suggestion was made to substitute cefoxitin, a less expensive drug, to save the hospital money. The incidence of side effects is similar for both therapeutic regimens, but the cure rate for intra-abdominal infections is higher with ampicillin-sulblactam than with cefoxitin.

Solution:

1. Institutional; 2. Cefoxitin or ampicillin-sulbactam; 3. Cost and outcomes; 4. CEA

Exercise 1: Evaluation of a pharmacoeconomic study

Before reading this section, the reader should obtain a copy of the following article:

McNabb JJ, Nightingale CH, Quintiliani and Niocolau DP. 2001. Cost-effectiveness of ceftazidime infusion versus intermittent infusion for nosocomial pneumonia. *Pharmacotherapy* 21(5):549–55.

This article is evaluated using the guidelines for conducting or evaluating a pharmacoeconomic evaluation discussed in this chapter.

DEFINITION OF THE STUDY QUESTION:

1. Is the environment for the study described? (Do the authors describe why the study was undertaken or important?)

   Yes: The authors explain that β-lactam antibiotics, specifically ceftazidime, are reliable therapy for nosocomial pneumonia. The primary determinant of ceftazidime efficacy is the ***duration of time*** that concentrations ***remain above the MIC***. The way to maintain optimal therapy is to take full advantage of antibiotic pharmacodynamics. Therefore, the study is important because the authors determine if continuous infusion ceftazidime is more cost effective and efficacious than intermittent infusion in patients with nosocomial pneumonia.

2. What perspective does the study take?

   Institutional perspective – Hartford Hospital

3. Are the alternatives clearly defined? Are they realistic?

Yes: There are two alternatives clearly defined and realisitic:

a. ***Continuous*** infusion ceftazidime + concomitant therapy with tobramycin

b. ***Intermittent*** infusion ceftazidime + concomitant therapy with tobramycin

The 'do nothing' alternative is missing; however, it would be considered unethical not to provide treatment.

4. Are pathways of clinical management, including decision nodes and chance nodes, clearly and logically specified? (In other words, does the decision tree follow logical and chronological sequence? How are probabilities determined?)

   The pathways of comparing continuous and intermittent infusion, including decision nodes and chance nodes, are clearly and logically specified. The probabilities are determined based on authors' study data. The results of the study are similar when one replicates the development of the decision tree using DATA 3.8, TreeAge Software. The cost effectiveness ratios at the terminal nodes (triangles) are explained in the Cost and Consequence section below.

5. Is the major study question or objective clearly stated? Are there any additional research questions being addressed in the study?

The purpose of the study was to determine if continuous infusion ceftazidime is more cost effective and efficacious than intermittent infusion in patients with nosocomial pneumonia.

COST AND CONSEQUENCE

1. What types of *costs* are considered?

Enumerated	***Measured***	***Value***	***Source***
Ceftazidime	Per gram	$9.46	Hartford Hospital pharmacy
Tobramycin	Per gram	$4.20	Hartford Hospital pharmacy

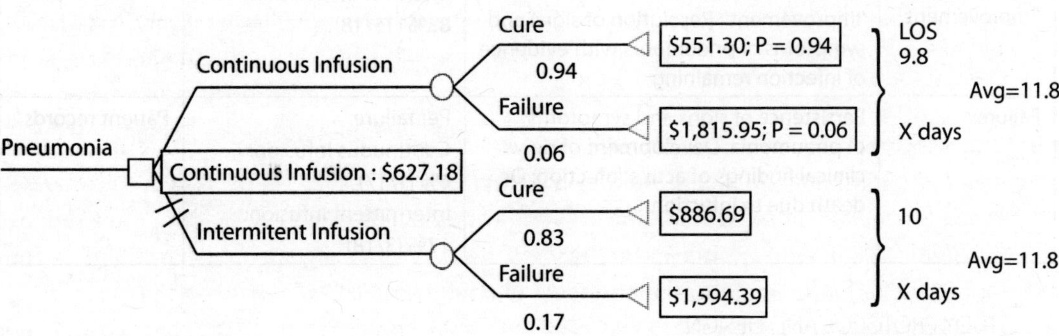

Drug preparation & administration	Per day	Continuous (Ceftazidime): 3g/day x \$9.46 = \$28.38/day Intermittent (Ceftazidime): 3 x 2g/day x \$9.46 = \$56.76/day Tobramycin: (Assume 70Kg. person) 70 x 7mg. x \$4.20/g = \$2.05	Hartford Hospital
Antibiotic related length of stay	Per length of stay (days)	*Continuous:* 11.8 = (9.8x16)+(X x1) 17 X = 43.8 days *Intermittent:* 15.3 = (10x15)+(X x 3) 18 X = 41.8 days	Hartford Hospital
Hospitalisation	Charge per medical service	Cost to charge ratio (not provided)	Hartford Hospital; 1999 Bureau of Labor & Statistics: Medical service charges
Physician charge		Excluded	Hartford Hospital
Outpatient expense		Excluded	Hartford Hospital

2. What types of ***consequences*** are considered? How are they enumerated? Measured? Valued? And, what using what sources?

Enumerated	***Measured***	***Value***	***Source***
Clinical cure was defined as combination of 'cure' and 'improvement'	'Cure': Complete resolution of signs and symptoms of pneumonia; or lack of progression of all abnormalities on chest radiograph 'Improvement': Resolution of signs and symptoms of pneumonia with evidence of infection remaining	Per Clinical Cure: Continuous Infusion: 94% (16/17) Intermittent Infusion: 83% (15/18)	Patient records
Failure	Persistence of signs and symptoms of pneumonia; Development of new clinical findings of active infection; Or death due to infection	Per failure: Continuous Infusion: 6% (1/17) Intermittent Infusion: 17% (3/18)	Patient records

STUDY PROTOCOL AND DESIGN

1. What type of economic evaluation technique is used: Is this the most appropriate for the study

   Cost effectiveness analysis was an appropriate technique used because study compares two alternative therapies (continuous vs. intermittent infusion) with varying levels effectiveness (clinical improvement, cure, and failure) and different costs.

2. What type of study design is used in the study? Is the design internally valid?

   A prospective, randomised study. The study appears internally valid due to the randomised control clinical trial comparing continuous infusion with intermittent infusion. There is no difference in demographic variables between the two groups. The total sample size of 35 is insufficient to fully evaluate differences in cost or effect parameter – the standard deviation at level II:

   Determination of sample size needed to achieve a stated precision: If we specify that $\alpha=0.05$, $t_{(0.05;\ 2\ tail;df=34)}=2.032$, s.d.(cost of continuous infusion)=387.84, and the small effect size of 0.1 which is 1/10 of the s.d.=38.78:

   $$n = \frac{(387.84)^2 \times (2.032)^2}{(38.78)^2} = \mathbf{412} \text{ per group} \leftarrow \text{sufficient sample size required}$$

   Even assuming a medium effect size of 0.2 requires a sample size of 103 per group.

DATA COLLECTION AND ADJUSTMENT

1. Are the future costs and consequences discounted? What was the rationale for the rate chosen?

   The authors suggest that 'All costs and outcomes and outcomes occurred during the same time period, so neither cost nor outcome is discounted'. This explanation is somewhat ambiguous. The clear explanation would state that the time period for the study was less than one year and hence, costs and outcomes are not discounted.

2. Is the sensitivity analysis conducted for the appropriate variables?

   Yes: A sensitivity analysis was conducted to test the robustness of results to variations in assumptions. The researchers performed a one- and two-way sensitivity analysis by varying each treatment arms probability of success from 50%–95% and varying acquisition cost of ceftazidime within 25%. The one-way analysis showed that intermittent infusion regimen would have to be 20% more clinically effective than continuous infusion to be cost effective. The two-way analysis showed that continuous infusion success would have to fall 64% and intermittent infusion would have to be 10–20% more clinically effective than continuous infusion before intermittent infusion would become more cost effective.

3. Is the marginal (or incremental) analysis conducted (if necessary)?

Articles reports that 'Incremental analysis was not performed because there was no statistically or clinically relevant difference in outcomes'. While the conclusion is correct, the rationale is weak. The authors could have stated that the comparison of costs and effectiveness measures indicate that continuous infusion is a dominant alternative (that is, lower cost and higher effect) as compared to intermittent infusion and hence, no incremental analysis is necessary.

Alternative	***Cost***	***Effectiveness (Clinical Cure)***	***Change in Cost***	***Change in Effectiveness***	***Incremental CE Ratio***
Intermittent Infusion	$18,083.52	83% (15/18)			
Continuous Infusion	$10,636.73	94% (16/17)			

DECISION RULES

1. How are the alternatives compared?

   Alternatives were compared using C/E. C/E is presented as cost per clinical cure and the preferred is the least costly regimen per cure. An additional relevant comparison is the least cost per day.

PRESENTATION AND INTERPRETATION OF FINDINGS

1. Are the results clearly presented? Does the presentation address the research question?

   The results were confusing to calculate, specifically the overall number of days of both treatments. The study does address the research question: To determine if continuous infusion ceftazidime is more cost effective and efficacious than intermittent infusion in patients with nosocomial pneumonia.
2. Based on the information provided in the study, can you replicate the study?

   Based on the information provided in the study, I would be able to replicate the study.
3. Are the conclusions based on the results? Or, are generalisations based on the results?

   The conclusions are based on the results. The results may not be generalisable because of the small sample size (35 patients).
4. Are comparisons with previous studies, implications and/or recommendations presented?

   There was a comparison to two previous studies that demonstrated cost-effectiveness of continuous β-Lactams: (1) Ambrose PG, et al., 1998 – Study showed no difference between in clinical cure rates between intermittent and continuous infusion of cefuroxime, but the continuous infusion regimen was associated with shorter length of treatment, decreased length of hospital stay, and overall cost savings; and (2) Zeisler JA, et al., 1992 – Study showed equivalent efficacy of intermittent and continuous infusion of β-Lactams and cost savings with continuous infusion.

5. Is the report unbiased and not affected by the source of funding for the study?

   The study does not seem to be biased. Even though the drug studied (ceftazidime) is a Glaxo Pharmaceuticals product and the study was supported by a grant by Glaxo Pharmaceuticals, the study design/model is appropriate.

Exercise 2: Evaluation of a pharmacoeconomic study

Before reading this section, the reader should obtain a copy of the following article:
Laohavaleeson S, Barriere SL, Nicolau DP, Kuti JL. 2008 Cost-effectiveness of telavancin versus vancomycin for treatment of complicated skin and skin structure infections. *Pharmacotherapy* 28(12):1471–1482.
This article is evaluated using the guidelines for conducting or evaluating a pharmacoeconomic evaluation discussed in this chapter.

DEFINITION OF THE STUDY QUESTION:

1. Is the environment for the study described? (Do the authors describe why the study was undertaken or important?)

   Yes, the authors state that the study was important because vancomycin is the standard of care for complicated skin and skins structure infections (c-SSSs) including suspected methicillin resistant *S. aureus* (MRSA). However, vancomycin is slow acting and not always effective. Therefore an antibiotic that is more potent is desirable. Authors report that telavancin is a new investigational drug, a lipoglycopeptide, that is 2–4 times more potent than vancomycin and can be administered once daily. Telavancin 10 mg/kg/day was well tolerated in phase II clinical trials in patients with MRSA and showed superior efficacy (effectiveness: 92 v 68%, FAST trial) supporting a cost effectiveness analysis.

2. What perspective does the study take?

   Institutional (hospital) perspective.

3. Are the alternatives clearly defined? Are they realistic?

   Two alternatives are provided they are.

   a. Telvancin 10 mg/kg IV once daily

   b. Vancomycin 1 g IV every 12 hours. Vancomycin monitoring was followed according to site protocol/renal function

   Drug dosing was continued for 7–14 days or until patient was cured (which could be more or less days of treatment).

   Alternatives are not realistic: (1) although vancomycin is regarded as the gold standard of care for MRSA (or suspected MRSA), blood level monitoring is important to ensure adequate efficacy and avoid toxicity. The standard of care is 48 hours after initiation of therapy and at least once after steady state has been reached. This basic standard was not included in the methods (and results showed that only 41% received at least one level), and (2) realistically a P&T committee would also consider linezolid and daptomycin. These two agents have excellent efficacy in c-SSSs. Furthermore, linezolid can be administered orally.

4. Are pathways of clinical management, including decision nodes and chance nodes, clearly and logically specified? (In other words, does the decision tree follow logical and chronological sequence? How are probabilities determined?)

   Yes. The pathways of comparing the two antibiotic treatments including decision nodes and chance nodes, are clearly and logically specified for the entire population study (all c-SSSs) but is not presented for the MRSA only subpopulation. However, it seems highly unusual that telavancin has a higher cure rate for non-MRSA (0.856) than MRSA (0.874) cases and the authors fail to explain this. The probabilities are determined based on authors' study data. The decision tree below was based on the base-case scenario (30% prevalence of MRSA and telavancin cost equal to vancomycin) using Data 3.8 Treeage software.

5. Is the major study question or objective clearly stated? Are there any additional research questions being addressed in the study?

   Yes. The purpose of the study was to determine if telavancin was more cost effective than vancomycin in the treatment of (a) c-SSSs (entire study population with evaluable microbiology data) and (b) the subpopulation of patients infected with MRSA, using patients from the ATLAS study.

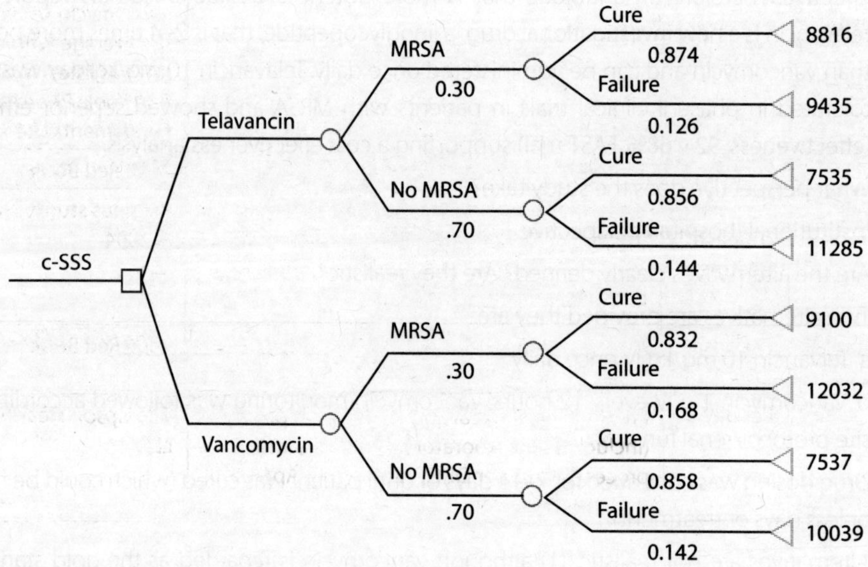

c-SSS: complicated skin and skin structure infection

The second objective raises questions, although readily estimated using software its value is clinically questionable. Treatment for c-SSSs is typically initiated empirically. Although Gram stain and organism susceptibility results present the ideal scenario, testing frequently does not always provide results (for example, in the ATLAS study, susceptibility was unavailable for 30% of patients, this is not unusual). Therefore, it is highly unlikely that a P&T committee would list an antibiotic on the formulary only for documented MRSA.

COST AND CONSEQUENCES:

1. What types of *costs* are considered?

   Direct costs are considered. Authors reported that patient-specific hospital costs were not available for all patients participating in the study, as a result cost data were extrapolated from the Solucient Explore Database (billing data). Total median hospital costs included bed, laboratory, radiology, antibiotic costs (telavancin and vancomycin), vancomycin monitoring costs, concomitant antibiotic costs and procedures (surgery related to infection care). For surgical patients the following diagnosis-related groups (DRGs) 213 (amputation), 217 (wound debridement), 263 (skin graft with complications), 264 (skin graft without complications), 271 (skin ulcers) and 277 (cellulitis) were grouped together to determine median daily costs. Hospital costs were prorated for each patient based on infection related length of stay (LOS_{IR}). Physician charges, drug preparation and administration costs appear to have been excluded from the study.

Enumerated	***Measured***	***Value US$2006***	***Source***
Telavancin	Per day	$13.44	Base case: set equal to vancomycin based on the average wholesale price as listed in 2006 Red Book: Pharmacy's Fundamental Reference
Vancomycin	Per day	$13.44	2006 Red Book
Vancomycin monitoring	Per course of treatment	Vancomycin monitoring= $18.93 x # levels (assay) + $32.32 (initial pharmacist consult) + $12.12 x #levels -1 (additional pharmacist consults)	Previous study: Shah et al 2004
Concomitant antibiotics	Per dose	Please see Appendix 2 of article	2006 Red Book:
LOS_{IR}	Per day	Prorated for surgical and nonsurgical patients (included bed, laboratory, radiology, and procedures as per DRG) –please see Appendix 1 of article	Thompson Healthcare LLC

$COST_{IR}$	Per patient	Total infection related cost included bed, laboratory, radiology, and procedures, antibiotics and vancomycin monitoring. Please see Appendix 1 of article	Thompson Healthcare LLC

LOS_{IR}: Infection related length of stay

$COST_{IR}$: Total infection related cost

2. What types of *consequences* are considered? How are they enumerated? Measured? Valued? And, using what sources?

Enumerated	*Measured*	*Value*	*Source*
Cured	Adequate clinical response to treatment 7–14 days after last dose of study drug.	Per cure: telavancin: 86.2% (443/514) vancomycin 84.9% (450/530)	Patient records (ATLAS study)
Failure	Inadequate response to treatment 7-14 days after last dose of study drug.	Per failure: telavancin: 13.8% vancomycin 15.1%	Patient records: (ATLAS study)

STUDY PROTOCOL AND DESIGN

1. What type of economic evaluation technique is used: Is this the most appropriate for the study?

   CEA was the most appropriate economic technique assuming telavancin was considered more effective than vancomycin at the time the study was conducted.

2. What type of study design is used in the study? Is the design internally valid?

   A prospective, randomised study. The study appears internally valid due to the randomisation of telavancin and vancomycin in a multi-center phase III clinical trial (ATLAS trial, Stryjewski et al. 2008[ref #20 of article]). There was no difference in baseline demographic variables between the two groups (listed in Table 1 of the article).

   This study was underpowered. The study was designed, assuming a 10% difference in efficacy between telvancin and vancomycin, with a probability of effectiveness for vancomycin=80%, power=0.86 and an alpha (1 tailed)=0.025 (Reported in Stryjewski et al. 2008). However, the actual difference was much less at 1.3%. Therefore the actual sample size needed to show a 1.3% difference was approximately 10,000 per group assuming the above parameters and assuming the difference is clinically meaningful! No standard deviation data is reported for cost; with only interquartile range data it is not possible to determine adequacy of sample size for cost ($N=SD^2 \times 1.96^2/error^2$).

DATA COLLECTION AND ADJUSTMENT

1. Are the future costs and consequences discounted? What was the rationale for the rate chosen?

The issue of discounting is not discussed. It is anticipated that no discounting was performed of costs or consequences given that hospitalisation lasted for an average of 8 days (less than 1 year).

2. Is the sensitivity analysis conducted for the appropriate variables?

A two-way sensitivity analysis was conducted for $COST_{IR}$ by varying the cost of telavancin (increased from \$50 to \$200) and MRSA rates (increased from 30% to 75%). The two-way analysis showed that telavancin was more cost effective (a) in the base case (when cost telavacin equal to vancomycin) for all MRSA rates tested (30%, 50% and 75%), and (b) when telavancin cost \$50 when the MRSA rate was equal to 75% for all patients.

Using the tree-diagram from above, the sensitivity analysis can be replicated for the base case in tree age software (where MRSA_rate is the varying rate of MRSA)

Given that there was no statistical difference in effectiveness (cure rate) between the two alternatives, a sensitivity analysis including effectiveness was warranted.

3. Is the marginal (or incremental) analysis conducted (if necessary)?

Yes, an incremental cost effectiveness (ICER) analysis was reported (Table 4 of article) assuming varying costs of telavancin (base-case to \$200) for the entire population and the subpopulation of MRSA patients. In addition, to determine the likelihood of ICER ratios, the authors performed a bootstrapping analysis. Bootstrapping is a non-parametric statistical method that is recommended for use to determine confidence intervals for ICER. However, in bootstrapping, confidence intervals cannot be interpreted directly, but are instead presented using the cost effectiveness plane. The C/E plane has four quadrants

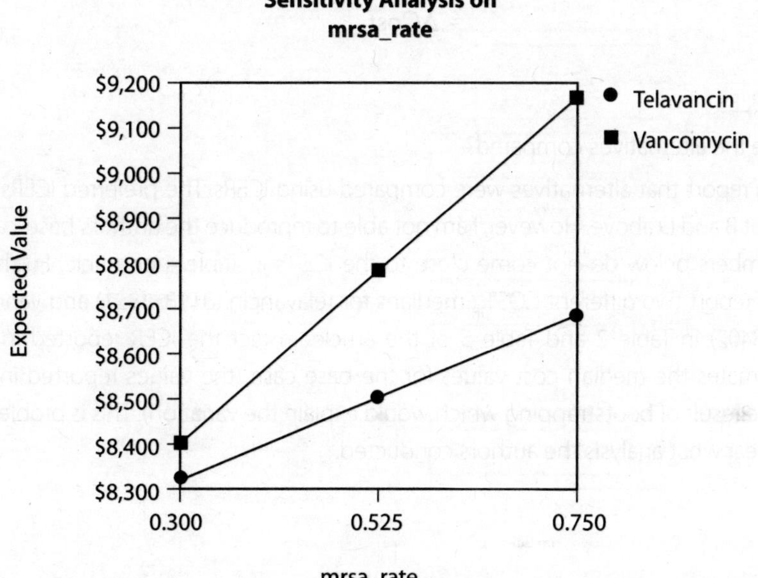

presented in the diagram (Please see Briggs, O'Brien and Blackhouse 2002 for a detailed explanation), where quadrant D is clearly desirable and quadrant B is desirable depending on if the increase in effectiveness is deemed worth the increase in cost.

The ICER analysis showed that telavancin was more cost effective in the base case for the entire c-SSS patient population and patients with MRSA only (negative ICER values in Table 4 of article). Telavancin was also more cost effective for MRSA patients with telavancin at a higher cost of $50.

Incremental cost-effectiveness plane showing four quadrants

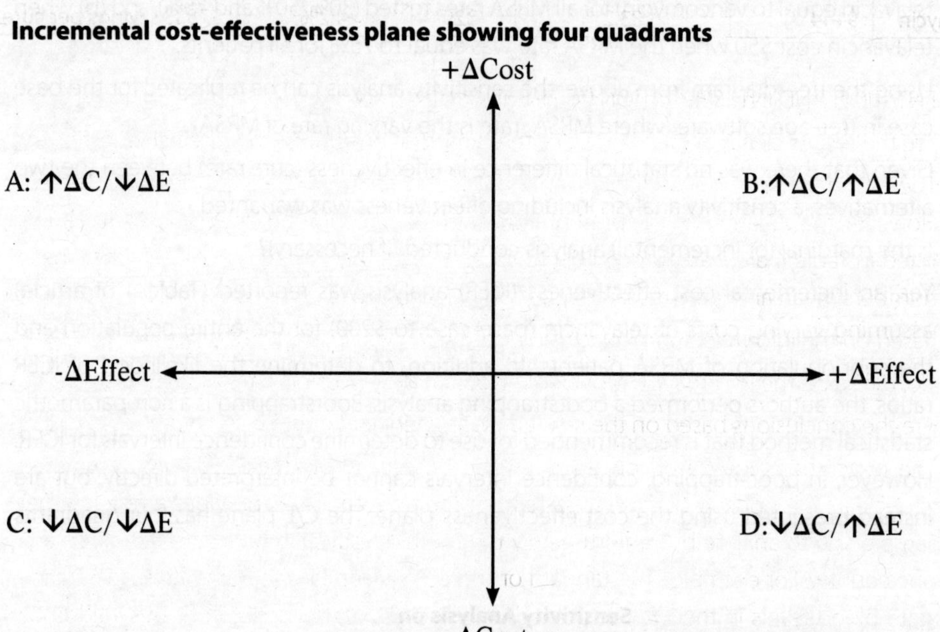

DECISION RULES

1. How are the alternatives compared?

   Authors report that alternatives were compared using ICERs. The preferred ICERs were in quadrant B and D above. However, I am not able to reproduce the authors' base-case ICER. The numbers below do not come close to the ICER's in Table 4 of article. Furthermore, authors report two different $COST_{IR}$ medians for telavancin (8118, 8321) and vancomycin (8185, 8402) in Table 2 and Table 5 of the article. In fact the ICER reported in Table 4 approximates the median cost values for the base case (the values reported in Table 4 were the result of bootstrapping which would explain the variation). This is problematic. It is not clear what analysis the authors conducted.

Population	Cost	Effectiveness %	ΔCost	ΔEffectiveness	ICER
Entire pop.					
Telavancin	8118,8321	86.2			
Vancomycin	8185, 8402	84.9	-67,-81	1.3%	$5154, $6230 savings per cure
MRSA					
Telavancin	8815	87.4			
Vancomycin	9144	83.2	-329	4.2%	$7833 savings per cure

PRESENTATION AND INTERPRETATION OF FINDINGS

1. Are the results clearly presented? Does the presentation address the research question?

   The cost data (appendices), effectiveness data and sensitivity data are clearly presented. However, the variations in the presentation of $COST_{IR}$ is confusing (listed above). The ICERs listed in Table 4 are not reproducible (the base case). Therefore it is not clear what these numbers mean and if the research question is addressed.

2. Based on the information provided in the study, can you replicate the study?

   No, based on the information provided it would not be possible to replicate the study.

3. Are the conclusions based on the results? Or, are generalisations based on the results?

   The conclusions are based on study results; however, how the ICERs were estimated is unclear. The pooling of study results from multiple countries provides a much larger sample size to analyse but unfortunately the pooled results are not generalisable to any one country. For example, the standard of care for vancomycin requires initial and steady state blood levels in the US. The pooled data showed levels for 41% of cases. Red Book drug prices and US hospitalisation costs may not be relevant to other countries: what is cost-effective in one country may not be cost effective in another. Lastly, the majority of MRSA cases were community acquired and where intravenous therapy in a hospital environment for at least a week was warranted. Since hospital acquired infections can respond differently to treatment these results are not generalisable to other nosocomial MRSA infections or other patient populations.

4. Are comparisons with previous studies, implications and/or recommendations presented?

   Yes. Authors conclude that telavancin and vancomycin length of stay and hospitalization costs due to infection were similar for patients with c-SSSs. Authors report that telavancin may be more cost effective in patients with MRSA. Authors do specify that other cheaper treatment options are available for c-SSSs; however, no discussion of other CEAs in MRSA are discussed.

5. Is the report unbiased and not affected by the source of funding for the study?

The inability to reproduce any of the ICERs listed in the study and conclusion that telavancin is more cost effective against MRSA brings to question the potential for bias in this study. In many cases (up to 50%) susceptibility testing for MRSA was not available: therefore, conducting a cost effective analysis for a clinical condition that is unidentifiable up to 50% of the time is questionable. As a result, this study appears to overstate the case.

KEY MESSAGES

- Pharmacoeconomics focuses on the description and analysis of the costs and outcomes of drug therapy to healthcare systems and to society.
- There are five major full economic evaluation techniques (in addition to partial economic evaluation techniques) that can be used to evaluate pharmaceutical programmes and services: cost minimisation (cost analysis when outcomes of the alternatives are the same, CMA); cost–benefit analysis (both cost and consequence are measured in monetary terms, CBA); cost effectiveness analysis (consequences are in natural units, CEA); cost utility analysis (consequences incorporate quantity and quality of life, CUA) and cost–consequences analysis (where decision criteria are specific to each decision maker for combining measures of costs and effectiveness).
- Conducting a pharmacoeconomic evaluation requires knowledge of various fields including research methods, statistics, epidemiology, psychometric theory and economics.
- The conduct or evaluation of a pharmacoeconomic study can be divided into six logical steps involving statement of the problem, identification and measurement of costs and consequences, designing the study and data collection, selecting decision criteria and presenting the results.
- Pharmacoeconomics is an important tool in decision making regarding various topics including drug product selection for formulary, comparison of alternative therapies, pricing a product and evaluating a drug product's expected quality-of-life improvement in relation to its cost.

Further Reading

Anon. 2001. Vision 2010: The strategy and the road map chart. *Vision 2010 statement*. *IDMA Bulletin* 24:560–561.

Berger, ML, Bingefors K, Hedblom E, Pashos CL and Torrance G. 2005. *Health care cost, quality, and outcomes: ISPOR book of terms*. International Society of for Pharmacoeconomics and Outcomes Research.

Bootman JL, Townsend RJ and McGhan WF. 1996. *Principles of Pharmacoeconomics*, 2nd ed. W Harvey Whitney Books Company: Cincinnati, OH.

Bootman JL, Wertheimer AI, Zaske D and Rowland C. 1979. Individualizing Gentamicin dosage regimens in burn patients with gram-negative septicemia: a cost-benefit analysis. *J Pharm Sci* 68(3):267–272.

Briggs A, O'Brien BJ and Blackhouse G. 2002. Thinking outside the box: recent advances in the analysis and presentation of uncertainty in cost-effectiveness studies. *Annu Rev Public Health* 23:337–401.

Briggs A, Sculpher M and Buxton M. 1994. Uncertainty in the economic evaluation of health care technologies: the role of sensitivity analysis. *Health Econ* 3:95–104.

Cook DJ, Guyatt GH, Laupacis A and Sackett DL. 1992. Rules of evidence and clinical recommendations on the use of antithrombotic agents. *Chest* 102(4): 305S–311S.

Coyle D and Tolley K. 1992. Discounting of health benefits in the pharmacoeconomic analysis of drug therapies. *Pharmacoeconomics* 2(2): 153–162.

Detsky AS. 1996. Evidence of effectiveness: evaluating its quality. In: Sloan FA (Ed) *Valuing health care: costs, benefits, and effectiveness of pharmaceuticals and other medical technologies,* 15–29 Chapter 2. Cambridge University Press: New York, NY.

Doubilet P, Weinstein MC and McNeil BJ. 1986. Use and misuse of the term "cost effective" in medicine. *N Eng J Med* 314(4):253–256.

Drummond ME, O'Brien B, Stoddart GL and Torrance GW. 1997. *Methods for the economic evaluation of health care programmes*, 2nd ed. Oxford University Press, Inc.: New York, NY.

Drummond MF, Schulpher MJ, Torrance GW and Stoddard GL. 2005. *Methods for the economic evaluation of health care programs.* 3rd ed. Oxford University Press, Inc: New York, NY.

Elixhauser A, Weschler JM, Kitzmiller JL et al. 1993. Cost-benefit analysis of preconception care for women with established diabetes mellitus. *Diabetes Care* 16(8):1146–1157.

Engel JF, Blackwell RD and Miniard PW. 1990. *Consumer Behavior*, 6th ed. The Dryden Press: Chicago, IL.

Food and Drug Administration. 2006. Guidance for Industry Patient-Reported Outcome Measures: Use in Medical Product Development to Support Labeling Claims. US Department of Health and Human Services, Rockville MD. February 2006. Available at: http://www.fda.gov/CDER/GUIDANCE/5460dft.pdf

Gold MR, Siegel JE, Russell LB and Weinstein MC. 1996. *Cost-effectiveness in health and medicine*. Oxford University Press: New York, NY.

Gold MR, Siegel JE, Russell LB and Weinstein MC. 1996. *Cost-effectiveness in health and medicine*. Oxford University Press: New York, NY.

Goldstein WM and Hogarth RM (eds). 1997. *Research on judgment and decision making*. Cambridge University Press: New York, NY.

Hakim Z, Pierson JF and Pathak DS. 1996. A proposed model for conducting institutional-specific cost-effectiveness analysis: a case study of lipid-lowering agents. *Pharm Pract Manag Q* 16(1):79–97.

Hurley SF. 1992. Indices of therapeutic outcome in pharmaceoeconomic evaluation of drug therapy. *Pharmacoeconomics* 1(3):155–160.

Johannesson M. 1996. *Theory and methods of economic evaluation of health care*. Kluwer, Kordrecht.

Kamlet MS, Paul N, Greenhouse J and Kupfer D et al 1995. Cost-utility analysis of maintenance treatment for recurrent depression. *Control Clin Trials* 16:17–40.

Kozma CM, Reeder CE, Schulz RM. 1993. Economic, clinical, and humanistic outcomes: a planning model for pharmacoeconomic research. *Clinl Ther* 15(6): 1121–1132.

Leidl RM. 1994. Some factors to consider when using the results of economic evaluation studies at the population level. *Int J Technol Assess Health Care* 10(3):467–478.

Levin HK and McEwan PJ. 2001. *Cost-effectiveness analysis: Methods and applications*, 2nd ed. Thousand Oaks, CA.

Logan A et al. 1981. Cost-effectiveness of a worksite hypertension treatment program. *Hypertension* 3:211–218.

Luce BR and Elixhauser A. 1990. *Standards for socioeconomic evaluation of health care products and services*. Springer-Verlag: New York.

MacKeigan LD and Pathak DS. 1992. Overview of health-related quality of life measures. *Am J Health Syst Pharm* 49:2236–45.

Mauskopf J. 1998. Prevalence-based economic evaluation. *Value Health* 1(4):251–259.

McGhan W, Rowland C and Bootman JL. 1978. Cost-benefit and cost-effectiveness: methodologies for evaluating innovative pharmaceutical services. *Am J Hosp Pharm* 35:133–140.

Mitchell RC and Carson RT. 1989. *Using Surveys to Value Public Goods: The Contingent Valuation Method.* Resources for the Future: Washington DC.

Nakahiro RK, Ho SS and Okamoto M. 1998. Concepts of Pharmacoeconomics, In Mirta Millares (Ed) *Applied Drug Information: Strategies for information management*. Applied therapeutics, Inc.: Vancouver, Canada.

O'Brien, BJ, Novisel S, Torrance G and Streiner D. 1995. Assessing the economic value of anew antidepressant. A willingness to pay approach. *PharmacoEconomics* 8(1): 34–45.

Oxford Centre for Evidence-Based Medicine. Levels of Evidence (March 2009). Available at URL www.cebm.net/levels_of_evidence.asp

Pashos CL, Klein EG and Wanke LA. 1998. *ISPOR Lexicon*, 1st ed. International Society for Pharmacoeconomics and Outcomes Research: Princeton, NJ.

Pathak DS and Boyer JG. 1995. Realities of conducting pharmacoeconomic evaluations as part of clinical trials: Introduction. *Pharm Prac Manag Q* 15(2):72–73.

Pathak DS. 1995. QALY in Health Outcomes Research: Representation of Real Preferences or Another Numerical Abstraction? *Journal of Research in Pharmaceutical Economics* 6(4):3–27.

Patrick DL and Erickson P. 1993. *Health status and health policy: Allocating resources to health care.* Oxford University Press.

Pizzi LT and Loftland JH. 2006. *Economic Evaluation in US Health Care: Principles and Applications.* Jones and Bartlett Publishers, Inc: Sudbury, MA.

Reardon G and Pathak DS. 1989. Contingent Valuation of Pharmaceuticals and Pharmacy Services - Methodological Considerations. *J Soc Adm Pharm* 6 (2):83–91.

Rothermich EA and Pathak DS. 1999. Productivity-Cost Controversies in Cost-Effectiveness Analysis: Review and Research Agenda. *Clin Ther* 21(1):255–67.

Sackett DL, Straus SE, Richardson WS, Rosenberg W and Haynes RB. 1997. Guidelines In: Evidence Based Medicine. 2nd ed. Churchill Livingston: 169–182.

Sackett DL. 1980. Evaluation of health services. In: Last JM (ed), *Health and Preventive Medicine,* 1800–1823. Appleton Century Croft: New York, NY.

Sanchez L. 1996. Pharmacoeconomics: Further practical considerations. In: Bootman JL, Townsend RJ and McGhan WF (eds), *Principles of Pharmacoeconomics*, 2nd ed. 290–301. W Harvey Whitney Books.

Sanchez LA and Lee J. 1994. Use and misuse of pharmacoeconomic terms: a definitions primer. *Top Hosp Pharm Manage* 13(4):11–22.

Tighe M and Goodman S. 1988. Carboplatin versus cisplatin. *Lancet* 1372–1373.

Torrance GW. 1987. Utility approch to measuring health-related quality of life. *J Chronic Dis* 40(6):593–600.

Townsend RJ. 1986. Post marketing drug research and development: an industry clinical pharmacist's perspective. *Am J Pharm Educ* 50:480–482.

Websites of Interest

NOTE: These websites provide further useful links.

Oxford Centre for Evidence-Based Medicine. Levels of Evidence
www.cebm.net/levels_of_evidence.asp

Center for Health Economics and Policy Analysis
www.chepa.org

International Health Economics Association
www.healtheconomics.com

Indian Drugs Manufacturers' Association
www.idma-assn.org

International Society of Quality of Life
www.isoqol.org

International Society of Pharmacoeconomics and Outcomes Research
www.ispor.org

Health Technology Assessment International
http://www.htai.org

Society of Medical Decision Making
www.smdm.org

Decision analysis by Treeage® software package
www.treeage.com

30

DEVELOPMENT OF THERAPEUTIC GUIDELINES

Renee Robinson and Milap C Nahata

Learning Objectives

Upon completion of this chapter, the reader should be able to:

- Discuss the meaning of a therapeutic guideline
- Understand the common definitions used when discussing therapeutic guidelines
- Be able to locate and give examples of guidelines from the medical literature
- Discuss the need for therapeutic guidelines focusing on quality, cost and consistency of practice
- List the steps involved in the development, review and implementation of therapeutic guidelines
- Discuss the potential limitations of therapeutic guidelines
- Identify the factors affecting the implementation and utilisation of guidelines in clinical practice
- Understand the skills needed to assist in the development, review and implementation of new guidelines

Rapid advances in clinical science and technology and the complexity of therapeutic regimens have made it difficult for healthcare practitioners to consistently provide high-quality care to patients. Guidelines are designed to help practitioners assimilate, evaluate and implement the ever-increasing amount of both evidence-based medicine and value judgments based on personal or organisational preferences regarding various risks and benefits. They assist in the clinical decision-making process and hence improve the quality of healthcare.

Interest in and utilisation of clinical or therapeutic practice guidelines have increased over the past 30 years, and today guidelines are available in many areas of therapeutics. However, the main goal of therapeutic guidelines remains the same: to provide consistent and high-quality care, reduce therapy costs through utilisation of substantiated means, and limit the number of adverse events and therapeutic misadventures.

What are Therapeutic Guidelines?

Lack of established terminology has led to confusion among practitioners. Practice guidelines, clinical guidelines or clinical practice guidelines, and physician-directed diagnostic and therapeutic plans are all terms that have been used interchangeably but are not necessarily equivalent.

Practice guidelines are systematically developed statements to assist practitioners in choosing the most appropriate means for diagnosis, monitoring and/or treatment based on predetermined clinical circumstances. Physicians, epidemiologists, dentists and pharmacists have all participated in the development of national, regional and institution-specific guidelines. In fact, over 1500 guidelines have been published in the United States alone. These were developed using a consensus method and published in booklet format and distributed to medical staff throughout the hospital.

Clinical practice guidelines are recommendations developed by healthcare providers to serve as a guide for diagnosis, evaluation and/or the treatment of a specific disease state.

They differ from standards, options and clinical pathways. Standards are more rigid than clinical practice guidelines and do not allow practitioner flexibility in deciding on patient care. Critical pathways are composed of many independent clinical practice guidelines. These guidelines can be used separately or together to provide comprehensive care based on the patient's disease state. *Therapeutic guidelines are clinical practice guidelines that focus on treatment recommendations.*

Where Can We Find Published Therapeutic Guidelines

Published and unpublished guidelines can be found in a number of sources such as medical databases (for example, Medline, Embase), pharmaceutical industry-sponsored websites (for example, Pfizer) and non-profit organisation websites (such as the American Heart Association). However, it is important to note that the guidelines and medical information provided on many of these sites is often in abbreviated or summarised form and may not accurately reflect the intended focus of the guidelines.

Internet sites of US government organisations such as the Centers for Disease Control and Prevention and the National Institutes of Health often include the unabridged versions of guidelines (see *Websites of Interest* at the end of the chapter). These guidelines are generally free and are often the most comprehensive resource for clinical practice guidelines. Organisations such as the American Medical Association (AMA), American College of Cardiology (ACC) and the American College of Clinical Pharmacy also offer clinical practice guidelines. However, these are often available only to active members, limiting accessibility to many clinicians.

Finally, many institutions publish their own guidelines for the treatment of specific disease states. These guidelines serve as the basis of treatment for clinicians throughout the institution (for example, a hospital) and are often provided to practitioners as a handbook or as a link on the institution's website.

The Need for Guidelines

Many governmental agencies and professional organisations have focused on improving the quality of patient care through the establishment of therapeutic guidelines. In 1989, the United States Congress adopted legislation and established a governing body (The Agency for Health Care Research and Quality or AHRQ) to improve healthcare and develop clinically relevant practice guidelines. Organisations such as the AMA, ACC, American Heart Association (AHA) and the American Society of Anesthesiologists (ASA) have developed and published principles for the development of both general and specific clinical practice guidelines.

Guidelines supported by professional organisations are commonly used by practitioners to guide treatment and patient monitoring. They allow practitioners to assess the efficacy and effectiveness of therapy, support and quantify patient outcomes, and develop links between the structure and process of caregiving with clinical outcomes. They assist practitioners in establishing monitoring parameters to assess the health status and quality of life.

Guidelines are also necessary to contain healthcare costs. Limited resources in both developed and developing countries are forcing policymakers to focus on cost-effective treatments shown to improve health outcomes. This is especially important in developing countries, where available funding sources for the healthcare system are often insufficient and conflicts of interest exist due to ownership of equipment by healthcare providers. Limited resources necessitate rationing of healthcare and demonstrate the importance of conveying information to appropriate policymakers, commissioning agencies and clinicians. Utilisation of published clinical guidelines allows practitioners to incorporate international research data into general practice and ensures that the standard of care is provided to all patients without the costs associated with individual practitioner investigation, clinical trials, bias and error.

In developed countries, guidelines decrease costs through standardisation of care. The recent growth in the development and implementation of practice guidelines is at least in part due to the cost containment efforts of government third-party payers and insurance providers. The focus of administrators and practitioners to control costs without adversely affecting patient care requires reduction in avoidable costs and emphasis on imperatives through regulatory efforts and utilisation review.

Lastly, guidelines are necessary to increase consistency of recommendations and treatment by practitioners. The establishment of guidelines allows practitioners to pool limited available data, especially in certain populations (such as paediatric patients, ethnic minorities and those residing in specific geographic regions) to evaluate and distribute resources in a more efficient manner. It enables practitioners to focus on established therapies and availability of services, while decreasing regional differences and improving quality of care. Organisations such as the AMA and the American Academy of Pediatrics (AAP) have played an active role in the establishment of guidelines for the identification, quantification and treatment of a variety of disease states (for example, hypertension, asthma, rhinitis, hypercholesterolaemia) and populations (for example, neonates, the elderly).

Examples of Guidelines

The Seventh Report of the Joint National Committee on Prevention, Detection, Evaluation and Treatment of High Blood Pressure (JNC 7) was developed by an executive committee, multidisciplinary healthcare team representing the fields of medicine, nursing, nutrition, pharmacy, public health and staff at the National Heart, Lung and Blood Institute (www.nhlbi.nih.gov/guidelines/hypertension/). Since the inception of JNC 7 awareness and control of hypertension has improved and the incidence of secondary disease such as end stage renal disease and coronary heart disease has decreased. The publication provides evidence-based guidance for the detection, prevention and treatment of hypertension, and is available on the NIH website (see *Websites of Interest* at the end of the chapter).

Guidelines to determine the presence and severity of hypertension, criteria for assessment of patient risk and treatment, identification of known causes, assessment of presence or absence of target organ damage and other cardiovascular risk factors to define the prognosis or guide treatment are provided. In addition, clinical clues to identifiable causes of hypertension are provided.

Patient-specific and general guidelines for the pharmacologic and non-pharmacologic management of hypertension are provided, and information pertaining to a variety of populations such as children, adolescents, the elderly, those with co-existing conditions and of various ethnic minorities is addressed. Numerous tables and figures stratifying risk and those treatment options are provided to the practitioner for quick reference based on identified risks (such as background, gender and age).

An algorithm for the treatment of hypertension is also provided to assist the clinician in patient care decisions. Note that the JNC 8 recommendations are set to

Table 30.1 Selection considerations for individualisation of anti-hypertensive drug therapy based on the Joint National Commission 7 Guidelines (www.nhlbi.nih.gov/guidelines/hypertension/)

Indication	***Initial therapy***
Diabetes mellitus (type 1) with proteinuria	Thiazides, beta blockers, angiotensin-converting enzyme inhibitor, angiotensin receptor blockers, aldosterone antagonists
Heart failure	Thiazides, beta blockers, angiotensin-converting enzyme inhibitor, angiotensin receptor blockers, calcium channel blockers
Chronic kidney disease	Angiotensin-converting enzyme inhibitor, angiotensin receptor blockers
Myocardial infarction	Beta blocker (without intrinsic sympathomimetic activity), angiotensin-converting enzyme inhibitor (with systolic dysfunction), aldosterone antagonists

be released in 2009 with full publication in 2010.

The Third Report of the National Cholesterol Education Program (NCEP) – Detection, Evaluation and Treatment of High Blood Cholesterol in Adults (Adult Treatment Panel III) was developed by a multidisciplinary panel composed of faculty in medicine, nursing, nutrition, pharmacy and public health with the assistance of many organisations such as the American Diabetic Association, AMA, Agency for Healthcare Research and Quality and the American Red Cross. The publication provides evidence-based guidance for the detection, primary target, prevention and treatment of hypercholesterolaemia; it is available on the NIH website (http://www.nhlbi.nih.gov/guidelines/cholesterol/).

The NCEP guidelines provide background information and discuss the risks of cardiovascular disease in patients with hypercholesterolaemia and address the primary target of therapy. Patient assessment, in particular the number of risk factors, estimation of 10-year coronary heart disease risk based on the Framingham Point Scores,

Table 30.2 An example of recommendations from the NCEP guidelines for the Detection, Evaluation and Treatment of High Blood Cholesterol in Adults. Low Density Lipoprotein (LDL) Goals Based On Underlying Risk Factors

Risk	LDL
CHD	<100 mg/dL
> 2 Risk factors[a]	<130 mg/dL
0 to 1 Risk	<160 mg/dL

[a] - Risk factors include smoking, hypertension, a low level of high density lipoprotein cholesterol, family history of premature CHD, age and diabetes.

and the utilisation of total cholesterol, high density lipoproteins (HDL) and low density lipoproteins (LDL) to assess individual patient risk are addressed. Practitioners are provided guidance for the assessment of secondary causes of increased LDL such as clinical and laboratory assessment for dyslipidemia secondary to diabetes, hypothyroidism and chronic renal failure (Table 30.2).

The guidelines include non-pharmacologic or lifestyle modifications and pharmacologic management based on the number of risk factors and the calculated 10-year risk. Special considerations for different populations based on underlying risk of coronary heart disease are also summarised for the practitioner. Essential therapeutic lifestyle changes and confirmation of the benefits of LDL-lowering agents on cholesterol have been confirmed with the utilisation of the ATP III guidelines.

Guidelines for the Diagnosis and Management of Asthma (EPR-3) provided by the expert panel from the National Asthma Education and Prevention Program (NAEPP) have served as the basis for the treatment of more than 22 million children and adults with asthma. Since the first NAEPP guidelines published in 1991, important gains have been made in reducing both morbidity and mortality due to asthma (www.nhlbi.nih.gov/guidelines/about/naepp/).

The first guidelines to be formulated by an expert body of Indian doctors were hypertension guidelines endorsed jointly by the Cardiology Society of India, the Hypertension Society of India, the Indian College of Physicians and the Association of Physicians of India in 2001. These guidelines closely follow the NIH hypertension guidelines discussed earlier, as well as the

WHO guidelines from 1999. The Indian guidelines have addressed specific dietary issues of relevance to the Indian population, such as a recommendation to reduce ghee intake and avoid processed foods such as pickles, chutneys and poppadums. Additional emphasis was given to the use of low-dose diuretics and beta blockers, and the use of fixed dose drug combinations is discouraged.

Development of Guidelines

Based on the literature, there are nine separate steps or stages that should be considered in the development and implementation of clinical practice guidelines (Table 30.3).

Identify group members for guideline development: Many investigators (for example, physicians, nurses and pharmacists) have written and/or published clinical practice guidelines. However, few investigators have studied what makes a guideline successful. When developing recommendations in the guidelines, it is always advisable to have a multidisciplinary group as individual's biases may be better balanced by such groups, and they may produce more valid guidelines. The ideal number of people involved in such a group is at least six but no more than 12–15; too few members limits adequate discussion and too many makes effective functioning of the team difficult.

The choice of medical specialists in the development group depends on the drug or disease being targeted. But it is always advisable to have three broad classes of relevant healthcare professionals (up to five general practitioners, up to two hospital consultants, a health authority medical adviser and a pharmacist); specialists (an epidemiologist and a health economist); and a specialist in guideline methodology and in leading small groups. Based on education and the skill sets available, pharmacists and pharmacy organisations can and should play an integral role in guideline development, implementation, monitoring and identification of problems and/or inefficiencies in our healthcare system.

The guideline development groups are intended to define important clinical questions, produce search criteria, draw up protocols for systematic review and, whenever necessary, to undertake an appropriate meta analysis. The group

Table 30.3 Steps in guideline development

1.	Identify group members for guideline development.
2.	Identify and refine the problem, focusing on the disease and published literature.
3.	Review the literature, organisational recommendations and internet resources to determine the present standard of care.
4.	Obtain opinions from experts in the field.
5.	Begin the information feedback process.
6.	Coordinate resources to avoid duplication of resources and time.
7.	Assess the quality, relevance, variability and strength of the information.
8.	Synthesise the information.
9.	Summarise and disseminate the information, focusing on measurable outcomes.

members in the development of guidelines should have sufficient skill in the following areas: literature searching and retrieval, epidemiology, biostatistics, health services research, writing and editing.

Identify and refine the problem focusing on the disease and published literature: Guidelines can be developed for a wide range of subjects. Given the large number of potential areas, priority subjects or topics for guideline development need to be determined. Potential areas can be identified based on the main causes of morbidity and mortality for a given population, uncertainty about the appropriateness of drug therapy or about the evidence for improving patient outcomes, or the need to conserve resources in providing care. For example, the first step in preparing a treatment guideline in a hospital setting is to select a drug/disease for guideline development and analyse the utilisation trends of the drug in the hospital to assess selection. For instance, treatment guidelines for smoking cessation may be more pertinent in an ambulatory care adult setting than in an inpatient paediatric ward.

After the topic is identified, it has to be refined before the evidence can be assessed in order to answer exact questions. The usual way of refining a topic is by having a dialogue among the potential users or evaluators of the guideline. Therefore, the group that is responsible for guideline development should be clear about which areas come within the scope of the topic and which do not, to avoid broadening the scope. Note, however, that it is possible to develop guidelines that are both broad in scope and evidence based but to do so may require considerable time and money, both of which are frequently underestimated by inexperienced developers.

Review the literature, organisational recommendations and internet resources to determine the present standard of care: Identification and assessment of the evidence is best done by performing a systematic review. The purpose of the systematic review is to collect all available evidence, assess its potential applicability to the clinical question under consideration, inspect the evidence for susceptibility to bias, and extract and summarise the findings.

Identifying the clinical questions of interest will help set the boundaries for admissible evidence (types of study designs, year of publication, etc). For example, questions concerning the efficacy of interventions usually mean that randomised controlled trials should be sought, while questions of risk usually mean that prospective cohort studies should be sought.

Methods of identifying and synthesising evidence include expert opinion, unsystematic literature review, graded systematic review and formal meta-analysis. Formal meta-analysis and graded systematic reviews have a high likelihood of scientific validity while ungraded and unsystematic reviews have only medium scientific validity. The least scientific validity is for expert opinion as this method is affected by individual bias.

The first step in gathering the evidence is to check if a suitable, recent systematic review has already been published. The Cochrane Library will also identify relevant Cochrane Review groups, which should be contacted to determine if a review is in progress. If a current systematic review is not available, a computer search of Medline and IOWA Drug Information Service may be a starting point, using search strategies tailored to appropriate types of studies (though such strategies have been validated only for randomised controlled trials).

Checking references in articles will show additional relevant articles not identified by the computer search, and having experts in the field examine the list of articles helps ensure there are no obvious omissions. Additional search strategies, including searches for articles published in languages other than English, computer searches of specialised databases, manual searching of relevant journals, and searching for unpublished material, will often yield additional studies, but the resources needed for such activities are considerable. The cost effectiveness of various search strategies has not been established. It is best to match the scope of the search strategy to the available resources.

Once studies have been identified, they are assessed for relevance to the clinical questions of interest and for bias. Screening for relevance is often possible from the abstract; it narrows the set of studies to those requiring a more detailed assessment. Using explicit rather than implicit criteria should improve the reliability of the process. Once the studies are assessed for relevance, they have to be summarised.

To ensure validity and reliability, the guidelines should be based on high-quality research studies. These should be identified during a comprehensive literature review conducted within the recent past. This may be 12 months for areas where the evidence has rapidly changed, but longer periods of time, say 24–36 months, may be acceptable where new evidence is produced more slowly. Data is extracted from the relevant studies on the benefits, harm and (where applicable) costs of the interventions being considered. This is usually presented in a form that allows comparison of the designs and results of studies. Where appropriate, meta-analysis can be used to summarise the results of multiple studies. After summarising, the evidence must be categorised.

Obtain opinions from experts in the field: The opinions of experts should be used to interpret evidence and to derive recommendations in the absence of evidence. When evidence is being interpreted, opinion is needed to assess issues such as generalisability of evidence, or to extrapolate results from a study in one population to the population of interest in the guideline. Recommendations based solely on clinical judgment and experience are likely to be more susceptible to bias and self-interest. Therefore, after deciding what role expert opinion is to play, the next step is to decide how to collect and assess expert opinion. Currently, there is no optimal method for this, but the process needs to be made as explicit as possible.

Begin the information feedback process: Information feedback refers to the provision of heath data information which may allow clinicians to compare their own practice with that of their colleagues or other hospitals. Feedback is most likely to influence the clinical practice of those who have already agreed to review their practice, and is most effective if it is accompanied by a standard setting exercise or discussion and presented to clinicians soon after the clinical decision-making process. Feedback is judged a clinical success if practice moves closer to what is believed to be the standard of care.

Coordinate resources to avoid duplication of resources and time: In addition to scientific evidence and the opinions of expert clinicians, practice guidelines must often take account of the resource implications and feasibility of interventions. Judgments about whether the costs of tests or treatments are reasonable depend on how cost effectiveness is defined and calculated, on the perspective taken and on the resource constraints of the healthcare system. Feasibility issues worth considering include the time, skills, staff and equipment necessary for the provider to carry out the recommendations and the ability of patients and systems of care to implement them.

Comparative studies conclude that internal guidelines are less likely to be scientifically valid because local groups require greater resources and lack the clinical, managerial and technical skills needed to develop guidelines. Therefore, the most attractive way for a local group to develop a guideline is to adapt published guidelines for local use, although by following this method, the quality of the guidelines may be variable.

Assess the quality, relevance, variability and strength of the information: Summarised evidence is categorised to reflect its susceptibility to bias. This is a shorthand method of conveying specific aspects of the evidence to a reader of the guideline. A number of such 'strength of evidence' classification schemes exist, but empirical evidence exists only for schemes that categorise effectiveness studies by study design. In addition, each recommendation should be linked to a specific reference, so readers can track the evidence back to its source.

Synthesise the information: Synthesis of study results is the most subjective area of guideline development and impacts on the presentation, acceptability and dissemination of results. Many methods have been used, by practitioners and investigators, to establish clinical practice guidelines. In meta-analysis, guidelines and recommendations are based on statistically significant differences found when patient information is pooled primarily from published data. The process is labour intensive and the statistical knowledge necessary limits its use. More commonly, factors such as efficacy, safety and cost are compiled and summarised from primary sources and literature reviews and the author provides recommendations based on this data.

Another option is the presentation and categorisation of results. This allows for presentation of all available data without overestimating the significance of these results. Utilisation of consensus rating to establish guidelines has not been as successful as expert panel reviews. An example of this is the chronic pain management guidelines developed by the directors of the Australian Pain Society. The management strategies presented were based more on clinical practice. The presented guidelines served as more of a review than management strategy for opioid use in patients with chronic non-malignant pain.

Newer methods of review such as logic software providing a systematic means of evaluating the data are becoming available and may be useful to practitioners and investigators to establish site-specific guidelines. These systems have the potential to manage large amounts of information; however, the work required may not balance the effect of these programs on quality of care, patient outcomes and the quality of the intervention.

Summarise and disseminate the information, focusing on measurable outcomes: The way in which the guideline is presented will determine how well it is accepted. Studies encourage developing guidelines as opposed to 'policy' (from the Greek word for 'to police'), which may be seen as too dictatorial and inflexible. There is little published evidence on the effect of style and format of guidelines on their adoption. Guidelines can be presented as the full version, summary sheets of all or part of it, or reminder sheets in patient records. Algorithmic styles of presenting the guideline are often perceived by the physicians to be too complex and lacking in flexibility.

Kahan et al. analysed the content of 24 consensus statements by the NIH and suggested that variations in style may affect their acceptance by physicians. Subsequently, the NIH encouraged consensus development conferences to produce guidelines, which were concrete (making specific recommendations), didactic (offering practical advice to the clinician) and divide the patients into subclasses. Whatever the format chosen, it is important that the guideline is both reader-friendly and comprehensive. Although more research is needed, it is reassuring to note that rigorously evaluated guidelines have achieved success with a wide range of styles and formats.

This 'plan, do, study, act' cycle is necessary to determine the effect of practice guidelines and to close the gap between practice and treatment. Evaluation of the failures in the present system is important to improve practitioner acceptance and utilisation. Is the information being received by the decision-makers of the institution? Are senior and junior staff in agreement? Are interventions occurring at the practice and consultant levels? These are all questions that must be addressed before dissemination of information begins.

Evidence for Effectiveness of Guidelines

Despite the inability of some published and unpublished guidelines to improve the quality and consistency of clinical practice and reduce the costs associated with treatment, they serve an important role in the evaluation and treatment of patients. Clinical practice guidelines provide an analytical framework for the diagnosis and treatment of patients. Structured guidelines may lead to improved patient outcomes. However, the success of a clinical practice guideline is dependent on many factors: clinical context, method used in the development of the guideline, means of dissemination of the information and method of implementation of the guideline. It must be valid, reproducible, reliable, representative of the population, clinically applicable, clear, based on documented assumptions, evidence and participation and must continually be updated.

The effectiveness of explicit clinical practice guidelines on the quality of patient care has not been proven. A review of 59 published guidelines found that if an appropriate evaluation mechanism was used to measure clinical improvement, the guidelines appeared to improve the quality and outcomes of care in most cases. Reports of individual guidelines also appeared to improve the quality of patient care.

The effectiveness of clinical guidelines on cost containment has been well documented. Clinical guidelines have been shown to be effective in decreasing costs associated with patient care. The effectiveness of clinical guidelines on consistency of practitioner management has shown mixed results. This may have occurred in part due to inconsistency of evaluation and the variability in evaluation criteria.

Adherence to guidelines has also been demonstrated. Kolla et al. found that clinicians adhered to the outlined bipolar protocol and that the General Psychiatric Management Adherence Scale (GPMAS) is a valuable measure for demonstrating adherence to therapies based on the American Psychiatric Association (APA) guidelines.

Potential Limitations and Harms of Guidelines

The potential limitations of the guidelines are as follows:

- Guidelines produced by governments or payers to control spiralling treatment costs may constitute responsible public policy, but may be resented by clinicians and patients for possibly compromising the quality of healthcare and as an invasion of personal autonomy.
- Guidelines developed by specialists may seem self-serving, biased and threatening to generalists.
- Guidelines developed without the input of specialists may not contain adequate expertise.
- Clinical guidelines make sense when practitioners are unclear about appropriate practice and when scientific evidence can provide an answer. They are a poor remedy when clinicians already know the information contained in guidelines or when scientific evidence for the recommendations is lacking.

Conclusion

Clinical practice guidelines contribute to consistency in practice and set the standard of care in healthcare centres throughout the world. In practice, students and clinicians need to be able to locate, implement, utilise and critically evaluate published guidelines. Clinicians should also be able to assist practitioners and other healthcare providers in developing their own guidelines.

KEY MESSAGES

- ❖ Clinical practice guidelines developed by healthcare providers serve as a guide for the diagnosis, evaluation and/or treatment of specific disease states.
- ❖ Structured guidelines provide an analytical framework for the diagnosis and treatment of patients and may lead to improved patient outcomes.
- ❖ Published and unpublished guidelines can be found in a variety of locations such as medical databases and internet sites.
- ❖ Pharmacy organisations and pharmacists can play an integral role in guideline development, implementation, monitoring and revision.

Further Reading

Angaran, DM. 1990. Measuring and monitoring health care. *Top Hosp Pharm Manage* 10(2):1–11.

Bousquet, J et al. 2009. Implementation of Guidelines for Allergic Rhinitis in Specialist Practices. A Randomized Pragmatic Controlled Trial. *Int Arch Allergy Immunol* 150(1):75–82.

Chesney, RW et al. 2001. The testing of antihypertensive medications in children: report of the Antihypertensive Agent Guidelines Subcommittee of the Pediatric Pharmacology Research Units. *Pediatrics* 107(3):558–61.

Clinical practice guideline: management of sinusitis. 2001. *Pediatrics* 108(3):798–808.

Eccles, M, Freemantle N and Mason J. 1998. North of England evidence based guideline development project: summary guideline for non-steroidal anti-inflammatory drugs versus basic analgesia in treating the pain of degenerative arthritis. The North of England Non-Steroidal Anti-Inflammatory Drug Guideline Development Group. *BMJ* 317(7157):526–30.

Eccles, M, Freemantle N and Mason J. 1998. North of England evidence based guidelines development project: methods of developing guidelines for efficient drug use in primary care. *BMJ* 316(7139):1232–5.

Eccles, M, Freemantle N and Mason J. 1998.North of England evidence based guideline development project: guideline on the use of aspirin as secondary prophylaxis for vascular disease in primary care. North of England Aspirin Guideline Development Group. *BMJ* 316(7140):1303–9.

Feder, G et al. 1999. Clinical guidelines: using clinical guidelines. *BMJ* 318(7185):728–30.

Furrow, BR. 1999. Broadcasting clinical guidelines on the Internet: will physicians tune in? *Am J Law Med* 25(2–3):403–21.

Garner, P et al. 1998. Getting research findings into practice: implementing research findings in developing countries. *BMJ* 317(7157):531–5.

Grabowski, BS. 1991. Practice guidelines and drug-usage evaluation. *Top Hosp Pharm Manage* 11(2):1–5.

Graziotti, PJ and Goucke CR. 1997. The use of oral opioids in patients with chronic non-cancer pain. Management strategies. *Med J Aust* 167(1):30–4.

Grimshaw, J and Russell I. 1993. Achieving health gain through clinical guidelines. I: Developing scientifically valid guidelines. *Qual Health Care* 2(4):243–8.

Grimshaw, JM and Hutchinson A. 1995. Clinical practice guidelines--do they enhance value for money in health care? *Br Med Bull* 51(4):927–40.

Grimshaw, JM and Russell IT. 1993. Effect of clinical guidelines on medical practice: a systematic review of rigorous evaluations. *Lancet* 342(8883):1317–22.

Grimshaw, JM and Russell IT. 1994. Achieving health gain through clinical guidelines II: Ensuring guidelines change medical practice. *Qual Health Care* 3(1):45–52.

Grundy, SM et al. 2004. Implications of recent clinical trials for the National Cholesterol Education Program Adult Treatment Panel III guidelines. *Circulation* 110(2):227–39.

Haynes, RB et al. 1986. How to keep up with the medical literature: V Access by personal computer to the medical literature. *Ann Intern Med* 105(5):810–6.

Haynes, RB et al. 1994. Performances of 27 MEDLINE systems tested by searches with clinical questions. *J Am Med Inform Assoc* 1(3):285–95.

Koch, KE. 1995. Opportunities for pharmaceutical care with critical pathways. *Top Hosp Pharm Manage* 14(4):1–7.

Kolla, NJ et al. 2009. Demonstrating adherence to guidelines for the treatment of patients with borderline personality disorder. *Can J Psychiatry* 54(3):181–9.

Medicine IOM. 1992. *Guidelines for clinical practice: from development to use*. National Academic Press: Washington, DC.

Merritt, TA et al. 1997. Clinical practice guidelines in pediatric and newborn medicine: implications for their use in practice. *Pediatrics* 99(1):100–14.

Morehead, MA, Lobach K and Lee J. 1987. Medication costs in different provider settings. *Qual Assur Util Rev* 2(3):71–8.

Mugford, M, Banfield P and O'Hanlon M, 1991. Effects of feedback of information on clinical practice: a review. *BMJ* 303(6799):398–402.

Murphy, MK et al.1998. Consensus development methods, and their use in clinical guideline development. *Health Technol Assess* 2(3):i–iv, 1–88.

Pierce, EC Jr. 1990. The development of anesthesia guidelines and standards. *QRB Qual Rev Bull* 16(2): 61–4.

Richardson, LP et al. 2000. Effectiveness of a vancomycin restriction policy in changing the prescribing patterns of house staff. *Microb Drug Resist* 6(4):327–30.

Shane, R. 1994. Development and implementation of practice guidelines (Part 1). *Hosp Formul* 29(10):711–4, 718–9.

Shane, R. 1995. Take the first step on the critical pathway. *Am J Health Syst Pharm* 52(10):1051–3.

Shekelle, PG et al.1999. Clinical guidelines: developing guidelines. *BMJ* 318(7183):593–6.

Shrank, WH et al.2009. Rationale and design of the Study Assessing the Effect of Cardiovascular Medications Provided as Low-cost, Evidence-based Generic Samples (SAMPLES) trial. *Am Heart J* 157(4):613–9.

Smith, EE. 1993. Variations in clinical guidelines, 3rd ed. *Ann Emerg Med* 22(7):1196–7.

Thomson, R et al. 2000. Decision analysis and guidelines for anticoagulant therapy to prevent stroke in patients with atrial fibrillation. *Lancet* 355(9208):956–62.

Tricoci, P et al. 2009. Scientific evidence underlying the ACC/AHA clinical practice guidelines. *JAMA* 301(8):831–41.

White, LJ and Ball, JR. 1990. Integrating practice guidelines with financial incentives. *QRB Qual Rev Bull* 16(2):50–3.

Websites of Interest

University of San Francisco
http://medicine/ucsf.edu/resources/

US Agency for Healthcare Research and Quality
http://www.guideline.gov/

US Department of Health and Human Services
www.ahcpr.gov/

National Institutes of Health (Guidelines)
http://www.nhlbi.nih.gov/guidelines/hypertension/
http://www.nhlbi.nih.gov/guidelines/cholesterol/

American Heart Association
http://www.heart.org

American Medical Association
www.ama-assn.org

American Colleges of Clinical Pharmacy
www.accp.com

Appendix I: Bibliography of Pharmacoepidemiologic Studies Done in India

Agrawal RP, Choudhary R, Sharma P, Sharma S, Beniwal R, Kaswan K and Kochar DK. 2007. Glyceryl trinitrate spray in the management of painful diabetic neuropathy: A randomized double blind placebo controlled cross-over study. *Diabetes Res Clin Pract* 77:161–167.

Balakrishnan S, Bambery P, Gupta N and Pandhi P. 2001. An audit of the use of antirheumatic drugs in a north Indian referral hospital. *Pharmacoepidemiol Drug Saf* 10:237–243.

Bapna JS, Tekur U, Gitanjali B, Shashindran CH, Pradhan SC, Thulasimani M and Tomson G. 1992. Drug utilization at primary health care level in southern India. *Eur J Clin Pharmacol* 43:413–415.

Biswas NR, Biswas RS, Pal PS, Jain SK, Malhotra SP, Gupta A and Pal SN. 2000. Patterns of prescriptions and drug use in two tertiary hospitals in Delhi. *Indian J Physiol Pharmacol* 44:109–112.

Biswas NR, Jindal S, Siddiquei MM and Maini R. 2001. Patterns of prescription and drug use in ophthalmology in a tertiary hospital in Delhi. *Br J Clin Pharmacol* 51:267–269.

Catalani E. 1999. Review of the Indian market of anti-tuberculosis drugs: focus on the utilization of rifampicin-based products. *Int J Tuberc Lung Dis* 3 (11 Suppl 3):S289–291, S317–321.

Chakraborty A. 1990. Psychotropic drugs in a new perspective. *J Indian Med Assoc* 88:333–334.

Datta SP, Srinivasa DK and Kale RV. 1971. A study on morbidity and drug costs in a primary health centre. *Indian J Med Sci* 25:690–695.

Dharnidharka VR and Kandoth P. 1999. Paediatric inpatient morbidity patterns and drug usage in a teaching hospital serving an underdeveloped area. *Indian J Public Health* 43:64–66.

Dimri S, Tiwari P, Basu S and Parmar VR. 2009. Drug use pattern in children at a teaching hospital. *Indian Pediatr* 46:165–167.

Dineshkumar B, Raghuram TC, Radhaiah G and Krishnaswamy K. 1995. Profile of drug use in urban and rural India. *Pharmacoeconomics* 7:332–346.

Dondorp A, Nosten F, Stepniewska K, Day N and White N, South East Asian Quinine Artesunate Malaria Trial (SEAQUAMAT) group. 2005. Artesunate versus quinine for treatment of severe falciparum malaria: A randomised trial. *Lancet* 366:717–725.

Gada MT, Agrawal BR, Pradhan PV, Shah LP and Bagadia VN. 1983. Report from a World Health Organization (WHO) Collaborative Centre for Psychopharmacology in India. Survey of antipsychotic drugs use. *Psychopharmacol Bull* 19:778–780.

Ghosh BN, Mitra J and Das KK. 1987. Prescription habits of physicians in an urban locality. *Indian J Public Health* 31:120–128.

Gogtay NJ, Mangalvedhekar SS and Kshirsagar NA. 2000. Adverse drug reaction (ADR) monitoring in India and the postal survey as a useful tool for ADR detection. *Pharmacoepidemiol Drug Saf* 9:235–236.

Gupta SK, Kaleekal T and Joshi S. 2000. Misuse of corticosteroids in some of the drugs dispensed as preparations from alternative systems of medicine in India. *Pharmacoepidemiol Drug Saf* 9:599–602.

Harugeri A, Joseph J, Parthasarathi G, Ramesh M and Guido S. 2010. Potentially inappropriate medication use in elderly patients: A study of prevalence and predictors in two teaching hospitals. *J Postgrad Med* 56:186–191.

Harugeri A, Joseph J, Parthasarathi G, Ramesh M and Guido S. 2010. Prescribing patterns and predictors of high-level polypharmacy in the elderly population: A prospective surveillance study from two teaching hospitals in india. *Am J Geriatr Pharmacother* 8:271–280.

Hazra A, Tripathi SK and Alam MS. 2000. Prescribing and dispensing activities at the health facilities of a non-governmental organisation. *Natl Med J India* 13:177–182.

International Collaborative Study of Severe Anaphylaxis. 2003. Risk of anaphylaxis in a hospital population in relation to the use of various drugs: An international study. *Pharmacoepidemiol Drug Saf* 12:195–202.

Jaiprakash H, Sarala N, Venkatarathnamma PN and Kumar TN. 2011. Analysis of different types of poisoning in a tertiary care hospital in rural south india. *Food Chem Toxicol* 49:248–250.

Jhaj R, Bhargava VK, Uppal R, Reeta KH, Kaur N and Kumar L. 2000. Drug prescribing in children in a North Indian referral hospital. *Pharmacoepidemiol Drug Saf* 9:423–427.

Jhaj R, Goel NK, Gautam CS, Hota D, Sangeeta B, Sood A and Sachdev A. 2001. Prescribing patterns and cost of antihypertensive drugs in an internal medicine clinic. *Indian Heart J* 53:323–327.

Jose J and Rao PG. 2006. Pattern of adverse drug reactions notified by spontaneous reporting in an indian tertiary care teaching hospital. *Pharmacol Res* 54:226–233.

Kohli K, Kela AK and Mehta VL. 1995. Rational drug therapy as evaluated from student's clinical case reports. *Indian J Physiol Pharmacol* 39:400–402.

Krishnaswami KV, Abdul Rahim M, Seshagiri K, Radhakrishna S, Satagopan MC, Somasundaram PR, Tripathy SP and Fox W. 1982. Study of a policy to minimise the prescription of medicaments at first attendance at chest clinics. *Lancet* 2(8296):483–486.

Krishnaswamy K, Kumar BD and Radhaiah G. 1985. A drug survey – precepts and practices. *Eur J Clin Pharmacol* 29:363–370.

Kshirsagar MJ, Langade D, Patil S and Patki PS. 1998. Prescribing patterns among medical practitioners in Pune, India. *Bull World Health Org* 76:271–275.

Kshirsagar NA, Karande SC and Potkar CN. 1993. Adverse reaction monitoring in India. *J Assoc Physicians India* 41:374–376.

Kumar A, Gogtay NJ and Kshrisagar NA. 2000. A survey of primaquine prescribing habits in the city of Mumbai. *J Assoc Physicians India* 48:660.

Kumar S and Sedgwick P. 2001. Can the factors influencing medication compliance reported from western populations be applied to an eastern Indian context? *J Mental Health* 10:267–277.

Kumar S and Sedgwick P. 2001. Non-compliance to psychotropic medication in eastern India: Clients' perspective, Part II. *J Mental Health* 10:279–284.

Lodha R, Gupta G, Baruah BP, Nagpal R and Kabra SK. 2004. Metered dose inhaler with spacer versus dry powder inhaler for delivery of salbutamol in acute exacerbations of asthma: A randomized controlled trial. *Indian Pediatr* 41:15–20.

Malhotra S, Grover A, Verma NK and Bhargava VK. 2000. A study of drug utilization and cost of treatment in patients hospitalized with unstable angina. *Eur J Clin Pharmacol* 56:755–761.

Malhotra S, Karan RS, Pandhi P and Jain S. 2001. Pattern of use and pharmacoeconomic impact of antihypertensive drugs in a north Indian referral hospital. *Eur J Clin Pharmacol* 57:535–540.

Manjula D, David J and Kulkarni C. 2002. Prescribing pattern of anti-seizure medications (ASMs): An evaluation of extent of xanthine co-medication. *Pol J Pharmacol* 54:285–291.

Mishra SK and Satpathy R. 2001. Physicians' attitudes about prescribing and knowledge of the costs of common medications. *Arch Intern Med* 161:1352–1353.

Mitra J, Saha JB and Chaudhuri RN. 1993. Drug consumption pattern in low socio-economic group in an urban community. *Indian J Public Health* 37:16–22.

Mundra VK, Rajkumar IR, Agrawal BR, Pradhan PV, Shah LP and Bagadia VN. 1984. Report from the World Health Organization Collaborative Centre for Psychopharmacy in India: Antianxiety drugs. *Psychopharmacol Bull* 20:178–179.

Oei PL and Ratnam SS. 1998. Hormone replacement therapy in the developing countries. *Aust N Z J Obstet Gynaecol* 38:141–144.

Phadke AR. 1996. The quality of prescribing in an Indian district. *Natl Med J India* 9:60–65.

Pradhan SC, Shewade DG, Tekur U, Zutshi S, Pachiappan D, Dey AK, Adithan C, Shashindran CH and Bapna JS. 1990. Changing pattern of antimicrobial utilization in an Indian teaching hospital. *Int J Clin Pharmacol Ther Toxicol* 28:339–343.

Prasad Rao DS. 1975. A sociological study of drug default in childhood tuberculosis. *Indian J Pediatr* 42(324):13–16.

Radhakrishnan K, Nayak SD, Kumar SP and Sarma PS. 1999. Profile of antiepileptic pharmacotherapy in a tertiary referral centre in South India: a pharmacoepidemiologic and pharmacoeconomic study. *Epilepsia* 40:179–185.

Ravikiran TN, Goel RC and Chaudhury RR. 1979. A study on drug usage on inpatients at the Nehru Hospital, PGI Chandigarh. *Hosp Adm (New Delhi)* 16:31–37.

Rewari S, Tekur U, Prabhu S and Ramchander X. 2000. Drug utilization patterns in sexually transmitted diseases and its economic considerations—a prospective study. *J Assoc Physicians India* 48:284–287.

Rupawala AH, Kshirsagar NA and Gogtay NJ. 2009. A retrospective analysis of adverse events in the elderly in a tertiary referral center in Mumbai (Bombay), India. *Indian J Med Sci* 63:167–173.

S RB, Narayan SS, Sharma GR, Rodrigues RJ and Kulkarni C. 2008. Pattern of adverse drug reactions to anti-epileptic drugs: A cross-sectional one-year survey at a tertiary care hospital. *Pharmacoepidemiol Drug Saf* 17:807–812.

Sehgal H. 1984. Use of diphenoxylate (Lomotil) in children. *Indian Pediatr* 21:582–583.

Sharma D, Reeta K, Badyal DK, Garg SK and Bhargava VK. 1998. Antimicrobial prescribing pattern in an Indian tertiary hospital. *Indian J Physiol Pharmacol* 42:533–537.

Sharma P, Gupta BD, Karkra A, Beg A, Arora V and Baso S. 1996. Prescribing practices of paediatricians in malaria. *Indian J Pediatr* 63:407–408.

Srishyla MV, Krishnamurthy M, Naga Rani MA, Clare SM, Andrade C and Venkataraman BV. 1994. Prescription audit in an Indian hospital setting using the DDD (defined daily dose) concept. *Indian J Pharmacol* 26: 23–38.

Srishyla MV, Naga Rani MA and Venkataraman BV. 1994. Drug utilization of antimicrobials in the in-patient setting of a tertiary hospital. *Indian J Pharmacol* 26: 282–287.

Thawani V, Motghare V, Purwar MB and Pagare A. 1997. Drug utilization in indoor ANC patients of Govt Medical College Hospital, Nagpur. *J Acad Hosp Adm* 9: 49–51.

Uppal R, Bhowmik SR, Malik SK, Jindal SK and Sharma PL. 1988. Drug usage in chest diseases. *Int J Clin Pharmacol Ther Toxicol* 26:33–35.

Uppal R, Bhowmik SR, Sharma PL, Kaur S and Arora R. 1988. Drug use in dermatology. *Int J Clin Pharmacol Ther Toxicol* 26:610–611.

Uppal R, Sarkar U, Giriyappanavar CS and Kacker V. 1993. Antimicrobial drug use in primary health care. *J Clin Epidemiol* 46:671–673.

Uppal R, Sarkar U, Giriyappanavar CS and Kacker V. 1994. Pharmacoepidemiology of drug use at two primary health care centres in northern India. *Int J Clin Pharmacol Ther* 32:284–285.

Uppal R, Singh A, Sharma PL and Sharma BK. 1987. Drug utilization studies in internal medicine. *Int J Clin Pharmacol Ther Toxicol* 25:216–217.

Appendix II: Steps Involved in Medication History Interview

Patient selection

Ideally, a patient medication history should be taken for all patients. If this is not possible, priority should be given to those patients where it is considered that maximum benefit is likely to accrue. For example, patients with polypharmacy, multiple and chronic diseases may benefit more compared to those on a single drug and/or treated for self-limiting diseases. A patient medication history interview may not be possible in certain cases; for example, patients with psychiatric disorders, impaired cognition or in acutely unwell patients. In these situations, useful information may be obtained from a family member or carer.

Self-preparation

Before commencing an interview, pharmacists should collect all relevant data from the various sources available and should have a thorough understanding of the patients' co-morbidities. A provisional list of medications based on information from medical notes or other sources is useful for helping patients recall their medications during the interview. A list of questions that are to be asked during the interview helps to focus on patient-specific questions and also saves time.

Privacy and confidentiality

Pharmacists must consider the factors relating to the privacy and confidentiality of interviews. In a hospital setting, this can be difficult as most interviews will be conducted at the patient's bedside. If the patient is unable to communicate appropriately, the patient's carer or family members can be involved in the discussion, preferably with permission from the patient. Pharmacists should maintain the confidentiality of the data collected during interview, except for exchange of information with other healthcare professionals caring for the patient.

Purpose of interview

It is essential for the pharmacist to introduce him or herself and to explain the purpose of conducting the interview and also the possible benefits that the patient might obtain from the interview. The pharmacist should respect the patient's right to decline an interview.

Conduct of interview

Use of communication skills such as listening, body language, voice intonation and history-taking skills is crucial to a successful patient interaction. It is important to adopt a suitable seated position to enable the conversation to take place comfortably and effectively. Pharmacists should use the patient's first language where possible. In the event that the patient is unable to communicate appropriately, the interview should be conducted with relevant persons such as a family member or carer after obtaining permission from the patient (if possible). Where possible, the pharmacist should ask open-ended questions. This technique encourages patients to reveal their knowledge and beliefs concerning medication use. Asking questions and receiving information in a non-judgmental way is also essential. ('Please tell me how you take your medications' rather than asking 'Do you take your medication as prescribed by your doctor?'). Close-ended questions may be useful to confirm details. All the questions asked should be appropriate and relevant to the patient's medical condition. Exhaustive interview and unimportant questions need to be avoided as these may tire the patient and be counter-productive.

Conclusion

At the end of the interview, check whether all the important and relevant information has been obtained (see *Table 13.1*). Ask the patient if he or she has any questions relating to their medications and also encourage them to provide more information which may be recalled after the interview.

Documentation and follow-up

All the information obtained during the medication history interview should be documented so that the gathered data can contribute to ongoing pharmaceutical care. The documented medications should be compared with information obtained from other healthcare professionals for any discrepancies (medication reconciliation). These should be brought to the attention of medical staff.

Appendix III: Laboratory Reference Ranges

Haematology	*Conventional Units*	*International Units*
Erythrocyte count, male	4.6–6.2 x 106/microliter	4.6–6.2 x 1012/L
Erythrocyte count, female	4.2–5.4 x 106/microliter	4.2–5.4 x 1012/L
Haematocrit	41–53%	
Haemoglobin	13.5–17.5 g/dL	2.09–2.71 mmol/L
HbA1C	5.3–7.5%	n/a
International Normalised Ratio (INR)	0.9–1.2	0.9–1.2
Leukocyte Count, total	4.5–11 x 103/microliter	4.5–11 x109/L
Segs	31–71%	n/a
Bands	0–12%	n/a
Lymphocytes	15–50%	n/a
Monocytes	0–12%	n/a
Eosinophils	0–5%	n/a
Basophils	0–2%	n/a
Mean Corpuscular Volume (MCV)	80–96 mcgm3	80–96 fL
Mean Corpuscular Haemoglobin (MCH)	27–31 pg	27–31 pg
Platelets	150–440 x 103/microliter	0.15–0.44 x 1012/L
Prothrombin time	10–13 secs	10–13 secs
Reticulocytes	0.5–1.5% of erythrocytes	n/a

Biochemistry	*Conventional Units*	*International Units*
Alanine aminotransferase (ALT, SGPT)	8–20 units/L	8–20 units/L
Albumin	3.7–4.7 g/L	37–47 g/dL
Alkaline phosphatase	30–75 units/L	30–75 units/L
Amylase	25–125 units/L	25–125 units/L
Aspartate aminotransferase (AST, SGOT)	8–20 units/L	8–20 units/L
B12	150–750 pg/mL	200–672 pmol/L
Bilirubin, total	0.2–1.0 mg/dL	3.4–17.1 mmol/L
Bilirubin, direct (conjugated)	0–0.2 mg/dL	0–3.4 micromol/L
Blood urea nitrogen (BUN)	8–20 mg/dL	2.9–7.1 mmol/L
Calcium	8.5–10.5 mL/dL	2.1–2.6 mmol/L
Carbon dioxide (bicarbonate)	22–28 mEq/L	22–28 mEq/L
Carbon dioxide (CO2)	22–29 mEq/L	22–29 mEq/L

Chloride	98–107 mEq/L	98–107 mmol/LC
Cholesterol, total	140–220 mg/dL	3.63–5.70 mmol/L
C-reactive protein (CRP)	< 8 mg/dL	
Creatinine	0.7–1.3 mg/dL	62–115 micromol/L
Creatinine clearance	90–130 mL/min	0.87–1.25 mL/s/m2
Creatinine kinase (CK), male	38–174 units/L	38–174 units/L
Creatinine kinase (CK), female	26–140 units/L	26–140 units/L
Ferritin	>10–20 ng/mL	20–300 micrograms/L
Folate,serum	2.8–40 ng/mL	6.5–45.0 nmol/L
Gamma-glutamyltransferase (GGT)	8–50 units/L	8–50 units/L
Glucose	60–110 mg/dL	3.3–6.1 mmol/L
Glucose, fasting	70–105 mg/dL	3.89–5.83 mmol/L
HDL cholesterol	30–85 mg/dL	0.78–2.20 mmol/L
Iron	65–170 mcg/dL	11.64–30.4 micromol/L
Iron binding capacity, total (TIBC)	250–450 mcg/dL	45–81 micromol/L
Lactate dehydrogenase (LDH)	110–210 units/L	110–210 units/L
LDL cholesterol	< 130 mg/dL	< 3.37 mmol/L
Lipase	18–180 units/L	18–180 units/L
Magnesium	1.8–3.0 mg/dL	0.75–1.25 mmol/L
Osmolality, urine	500–800 mOsm/kg	
Osmolality, serum	289–308 mOsm/kg	
Phosphorus, inorganic, male	2.3–3.7 mg/dL	0.74–.20 mmol/L
Phosphorus, inorganic, female	2.8–4.1 mg/dL	0.90–1.32 mmol/L
Potassium	3.5–5.1 mEq/L	3.5–5.1 mmol/L
Protein, total, ambulatory	6.2–8.1 g/dL	62–81 g/L
Protein, total, recumbent	5.8–7.6 g/dL	58–81 g/L
Sodium, serum	136–146 mEq/L	136–146 mmol/L
TSH	0.3–5.0 micro units/mL	0.3–5.0 munits/L
Thyroxine, total	5–10 mcg/dL	65–129 nmol/L
Transferrin	180–380 mg/dL	1.80–3.80 g/L
Triglycerides	40–160 mg/dL	0.45–1.81 mmol/L
Urea nitrogen (BUN)	8–21 mg/dL	1.3–3.5 mmol/L
Uric acid	3.5–7.2 mg/dL	0.21–0.42 mmol/L
Vitamin B12	200–900 pg/mL	140–700 pmol/L

GLOSSARY

Absolute risk reduction: The difference between how often an outcome occurs in the treatment group compared to the control group.

Absolute risk: The probability that an individual will experience a specified outcome during a specified time period.

Academic detailing: A programme of structured, one-to-one educational visits with the aim of modifying behaviour in a targeted area of clinical practice.

Adherence: The extent to which the patient's actual history of medicine intake corresponds to the prescribed regimen.

Adverse drug event: Injury resulting from medical interventions related to a medicine.

Adverse drug reaction: Any response to a medicine that is noxious and unintended, and that occurs at doses used in humans for prophylaxis, diagnosis or therapy of a disease, or for the modification of physiologic function.

Adverse event/Adverse experience: Any untoward medical occurrence that may present during treatment with a pharmaceutical product but which does not necessarily have a causal relationship with this treatment.

Allergic reaction: An immunological hypersensitivity, occurring as the result of unusual sensitivity to a drug.

Allocation: Allotment; apportioning, in this context: to assign funding to.

Anaemia: The term used to describe a condition characterised by an abnormally low concentration of haemoglobin in peripheral blood.

Anti-HBc: Antibody to hepatitis B core antigen.

Anti-HCV: Antibody to the hepatitis C virus.

Assessor: Any person involved in assessing the outcomes of an intervention in a clinical trial.

Assistant: A resident who acts as assistant to the chief or attending specialist.

ATC system: The Anatomic-Therapeutic-Chemical system, developed and used by the World Health Organization to categorise drugs in a systematic fashion.

Attributable risk: Also known as the risk difference. It is the rate of an adverse drug event or reaction that occurs in excess of the rate observed in non-exposed individuals.

Basal–bolus insulin: An intensive insulin regimen using a combination of a long-acting insulin given once daily and ultra-fast acting insulin given immediately before meals.

Bias: Systematic deviation of study results from the true results, because of the way in which the study was conducted.

Bioavailability: The fraction of an administered dose that reaches systemic circulation.

Birth defect: Abnormality present at birth.

Breast pump: A device used to extract milk from the breast during lactation.

Case notes: Medical information collected on a patient by health professionals to record examinations, investigations, diagnoses made, observations, treatment, etc.

Case-control study: A research study in which a group of patients having an outcome are identified, and another group not having the outcome are identified; then rates of exposure to a drug are determined and compared in an odds ratio.

Clearance: The pharmacokinetic parameter that describes the efficiency of elimination from the body.

Clinical pharmacokinetics: The process of using pharmacokinetic principles and pharmacodynamic criteria to assist in the selection of appropriate drug dosage regimens for individual patients.

Clinical pharmacologist: A medical specialist who studies how drugs work, how they interact with other drugs, how their effects can alter the disease process and how disease can alter their effects.

Clinical pharmacology: Links basic pharmacology with the therapeutic use of drugs and involves the study of pharmacodynamics and pharmacokinetics in humans.

Clinical pharmacy practice: The practice of pharmacy in a multidisciplinary healthcare team directed at achieving patient treatment goals.

Clinical practice guidelines: Systematic recommendations developed by healthcare providers to serve as a guide for diagnosis, evaluation and/or treatment of a specific disease state.

Closed body position: Where the arms and legs are crossed in front of the body.

Closed questions: Questions that require a one-word answer.

Cochrane Library: A well-known and respected database for evidence-based medicine.

Cockcroft–Gault equation: A numerical equation used to estimate the GFR.

Cognitive impairment: Impairment of mental activities such as thinking, learning and remembering.

Cohort study: A comparative research study involving a group of individuals exposed to a drug and a comparison group of individuals not exposed to the drug. Both groups are monitored, usually prospectively over time, to note the development of outcomes, which are compared using the relative risk.

Cohort: A group of people studied, usually over time, to determine the outcome after exposure to a drug or other substance.

Colonisation: Invasiveness of an organism without disease in the host.

Comparison group: A group of (usually) non-exposed individuals whose rate of use (or other outcome) is used as the basis against which observed rate in exposed individuals is compared, assuming that the comparison group rate represents that of the population to whom results are to be extrapolated.

Complete blood picture (CBP): A panel of investigations that provides information about the characteristics of blood cells in peripheral circulation.

Compliance (adherence): The extent to which a person's behaviour (in terms of taking medications, following diets or executing lifestyle changes) coincides with medical or health advice.

Conception: Fertilisation, which is the union of a male sperm with a female ovum.

Confidence interval: A measure of the precision of an estimated value. Wider intervals indicate lower precision.

Confounding factors: Variables which may offer alternative explanations for the results of a research study.

Congenital: A condition present at birth.

Consultant: A senior physician or surgeon.

Contingent valuation (CV): Survey-based approach to acquire respondent utility values for a non-market good or service contingent on a hypothetical market to purchase the good. The term CV and WTP are frequently used interchangeably.

Controls: Subjects in a comparison group in an RCT. They are allocated to receive placebo, no treatment or standard treatment.

Co-payment: A nominal fee charged to members of a managed care organisation or insurance to offset costs not covered in health plan dues. Typical co-payments are fixed or variable flat amounts for physician office visits, prescriptions or hospital services.

Cost effectiveness analysis (CEA): Ratio of costs measured in monetary units to health effects measured in natural units. For example, cost per additional life year.

Cost utility analysis (CUA): Ratio of costs, measured in monetary units to benefits measured in QALYs, that is, cost per additional QALY.

Cost–Benefit analysis (CBA): Both costs and outcomes are measured in monetary units.

Costs versus charges: Costs are incurred by an organisation in delivery of services while charges are billed to the buyer for delivered services.

C-reactive protein: An acute phase reactant indicating tissue damage from infection, infarction, inflammation or trauma.

Critical appraisal: The reading of original research papers in a way that allows us to judge their scientific value, and to consider how the results can be applied in practice.

Cytochrome P450: A mitochrondial enzyme family which metabolises a wide range of endogenous and exogenous compounds including drugs.

Defined daily dose (DDD): The average amount of a drug ingested daily when used in its most common indication.

Delirium: An altered state of consciousness, consisting of confusion, distractibility, disorientation, disordered thinking and memory, defective perception, hyperactivity and agitation; caused by a number of toxic structural and metabolic disorders.

Dementia: The loss, usually progressive, of cognitive function, without impairment of perception or consciousness; characterised by disorientation and impairment of memory, judgement and intellect; caused by a variety of disorders.

Dialysis: A mechanical process that is used to remove soluble metabolic waste and to some extent, electrolytes, from blood in the context of severe renal dysfunction.

Differential: The proportion of the total leucocyte count contributed by neutrophils, lymphocytes, basophils, monocytes and eosinophils.

Dipstick: A colourimetric indicator strip used to detect the presence of various substances in biological fluids.

Direct costs: They include the cost of resources directly involved in the delivery of services and include capital costs (property, plant and equipment) and variable costs (such as supplies, lab tests, hourly wage and personnel). For example, cost of inpatient care to the institution could include cost of medication (acquisition), personnel costs and hospital day costs.

Discounting: The process of reducing the value of cost or outcomes occurring in the future to reflect the time preference. Most researchers (but not all) assume that persons would rather receive a health benefit sooner than later, implying a positive discount rate. As a result, benefits and costs incurred in future years are weighted less heavily than those incurred earlier by discounting.

Disposition: A term used to describe collectively the processes of drug distribution and elimination that occur upon entry of a drug into the body.

Drug metabolite: A chemical derivative of a drug molecule that is produced through transformation (metabolism) by one or more organ systems including the liver, gut wall and kidneys.

Drug transporters: Energy requiring systems which carry molecules across extra and intracellular membranes.

Drug–drug interactions: Occur when two (or more) therapeutically active substances produce enhancement or diminution of the therapeutic effect or side effects of one or both drugs.

Drug–food interactions: Occur when food or a food constituent interferes with a drug and the expected effect of the medicine is modified.

Drug-related problem: Any event or circumstance involving drug treatment that interferes or potentially interferes with the patient achieving an optimum outcome of medical care.

Effectiveness: How well a programme or a drug works under real-life conditions.

Efficacy: How well a programme or drug works under ideal or optimal conditions; for example, in a randomised clinical trial.

Empathy: The ability to see and feel the way another person does.

Epidemiology: The study of the distribution and determinants of health-related states or events in specified populations, and the application of this study to the control of health problems.

Erythrocyte sedimentation rate (ESR): An acute phase reactant often markedly elevated in acute and chronic infections and inflammation.

Essential medicine: A medicine that satisfies the priority healthcare needs of a population.

Evidence-based medicine: The conscientious, explicit and judicious use of current best evidence in making decisions about the care of individual patients.

External costs: The costs external to the provision of a programme or a service; for example, the cost of homemaker services.

External validity: The extent to which trial results can be correctly generalised to other patients or settings.

Extrapyramidal effects: Adverse effects characterised by disorders of movement, such as Parkinsonian symptoms (rigidity, akinesia and tremor), dystonias or tardive dyskinesia; caused by blockade of dopamine receptors in the extrapyramidal motor system of the brain.

First-line therapy: A therapy for which there is evidence and/or consensus of opinion that it is an appropriate first choice for the disease/condition in question (that is, the therapy is among those with the greatest benefit to risk ratio).

Floor stock system: Bulk supplies of medications are kept in stock in patient care areas. These medicines are not labelled for individual patients. Doses are taken from these bulk supplies to administer to patients without a check by the pharmacist.

Formulary: A listing of drugs that a physician may prescribe. The physician is requested or required to prescribe only formulary drugs unless there is a valid medical reason to prescribe non-formulary drugs.

Genetic polymorphism: Variation in genetic (DNA) sequence to produce inter-individual differences, for example, in drug metabolising enzyme activity.

Geriatrics: The branch of general medicine concerned with the clinical, preventive, remedial and social aspects of health and illness in the elderly.

Gestation: The period of time from conception in pregnancy.

Glomerular filtration rate (GFR): Estimated by calculation of the creatinine clearance, the GFR is a surrogate marker of renal function.

Gram stain: A differential stain used for determining bacterial cell morphology.

Haemolysis: Lysis or rupture of erythrocytes (red blood cells). This may occur intravascularly, or after a blood sample has been taken from the patient for use in laboratory tests. Haemolysis may significantly affect the results of certain laboratory tests, such as the plasma haemoglobin and serum potassium concentration.

Half-life: The time necessary for the plasma concentration of a drug to decline to half of its existing value.

HBsAg: The hepatitis B surface antigen, which is the outer surface of the hepatitis B virus that triggers an antibody response.

Hemiplegia: Paralysis of one side of the body.

High power field (hpf): Represents a level of magnification under the microscope.

Home medicines review: A service provided by pharmacists which involves the pharmacist visiting the patient at home to identify medication-related problems, and then providing a written report to the patient's doctor.

Homeostasis: The state of equilibrium (balance between opposing processes) that exists in the body with respect to various functions, and the processes through which such equilibrium is maintained.

Hypercalcaemia: Used to denote a finding where the serum calcium concentration is above the upper limit of the reference range.

Hyperglycaemia: Used to denote a finding where the serum glucose concentration is above the upper limit of the reference range.

Hyperkalaemia: Used to denote a finding where the serum potassium concentration is above the upper limit of the reference range.

Hypernatraemia: Used to denote a finding where the serum sodium concentration is above the upper limit of the reference range.

Hypocalcaemia: Used to denote a finding where the serum calcium concentration is below the lower limit of the reference range.

Hypoglycaemia: Used to denote a finding where the serum glucose concentration is below the lower limit of the reference range.

Hypokalaemia: Used to denote a finding where the serum potassium concentration is below the lower limit of the reference range.

Hyponatraemia: Used to denote a finding where the serum sodium concentration is below the lower limit of the reference range.

Iatrogenic illness: Any adverse condition in a patient occurring as the result of treatment by a physician, surgeon or other health professional (adverse drug reaction).

Icterus/icteric: Terms used to refer to a patient who is jaundiced because of an elevated serum bilirubin concentration. A common finding is a yellowing of the sclera.

Idiosyncratic reaction: An abnormal susceptibility to a drug that is peculiar to the individual. These are also considered ADRs.

Incidence: Usually defined in epidemiology as the number of new cases of a disease in a population over a period of time.

Indirect costs: The costs that are not directly incurred due to the provision of care but yet impact the total costs.

Inpatient: A patient who remains in a hospital while under medical treatment.

Inputs: Resources, costs

Intangibles: Costs that are subjective in nature and hence more difficult to measure.

Intelligent non-adherence: Non-adherence by patients who alter their therapy without suffering any adverse events, and the patient's non-adherence appears rational when analysed without any bias; for example, misdiagnosis, inappropriate prescribing.

Intention to treat analysis: Analysis of data for all subjects based on the group to which they were originally randomised, and not based on the actual treatment they received.

Interactive communication: Where people communicating take turns at speaking and listening to each other.

Intern (or house surgeon): A medical graduate serving in a hospital preparatory to being licensed to practice medicine.

Interviewee: The person being interviewed.

Interviewer: The person conducting the interview.

Intrinsic clearance: The efficiency of the actual elimination mechanisms in the kidney and liver without the influences of plasma protein binding or blood flow to the organs.

Korsakoff's syndrome: A condition frequently encountered in chronic alcoholics, largely due to thiamine deficiency, characterised by confusion and short-term memory impairment. Often co-exists with Wernicke's syndrome (characterised by disturbances in ocular motility, nystagmus, ataxia and tremors).

Laboratory data: Information about a patient that is generated by the use of tests or investigations that are traditionally performed in biochemistry, haematology or other laboratories.

Leucopaenia: Used to refer to the situation when the total white blood cell count is significantly lower than the reference range.

Lewy body dementia: A type of dementia characterised by the pathologic finding of Lewy bodies in the cerebral cortex and brainstem and the presence of symptoms of mild Parkinsonism, hallucinations and/or altered alertness or attention; such patients may be very sensitive to the adverse effects of anti-psychotics drugs.

Loading dose: The initial dose required to achieve a desired plasma concentration.

Mail order: A pharmacy service that allows members to order prescriptions by telephone and receive their prescriptions through the mail.

Maintenance dose: The dose that is required to replace a drug that is being cleared from the body while maintaining a desired average concentration.

Managed care: A system of healthcare delivery that influences utilisation and cost of services and measures performance. The goal is a system that delivers value by giving people access to quality healthcare in a cost-effective way.

Medication adherence: The extent to which a patient's behaviour coincides with the intention of the health advice given.

Medication chart review: A systematic review of an inpatient's drug therapy orders to ensure that the prescribed medication is appropriate for the patient.

Medication chart: Hospital chart on which orders for medication are written for a particular patient (also called treatment chart)

Medication counselling: An advisory session to educate a patient on the medicines they are taking.

Medication error: Any preventable event that may cause or lead to inappropriate medication-use or patient harm while the medicine is in the control of the healthcare professional, patient or consumer.

Medication history interview: An interview conducted by a pharmacist to obtain accurate information on a patient's medication use that may assist in the overall healthcare of the patient.

Medication history: Information on the medicines a patient is currently taking, has taken in the past and their experience of these medicines.

Medication reconciliation: A process where the drugs prescribed for a patient on admission are compared to a complete and accurate medication history obtained by the pharmacist, in order to identify discrepancies.

Medication review: The review of a patient's medication regimen to ensure that the medication is appropriate for the patient and is effective, safe and cost-effective.

Medication use system: A series of inter-related steps, including prescribing, dispensing, administration and monitoring drug therapy intended to improve symptoms, prevent or cure a disease.

Medication-related problem: Any event or circumstance involving medication use that interferes or potentially interferes with the patient achieving an optimum outcome of medical care.

Medicine reconciliation: A process to identify an accurate list of the medicines currently being taken by a patient, to compare this to their current prescription and then identify discrepancies and omissions.

Meta analysis: A statistical technique which summarises the results of several studies into a single estimate, giving more weight to results from larger studies.

Metabolic induction: A process whereby a compound increases the amount of a metabolising enzyme to increase the rate of metabolism.

Metabolic inhibition: A process where a compound binds to an enzyme to reduce the action of the enzyme and decrease the rate of metabolism.

Milk:plasma concentration ratio: Ratio of the concentration of medication in breast milk to the concentration in the mother's plasma.

Minimum bactericidal concentration (MBC): Lowest concentration of a drug that results in a 99.9% reduction in the initial bacteria density.

Minimum inhibitory concentration (MIC): The lowest concentration of an anti-microbial agent capable of preventing the growth of a particular organism.

Morbidity: Disease burden; or the proportion of patients with a particular disease.

Morning sickness: A common condition of nausea and vomiting experienced by pregnant women upon wakening, typically in the early stages of pregnancy.

Mortality: Fatal outcome; death rate.

Net present value: Discounted value of income or expenditure generated in the future years.

Non-adherence: Failure to adhere to a therapeutic regimen.

Non-teaching hospital: Any hospital other than a teaching hospital.

Non-verbal messages: Information conveyed by methods other than through words.

Nosocomial: Relating to the hospital; usually used to denote a new disorder associated with the patient being treated in a hospital (a hospital-acquired infection).

Number needed to treat: The number of patients who need to be treated over a defined period of time for one person to benefit in the outcome of interest.

Observation chart: Hospital chart on which the patient's vital signs are recorded, including blood pressure, heart rate and body temperature.

Odds ratio: An effect size used in case control studies to represent the relative risk.

Open body position: Where the arms and legs are relaxed and not crossed in front of the body.

Open questions: Questions that allow a wide range of responses.

Orthostatic hypotension: (see postural hypotension)

Outpatient: A patient who receives treatment at a hospital without being admitted.

Output: Consequences, outcomes

Over-the-counter drugs: Drugs which can be legally purchased without a prescription.

Oximetry: A simple non-invasive method of monitoring the percentage of haemoglobin which is saturated with oxygen.

Pancytopaenia: Used to refer to the situation where the plasma haemoglobin, total white cell count and platelet count are simultaneously lower than the reference range.

Parent drug: The active drug compound before it undergoes metabolism or transformation.

Passive communication: Where one person speaks and others listen.

Patient counselling: The provision of information, advice and assistance to help patients use their medications appropriately.

Patient information leaflet: Information written for patients on a particular medicine.

Patient medication record: Tabulated information of the medicines a patient is currently taking.

Pharmaceutical care: A patient-centred practice in which the pharmacist assumes responsibility for a patient's medicine-related needs and is accountable for this commitment.

Pharmacodynamics: The study of the relationship between drug concentration and pharmacologic and toxicological responses.

Pharmacoepidemiology: The study of the use of drugs in populations.

Pharmacokinetics: The study and understanding of the factors that determine the time-course of a drug within the body, including the absorption, distribution, metabolism and excretion of the drug.

Pharmacovigilance programmes: National or international (such as the World Health Organization) programmes that collect and interpret information on adverse drug reactions, including drug interactions, to define, advise and educate people about the adverse effects of medicinally active substances.

Pharmacovigilance: The science and activities related to the detection, assessment and prevention of adverse effects and other possible drug-related problems.

Pharmacy intervention: Any action by a pharmacist that directly results in a change in patient management or therapy.

Pictogram: A picture that presents a concept or object.

Placebo effect: Positive or negative clinical outcomes following the administration of a placebo ('dummy') medication.

Placenta: The organ that develops from the uterine lining during pregnancy. Through diffusion of substances between the mother and foetus, the placenta provides nourishment to the foetus and allows for elimination of foetal waste.

Pneumonia severity index (PSI): A rating scale used to assess the severity and prognosis of community-acquired pneumonia.

Polymerase chain reaction (PCR): A technique for cloning DNA for a single molecule in a test tube.

Polypharmacy: Prescription or use of multiple medications (definition varies, but usually refers to four or more medications).

Population: Large groups of people

Postural hypotension: A fall in systolic BP of at least 20 mmHg or a fall in diastolic BP of at least 15 mmHg when a patient moves from a lying to a standing position (the fall in BP may take 3–5 minutes to occur); may result in dizziness, syncope or falls.

Pre-eclampsia: A condition in pregnancy characterised by abrupt hypertension, albuminuria and oedema.

Prevalence: Usually defined in epidemiology as the number of people taking a specific drug or with a particular condition or disease in a given population, as measured in a cross-sectional survey.

Prodrug: An inactive pharmacological compound which must be modified in the body to form the active drug.

Prospective study: A study planned to observe events that have not yet occurred. Usually, these studies involve looking forward from cause to effect.

Quality adjusted life years (QALYs): A health index measure that incorporates quality of life (Q) and quantity of life (Y) in order to provide a common set of units to describe health effects. The health index is a weighting scheme where Q or utility is measured on a scale from worst possible health to perfect health, which are usually predefined as zero and one, respectively. And Q is weighted by the duration of life, Y, typically measured in years.

Randomised controlled trial: A trial in which subjects are randomly assigned to two or more groups, with one group acting as a control or comparison group and the other group(s) receiving the treatment(s) under investigation.

Rapport: A sympathetic relationship based on understanding.

Recall bias: Bias or inaccuracy in information as a result of patients being able to remember and give accurate information only for short periods of time.

Reference range: The range of values for a particular variable that is intended to encompass the majority of results that would be expected in approximately 95% of cases where the investigation is performed for a group of normal individuals in the absence of significant disease or pathology.

Reflective practice: Reviewing a situation and through critical evaluation to consider approaches which could have had a more successful outcome; also learning from good practice.

Registrar: A resident specialist-in-training who acts as assistant to the chief or attending specialist.

Relative risk reduction: The difference between the relative risk and there being no effect (1.00 – RR), often expressed as a percentage.

Relative risk: Also called the risk ratio. The percentage of an outcome in an exposed group of individuals divided by the percentage in a group of non-exposed individuals.

Renal function: A generic term used to describe the functional capacity of the kidneys as organs of excretion (and to a lesser extent, as endocrine organs).

Resident: A graduate and licensed physician receiving training in a hospital.

Retrospective study: A study conducted using data that has already been collected; for example, data from published studies or from medical records. Usually, these studies require looking backward from effects to preceding causes.

Role play: A situation where people imitate and practice situations they are not familiar with.

Salt form factor: The fraction of an administered salt form of a drug which is the active moiety.

Sepsis: A systemic illness caused by microbial invasion of normally sterile parts of the body.

Serotonin syndrome: A clinical condition characterised by fever, shivering, sweating, diarrhoea, mental state changes, hypereflexia or myoclonus, and most commonly caused by a combination of two or more drugs which increase synaptic serotonin levels.

Side effect: Any unintended effect of a pharmaceutical product occurring at doses normally used in humans, which is related to the pharmacological properties of the drug.

Signal: Reported information on a possible relationship between an adverse event and a drug, the relationship being unknown or incompletely documented previously. Usually, more than a single report is required to generate a signal, depending on the seriousness of the event and the quality of the information.

Standard Treatment Guidelines (STGs): A systematically developed statement designed to assist practitioners and patients in making decisions about appropriate healthcare for specific clinical circumstances.

Statistical significance: Describes the likelihood of a study's results occurring by chance.

Steady state: Occurs when the rate at which a drug enters systemic circulation is equal to the rate at which drug is eliminated from the body.

Stroke: A sudden, non-convulsive loss of neurologic function due to an ischaemic or haemorrhagic intracranial vascular event, resulting in permanent damage to brain tissue and long-term neurological deficits. Also known as 'cerebrovascular accident' or 'CVA'.

Surrogate end points (markers): Indirect measures of treatment efficacy which are relatively easily measured.

Syndrome of Inappropriate Anti-diuretic Hormone (SIADH): A condition where an inappropriate amount of anti-diuretic hormone (ADH) is produced, or where the kidneys become abnormally responsive to ADH. The most obvious abnormal laboratory finding is hyponatraemia.

Systematic review: An overview of primary studies undertaken for a specified purpose (aim) and which adopts a comprehensive search strategy, criteria for inclusion and exclusion of studies and an explicit grading of study quality.

Teaching hospital: A hospital affiliated with a medical school or university, where medical students are instructed.

Teratogen: An agent with known potential to harm the embryo or foetus.

Therapeutic drug monitoring: The measurement and interpretation of a drug concentration in biological fluids for the purpose of optimising a patient's drug therapy and clinical outcome.

Therapeutic goal: The desired outcome of medical treatment.

Therapeutic guidelines: A systematically developed statement of recommendations to assist clinicians in choosing the most appropriate treatment in specific clinical circumstances.

Therapeutic index: The ratio of the toxic dose to the minimally effective dose of a drug.

Therapeutic range: In TDM, the range of drug concentrations that is effective for a particular indication in the majority of patients, with a minimal risk of toxicity.

Thrombocytopaenia: Used to refer to a finding where the platelet count in peripheral blood is significantly lower than 15 0 x 103 /microL.

Total costs: Addition of all costs relevant to the service: direct, indirect and intangible costs.

Transient ischaemic attack (TIA): Brief, reversible episode of focal, non-convulsive ischaemic dysfunction of the brain lasting less than 24 hours, and usually less than one hour; caused by transient thrombotic or embolic blood vessel occlusion or stenosis. Sometimes also called 'mini-stroke'.

Triple whammy: A term used to describe the high risk for renal toxicity associated with the combination of a diuretic, an NSAID and either an ACE inhibitor or AN angiotensin receptor blocker.

Unexpected adverse reaction: An adverse reaction, the nature or severity of which is not consistent with domestic labelling or market authorisation, or expected from characteristics of the drug.

Unit dose drug distribution system: Medicines are contained in single unit packages. They are dispensed in an as ready-to-administer form as possible. Not more than a 24-hour supply is delivered or available at any time. Medicines are provided in a patient-specific container.

Utilisation: The utilisation of healthcare services by the patient including setting appointments and also for looking after them.

Utility: The desirability or preference of the health state. Utility incorporates two concepts, preference and value. Preference indicates a scenario where good A is favoured over good B. Preference indicates direction of desirability of good (A is preferred over B). Value indicates the intensity or magnitude of that preference. Utility captures both of these components.

Verbal messages: Information conveyed through words.

Volume of distribution: A measure of the extent of distribution of a drug within the body.

Ward pharmacy: A service where the pharmacist visits hospital wards regularly to monitor for completeness and accuracy of prescriptions, is available for consultation by medical and nursing staff and ensures that the drug distribution system is operating correctly.

Ward round: A visit made by a medical practitioner, alone or with a team of health professionals and medical students, to each hospital inpatient at their bedside to review and follow up the progress in their health.

Western blot: An immunoelectrophoretic procedure for identifying antibodies to specific viral proteins separated by their molecular weight.

Willing to pay (WTP): The maximum amount of money a person is willing to give up (pay) to obtain a health benefit and still consider him/herself as well off as with his previous entitlement. In economics, this is also commonly known as contingent valuation.

INDEX

D

E

F

G